Orthopedic/Neurology Words and Phrases

A Quick-Reference Guide

Orthopedics
Neurology
Neurosurgery
Podiatry
Rehabilitation
Chiropractic

Health Professions Institute • Modesto, California • 1994

Orthopedic/Neurology Words and Phrases
A Quick-Reference Guide

Orthopedics, Neurology, Neurosurgery, Podiatry, Rehabilitation, Chiropractic

H·E·A·L·T·H PROFESSIONS INSTITUTE

Sally C. Pitman
Editor & Publisher
Health Professions Institute
P. O. Box 801
Modesto, CA 95353
Phone (209) 551-2112
Fax (209) 551-0404

Printed by
Parks Printing & Lithograph
Modesto, California

ISBN 0-934385-55-6
Last digit is the print number: 9 8 7 6 5

Preface

Orthopedic/Neurology Words and Phrases is an update of the 146-page *Orthopedic Words and Phrases: A Quick-Reference Guide*, a 1988 publication. This new book, however, with over 50,000 entries in 623 pages, is far more than a mere revision of the earlier book.

When we decided to update the orthopedic book in 1993, we thought it would be useful to include neurology and neurosurgery words since the terminology overlaps with orthopedics. Then we decided to include podiatry and rehabilitation medicine and chiropractic terms since available word books don't cover those specialties, and the terminology overlaps with orthopedics and neurology. What we didn't expect was a new book four times as large as the old! And we could have had thousands more entries . . . but we finally had to stop and go to press—months later than we had planned.

We think we have produced a very useful and usable book for medical transcriptionists and other healthcare professionals who need quick and easy access to the spelling of orthopedic, neurologic, podiatric, rehabilitation, and chiropractic terms. Extensive cross-referencing assures the user greater success in finding a desired word or phrase.

The primary research for the new terminology was done by Bron Taylor of San Francisco and Susan Turley, MA, CMT, of Baltimore, experienced medical transcriptionists, writers, researchers, and long-term associates of Health Professions Institute. They culled words and phrases from hundreds of medical journals, respected textbooks in the field, and transcripts of medical reports in all relevant specialties. We appreciate the fine quality of their research and scholarship, coupled with their knowledge of medical transcription, operative procedures, and diagnostic tests.

Other medical transcriptionists contributed useful specialty word lists, and our thanks go especially to Catherine Baxter, CMT, Houston, for her fine research in all specialties, and to Sheryl Mustain, CMT, San Diego, for providing chiropractic terminology.

Invaluable assistance in verifying the accuracy of entries and reconciling discrepancies from various authoritative references was provided by John H. Dirckx, M.D., medical editorial consultant, Dayton, Ohio, and Vera Pyle, CMT, editorial consultant, San Francisco. Special thanks go to our director of education Ellen Drake, CMT, who joined Health Professions Institute in mid-1993 just in time to review the galleys many times and catch numerous errors.

This reference book was produced by the professional staff of Health Professions Institute, including Elaine Aamodt, Linda Campbell, CMT, Randy Drake, Dianna McElroy, and Laraine Sookhoo.

My warmest gratitude to all.

Sally C. Pitman, MA, CMT
Editor & Publisher

How to Use This Book

The words and phrases in this book are alphabetized letter by letter of all words in each phrase, and the possessive form ('s) is omitted from eponyms for accuracy in alphabetizing. Numbers are alphabetized as if written out.

Eponyms may be located alphabetically as well as under the nouns they modify. For example, *Ogden classification of epiphyseal fracture* may be found under *Ogden* as well as under *fracture* and *classification*.

The main entry *drugs* includes descriptive terms related to drugs, not the names of pharmaceuticals. The names of hundreds of medications commonly used in orthopedics and neurology appear under the entry *medications*. The main entry *muscles* includes phrases and descriptive terms related to muscles rather than the names of muscles which are readily available in medical dictionaries. Physicians frequently dictate many abbreviations, especially for muscle groups, and those muscles frequently abbreviated in medical dictation are listed as subentries under *muscles*.

In medical dictation physicians may arbitrarily refer to an operative procedure as an *approach*, *method*, *operation*, *procedure*, *repair*, or *technique*, or by the type of procedure, such as *arthroplasty*. Thus, all procedures are listed alphabetically by the eponym, under the type of procedure, and under the main entry *operations*.

Instruments used in operative and diagnostic procedures may also be referred to variously as an *apparatus*, *device*, *instrument*, *system*, or a particular type of instrument, such as *forceps*. Thus, instruments are listed under the type of instrument when there are many examples given, and those devices or instruments or machines that do not fit neatly in their own categories are listed under the general terms *device* and *system*.

A few main entries with extensive subentries include the following:

brace
cast
cerebrospinal fluid
classification
device
disease
drugs
electrode
electroencephalogram
electromyogram
epilepsy
forceps
fracture
graft
medications
muscles
operations
orthosis
prosthesis
reflex
retractor
rongeur
screw
sign
splint
suture
syndrome
system
test

A, a

AAA (diagnostic arthroscopy, operative arthroscopy, and possible operative arthrotomy)
AAA bone
AAO (awake, alert, and oriented)
AAOS (American Academy of Orthopaedic Surgeons)
AAOS classification of acetabular abnormalities
AAROM (active ankle joint complex range of motion)
AARP (American Association of Retired Persons)
abasia
abate, abated
abatement
Abbe operation
Abbott brace
Abbott-Fisher-Lucas arthrodesis
Abbott-Gill epiphyseal plate exposure
Abbott-Lucas shoulder operation
Abbreviated Injury Scale (AIS)
ABD (abdominal) dressing
ABD pad
abdominal epilepsy
abdominal migraine
abdominal reflex
abdominis rectus muscle
abducens (or abducent) nucleus
abducens nerve (sixth cranial nerve)
abducens nerve palsy
abducens nerve paresis
abduct, abductor
"a-b-duction" (as dictated)
abduction fracture
abduction stress test
abductor digiti minimi manus musculus
abductor digiti minimi pedis musculus
abductor digiti quinti (ADQ) muscle
abductor digiti quinti (ADQ) tendon
abductor hallucis muscle
abductor lurch (gluteus medius gait)
abductor pollicis brevis (APB) muscle
abductor pollicis brevis (APB) tendon
abductor pollicis longus (APL) muscle
abductor pollicis longus (APL) tendon
abductovalgus, hallux
Abercrombie neuronal cell count formula
aberrant patterns (of sweating, hair distribution, color)
aberrations, intersegmental
abet, abetted, abetting
ABGs (arterial blood gases)
ABI (ankle/brachial index)
ability (pl. abilities)
    bathing and dressing
    abstracting
    conceptual
    constructional
    following (of the eyes)
    positive
ability to abstract
ability to attend
ablation
    radical nail bed
    stereotactic or stereotaxic
    surgical

ablation *(cont.)*
  total pituitary
  Zadik total nail bed
ablative arthroplasty
ABLB (alternate binaural loudness balance) test
Abnormal Involuntary Movement Scale (AIMS)
abnormality
  bony
  bulbar
  cranial nerve
  cytoarchitectonic
  frontal plane growth
  soft tissue
  torsional
ABOS (American Board of Orthopaedic Surgery)
abrader, cartilage
Abramson catheter
abrasion arthroplasty
abrasions and contusions
abscess
  actinomycotic brain
  arthrifluent
  Aspergillus cerebral
  bone
  brain
  Brodie metaphyseal
  cerebral
  collar-button
  daughter
  encapsulated brain
  epidural
  extradural
  frontal
  growth plate
  horseshoe (in the hand)
  intradural
  intraosseous
  metaphyseal
  midpalmar
  Pott
  psoas

abscess *(cont.)*
  serous
  spinal epidural (SEA)
  subaponeurotic
  subdural
  subgaleal
  subperiosteal
  subungual
  suture
  thecal
  thenar space
absence attack
absence seizure (see *seizure*)
absence status (seizure)
absent ataxia
absent consensual constriction (pupil)
absolute scotomata
absorbable polyparadioxanone pin
absorption cavity
absorption, lysosomal (of cartilage in rheumatoid arthritis)
abstraction
abstract thinking
abulia
abulic mental changes
abut, abutted, abutment
AC (acromioclavicular) joint separation
AC (anterior commissure)
ACA (anterior cerebral artery)
ACA (anterior choroidal artery)
acalculia
  aphasic
  visual-spatial
Acanthamoeba meningitis
ACAT (automated computed axial tomography)
ACB (asymptomatic carotid bruit)
accelerator
  Bevatron
  linear
  Philips linear
acceptance, weight (of gait)
accessory atlantoaxial ligament

accessory bones (sesamoid bones of foot or hand)
accessory oculomotor nucleus
accident
  ATV (all-terrain vehicle)
  cerebrovascular (CVA) (stroke)
  compensable
  horseback riding
  motorcycle (MCA)
  motor vehicle (MVA)
  skateboarding
  vascular
  vehicular
acclivity
accommodation reflex
Accommodator arch support
Accucore II
Accuflate tourniquet
Accu-Flo CSF reservoir
Accu-Flo dura film
Accu-Flo polyethylene bur hole cover
Accu-Flo silicone rubber bur hole cover
Accu-Flo ventricular catheter
Accu-Line dual pivot
Accu-Line femoral resector
Accu-Line guide
Accu-Line knee instrumentation
Accu-Line tibial resector
Accu-Tron microcurrent machine
Ace bandage
Ace-Colles fixator
Ace-Colles frame technique
Ace-Colles half ring
Ace-Fischer external fixator
Ace screw
Ace Unifix fixation device
Ace wrap
acetabular cup (see *cup*)
acetabulectomy
acetabuloplasty
acetabular
acetabulum (pl. acetabula)
  deep-shelled
  dysplastic
acetylcholine esterase
acetylcholine receptor antibody (AChRab)
ACF (anterior cervical fusion)
ACh (acetylcholine) receptor
achalasia, cricopharyngeal
ache, achy
acheiria
aches and pains
Achilles bulge sign
Achilles jerk
Achilles paratendinitis
Achilles squeeze test
Achilles tendon
Achilles tendon lengthening
Achilles tendon reflex
Achilles tendon shortening
Achillis, tendo
achillodynia
achillorrhaphy
achillotenotomy
aching, interscapular
aching pain
achondroplasia
achondroplastic dwarfism
AChR (acetylcholine receptor) antibody
AChRab (acetylcholine receptor antibody)
achromatopsia
acid, arachidonic
acid class, pyranocarboxylic
acidophilic pituitary tumor
aciduria
  argininosuccinic
  methylmalonic
Ackerman criteria for osteomyelitis
ACL (anterior cruciate ligament)
ACL drill guide
ACL graft
ACL guide set
ACL repair
Acland clamp or clip
Acland clamp-applying forceps
Acland double-clamp approximator

ACLR (anterior capsulolabral reconstruction)
ACM (acute confusional migraine)
ACoA (anterior communicating artery)
Acor Quikform I shoe
Acor Quikform II shoe
acorn, Midas Rex
acoustic nerve
acoustic nerve tumor
acoustic neurinoma
acoustic neuroma
acoustical shadowing
AC-PC line (anterior commissure-posterior commissure)
AC-PC plane
acquired (posttraumatic) syringomyelia
acquired flatfoot
acquired myopathy
acquired nystagmus
acquired toxoplasmosis
acquisition time
Acra-Cut cranial perforator
Acra-Cut cranioblade
Acra-Cut wire pass drill
Acrel ganglion
ACRM (American Congress of Rehabilitation Medicine)
acrocephalosyndactylism
acrocephalosyndactyly
acromacria
AcroMed plate
AcroMed screw
AcroMed VSP (variable screw placement) fixation system
acromegaly
acromioclavicular (AC) joint
acromiohumeral interval (AHI)
acromion
acromionectomy, Armstrong
acromioplasty
  anterior
  arthroscopic
  decompressive
  McLaughlin
  Neer
acro-osteosclerosis
acropachy
acroparesthesia of limbs
acro-pectoro-vertebral dysplasia
acrosyndactyly
Acrotorque hand engine
acrylic cement
ACS acetabular liner
ACTH (adrenocorticotrophic hormone) antibody
ACTH-producing pituitary adenoma
ACTH-producing pituitary tumor
actinomycotic brain abscess
action
  scotomata of
  tenodesis
  viscoelastic
action myoclonus
action potential
Action Research Arm (ARA) Test
activating procedures on EEG
activating techniques
  hyperventilation
  photic stimulation
  stroboscopic light
  sleep
activator table
active-assistive range of motion
active deformers (muscle action in arthritis)
active range of motion (AROM) exercise
activities
  high-impact
  instrumental activities of daily living (IADL)
activities of daily living (ADLs)
activity on EEG
  alpha
  asymmetrical epileptiform
  asymmetrical generalized epileptiform
  background
  barbiturate-induced spindle-like

activity on EEG *(cont.)*
beta
bilateral
burst of
burst of delta
burst of slow wave
burst of theta
cerebral
delta
desynchronization
diffuse distribution of
discontinuous
distribution of
electrocerebral
electrographic seizure
epileptiform
excessive diffuse low and medium wave beta
extracerebral
focal delta slow wave
focal epileptiform
focal interictal epileptiform
frontal intermittent rhythmic delta (FIRDA)
frontal rhythmic theta
generalized delta
generalized distribution
generalized epileptiform
generalized paroxysmal fast
high voltage slow and sharp
ictal epileptiform
interictal epileptiform
interictal localized
intermittent rhythmical delta activity (IRDA)
lateralized
lateralized epileptiform
level of
localized delta
localized epileptiform
low-amplitude
low-voltage
medium-voltage beta
monomorphic

activity on EEG *(cont.)*
monorhythmic frontal delta (MFD)
monorhythmic sinusoidal delta
noncerebral
nonepileptiform
occipital dominant intermittent rhythmic delta
occipital intermittent rhythmical delta (OIRDA)
paroxysmal alpha
paroxysmal beta
paroxysmal delta
paroxysmal theta
polymorphic delta
polyrhythmic
posterior dominant
posttraumatic epileptiform
propagation of
pseudoepileptiform
reflex neurologic
rhythmic
rhythmical spindle-shaped
runs of
scattered dysrhythmic slow
serotonergic
sleep
slow wave
spectral peak frequency of
spiking
spindle-like
theta
triphasic slow wave
unilateral epileptiform
unilateral focus of
widespread distribution
Activity Losses Assessment (ALA)
activity restriction
actual leg length test
ACU-derm wound dressing
ACU-dyne antiseptic
Acufex ankle distractor
Acufex arthroscopic instruments
Acufex bioabsorbable fixation device
Acufex curet

Acufex distractor pin
Acufex gouge
Acufex knee laxity arthrometer
Acufex mallet
Acufex meniscal basket
Acufex osteotome
Acufex probe
Acufex rasp
Acufex tibial guide
acuity, central visual
Acumeter
acupuncture
acute acquired hemiplegia
acute aphonia
acute ascending motor paralysis
acute avulsion fracture
acute brain syndrome
acute cerebellar hemispheric lesion
acute chorea
acute confusional state
acute exogenous reaction
acute foot strain
acute gout
acute hematogenous arthritis
acute hematogenous osteomyelitis (AHO)
acute inflammatory polyradiculopathy
acute labyrinthine disorder
acute meningitis
acute purulent meningitis
acute spinal arthritis
acute stretch injury
acute stroke
acute whiplash
ACUTENS
AD (Alzheimer disease)
adactyly (adactylia)
Adam and Eve splint
adamantinoma
Adamkiewicz (also Adamkiewitz)
  artery of
  syndrome of the great radicular artery of
Adams position test
Adams procedure
Adams saw
Adams splint
Adapta physical therapy table
adapter
  Christmas tree
  chuck
  collet screwdriver
  French
  Hudson chuck
  Jacobs chuck
  Lloyd
  Mayfield
  Trinkle chuck
Adaptic dressing
Adaptic gauze
Adaptic packing
Adaptic sponge
adaptive equipment
ADAS (Alzheimer's Disease Assessment Scale)
ADAS noncognitive subscale
ADC (AIDS dementia complex)
ADD (attention deficit disorder)
Addis test
adduct
"a-d-duction" (as dictated)
adduction, Edgarton-Grand thumb
adduction fracture
adduction stress to fingers
adduction to neutral
adductor magnus
adductor sweep of thumb
adductor tendon
adductor tendon and lateral capsular release
adductor tenotomy and obturator neurectomy (ATON)
adductus
  metatarsus (MTA)
  true metatarsus (TMA)
adenohypophysectomy
adenohypophysial
adenohypophysis

adenoma
  acidophilic
  ACTH-producing pituitary
  basophilic
  chromophobic
  cutaneous
  eosinophilic
  glycoprotein-secreting
  gonadotropin-secreting
  intraspinal
  null cell
  pituitary
  prolactin-secreting
  sebaceum
  suprasellar
adenopathy
ADH (antidiuretic hormone) secretion, inappropriate
ADHD (attention deficit/hyperactivity disorder)
adherent tape, benzoin
adhesed
adhesion
  capsular
  fibrous
  intra-articular
  subacromial bursal
  subdeltoid bursal
adhesive (see also *cement*)
  APR cement fixation
  Aron Alpha
  benzoin
  Biobrane
  Coe-pak paste
  Cover-Roll gauze
  Coverlet
  cyanoacrylate
  fibrin glue
  Histoacryl glue
  hydroxyapatite
  Implast bone cement
  ligand
  LPPS hydroxyapatite
  medical
adhesive *(cont.)*
  methyl methacrylate
  Palacos cement
  Simplex
  Superglue (cyanoacrylate)
  Surfit
  Surgical Simplex P
  Zimmer low viscosity
adhesive arachnoiditis
adhesive capsulitis
ADI (atlanto-dens interval)
adiabatic fast passage
adiadochokinesia
Adie-Holmes pupil
Adie pupils
Adie syndrome
Adie tonic pupil
adipose tissue
adiposogenital dystrophy
Adjustable Leg and Ankle Repositioning Mechanism (ALARM)
adjustive treatment (chiropractic)
adjustment, chiropractic spinal
adjustment of the articulations and adjacent tissues
adjuvant therapy
Adkins arthrodesis
Adkins spinal fusion
ADL (adrenoleukodystrophy)
ADL indices
ADLs (activities of daily living)
  extended
  hierarchical scales of
  indices of
  instrumental
adolescent hallux valgus
ADQ (abductor digiti quinti) muscle
ADRDA (Alzheimer's Disease and Related Disorders Association)
adrenal medullary tissue, autologous
adrenaline
adrenergic neurotransmission
adrenocortical coma

adrenoleukodystrophy (ADL), X-linked recessive
ADROM (ankle dorsiflexion range of motion)
Adson-Anderson cerebellar retractor
Adson aneurysm needle
Adson bipolar forceps
Adson brain-exploring cannula
Adson brain retractor
Adson brain suction tip
Adson brain suction tube
Adson-Brown tissue forceps
Adson bur
Adson cerebellar retractor
Adson chisel
Adson clip-introducing forceps
Adson conductor
Adson cranial rongeur
Adson dissecting hook
Adson dressing forceps
Adson drill
Adson drill guide
Adson dural hook
Adson dural knife
Adson dural needle holder
Adson dural protector
Adson elevator
Adson enlarging bur
Adson exploring cannula
Adson forceps
Adson ganglion scissors
Adson hemilaminectomy retractor
Adson hemostatic forceps
Adson hypophyseal forceps
Adson knife
Adson knot tier
Adson laminectomy chisel
Adson maneuver
Adson-Mixter neurosurgical forceps
Adson modified maneuver
Adson needle
Adson needle holder
Adson nerve hook
Adson perforating bur
Adson periosteal elevator
Adson retractor
Adson right-angle knife
Adson-Rogers cranial bur
Adson rongeur
Adson saw
Adson saw guide
Adson scalp clip
Adson scalp needle
Adson scissors
Adson sign
Adson suction tube
Adson test
Adson tissue forceps
Adson twist drill
Adson wire saw
ADT (anterior drawer test)
AdTech electrode grid
AdTech electrode strip
advanced cortical disease
advancement
  fronto-orbital
  heel-cord
  tendon
  transcranial frontofacial
  VMO (vastus medialis obliquus)
advancer
adventitia
adventitial forceps
adventitious bursa
adventitious movements
adversive (visual) fields
adversive attack
adversive fields (visual)
adversive motor seizure
AE (above-elbow) amputation
AE1 antibody
AE3 antibody
AER (apical ectodermal ridge)
aerate, aerated, aeration
aerobe
aerobic dance
  high-impact (HIAD)
  low-impact (LIAD)

Aeroplast dressing
Aesculap bipolar cautery forceps
Aesculap forceps
Aesculap head holder
Aesculap-PM noncemented femoral prosthesis
Aesculap screw
aesthetic, aesthetically
aesthetic surgery
AF (anterior frontal) electrode (AF_3, AF_4, AF_7, AF_8, AF_z)
AF (arcuate fasciculus)
affect
  blunted
  flat
  inappropriate
  infantile
  labile
  normal
  shallow
affective prodrome of epilepsy
affective prodrome of migraine
affective symptoms of seizures
afferent digital lesion
afferent digital nerves
afferent nerve lesion
afferent neuron
afferent pupillary defect
AFI total hip replacement prosthesis
AFO (ankle-foot orthosis)
  articulated
  molded
  posterior leaf spring
  standard shell
AFP (alpha-fetoprotein) test
A-frame electrode
after-discharge on EEG
after-nystagmus, cycles of
AG (angular gyrus)
AGC (anatomically graduated component)
AGC Biomet total knee system
AGC femoral prosthesis
AGC knee prosthesis
AGC tibial prosthesis
age
  biologic
  bone
  chronologic
AGE (angle of greatest extension)
Agee endoscope
Agee-WristJack fracture reduction system
agenesis of corpus callosum
agenesis, sacral
agenetic
agent
  fibrinolytic
  keratolytic
  nociceptor
AGF (angle of greatest flexion)
aggregate
  epileptic neuronal
  gaze coordinating
  neuronal
aggressive behavior
aggressive outbursts
agitation
Agnew splint
agnosia
  apperceptive visual
  associative visual
  auditory
  autotopagnosia
  color
  corporal
  facial
  finger
  generalized auditory
  object
  selective auditory
  somatagnosia
  tactile
  topographical
  verbal auditory
  visual

agonist-antagonist contraction
agonist, dopamine
agonist muscle groups
agrammatic speech
agrammatism
agranular chromophobe cells in adenohypophysis
agraphia
  agrammatism
  alexia with
  alexia without
  aphasic
  apractic
  lexical
  phonological
  pure
  spatial
agrypnodal coma
agyria
AH (ataxic hemiparesis)
Ahern trochanteric debridement
AHI (acromiohumeral interval)
AHI (Arthritis Helplessness Index)
AHO (acute hematogenous osteomyelitis)
AHP (American Hand Prosthetics)
AHP digital prosthesis
AHSC (Arizona Health Science Center) elbow prosthesis
AICA (anterior inferior cerebellar artery)
AICA (anterior inferior cerebral artery)
AICA (anterior inferior communicating artery)
Aicardi syndrome
AICS (artery of inferior cavernous sinus)
aid, external memory
AIDP (acute inflammatory demyelinating polyradiculopathy)
aids
  external memory
  walking
AIDS dementia complex (ADC)
AIDS encephalopathy
AIDS myelopathy
Aiken osteotomy
AIM CPM (continuous passive motion) for hand and legs
aimer
  femoral
  tibial
AIMS (Abnormal Involuntary Movement Scale)
AIMS (Arthritis Impact Measurement Scale)
Ainsworth modification of Massie nail
Aircast Air-Stirrup brace
Aircast pneumatic air stirrup
Aircast Swivel-Strap brace
Aircast walking brace
air contrast studies
Air-Dyne bicycle
air embolism of the brain
air hunger
air plethysmography
air pressure splint
air splint
AIROM (active integral range of motion)
airplane cast
airplane splint
Air-Stirrup Ankle Training Brace
AIS (adolescent idiopathic scoliosis)
Aitken classification of epiphyseal fracture
Aitken femoral deficiency
AJ (ankle jerk)
AJC (ankle joint complex)
AK (above-knee) amputation (AKA)
akathisia, tardive
Akin bunionectomy
Akin osteotomy
akinesia
akinesthesia
akinetic drop attack
akinetic drop spell

akinetic mutism
  alert
  apathetic
akinetic seizure
akinetic spell
Akros extended care mattress
Akros pressure mattress
ala, sacral
ALA (Activity Losses Assessment)
alalia
Alanson amputation
alar ligament
alarm clock headache
ALARM (Adjustable Leg and Ankle Repositioning Mechanism)
Albee bone graft
Albee-Compere fracture table
Albee-Delbert operation
Albee hip arthrodesis
Albee lumbar spinal fusion
Albee olive-shaped bur
Albee shelf procedure
Albers-Schönberg disease (Schoenberg)
Albert knee operation
Alberts Famous Faces Test
albicans, Candida
Albright-Chase arthroplasty
Albright-McCune-Sternberg syndrome
albumin, radioiodinated serum (RISA)
albuminocytologic dissociation in Guillain-Barré disease
Alcock canal
alcohol, blood levels of
alcoholic amnesia
alcoholic epilepsy
alcoholic hallucinosis
alcoholic intoxication
alcoholic myopathy
alcoholic stupor
alcohol-precipitated epilepsy
alcohol-related seizure
alcohol withdrawal
alcohol withdrawal seizures
alcohol withdrawal syndrome
Alden CDI orthotic
alert and oriented x 3 (to person, place, and time)
alert and oriented x 4 (to person, place, time, and future plans)
alerting maneuver on EEG
alerting stimulus on EEG
alertness
  level of
  state of
Alexander chisel
Alexander costal periosteotome
Alexander disease
Alexander-Farabeuf periosteotome
Alexander-Farabeuf rasp
alexia
  anterior
  central
  posterior
  tactile
alexia with agraphia
alexia without agraphia
Alexian Brothers overhead frame
algesimeter
  Aly
  Björnström
algodystrophy
aliasing on EEG
alien hand sign
align, aligned
aligner
  Charnley femoral inlay
  femoral
  patellar
  tibial
alignment
  anatomic
  angular
  integrity and
  lower extremity
  poor
  rotational
  torsional
  transverse-plane
alignment of fracture fragments

alignment of vertebral bodies
alignment rod
Alimed insert
Alimed wrist/thumb support
alimentary seizure
Aliplast insoles
aliquorrhea (low CSF production)
Alivium implant metal
all-median nerve hand
all-terrain vehicle (ATV)
all-ulnar nerve hand
ALL (anterior longitudinal ligament)
allachesthesia
Allen arm/hand surgery table
Allen arthroscopic elbow positioner
Allen arthroscopic knee positioner
Allen arthroscopic wrist positioner
Allen maneuver
Allen open reduction of calcanea fracture
Allen shoulder/wrist arthroscopy traction system
Allen sign
Allen stirrups
Allen test
Allen wrench
Allender vertical laminar flow room
Allevyn dressing
Allis clamp
Allis forceps
Allis sign
Allis tissue forceps
Allman classification of acromioclavicular injury
Allman modification of Evans ankle reconstruction
allochiria (allocheiria)
allocortex
allodynia
alloesthesia
allogeneic bone graft
allogenous bone graft
allograft
  bone
  bone-tendon-bone

allograft *(cont.)*
  fresh frozen
  osteochondral
  Red Cross freeze-dried
allograft transplantation
AlloGrip bone vise
alloy
  cobalt-chromium
  stainless steel
  Ti-Nidium
  Ti6A14V
  Wood
Allport retractor
Alm wound retractor
Alouette amputation
ALP (ankle ligament protector)
Alpers disease
Alpers syndrome
alpha activity
alpha band on EEG
alpha blocking on EEG
alpha-fetoprotein
alpha frequency band on EEG
alpha frequency coma
alpha frequency range
alpha index
alpha motor neuron
alpha pattern on EEG
alpha rhythm on EEG
alpha spindles on EEG
alpha wave on EEG
ALPS (anterior locking plate system), Amset
ALS (amyotrophic lateral sclerosis), carcinomatous
ALS-like syndrome
alta, patella
alterations in consciousness
altered mental status
alternans, hemiplegia
alternate binaural loudness balance (ABLB) test
alternate hemiplegia
alternating motion rate (AMR)

alternating single-leg support (running gait)
altitudinal anopsia
altitudinal hemianopsia
Alumafoam splint
aluminum oxide ceramic coating
Alvar condylar bolt
Alvarado collateral ligament protector
Alvarado knee holder
Alvarado leg holder
alveolar bone fracture
alveolar rhabdomyosarcoma
Aly algesimeter
Alzheimer disease (presenile dementia)
Alzheimer's Disease Asssessment Scale (ADAS)
Alzheimer neurofibrillary degeneration
Alzheimer-type, senile dementia (SDAT)
AM-MI orthopedic table
AMA Guide to Evaluation of Permanent Impairment
amalgam
amaurosis
  central
  cerebral
  uremic
amaurosis centralis
amaurosis fugax
AMBI hip screw
ambidexterity
ambidextrous
ambient cistern
ambifixation
ambiguus, nucleus
ambilevosity
ambilevous
amblyaphia
amblyopia ex anopsia (lazy eye)
amblyopia, toxic (toxic retino-neuropathy)
ambon
ambulant
ambulate with assistance
ambulate with support
ambulate without assistance
ambulate without support
ambulation, brace-free
ambulation skills
Ambulators shoe
ambulatory EEG recording
ambulatory patient
ambulatory status
ambulatory with a cane
ambulatory with assistance
AMC total wrist prosthesis
AMD (arthroscopic microdiskectomy)
AMD (articular motion device)
AME (American Medical Electronics)
AME (Austin Medical Equipment)
AME bone growth stimulator
AME microcurrent TENS unit
AME PinSite Shield
amebiasis (see *amoebiasis*)
amelia
amenorrhea, exercise-induced
amentia
American Academy of Orthopaedic Surgeons (AAOS)
American Association of Homes for the Aging
American Association of Mental Deficiency
American Association of Retired Persons (AARP)
American Board of Orthopaedic Surgery (ABOS)
American Congress of Rehabilitation Medicine (ACRM)
American Dietetic (not Diabetic) Association diets for athletes
American EEG Society
American Foundation for the Blind
American Geriatrics Society
American Musculoskeletal Tumor Society rating scale
American Nursing Home Association
American Parkinson's Disease Association

American Physical Therapy
  Association (APTA)
American Rheumatism Association
  (ARA)
American Seating Access-O-Matic bed
American shoulder and elbow system
  (ASES)
American Spinal Cord Injury
  Association classification
Americans with Disabilities Act
Amigo mechanical wheelchair
aminoaciduria
  arginase deficiency
  argininosuccinic
  Baló
  carnosinemia
  citrullinemia
  cystathioninuria
  Devic
  Hartnup disease
  histidinemia
  homocystinuria
  hydroxyisovaleric
  hyper-ß-alaninemia
  hyperlysinemia
  hyperprolinemia
  hypersarcosinemia
  hypervalinemia
  isovaleric acidemia
  maple-syrup urine disease
  Marchiafava-Bignami
  methylmalonic
  neonatal tyrosinemia
  oasthouse urine disease
  Pelizaeus-Merzbacher
  phenylketonuria (PKU)
  primary
  saccharopinuria
  Schilder
  sulfite oxidase deficiency
  tyrosinemia
AML (amyotrophic lateral sclerosis)
AML (anatomic medullary locking)
AML hip prosthesis
AML Tang femoral prosthesis
Ammon horn (mesial temporal)
  sclerosis
amnesia
  alcoholic
  amnesic
  antegrade
  anterograde
  auditory
  Broca
  circumscribed
  concussion
  continuous
  dissociative
  emotional
  episodic
  generalized
  global
  hippocampal
  hysterical
  infantile
  ictal
  Korsakoff
  lacunar
  localized
  olfactory
  organic
  partial
  patchy retrograde
  postconcussive
  posthypnotic
  posttraumatic
  psychogenic
  retroactive
  retrograde
  selective
  shrinking retrograde
  tactile
  transient
  transient global (TGA)
  traumatic
  verbal
  visual
amnesiac

amnesic aphasia
amnestic state
amnestic syndrome
amobarbital sodium test
amoebiasis, cerebral (or amebiasis)
  Entamoeba histolytica
  Iodamoeba buetschlii
amorphosynthesis
Amoss sign
amphiarthrosis
amplifier drift on EEG
amplitude (on EEG)
  absolute band
  absolute EP (evoked potential)
  asymmetry
  local reduction in
  peak-to-peak
  reduction of
  relative band
  SNAP (sensory nerve action potential)
  very low
  waveform
amputation
  above-elbow (AE)
  above-knee (AK) (AKA)
  Alanson
  Alouette
  Beclard
  below-knee (BK) (BKA)
  Berger interscapular
  Bier
  Boyd ankle
  Bunge
  Burgess below-knee
  button toe
  Callander
  chop
  Chopart hindfoot
  circular supracondylar
  closed flap
  complete
  congenital
  digital
amputation *(cont.)*
  femoral head
  fingertip
  fish-mouth
  forearm
  forefoot digital
  forequarter
  Gritti-Stokes distal thigh
  guillotine
  hindquarter
  incomplete
  index ray
  interinnominoabdominal
  interphalangeal
  interscapular
  interscapulothoracic
  Jaboulay
  Kirk distal thigh
  Lisfranc
  midthigh
  nonreplantable
  one-stage
  Pirogoff
  ray
  replantable
  supramalleolar open
  Syme
  Syme ankle disarticulation
  toe
  transcarpal
  transcondylar
  translumbar
  transmetatarsal (TMA)
  traumatic
  two-stage
amputation neuroma
amputation stump
amputee
AMR (alternating motion rate)
Amrex muscle stimulator
Amset ALPS (anterior locking plate system)
Amset R-F fixation system
Amset R-F rod

Amset R-F screw
Amsler grid visual test
Amspacher-Messenbaugh technique
Amstutz resurfacing procedure
Amstutz total hip replacement
Amstutz-Wilson osteotomy
AMTR (anteromedial temporal lobe resection)
amusia
amyelination
amygdala of cerebellum
amygdalofugal pathway
amygdalohippocampectomy
amygdaloid area
amygdaloid nuclear complex
amygdalotomy
amyloid
amyloidoma
amyloidosis, skeletal
amyoplasia congenita
amyostatic syndrome
amyotonia congenita
amyotrophic lateral sclerosis (ALS)
amyotrophic type of spongiform encephalopathy
amyotrophy
  Aran-Duchenne
  asthmatic
  brachial
  diabetic
  dystonic
  neuralgic
  neuritic
  primary progressive
  progressive nuclear
  syphilitic
ANA (antinuclear antibody) test
anachronism on EEG
anaerobe, anaerobic
anal reflex
anal wink
anal wink reflex
analgesia, patient controlled (PCA)
analog to digital converter
analogous
analysis
  biomechanical
  cephalometric
  computer-assisted EEG signal
  computerized EEG signal
  EEG autoregressive model for signal
  EEG digital signal
  EEG spectral
  electro-oculographic
  footprint
  force plate foot
  gait
  power spectral (PSA)
  quantitative EEG
  Sassouni
  short EEG epoch FFT
  signal
  total body neutron activation (TBNAA)
Anametric total knee system
anaplastic astrocytoma
anaplastic glioma
anarithmetria
anarthria
anastomosis
  extradural
  intradural
  Ma-Griffith end-to-end
  Ma-Griffith tendon
  Martin-Gruber
  Riche-Canieu
anatomic landmarks
anatomic medullary locking (AML)
anatomic snuffbox
ANB cephalometric measurement
anchor
  Mitek bone
  traction
anchor hole
anchor plate
anchor splint
anchorage-dependent growth

anchoring fibers of hand
anchoring system, bone
anchovy, tensor fasciae latae
anconeus, anconeal, anconoid
Anderson acetabular prosthesis
Anderson-Adson scalp retractor
Anderson classification of tibial pseudoarthrosis
Anderson-D'Alonzo classification
Anderson distractor
Anderson fixation apparatus
Anderson fixation device
Anderson-Fowler procedure
Anderson-Green growth prediction
Anderson-Hutchins tibial fracture
Anderson-Neivert osteotome
Anderson screw placement technique
Anderson splint
Anderson traction
andersoni, Dermacentor
Andersson hip status system
André hook
Andrews iliotibial band reconstruction
Andrews osteotome
Andrews spinal surgery frame
Andrews SST-3000 spinal surgery table
anemic hypoxia
anencephaly
anesthesia
  ankle block
  axillary block
  Bier block
  bulbar
  compression
  continuous intravenous regional (CIVRA)
  crash induction of
  doll's head
  dolorosa
  epidural block
  gauntlet
  general
  general endotracheal

anesthesia *(cont.)*
  general orotracheal
  glove
  glove and stocking
  hysterical
  inhalation, inhalant
  intrathecal
  intravenous regional (IVRA)
  local standby
  Mayo block
  peripheral nerve block
  regional ankle block
  ring block
  saddle
  segmental
  short-acting block (SAB)
  spinal
  supraclavicular brachial block
  tactile
  thalamic hyperesthetic
  thermal
  traumatic
anesthesic region
anesthetic block
aneurysm
  arteriovenous
  aspergillotic
  basilar artery
  berry
  brain
  carotid
  cavernous carotid
  cavernous sinus
  cerebral
  Charcot-Bouchard intracerebral
  circle of Willis
  clinoid
  clip ligation of
  clipping of
  coating of
  congenital arteriosclerotic
  cranial
  de novo
  dissecting

aneurysm *(cont.)*
- dissecting intracranial
- dome of
- extracerebral
- extracranial
- feeding artery of
- fundus of
- fusiform
- giant
- great cerebral vein of Galen
- hunterian ligation of
- internal carotid artery
- intracranial
- M1 segment
- miliary
- mycotic intracranial
- neck of
- neoplastic
- PICA (posterior inferior cerebellar artery)
- posterior communicating artery
- precursor sign to rupture of
- prerupture of
- rebleeding of
- rerupture of
- ruptured intracranial
- saccular
- suprasellar
- thrombosed
- thrombotic
- trapping of
- traumatic intracranial (TICA)
- unruptured
- wrapping of

aneurysmal bone cyst
aneurysmal bruit
aneurysmal bulging
aneurysmal dilatation
aneurysmal hemorrhage
aneurysmal rebleed
aneurysmal vein
aneurysm clip applicator
aneurysmectomy
aneurysm needle
aneurysmoplasty
aneurysmorrhaphy
aneurysmotomy
Angelchik anti-reflux prosthesis
Angell James dissector
Angell James hypophysectomy forceps
Anghelescu sign
angiitis, granulomatous giant cell
angiofibroblastic proliferation
angiogram, angiography
- biplane
- blush of dye on
- carotid
- cerebral
- digital subtraction cerebral
- four-vessel cerebral
- innominate
- intercostal artery
- internal carotid
- intra-arterial digital subtraction (IADSA)
- postembolization
- postoperative
- preoperative
- Seldinger
- small angle-double incidence (SADIA)
- spinal
- stereotactic cerebral
- stereotaxic cerebral
- superselective
- vertebral

angiographic catheter
angiographic finding
angiographic recanalization
angiographic targeting
angiographically confirmed
angiographically occult intracranial vascular malformation (AOIVM)
angiography (see *angiogram*)
angiolipoma
angioma
- arteriovenous
- cavernous

angioma *(cont.)*
- cutaneous
- intracranial cavernous
- intradermal
- venous

angiomatosis
- cerebroretinal
- corticomeningeal
- Divry-van Bogaert familial
- encephalotrigeminal
- leptomeningeal
- retinocerebral

angiomatosis of retina
angioparalytic blockade
angiopathy, cerebral amyloid
angioplastic meningioma
angioplasty, transluminal
angiosarcoma
angiotomomyelography
angle
- acetabular
- acromial (of scapula)
- antegonial
- anteroposterior talocalcaneal (APTC)
- arch
- Bauman
- Beatson combined ankle
- bimalleolar
- Boehler calcaneal (Böhler)
- Boehler lumbosacral (Böhler)
- C
- calcaneal pitch
- calcaneoplantar
- carrying
- CE (capital epiphysis)
- central collodiaphysial (CCD)
- cephalic
- cephalometric
- cerebellopontile
- Citelli
- Clarke arch
- Cobb lumbar
- Cobb scoliosis

angle *(cont.)*
- Codman
- condylar
- costal
- costolumbar
- costophrenic
- costosternal
- costovertebral
- craniofacial
- distal articular
- dorsoplantar talometatarsal
- dorsoplantar talonavicular
- Drennan metaphyseal-epiphyseal
- femorotibial (FTA)
- first-fifth intermetatarsal
- first metatarsal
- foot-progression (FPA)
- first-second intermetatarsal
- Garden
- Gissane
- gonial
- hallux dorsiflexion (DFA)
- hallux interphalangeus
- hallux valgus (HVA)
- hallux valgus interphalangeus
- Hibbs metatarsocalcaneal
- Hilgenreiner
- IM (intermetatarsal)
- increased carrying
- intermetatarsal (IMA)
- intermetatarsal I or II
- Kite
- Konstram
- lateral plantar metatarsal
- lateral talocalcaneal (LATC)
- lateral tarsometatarsal
- Laurin
- lumbosacral joint
- mandibular
- Meary metatarsotalar
- mediolateral radiocarpal
- Merchant
- metaphyseal-epiphyseal
- metatarsocalcaneal

angle *(cont.)*
  metatarsotalar
  metatarsus adductus
  metatarsus primus
  Mikulicz
  navicular to first metatarsal
  neck shaft
  occipitocervical
  Pauwels
  pelvic femoral
  plantar metatarsal
  proximal articular set (PASA)
  Q
  radiocarpal
  resting forefoot supination
  sacrohorizontal
  sacrovertebral
  set
  slip
  spinographic
  sulcus
  talar-tilt
  talocalcaneal (subtalar)
  talocrural
  talometatarsal
  talonavicular
  tarsometatarsal
  TC
  thigh-foot (TFA)
  tibiofemoral (TFA)
  tibiotalar
  TMA-thigh (transmalleolar axis)
  transmetatarsal (TMA)
  valgus
  varus
  varus metatarsophalangeal (MTP)
  Wiberg
  Wiltze
angle of anteversion
angle of declination of metatarsal
angle of greatest extension (AGE)
angle of greatest flexion (AGF)
angle of incongruity
angular frequency
angular gyrus (AG)
angular momentum
angular process of orbit
angulation
  anterior
  cephalic
  degrees of valgus
  degrees of varus
  forefoot
  posttraumatic
  spinal
anhidrosis
animation, suspended
anisocoria
ankle
  autologous reverse graft to
  eversion sprain of the
  footballer's
  fused
  giving way of
  inversion injury of the
  neuropathic
  sprained
  syndesmosis sprain of the
  synthetic graft bypass to
  tailor's
  transmalleolar
  twisted
  Wiltse osteotomy of
ankle Air-Stirrup
ankle/arm blood pressure index
ankle/arm index
ankle block
ankle brace
ankle/brachial blood pressure index
ankle/brachial pressure ratio
ankle disk
ankle dorsiflexion range of motion
  (ADROM)
ankle dressing, Cryo/Cuff
ankle eversion
ankle-foot orthosis (AFO)
ankle fracture
ankle fusion
ankle instability
ankle inversion-eversion range of motion

ankle jerk (AJ)
ankle jerk reflex
ankle joint complex (AJC)
ankle-level arteriotomy
ankle ligament protector (ALP)
ankle mortise
ankle orthosis, Malleoloc anatomic
ankle sprain
ankle systolic pressure
anklet, elastic
ankylodactyly
ankylosing spondylitis
ankylosis, ankyloses
  bony
  extracapsular
  false
  fibrous
  intracapsular
  ligamentous
  shoulder
  spurious
  vertebral
anlage (pl. anlagen)
  cartilaginous
  radial head
  ulnar
anlage à priori
anneal, annealed
annular
annular ligament of finger
annuli (pl. of annulus)
annulospiral fibers
annulotomy
annulus (also anulus)
annulus fibrosus
annulus fibrosus disci intervertebralis
annulus, fissure of
annulus of Vieussens
anode
anoia
anomalous insertion
anomalous movement
anomaly, anomalies
  congenital
  cranial

anomaly *(cont.)*
  multiple congenital (MCA)
  vascular
anomia
  color
  finger
  tactile
anomic aphasia
anomie
anopsia, altitudinal
anosmia, anosmic
anosodiaphoria
anosognosia
anosognosis
anosteoplasia
anostosis
anoxemia
anoxia
  acute
  birth
  cerebral
  consumptive
  perinatal
anoxic damage
anoxic encephalopathy
anoxic hypoxia
anoxic ischemia
ansa (pl. ansae)
ansae nervorum spinalium
ansa cervicalis
ansa et fasciculus lenticulares
ansa hypoglossi
ansa lenticularis
ansa of Vieussens
ansa peduncularis
ansa subclavia
anserinus, pes
Anspach Cement Eater
Anspach craniotome
Anspach power drill
Anspach reamer
antagonist muscle groups
antalgic gait
antalgic limp
anteater sign

antebrachial fascia
antebrachium
antecubital fossa
anteflexion
antegrade amnesia
antenna
anterior cerebellar artery syndrome
anterior cingulate gyrus tumor
anterior circulation stroke
anterior colliculus
anterior column of spine
anterior communicating artery distribution infarction
anterior compartment syndrome
anterior corpus
anterior corticospinal tract
anterior cruciate instability with pivot shift
anterior cruciate ligament (ACL) drill guide
anterior cruciate ligament (ACL) repair
anterior fibular ligament
anterior foot draw sign
anterior gray column of cord
anterior head region
anterior horn-cell disease
anterior horn-cell motor impairment
anterior horns of spinal cord
anterior hypothalamus
anterior inferior cerebellar artery (AICA)
anterior inferior cerebral artery (AICA)
anterior inferior communicating artery (AICA)
anterior innominate test
anterior lobe, midline tumor of the
anterior medial ankle ligament
anterior median fissure of cord
anterior metatarsal arch
anterior shear
anterior shin splints
anterior spinal artery syndrome
anterior spinocerebellar tract
anterior spinothalamic tract
anterior superior iliac spine (ASIS)
anterior talar dome
anterior talofibular ligament
anterior tibial compartment syndrome
anterior tibiofibular ligament
anterior tibiotalar ligament
anterocollis
anterograde amnesia
anterolateral white matter of cord
anterolisthesis
anteromedial
anteromesial temporal discharge on EEG
anteroposterior (AP)
antetorsion, femoral
anteversion
  angle of
  femoral
  Magilligan technique for measuring
  neutral
anteversion determination, Budin-Chandler
anteverted
anti-AChR (antiacetylcholine receptor) antibody
antibiotic and saline solution
antibiotic-impregnated beads
antibiotic-impregnated polymethyl methacrylate (PMMA)
antibody
  AChR (acetylcholine receptor)
  ACTH
  AE1
  AE3
  anti-ACh receptor
  anti-AChR (antiacetylcholine receptor)
  antistriated muscle
  beta-endorphin
  Borrelia burgdorferi
  CAM 5.2
  cytokeratins

antibody *(cont.)*
  EMA (epithelial membrane antigen)
  GFAP (glial fibrillary acidic protein)
  glutinin 1
  growth hormone
  kinase C antiglioma monoclonal
  lectins
  luteinizing hormone
  MG (myasthenia gravis)
  monoclonal
  neuron-specific enolase (NSE)
  neutralization
  NSE (neuron-specific enolase)
  prealbumin
  prolactin hormone
  RCA (*Ricinus communis* agglutinin 1)
  S-100 protein
  St. Louis encephalitis
  thyrotropin hormone
  UE (Ulex europaeus)
  vimentin
  VZ (varicella-zoster)
anticonvulsant drugs
anticonvulsant intoxication, hypersensitivity reaction
anticonvulsants
  blood levels of
  hypersensitivity reaction to
antidepressants, tricyclic
antidromic (sensory) conduction studies
antiembolism hose
antiembolism stockings, Orthawear
antiepilepsirine
antiepileptic effect of drug
antigen
  antiproliferating cell nuclear
  carcinoembryonic (CEA)
  epithelial membrane (EMA)
antiglioma monoclonal antibody kinase C
antigravity muscles
anti-inflammatory drug
anti-Ki-67
antimalarial
antimyoclonic effect of drug
antineurofilament
antinuclear antibody (ANA) test
antiparkinsonism
antirotation device
antiseptic, ACU-dyne
Anti-Shox foot cushion
antistreptolysin O (ASO) titer
Anton syndrome
Antoni A cell
Antoni B cell
Antoni-A classification of neurinoma
antrum, Malacarne
anulus (annulus)
anvil
  Bunnell
  Hurteau skull plate
anvil sign
anvil test
anxietas tibiarum
AO-ASIF compression technique
AO-ASIF implant
AO-ASIF screw
AO blade plate
AO classification of ankle fracture
AO cortical screw
AO-Danis-Weber classification of ankle fractures
AO drill bit
AO nail
AO plate
AO pseudoisochromatic color plate test
AO reconstruction plate
AO reduction forceps
AO semitubular plate
AO spongiosa screw
AO spoon plate
AO technique
AOA halo traction
AOIVM (angiographically occult intracranial vascular malformation)
aortic valve prosthesis
AOVM (angiographically occult vascular malformation)

AP (anteroposterior)
APACHE II measure of disease severity
apallic patient
apallic state
apallic syndrome
apathy
APB (abductor pollicis brevis) muscle
A-P cutter
ape hand (simian griffe)
ape hand of syringomyelia
ape-like hand
aperiodic complex
aperiodic wave
Apert disease
Apert syndrome
aperta, rhinolalia
aperture
apex
  orbital
  petrous
apex of head of femur
apex of head of fibula
apex of head of patella
apex of horn of spinal cord
apex of petrous portion of temporal bone
Apfelbaum mirror
aphagia
aphalangia
aphasia
  acoustic
  acquired epileptic
  acquired fluent
  ageusic
  amnemonic
  amnesic
  amnestic
  anomic
  associative
  ataxic
  auditory
  Benson-Geschwind classification of
  Broca

aphasia *(cont.)*
  combined
  commissural
  complete
  conduction
  cortical
  dynamic
  expressive
  expressive-receptive
  fluent
  frontocortical
  frontolenticular
  functional
  gibberish
  global
  graphomotor
  Grashey
  hypophonic
  impressive
  intellectual
  jargon
  Kussmaul
  lenticular
  Lichtheim
  major motor
  mixed
  motor
  nominal
  nonfluent
  optic
  parieto-occipital
  partial nominal
  pathematic
  pictorial
  psychosensory
  receptive
  semantic
  sensory
  subcortical
  syntactical
  tactile
  temporoparietal
  total
  transcortical (motor)

aphasia *(cont.)*
  transcortical (sensory)
  transcortical mixed
  true
  verbal
  visual form of Wernicke
  Wernicke
Aphasia Screening Test, Halstead-Wepman
aphasic error
aphasic patient
aphasic seizure
aphasic speech
  fluent
  nonfluent
aphasiology
aphemia
aphonia
  acute
  functional (hysterical)
  hysterical (functional)
apical corn
apical ligament
apiculate waveform
APL (abductor pollicis longus) muscle
APL (abductor pollicis longus) tendon
aplasia, cerebellar
APLD (automated percutaneous lumbar diskectomy)
Apley grinding test
Apley scratch test
Apley sign
Apley test, two-part
apnea
  central
  central sleep
  mixed sleep
  obstructive
  obstructive sleep
  sleep
apneic seizures
apneustic breathing
apneustic period
apodia
apogeotropic nystagmus
aponeurectomy
aponeurorrhaphy
aponeurosis
  digital
  palmar
  plantar
aponeurosis of tendon
aponeurotic band
aponeurotic triangle
aponeurotic troika
aponeurotomy
apophysis, apophyseal
apophysitis
  calcaneal
  iliac
apoplectic
apoplexy
  delayed
  pituitary
  posttraumatic (of Bollinger)
apotentiality, cerebral
apparatus (see *device*; *orthosis*)
appearance
  beaten-silver (of the skull)
  disheveled
  isodense
  onion peel (on x-ray)
  unkempt
appendicular ataxia
apperceptive disorder
appliance (see *device*; *orthosis*)
application of traction device
applicator
  aneurysm clip
  scalp clip
applier
  bayonet clip
  clip
  Ligaclip
  Mayfield miniature clip
  Mayfield temporary aneurysm clip
  mini
  vari-angle clip

apposing articular surfaces
apposition
  bone-to-bone
  fracture in close
apprehension shoulder
apprehension test
approach (see *incision*; *operation*)
  holistic
  ipsilateral
  lateral
  posterolateral
  transsylvian
  transventricular
  veterinary
approximator (also see *contractor*)
  Acland double-clamp
  double-clamp
  Lalonde tendon
  Lemmon sternal
  sternal
  Van Beck nerve
APR (anatomic porous replacement)
APR acetabular prosthesis
APR cement fixation
APR femoral prosthesis
APR II hip prosthesis
APR total hip system
apractognosia
apractic (or apraxic)
apraxia
  akinetic
  amnestic
  Bruns gait
  buccofacial
  callosal
  cerebral mapping of
  classic
  constructional
  cortical
  disconnection
  dressing
  ideational
  ideokinetic
  ideomotor
apraxia *(cont.)*
  innervation
  Liepmann
  limb-kinetic
  magnetic
  motor
  ocular
  oculomotor
  oral
  pure limb
  sensory
  transcortical
apraxic disorder (or apractic)
apraxic dysarthria (or apractic)
APRL (Army Prosthetics Research Laboratory) prosthesis
apron, quadriceps
APS (air plasma spray) hydroxyapatite
APTA (American Physical Therapy Association)
APTC (anteroposterior talocalcaneal) angle
Aquaphor gauze dressing
Aquaplast splint
AquaShield orthopedic cast cover
Aquatech cast padding
aquatic exercise program
aquatic rehabilitation
aqueduct
  cerebral
  forking of sylvian
  gliosis of
  mesencephalon
  midbrain
  Monro
  Sylvius
  ventricular
aqueductal occlusion
aqueductal stenosis
ARA (Action Research Arm Test)
ARA (American Rheumatism Association)
arachidonic acid

arachnodactyl
  congenital
  contracture
arachnodactyly
arachnoid canal
arachnoid cyst
arachnoid of uncus
arachnoid-shape Beaver blade
arachnoid villi
arachnoiditis
  adhesive
  basilar
  fibrosing
  spinal
arachnoiditis of opticochiasmatic cistern
Arafiles elbow arthrodesis
Arafiles prosthesis
Arana-Iniquez intracranial cyst removal technique
Aran-Duchenne amyotrophy
arborization
arborize
arbovirus (arthropod-borne)
arbovirus meningo-encephalitis
arboviruses, group b (causing encephalitis)
arc
  monosynaptic reflex
  stereotactic
arc of motion
arcade
  Frohse ligamentous
  Struthers
  superficialis
arch
  anterior atlas
  anterior metatarsal
  articular
  carpal
  coracoacromial
  deep
  flat
  flattened longitudinal (of foot)

arch *(cont.)*
  Hapad metatarsal
  Hapad scaphoid
  high
  Hillock
  longitudinal (of foot)
  metal
  neural
  neural vertebral
  palmar arterial
  plantar
  plantar arterial
  posterior metatarsal
  pubic
  superciliary
  superficial palmar arterial
  tarsal
  transverse (of foot)
  vertebral
archicortex
archimedean hand drill
arch index
architectural alterations of bone (seen on x-ray)
architecture, bony
architecture of brain
architecture of foot
arch of atlas
archplasty
arch support
  plantar
  Plastizote
  Whitman
arcuate complex
arcuate fasciculus (AF)
arcuate ligament
arcuate movement
arcuate nucleus
arcuatus, pes
arcus atlantis
arcus palmaris profundus
arcus palmaris superficialis
arcus parieto-occipitalis
arcus pedis transversalis

arcus plantaris
arcus plantaris profundus
arcus pubicus
arcus vertebrae
arcus vertebralis
arcus volaris profundus
arcus volaris superficialis
area (see also *region*)
  Broca
  Brodmann
  callosal (parolfactory nerve)
  language
  olfactory
  parietal association
  parietotemporal
  premotor
  sclerotic
  sclerotome
  septal
  watershed
  Wernicke
areflexia, pupillary
areflexic dystasia, Roussy-Levy hereditary
areolar plane
areolar tissue, dorsum of hand
arginase deficiency
argininosuccinic aciduria
argon laser
Argyll Robertson pupils of tabetic neurosyphilis
argyrophil plaque
arhinencephaly
Ariel computerized exercise system
arithmetical epilepsy
Arizona Health Science Center-Volz elbow prosthesis
Arizona leg support
arm
  abductor lever
  flail
  Leyla
  linebacker's
  outrigger

arm *(cont.)*
  popeye
  tackler's
  Utah artificial
  Yasargil Leyla retractor
arm abduction test
armboard, Flexisplint flexed
arm cuff
arm drift
Armistead technique
arm sling
Armstrong acromionectomy
Armstrong plate
arm swing, synkinetic
arm swing with gait
Army bone gouge
Army-Navy retractor
Army osteotome
Arnold-Chiari deformity
Arnold-Chiari malformation
Arnold-Chiari syndrome
Arnold lumbar brace
AROM (active range of motion exercises)
Aron Alpha adhesive
arousable patient
arousal from sleep
array
  compressed spectral (on EEG)
  linear electrode
  educed EEG electrode
array of electrodes
array processor
arrest, epiphyseal
arrest of speech
arrest reaction
arrested derotation of foot position as cause of foot deformities
arterial blood gases (ABGs)
arterial tonus
arteriogram, arteriography
  arch and carotid
  cerebral
  contrast

arteriolar muscle tone
arteriosclerotic intracranial aneurysm
arteriotomy, ankle-level
arteriovenous angioma
arteriovenous fistula (AVF)
arteriovenous interhemispheric
  angioma
arteriovenous malformation (AVM)
arteritis
  cranial
  Horton giant cell
  spinal cord
  Takayasu
  temporal
  viral intracerebral
artery
  A1-A5 segments of anterior cerebral
  aberrant
  Adamkiewicz (Adamkiewitz)
  aneurysm of internal carotid
  aneurysm of posterior communicating
  angular MCA (middle cerebral
    artery)
  anterior cerebral (ACA)
  anterior choroidal (ACA or AChA)
  anterior communicating (ACoA)
  anterior inferior cerebellar (AICA)
  anterior inferior cerebral (AICA)
  anterior inferior communicating
    (AICA)
  anterior spinal
  anterior spinal canal
  anterior temporal branch of
    posterior cerebral
  ascending frontoparietal (ASFP)
  basal perforating
  basilar
  bifurcation of anterior communicating
  bifurcation of common carotid
  bifurcation of internal carotid artery
  bifurcation of middle cerebral
  brachiocephalic
  branch of
  C1-C5 segments of internal carotid

artery *(cont.)*
  calcarine
  callosomarginal
  carotid
  choroidal
  choroidal branch of internal carotid
    artery
  choroidal pericallosal
  circumflex
  common carotid (CCA)
  compression of
  cortical branch of middle cerebral
  costocervical
  course of
  deltoid branch of posterior tibial
  dissection of
  dorsal spinal
  dural
  dynamic entrapment of vertebral
  en passage feeder
  external carotid (ECA)
  extracranial vertebral
  extradural
  feeder
  feeding
  friable
  frontopolar (FPA)
  internal carotid (ICA)
  intracavernous internal carotid
  intracranial vertebral
  lateral posterior choroidal (LPCh)
  lenticulostriate
  leptomeningeal
  M1-M5 segments of middle cerebral
  MCA (middle cerebral)
  medial posterior choroidal (MPCh)
  meningeal
  meningohypophyseal trunk (MHT)
  mesencephalic
  middle cerebral (MCA)
  middle meningeal
  nodular induration of temporal
  nutrient
  occipital branch of external carotid

artery *(cont.)*
- occlusion of
- ophthalmic
- P1-P4 segments of posterior cerebral
- paramalleolar
- paramedian thalamopeduncular
- parietal MCA
- parieto-occipital branch of posterior cerebellar
- peduncular segment of superior cerebellar
- pericallosal
- petrous segment of carotid
- plantar metatarsal
- pontine
- post-temporal MCA
- posterior cerebral (PCA)
- posterior choroidal
- posterior communicating (PCA)
- posterior inferior cerebellar (PICA)
- posterior parietal
- posterior spinal
- posterior temporal
- posterolateral spinal (PLSA)
- precommunicating segment of anterior cerebral
- primitive trigeminal (PTA)
- proximal digital
- radial digital
- radicular
- radiculomedullary
- radiculospinal
- recurrent (of Heubner)
- retinal
- scalp branch of external carotid
- segmental branch of vertebral
- splenial branch of posterior cerebral artery
- subclavian
- superficial temporal (STA)
- superior cerebellar (SCA)
- supraclinoid carotid
- thalamocaudate
- thalamogeniculate

artery *(cont.)*
- thalamoperforating
- thyrocervical trunk of subclavian
- trifurcation of middle cerebral
- twig of
- ulnar anesthetic
- ulnar digital
- vertebral basilar

Arthopor cup prosthesis
Arthopor pad
Arthopor II acetabular prosthesis
arthralgia
- migratory
- subtalar
- temporomandibular joint

arthrectomy
arthrempyesis
Arthrex arthroscopy instruments
arthrifluent abscess
arthritic talonavicular changes
arthritis (pl. arthritides)
- acute hematogenous
- acute spinal
- allergenic
- assignment criteria for rheumatoid
- Bekhterev
- Brucella
- cervical
- Charcot
- degenerative
- Fries score for rheumatoid
- gold therapy for rheumatoid
- gonococcal
- gouty
- inflammatory
- juvenile rheumatoid (JRA)
- Marie-Strümpell
- migratory
- NewYork diagnostic criteria for rheumatoid
- osteoarthritis
- Outerbridge staging of degenerative
- pantalocrural
- pauciarticular

arthritis *(cont.)*
polyarticular
posttraumatic
psoriatic
pyogenic
rheumatoid (RA)
Rome criteria for rheumatoid
Salmonella
septic
seronegative
seropositive rheumatoid
spinal
Steinbrocker classification of rheumatoid
suppurative
traumatic
tuberculous
ulnar deviation of hand in rheumatoid
Arthritis Foundation
Arthritis Helplessness Index (AHI)
Arthritis Impact Measurement Scales (AIMS)
Arthrobot-Zimmer
arthrocele
arthrocentesis
arthrochalasis
arthrochondritis
arthroclasia
arthrodesed digit
arthrodesis (see also *operation*)
Albee hip
anterior slot graft arthrodesis
atlantoaxial
Baciu-Filibiu dowel ankle
Badgley
Benyi modification of Lambrinudi triple
bimalleolar approach to ankle
Blair tibiotalar
Brett
Brockman-Nissen
Brooks atlantoaxial
calcaneocuboid

arthrodesis *(cont.)*
Campbell
Carroll
Chandler
Chapchal knee
Charcot hip
Charnley ankle
Charnley-Houston
Chuinard-Petersen ankle
closing wedge
Compere-Thompson
compression screw
cone
distraction-compression bone graft
dowel
extra-articular subtalar
fused
Gallie ankle
Gallie atlantoaxial
Gant hip
Gill-Stein
Grice extra-articular subtalar
Grice-Green extra-articular subtalar
Grice-Green subtalar
Guttmann subtalar
hallux interphalangeal (IP) joint
hindfoot
Ilizarov ankle
interbody
internal fixation compression
intertransverse process
intra-articular
Lambrinudi triple
lesser tarsal
Mann-Coughlin
Mann-Thompson-Coughlin
McKeever
metatarsocuneiform
metatarsophalangeal joint
midfoot
Moberg
Müller (Mueller)
Nalebuff
naviculocuneiform joint

arthrodesis *(cont.)*
  nonfused
  occipitocervical
  pantalar
  Potenza
  Potter
  Schneider
  sliding
  spinal
  Stone
  subtalar
  talonavicular
  tibiotalar
  transfibular
  transmalleolar ankle
  triple
  Uematsu shoulder
  ulnocarpal
arthrodiastasis
arthrodynia
arthrodysplasia
arthroempyesis
arthroendoscopy
arthroereisis, staple
arthrofibrosis
Arthro-Flo arthroscopic irrigation system
Arthro-Flo irrigator
Arthro-Flo system
arthrogram
arthrography
  Brostrom-Gordon
  coronal computed tomographic (CCTA)
  double-contrast
  Gordon-Brostrom single-contrast
  single-contrast
arthrogryposis multiplex congenita
arthrokatadysis
arthrokleisis
arthrolith
Arthro-Lok blade
Arthro-Lok system
arthrolysis
arthromeningitis
arthrometer
  Acufex knee laxity
  Genucom
  joint
  KT-1000 joint
  KT-1000 knee
  Medmetric KT-1000 knee laxity
  Robinson
  stress-testing
  Stryker knee laxity
arthroncus
arthroneuralgia
arthronosos
arthro-onychodysplasia
arthro-ophthalmology, hereditary progressive
arthropathology
arthropathy
  Charcot
  crystal-related
  inflammatory
  Jaccoud
  midfoot
  neuropathic (NA)
  systemic lupus erythematosus (SLE)
arthrophyma
arthrophyte
arthroplasty (see also *operation*)
  ablative
  abrasion
  Albright-Chase
  ankle
  Aufranc-Turner
  Bowers radial
  capitellocondylar total elbow
  Carroll and Taber
  cemented total hip
  cementless total hip
  Clayton resection
  constrained ankle
  Cracchiolo-Sculco implant
  Crawford-Adams acetabular cup
  cuff-tear
  cup

arthroplasty *(cont.)*
- ELP stem for hip
- excision
- extensor brevis
- failed implant
- fascial
- forefoot
- four-in-one
- Girdlestone
- Global total shoulder
- Gustilo-Kyle cementless total hip
- hemijoint
- hip (cup on cup)
- implant
- interpositional elbow
- Irvine ankle
- Johnson resection
- Kates forefoot
- Keller
- Keller resection
- Kocher-McFarland hip
- Koenig metatarsophalangeal joint
- Koenig MPJ implant and
- LICA (laser image custom)
- Mann resection
- Mark II Sorrells hip
- Mayo ankle
- Mayo resection
- McAtee Tharias-Blazina
- McKee-Farrar total hip
- modified mold and surface replacement
- monospherical total shoulder
- Mumford-Gurd
- Neer hemiarthroplasty
- New England Baptist
- primary
- Putti-Platt
- resection
- revision
- Schlein elbow
- silicone implant
- Stanmore shoulder
- surface replacement

arthroplasty *(cont.)*
- Swanson interpositional wrist
- Swanson metatarsophalangeal joint
- Swanson PIP joint
- tendon interposition
- total ankle
- total articular resurfacing (TARA)
- total hip (THA)
- total knee (TKA)
- triaxial total elbow
- Tupper
- UCLA anatomic shoulder
- Vainio
- Valenti
- Volz total wrist

arthroplasty implant technique, great toe (GAIT)

ArthroProbe arthroscopic laser

ArthroProbe laser system

arthropyosis

arthrorheumatism

arthroscope
- angled
- Baxter angled
- Dyonics
- Eagle straight-ahead
- panoview
- Storz oblique
- Stryker viewing
- Wolf

arthroscopic examination

arthroscopic resection, screw fixation

arthroscopic sheath

arthroscopic system, McCain TMJ

arthroscopically

arthroscopy
- Allen shoulder
- ankle
- diagnostic and operative
- Gilquist
- knee
- second-look
- wrist

arthroscopy-assisted patellar tendon substitution

arthroscopy entry portal, stab wound
arthrosis
  crystal-induced
  degenerative
  IRM spiral
arthrosynovitis
arthrotome
arthrotomy
  Magnuson-Stack shoulder
  medial parapatellar
  subtalar
arthroxerosis
arthroxesis
articular cartilage degeneration
articular cortex
articular disk
articular fragment
articular surfaces
  apposing
  contiguous
articulate
articulating bone ends
articulation
  acromioclavicular
  atlantoaxial
  calcaneocuboid
  carpometacarpal
  carporadial
  condylar
  costovertebral
  DIP (distal interphalangeal)
  humeroradial
  humeroulnar
  intercarpal
  intermetacarpal
  interphalangeal
  metacarpophalangeal
  occipitocervical
  patellofemoral
  PIP (proximal interphalangeal)
  radiocarpal
  radiohumeral
  radioulnar
  scapuloclavicular
articulation *(cont.)*
  subtalar
  talocalcaneal
  talocalcaneonavicular
  tarsometatarsal
  tibiofibular
articulation disturbance
articulatory skills
articulatory tics
artifact, asymmetric
artifact-free EEG
artifact on EEG
  asymmetric
  blink
  cardiac pacemaker
  electrode-popping
  eye blink
  glossokinetic
  lateralized
  movement
  muscle
  nonbiological
  nonphysiologic
  paper stop
  perspiration
  physiologic
  pikelike
  pulse wave
  spikelike
  rhythmic
  stimulus
artifact on x-ray
artificial limb, Utah
ascending activating system
ascending reticular activating system
ascending tract
Asch forceps
Asch splint
ASD (antisiphon device), Heyer-Schulte
ASE (axilla, shoulder, elbow) bandage
aseptic fashion
aseptic felon (herpetic whitlow)
aseptic meningitis
aseptic necrosis

aseptic uremic meningitis
ASES (American shoulder and elbow system)
ASFP (ascending frontoparietal) artery
Asher physical build assessment technique
Ashhurst fracture classification system
Ashhurst sign
Ashhurst splint
Ashworth implant arthroplasty
Ashworth scale
Ashworth score of muscle spasticity
ASIF (Swiss Association for the Study of Internal Fixation)
ASIF blade plate
ASIF chisel
ASIF plate
ASIF screw
ASIS (anterior superior iliac spine)
Asnis 2 guided screw
Asnis cannulated screw
ASO (antistreptolysin O) titer
Aspen electrocautery
Aspen laparoscopy electrode
aspergillosis, intracranial
aspergillosis of the central nervous system
aspergillotic aneurysm
Aspergillus fumigatus
Aspergillus niger
Aspergillus invasion of the nervous system
asphyxia
  neonatal
  perinatal
aspiration
  bone marrow
  joint
  joint fluid
  therapeutic
aspirator
  Cavitron ultrasonic surgical (CUSA)
  Sharplan ultrasonic
  Sonocut ultrasonic
assay, radioisotope clearance
assessment
  Activity Losses (ALA)
  BFM arm (Brunnstrom-Fugl-Meyer)
  Brunnstrom-Fugl-Meyer (BFM) arm impairment
  CFQ-for-others
  closed-chain functional
  environmental
  functional
  Glasgow Assessment Schedule
  global assessment of sensory disturbance
  home
  quality of life
  rehabilitation
  Rivermead Motor Assessment
  Stone and Neale Daily Coping
ASSI coagulator (ASSI, Accurate Surgical and Scientific Instruments Corp.)
assignment criteria for rheumatoid arthritis
assist
  hand-held
  maximal assist of one or more
  minimal
  standby
assistant, chiropractic (C.A.)
Association
  American Dietetic Association diet for athletes
  American Association of Mental Deficiency
  American Rheumatism (ARA)
  National Collegiate Athletic (NCAA)
  National Association for Mental Health
  National Association for the Deaf
  National Association for the Visually Handicapped
  Visiting Nurse
associational thalamic nuclei
association cortex of parietal lobes

associations
  clang
  loose
associative visual agnosia
astasia
astasia-abasia
astatic seizures
astereognosis (tactile agnosia)
asterixis (hepatic encephalopathy tremor)
asthenia, asthenic
ASTM designation of Biophase
Aston cartilage reduction
astragalectomy
astragalus (talus), aviator's
astroblast
astrocyte
  fibrous
  gemistocytic
  plasmatofibrous
  protoplasmic
astrocytic gliosis
astrocytic tumor
astrocytoma
  anaplastic
  fibrillary
  gemistocytic
  grades 1-4
  high-grade (glioblastoma multiforme)
  intracranial
  low-grade (LGA)
  pilocytic
  protoplasmic
  supratentorial
astrocytoma tumor
astrocytosis
astroglial tumor
asymmetric hyperreflexia
asymmetric tonic neck reflex (ATNR)
asymmetrical
asymmetry
  amplitude
  facial
  interhemispheric

asymmetry *(cont.)*
  limb length
  skull
asyndesis
asyndetic communication
asynergia, asynergic
Atasoy-Kleinert flap
Atasoy palmar flap
Atasoy triangular advancement flap
Atasoy V-Y technique
atavicus, metatarsus
ataxia
  absent
  appendicular
  atactic
  Bruns
  cerebellar
  crural
  equilibratory
  familial paroxysmal kinesigenic
  familial spastic
  Friedreich
  frontal
  gait
  Greenfield classification of spinocerebellar
  hereditary spastic
  ipsilateral cerebellar
  kinesigenic
  limb
  limb-gait
  locomotor
  Marie hereditary spastic
  mild
  moderate
  sensory
  severe
  truncal
ataxia of cerebellar origin
ataxia of posterior column origin
ataxia-telangiectasia
ataxic breathing
ataxic gait
ataxic hemiparesis (AH)

ataxic respiration
ataxic speech
ATD (assistive technology devices)
Aten olecranon screw
ATF (anterior talofibular ligament)
atheroma, carotid bifurcation
atherostenosis
athetoid palsy, pure
athetosis, double congenital
athetotic
athlete
  differentially-abled
  high-power
athlete's diet, American Dietetic Association
athlete's foot
athlete's pseudonephritis
athletic caloric requirements
Atkinson endoprosthesis
ATL (anterior temporal lobectomy)
ATL real-time Neurosector scanner
Atlanta brace orthosis
atlantoaxial arthrodesis
atlantoaxial fixation
atlantoaxial instability
atlantoaxial posterior membrane
atlantoaxial interval
atlantoaxial joint
atlantoaxial separation
atlantoaxial stabilization
atlantoaxial subluxation
atlantomastoid
atlanto-occipital fusion
atlanto-occipital junction
atlanto-occipital membrane
atlanto-odontoid
atlas (C1, first cervical vertebra)
  arch of
  burst fracture of the
  compression fracture of the
  transverse ligaments of the
ATNR (asymmetric tonic neck reflex)
ATON (adductor tenotomy and obturator neurectomy)
atonic bladder
atonic seizure
atony (atonia)
atopognosia
atraumatic
atretic
atrium of ventricle
atrophic dementia
  Alzheimer
  Pick
  senile
atrophic lesion of the brain
atrophic neuroarthropathy
atrophied muscle
atrophy
  brachial muscular
  brain
  cerebral
  cerebral surface
  cortical
  dentatorubral
  dentatorubropallidoluysian
  disuse
  dorsum sellae
  divopontocerebellar
  Duchenne-Aran spinal muscular
  Duchenne muscular
  frontotemporal
  Gudden
  hemisphere
  Kugelberg-Welander juvenile spinal muscle
  Leber optic
  lesser (of disuse)
  lobar (of Pick)
  localized muscular
  Marie-Foix-Alajouanine cerebellar
  Menzel olivopontocerebellar
  muscle
  neurogenic
  olivopontocerebellar
  parenchymatous
  peroneal muscular
  postneuritic

atrophy *(cont.)*
primary optic
progressive neuropathic muscle
progressive post-polio muscle (PPPMA)
quadriceps
scapuloperoneal muscular
spinal muscular (SMA)
subcortical
Sudeck
sulcal
temporal horn
Vulpian-Bernhardt spinal muscular
Welander distal muscular
Werdnig-Hoffmann spinal muscular
attachment
capsular
cerebellar
dural
fibrous
Hudson cerebellar
ligamentous
Pearson
tendinous
attack
adversive
akinetic drop
cataleptic
cephalalgic
cephalgic
cryptogenic drop
decerebrate
drop
epileptic drop
factitious
falling
jackknife
kinesigenic
masticatory
motor jacksonian
psychomotor
salaam
sensory jacksonian
sleep

attack *(cont.)*
Stokes-Adams
transient hemisphere (THA)
transient ischemic (TIA)
vagal
vasospastic
waking
attack absence
Attenborough knee prosthesis
attend, ability to
attention
fix and focus
heightened
raptus of
attention deficit
attention deficit disorder (ADD)
attention deficit/hyperactivity disorder (ADHD)
attention span
attentuate, attentuated
attentuating
attenuation coefficient on MRI scan
attenuation of alpha rhythm on EEG
attenuation of tendons
attenuation value on MRI scan
attitude, over-dependent
Atton disease
attrition rupture of tendon
ATV (all-terrain vehicle) accident
ATV (anterior terminal vein)
atypical absence seizure (petit mal variant)
atypical giant cell tumor
auditory agnosia
auditory cortex, primary
auditory division of eighth cranial nerve
auditory evoked potential
auditory evoked response
auditory radiation
auditory seizure
auditory symptoms
Aufranc cobra hip prosthesis
Aufranc cobra retractor
Aufranc modification of Smith-Petersen cup

Aufranc osteotome
Aufranc retractor
Aufranc-Turner acetabular cup
Aufranc-Turner arthroplasty
Aufranc-Turner hip prosthesis
Aufricht glabellar rasp
auger
augmenting response on EEG
Augustine boat nail
aula
auliplexus
aulix
aura
  auditory
  déjà vu
  epigastric
  epileptic
  gustatory
  hysterical
  intellectual
  jamais vu
  kinesthetic
  migraine
  migrainous
  motor
  olfactory
  reminiscent
  sensory
  shimmering light with
  status
  tactile pricklings with
  tingling with
  uncinate
  visual shimmering with
  visual shining with
  visual sparkling with
  wavering light with
aura of migraine
aura procursiva
aura symptoms in migraine
Aussies-Isseis unstable scoliosis
Austin bunionectomy
Austin Moore chisel
Austin Moore hemiarthroplasty
Austin Moore hip prosthesis
Austin Moore hook
Austin Moore impactor
Austin osteotomy
Australian X viral encephalitis
autism
  akinetic
  infantile
autistic thinking
auto-reinforced polyglycolide rods
Auto-Implant procedure
autochthonous graft
autoecholalia
Autoflex II CPM (continuous passive motion) unit
autofusion
Autogenesis automator for Ilizarov screws
autogenous bone graft
autograft
  bridge
  free revascularized
  iliac crest
  tendon-bone
autoimmune response
autologous adrenal medullary tissue
autologous blood transfusion
autologous reverse graft to ankle
automated computerized axial tomography (ACAT)
automatic behavior
automatic bladder, in spinal cord syndromes
automatic bladder reflex
automatic phrase level
automatism
  chewing
  epileptic
  facial expression
  gestural
  ictal
  lip smacking
  mumbling
  patting

automatism *(cont.)*
scratching
swallowing
Automator device
autonomic denervation
autonomic dysfunction
autonomic hyperactivity
autonomic hyperreflexia
autonomic hyperventilation
autonomic nervous system
autonomic neuropathy
autonomic or accessory oculomotor or Edinger-Westphal nucleus
Autophor ceramic hip prosthesis
Autophor femoral prosthesis
autoregulation, cerebral
autosomal
autosympathectomization, spontaneous
autosympathectomy secondary to diabetic neuropathy
autotopagnosia
avascular necrosis (AVN)
AVDO2 (cerebral arteriovenous oxygen content difference)
AVEEG (audiovisual electroencephalogram)
Avellis syndrome
averaging, spike
Averett hip prosthesis
Averill total hip replacement
aviator's astragalus
Avila technique
A-V Impulse System
Avitene
AVM (arteriovenous malformation)
AVN (avascular necrosis)
avulse, avulsed, avulsion
avulsed fracture fragment
avulsion
coracoid tip
ligament
avulsion chip fracture
avulsion fragment
avulsion of nail plate
avulsion of spinal nerve root
AVVM (angiographically visualized vascular malformation)
A wave form on ICP monitor
awareness
heightened
lapse of
postural
awl
angled
Aufranc
bone
curved
DePuy
Ender
Küntscher
pointed
reaming
rectangular
Rush
square-shaped
Swanson lunate
Swanson scaphoid
T-handled
Zuelzer
Axer-Clark procedure
Axer varus derotational osteotomy
axial compression forces
axial compression of foot
axial loading, spinal
axial manual traction test
axial musculature
axial neuritis
axial spinal system
axial traction
axillary block anesthesia
axis (C2, second cervical vertebra)
anatomic
ankle mortise
bimalleolar-foot
cortical hinge
distal reference (DRA)
eccentric axis of ankle rotation
eccentric axis of rotation of the ankle

axis *(cont.)*
  femoral shaft
  flexion-extension
  hypothalamic-pituitary
  hypothalamic-pituitary-adrenal
  hypothalamoneurohypophyseal (HNA)
  leg
  long
  longitudinal
  mechanical
  metatarsal
  proximal reference (PRA)
  rotation
  single (on knee prosthesis)
  spinal
  subtalar
  transcondylar (TCA)
  vertical
  weightbearing
axle lock and bumper
axodendritic synapse
axoid
axon
  centrally directed
  distally directed
axonal
axon degeneration
axon flare
axon hillock
axon loss
axon regeneration
axon regrowth
axon sprouting
axon terminal
axon transport
axonapraxia
axonopathic neurogenic thoracic outlet syndrome
axonopathy
axonotmesis
axoplasm
axoplasmic flow and papilledema
Axostim nerve stimulator
Ayers needle holder
Azorean disease
azotemic osteodystrophy

B, b

Baastrupi syndrome
Babcock scissors
Babcock sentences
Babcock stainless steel wire
Babcock wire-cutting scissors
"babies" the injured part
Babinski-Fröhlich syndrome
Babinski-Nageotte syndrome
Babinski percussion hammer
Babinski reflex
Babinski sign
bacitracin solution
Baciu-Filibiu dowel ankle arthrodesis
back
  arching of
  industrial
backache
Backbiter
Back Bubble gravity traction unit
back crease
Back-Huggar lumbar support cushion
backfire fracture
background activity on EEG
background disorganization on EEG
Backhaus towel clamp
Backhaus towel forceps
Backlund biopsy needle
back manipulation
backpack palsy
backpack paralysis
back school
Back Specialist chiropractic table
Bacon bone rongeur
Bacon cranial rongeur
Bacon raspatory
Bacon rongeur
Bacon rongeur forceps
Bacon thoracic shears
bacterial cerebritis
bacterial meningitis
Bacterium anitratum meningitis
bactogen (slang for bacterial antigen in CSF)
Badgley arthrodesis
Badgley laminectomy retractor
Badgley resection of iliac wing
Badgley retractor
BAEP (brain stem auditory evoked potential)
Baer bone-cutting forceps
Baer bone rongeur
Baer rib shears
BAER (brain stem auditory evoked response)
bag, stereotactic
Bagby angled compression plate
Bahler hinge
BAI (Barthel ADL Index)
bail-lock knee joint
Bailey-Badgley cervical spine fusion
Bailey conductor
Bailey-Dubow technique
Bailey-Gibbon rib contractor
Bailey-Gigli saw guide
Bailey rib contractor
Bailey rib spreader
Bailey saw guide
Bailey wire saw

Baillinger, inner stripe of (in brain)
baked brain phenomenon
Baker cyst
Baker-Hill osteotomy
Baker lateral semitendinosus transfer
Balacescu-Golden technique
balance
  dopaminergic-cholinergic
  dynamic ambulatory
  dynamic standing balance
  homeostatic
  sitting
  standing
  static and dynamic sitting
  static and dynamic standing
  static standing
balance padding
balanced suspension
Balint syndrome
Balkan fracture frame
Balkan splint
ball
  cold-weld femoral
  Gymnic
  Jurgan pin
  Silastic
  therapy
ball-and-socket joint
Ballantine hemilaminectomy retractor
ball-bearing eye sign
ball bearing, Steinmann pin with
Ballenger-Hajek chisel
Ballenger knife
Ballenger periosteotome
Ballenger swivel knife
ballism
ballistic injury
ballistic wound
ball of foot
balloon, Spiegelberg epidural
ballooned floor of ventricle
ballooning of the sella (on x-ray)
ballooning of vertebral interspace
ballottement of patella
ball-valve tumor
balmoral laced shoe
balneotherapy
Baló disease
Baló sclerosis
balsa wood filler block
Baltic myoclonus syndrome
Baltimore Therapeutic Equipment Work Simulator
banana Beaver blade
Bancaud phenomenon on EEG
Bancroft sign
band
  alpha
  alpha frequency
  AO tension
  aponeurotic
  arm
  beta
  beta frequency
  Broca diagonal
  calf
  constriction
  delta frequency
  external
  fascial
  frequency band on EEG
  iliotibial (IT)
  internal
  lateral
  lucent
  oligoclonal band in CSF
  Parham
  Parham-Martin
  Partridge
  pretendinous band of hand
  scar
  tennis elbow arm
  theta frequency
bandage (see also *dressing*)
  Ace adherent
  adhesive
  ASE (axilla, shoulder, elbow)
  Barton

bandage *(cont.)*
- capeline
- Champ elastic
- Comperm tubular elastic
- Fabco gauze
- gum rubber Martin
- Hamilton
- Helenca
- Heliodorus
- Hippocrates
- Hueter
- Hydron Burn Bandage
- compression
- Conco elastic
- cotton elastic
- cravat
- crepe
- demigauntlet
- Desault
- Dressinet netting
- E Cotton
- elastic
- elastic wrap
- Elastic Foam
- Elastomull
- Elastoplast
- Esmarch
- Fabco gauze
- figure-of-8 interscapular
- Flex-Foam
- Flex-Master
- Flexilite conforming elastic
- Fractura Flex
- gauntlet
- Gibney
- Gibson
- immobilizing
- Kerlix
- Kling elastic
- malleable metal finger splints
- Martin sheet rubber
- nonadhesive
- Nu Gauze sterile gauze
- Ortho-Trac adhesive

bandage *(cont.)*
- Ortho-Vent nonadhesive
- Pavlik
- plaster of Paris (POP)
- PRN
- Redigrip pressure
- replantation
- restrictive
- Ribble
- Richet
- Sayre
- scultetus
- self-adhering
- sling-and-swathe
- spica
- spiral
- starch
- stockinette
- Tricodur compression support
- Tricodur Epi (elbow) compression
- Tricodur Omos (shoulder) compression
- Tricodur Talus (ankle) compression
- Tru-Support
- Tru-Support EW (elastic wrap)
- Tru-Support SA (self-adhering)
- Tubigrip
- tubular elastic
- two-inch gauze
- Velpeau
- Webril

Bandage Gard cast protector
band around head, feeling of
B&L pinch gauge
band of Gennari
Bandi procedure
Bane bone rongeur
Bane-Hartmann bone rongeur
Bane rongeur forceps
Bangerter muscle forceps
banjo cast
banjo splint
bank, bone
Bankart procedure for shoulder dislocation

Bankart-Putti-Platt operation
Bankart retractor
Bankart shoulder prosthesis
Banks-Laufman approach
Bantam wire-cutting scissors
bantenadesis
bar
  bony
  cartilaginous
  congenital
  Denis Browne (DB)
  distraction
  fibrous
  Fillauer
  Gerster traction
  intramedullary
  L
  Leyla
  Livingston
  lumbrical
  metatarsal flatfoot
  opponens
  parallel
  patellar
  quad
  rigid
  spacer
  spondylitic
  spondylotic
  spreader
  Stephen spreader
  supraorbital
  tarsal
  Thornton
  Tommy trapeze
  torsion
  traction
  trapeze
  unsegmented vertebral
barber's chair sign
barbiturate poisoning
barbiturates, blood screen for
barbotage
Bard-Parker blade
Bard-Parker scalpel
Bardeen disk
Bardeleben bone-holding forceps
Bardeleben rasp
Bareskin knee positioner
baresthesia
bar-like ventral defect on myelography
Barlow hip instability test
Barlow maneuver
Barlow sign
Barlow splint
Barlow test
barognosis
Baron suction tube
baroreceptors in the carotid bulb
Barouk button space for hallux valgus deformity
Barouk cannulated bone screw
Barouk microscrew with shortening osteotomy
Barouk microstaple
Barouk spacer
Barr-Record ankle arthrodesis
Barraquer needle holder
Barrasso-Wile-Gage arthrodesis
Barré-Lieou syndrome
barrier, blood-brain
Barsky procedure
Barthel ADL Index (BAI)
Bartlett nail fold excision
Barton-Cone tong traction
Barton fracture
Barton skull traction tongs
basal caloric requirements
basal cistern
basal endothelium-derived relaxing factor
basal ganglia
basal ganglia calcifications (on x-ray)
basal ganglia of cerebellum
basal joint of thumb
basal part of brain
basal part of temporal lobe
basal skull fracture

basal vein of Rosenthal
base
  cranial
  dorsal spinal cord horn
  Dycal
  posterior spinal cord horn
  skull
baseball elbow
baseball finger
baseball shoulder
baseball splint
baseline distortion on EEG
base of brain
base of fingernail
base of metacarpal
base of nail
base of phalanx
base of skull
base of toe
base wedge osteotomy
basiarachnitis
basiarachnoiditis
basicranial
basilar artery migraine headache
basilar cistern
basilar ectasia
basilar insufficiency
basilar invagination
basilar occlusion
basilar skull fracture
basilar suture
basilar syndrome
basilar-vertebral artery disease
Basile screw
basioccipital
basiocciput tumor
basis pedunculi
basis pontis
basket
  Acufex meniscal
  shovel-nose Schutte
basket-weave ankle taping
basocervical fracture
basophilic adenoma
basophilic pituitary tumor
basophilism
  Cushing
  pituitary
Bassen-Kornzweig disease
Bassen-Kornzweig syndrome
Basser syndrome
Bassett electrical stimulation device
basswood splint
Batch-Spittler-McFaddin knee
  disarticulation
Batchelor-Brown arthrodesis
Bateman shoulder procedure
Bateman UPF (universal proximal
  femur)
Bateman UPF II bipolar endoprosthesis
Bateman UPF II bipolar hip prosthesis
Bateman UPF II shoulder prosthesis
bath, baths
  contrast
  hot and cold contrast
  hot sulfur
  mud pack
  paraffin (PB)
  paraffin-oil
  sitz
  whirlpool
bathing and dressing ability
batrachian (frog) gait or posture
Batson plexus
Batson vertebral brain system
Batten disease
Battery
  Cambridge Test
  Halstead-Reitan
  Rand Functional Limitations
  Rand Physical Capacities
  Rand Social Health
  Rivermead Perceptual Assessment
    (RPAB)
battery of tests, neuropsychologic
Battle sign
battledore incision
Batzdorf cervical wire passer

Batzdorf cervical wire twister
Bauer-Tondra-Trusler technique
Bauman angle
Baumgard-Schwartz tennis elbow
  technique
Bavarian splint
Baxter angled arthroscope
Baylor splint
Bayne classification of radial agenesis
bayonet dislocation
bayonet-point wire
bayonet position of fracture
BB shot
BBC (biceps, brachialis, coraco-
  brachialis) muscles
B-cell surface marker of CNS
  neoplasm
BDD (blistering distal dactylitis)
BDH (biologically designed hip)
  prosthesis
BDRS (Blessed Dementia Rating
  Scales)
BDRS, information-memory-concen-
  tration test (of impairment)
beach chair position
beads
  antibiotic-impregnated
  gentamicin
  methyl methacrylate
  PMMA
  targeting
beaked cervicomedullary junction
beaking of head of talus
beaking, talonavicular
beaklike osteophyte formation
Beall-Webel-Bailey technique
BEAM (brain electrical activity map)
  (or mapping)
beanbag
bear's paw hand
beaten silver appearance of skull
Beath needle
Beath pin
Beath view
Beatson combined ankle angle
Beau line
Beaver blade
  arachnoid-shape
  banana
  cataract knife
  discission knife
  keratome
  retrograde
  rosette
  sickle-shape
Beaver cataract knife
Beaver DeBakey blade
Beaver keratome blade
Bebax shoe for forefoot deformity
Bechtol acetabular component
Bechtol hip prosthesis
Bechtol shoulder prosthesis
Beck Questionnaire
Beck-Steffee total ankle prosthesis
Beckenbaugh technique
Becker external drain
Becker-Kiener dystrophy
Becker muscular dystrophy (BMD)
Becker tendon repair
Becker-type of muscular dystrophy
Becker variant of Duchenne dystrophy
Beckman-Adson laminectomy blade
Beckman-Eaton laminectomy retractor
Beckman EEG instrument, 20-channel
Beckman laminectomy retractor
Beckman-Weitlaner laminectomy
  retractor
Beclard amputation
Becton technique
bed
  American Seating Access-O-Matic
  BioDyne
  Borg-Warner orthopedic
  Burke Bariatric
  Cardiopulmonary Paragon 8500
  Carrom orthopedic
  Chick-Foster orthopedic
  circle

bed *(cont.)*
- CircOlectric
- Clinitron air
- DMI orthopedic
- Flexicair
- FluidAir
- Foster
- fracture
- Gatch
- gatched
- Goodman orthopedic
- Hausted orthopedic
- high-air-loss
- high muscular resistance
- Hill-Rom orthopedic
- Hollywood
- Inland Super Multi-Hite orthopedic
- Inter-Royal frame orthopedic
- Joerns orthopedic
- Keane Mobility
- KinAir
- Lapidus
- low-air-loss
- Magnum 800
- Medicus
- Mega-Air
- Mega Tilt and Turn
- nail
- orthopedic
- primary tumor
- Pulmonair 40
- Restcue
- RotoRest
- Simmons Multi-Matic orthopedic
- Simmons Vari-Hite orthopedic
- skeletal
- Skytron
- SMI 3000
- SMI 5000
- Smith-Davis Converta-Hite orthopedic
- Stryker
- Superior Sleeprite Hi-Lo orthopedic
- TheraPulse

bed *(cont.)*
- Tilt and Turn Paragon
- tumor
- Ultra-Flex orthopedic

bed cradle
bed mobility skills
bed of nail
bed of rib
bedrest
bedridden
bed wedge, Duo-Cline (by Bodyline)
Beebe wire-cutting scissors
beefy tongue
bees' nest (in angiomatous malformations of the retina)
Beeson cast spreader
Beeson plaster spreader
Beevor sign
behavior
- aggressive
- automatic
- explosive
- explosivity of
- hyperactive
- illness
- impulsive
- impulsivity of
- inappropriate
- infantile
- interictal
- pain
- rehabilitation
- repetitive
- semipurposeful (in petit mal seizures)
- stereotypical
- ticlike

behavioral changes
Behavioral Inattention Test (BIT)
behavioral mapping
Behr syndrome
Bekhterev arthritis
Bekhterev layer
Bekhterev-Mendel reflex

Bekhterev sitting test
Bell-Dally cervical dislocation
Bellemore-Barrett-Middleton-Scougall-Whiteway technique
Bell-Magendie law
Bell palsy
Bell phenomenon
Bell suture
Bell-Tawse open reduction technique
Bellucci alligator scissors
belly of muscle
belt
  cast
  Meek pelvic traction
  MicroTeq portable
  pelvic traction
  Posey
  Reed cast
  rib
  Silesian
  test
  tub
  waist suspension
  Zim-Zap rib
Bence Jones protein
bench examination
bench, tub
bender
  French rod
  Rush
Bendixen-Kirschner traction
bends, the (caisson disease)
benediction posture (of hand)
Benedikt ipsilateral oculomotor paralysis
Benedikt syndrome
benign capillary hemangioblastoma
benign essential tremor
benign functional vertigo
benign lymphocytic choriomeningitis
benign pain syndrome
benign paroxysmal positional vertigo
benign raised intracranial pressure
benign senescent forgetfulness
benign X-linked recessive muscular dystrophy
Benink tarsal index
Bennett basic hand dislocation
Bennett basic hand fracture
Bennett basic hand splint
Bennett bone elevator
Bennett bone retractor
Bennett fracture
Bennett lesion
Bennett posterior shoulder approach
Bennett quadriceps plastic procedure
Bennett tibial retractor
Benson-Geschwind classification of aphasia
bent knee pelvic tilts
Benton Visual Retention Test
bentonite flocculation test (BFT)
Benyi modification of Lambrinudi triple arthrodesis
benzoin adherent tape
BeOK hand exercise putty
Berens muscle clamp
Berens muscle forceps
Berger interscapular amputation
Berger rhythm (on EEG)
Bergeron chorea
Bergman mallet
Bergstrom cannula
Berliner percussion hammer
Berman-Gartland metatarsal osteotomy
Berman-Moorhead metal locator
Bermuda spica cast
Bernard-Horner syndrome
Berndt-Hardy classification of transchondral fracture
Berndt-Hardy talar lesion staging
Berndt hip ruler
berry aneurysm
Berstein cast table
Bertillon cephalometer
beta activity
beta frequency band on EEG
beta index
beta pattern on EEG
beta rhythm on EEG

beta spindles on EEG
beta wave on EEG
Betadine Helafoam solution
Betadine scrub solution
Betadine soak
Bethesda bone
Bethune-Coryllos rib shears
Bethune periosteal elevator
Bethune rib shears
BETS (benign epileptiform transients of sleep)
Betz giant pyramidal cell
Bevatron accelerator
bevel, beveled, beveling
Bevin shoe
Beyer rongeur forceps
Beyer-Stille bone rongeur
BFM arm assessment (Brunnstrom-Fugl-Meyer)
BFT (bentonite flocculation test)
B.H. Moore procedure
Bi-Angular shoulder prosthesis
bias potential
Bias hip prosthesis
BICAP (bipolar cautery probe) unit
biceps
  long head of (LHB)
  short head of
biceps femoris
biceps jerk (BJ), stretch reflex
biceps stretch reflex
bicerebral infarction
Bichat canal
bicipital groove
bicipital tendinitis
Bickel intramedullary rod
Bickel leg holder
Bickel-Moe procedure
Bickerstaff migraine
bicondylar fracture
bicorrectional Austin osteotomy
bicortical iliac bone graft
bicortical screw
bicycle
  Air-Dyne
  FES exercise
bidirectional traction
Bielschowsky-Jansky disease
Biemer-Clip aneurysm clip
Bier amputating saw
Bier block anesthesia
Bier lumbar puncture needle
Bier saw
bifida, spina
bifocal manipulation with distraction
bifrontal headache
bifurcation
  basilar artery
  carotid
  common carotid artery
  middle cerebral artery
Bigelow calvarium clamp
Bigelow maneuver, reverse
BIH (benign intracranial hypertension)
bihemispheral insult
bikini skin incision
bilateral Babinksi sign
bilateral carotid artery occlusion
bilateral carotid stenosis
bilateral cerebral dysfunction
  metabolic
  structural
bilateral corticobulbar disease
bilateral decortication
bilateral frontal lobe disease
bilateral hallux valgus (HV)
bilateral hemisphere dysfunction
bilateral hyperreflexia
bilateral orbital frontal cortex
bilateral paralysis
bilateral pyramidal sign
bilateral simultaneous stimulation
bilateral synchrony on EEG
bilateral theta slowing (on EEG)
bilateral upper motor neuron (supranuclear) dysfunction
Bill bar (bone)

Bilos pin
bimalleolar ankle fracture
bimalleolar approach to ankle
  arthrodesis
Bi-Metric hip prosthesis
binder (see also *bandage*; *dressing*)
  Dale abdominal
  Helenca
  scultetus
binding, biological
Bing-Horton syndrome
binocular acuity change
Binswanger dementia
Binswanger disease
Bio-Boot
Biobrane adhesive
Biobrane glove
biocalibration of EEG
bioceramic joint replacement material
Bio-Chromatic hand prosthesis
Bioclad acetabular prosthesis
Bioclusive transparent dressing
biocompartmental replacement of knee
Biocoral
biodegradable fixation device
biodegradable implant
biodegradable pin
biodegradable plate
biodegradable rod
biodegradable screw
biodegradable synthetic polymer
Biodel
Biodex dynamometer
Biodex isokinetic exercise system
BioDyne bed
bioelectrical repair of delayed union or
  nonunion
biofeedback
Biofit acetabular prosthesis
Biofix absorbable fixation
Biofix biodegradable implant
Biofix system pin
Bio-Groove acetabular prosthesis
Bio-Groove Macrobond HA femoral
  prosthesis
Biokinetics pedobarograph
biologic age
biological osteosynthesis
Biolox ball head for hip replacement
Biolox ceramic coating
biomechanical analysis
biomechanical imbalance
biomechanical stress
biomechanics, gait
biomechanics of limb length
  discrepancy
Biomet acetabular cup
Biomet AGC knee prosthesis
Biomet button
Biomet hip prosthesis
Biomet Ultra-Drive cement remover
Bio-Modular shoulder prosthesis
Bio-Moore endoprosthesis
Bio-Oss synthetic bone material
Biophase, ASTM designation of
Biophase implant metal
BioPolyMeric graft
biopsy
  bone
  bone marrow
  brain
  channel and core
  cone
  Dunn
  forage core
  freehand CT-guided
  Michele vertebral
  muscle
  nerve
  onion bulb changes on
  open brain
  punch
  stereotactic brain
  sural nerve
  synovial
  targeted brain
  temporal artery
  transnasal
  Tru-Cut needle (TCNB)

biopsy *(cont.)*
  ultrasound-guided echo
  ultrasound-guided stereotactic
biopsy specimen
biopsy trephine
Biotex implant metal
Bio-Thesiometer
Biothotic foot orthosis
BIOWARE software for Biodex isokinetic exercise system
biparietal hump wave on EEG
biparietal suture
bipartite sesamoid
bipenniform muscles of hand
biphasic wave on EEG
biplaning of osteotomy
BIPLED (bilateral independent periodic lateralizing epileptiform discharge) on EEG
bipolar EEG recording
bipolar hip replacement
bipolar montage
Bircher bone/cartilage clamp
Bircher-Ganske cartilage forceps
Bircher meniscotome
Bircher meniscus knife
Bircher-Weber technique
birdcage splint
birdlike facies
birefringent lipid crystals in tendinitis
birth fracture
bisection, AP malleolar
Bishop-Black tendon tucker
Bishop chisel
Bishop clamp
Bishop-DeWitt tendon tucker
Bishop-Peter tendon tucker
bit (see *drill bit*)
BIT (Behavioral Inattention Test)
bitemporal hemianopsia
biter, Stille bone
bivalved cylinder cast
BJ (biceps jerk)
Björnström algesimeter
BKA (below-knee amputation)
black dot heel
black eye
Black and Decker drill
Black-Broström staple technique
Black rasp
Blackburn traction
blackout, alcoholic
bladder
  atonic
  automatic bladder in spinal cord syndromes
  centrally uninhibited
  motor paralytic
  neurogenic
  refluxing spastic neurogenic
  sensory paralytic
  spastic neurogenic
  uninhibited
bladder knock in distance runners
blade (see also *knife*)
  arachnoid-shape
  arthroscopic
  banana
  Bard-Parker
  Beaver cataract
  Beaver DeBakey
  Beaver discission
  Beaver keratome
  Beckman-Adson laminectomy
  Beckman-Eaton laminectomy
  carotid
  cartilage shaver
  Caspar
  cataract
  chisel
  chondroplasty
  copper
  craniotome
  crescentic
  Curdy
  deep
  discission
  double-edged razor

blade *(cont.)*
- drill
- Dyonics arthroscopic
- Feild (*not* Field)
- full-curve
- Gigli saw
- Hebra
- Hibbs
- Incisor arthroscopic
- K
- keratome
- knife
- laminectomy
- malleable
- meniscal trimmer
- meniscectomy
- Meyerding laminectomy
- Meyerding-Scoville
- Micro-Aire
- mini-meniscus
- MVR
- notchplasty
- oscillating
- partial-curve
- Paufique
- PowerCut drill
- razor
- retractor
- Scoville
- sickle-shape
- skin
- spinal retractor
- Superblade
- Swann-Morton surgical
- Synovator arthroscopic
- synovectomy
- Taylor spinal retractor
- Temperlite saw
- 3 M Maxi Driver
- tracheal
- tri-radial resector

blade plate (see also *plate*)
- ASIF
- Giebel
- 10-hole

Blair ankle fusion
Blair-Brown skin graft
Blair chisel
Blair elevator
Blair-Morris-Dunn-Hand arthrodesis
Blair talar body fusion
Blair tibiotalar arthrodesis
blanch
Blanchard traction device
blanching
Blazina prosthesis
bleb, myelin
Bleck classification of metatarsus adductus
Bleck recession technique
Bledsoe fracture brace
bleed (noun) (see *hemorrhage*)
bleeders, persistent
blennorrhagic swelling
blepharospasm
Blessed Behavior Scale
Blessed Dementia Rating Scales (BDRS)
Blessed information-memory-concentration test
Blessed-Roth Dementia Scale (BRDS)
blind headache (preceded by visual phenomena)
blindness
- cortical
- hysterical
- ipsilateral monocular
- monocular
- total cortical
- transient cortical
- transient monocular (TMB)
- word

blind spot in visual field
blind spots (from multiple sclerosis)
blind spots, migrainous
blink artifact
blink reflex to corneal stimulation
blinking, reflex
Bliskunov implantable femoral distractor
blister (vesicle)

blister, fracture
blister of bone
blistering distal dactylitis (BDD)
Bloch equation
block (see also *anesthesia*)
  anesthetic
  axillary
  axillary anesthetic
  balsa wood filler
  Bier anesthetic
  bone
  Campbell posterior bone
  cutting
  digital nerve
  epidural steroid
  filler
  Gill posterior bone
  Howard bone
  Inclan posterior bone
  Kohs
  median nerve anesthetic
  Mikhail bone
  nerve
  peripheral nerve
  phenol nerve
  radial nerve anesthetic
  regional
  regional ankle
  scalene
  sphenopalatine ganglion
  spinal (by cord compression)
  stellate sympathetic ganglion
  Styrofoam filler
  subarachnoid
  supraclavicular anesthetic
  sympathetic ganglion
  ulnar nerve anesthetic
  ventricular
blocker's exostosis
blocking, alpha
Block-Sulzberger syndrome
blood (see *hemorrhage*)
  autologous
  intraparenchymal
blood *(cont.)*
  intraventricular
  new
  old
  subdural
blood behind tympanic membrane
blood-brain barrier
blood flow (see *flow*)
blood gases, arterial (ABGs)
blood patch for post-LP headache
blood pool imaging
blood supply, longitudinal
blood vessel tumor
bloody cerebrospinal fluid (CSF)
bloody tap
Bloom-Raney modification of Smith-Robinson technique
Bloom splint
Blount disease
Blount displacement osteotomy
Blount lamina spreader
Blount retractor
Blount-Schmidt Milwaukee brace
blow-in fracture
blow-out fracture
blucher laced shoe
blue toe syndrome
Blumensaat line
Blumenthal bone rongeur
Blumer shelf
Blundell Jones hip osteotomy
blunt spike-and-wave complex on EEG
blur, saccadic
blurring of disk margins
blurring of vision in multiple sclerosis
blush
  tumor blush on cerebral angiography
  vascular blush of tumor on carotid angiography
BMC (bone mineral content)
BMD (Becker muscular dystrophy)
BMD (bone mineral density)
BMP (bone marrow pressure)
BNMSE (Brief Neuropsychological Mental Status Examination)

board
- arm
- Euroglide MKII slide
- Flexisplint flexed arm
- Hadfield hand
- hand
- slide
- spine
- Spri Xercise
- Tegtmeier hand
- vertical foot
- Yucca

boathead
bobbing
- head
- ocular

Bobechko hook
Bobechko spreader
Bobrath technique
Bock knee prosthesis
Bodenstab tourniquet
BODI knee extension orthosis
Bodnar retractor
body, bodies
- alignment of vertebral
- carotid
- Cowdry-type intranuclear inclusion
- foreign (retained)
- geniculate
- Hirano
- height of vertebral
- inclusion
- intra-articular
- juxtarestiform
- Lafora
- Lewy
- loose bodies of knee
- Luys
- mamillary
- navicular
- Negri
- nemaline
- ossified
- osteochondritic loose

body *(cont.)*
- pacchionian
- Pick
- psammoma
- restiform
- retained foreign
- rhinencephalic mamillary
- rice
- Schwann cell
- trapezoid
- Vater-Pacini
- Verocay
- vertebral

body dystonia
body fat calipers
body jacket cast
body mechanics
body of scapula
body of vertebra
Body Gard neoprene support
Boeck sarcoid
Boehler (Böhler)
Boehler angle
Boehler-Braun leg frame
Boehler-Braun splint
Boehler extension bow
Boehler guidelines
Boehler-Steinmann pin holder
boggy synovitis
boggy synovium
Bohlman cervical vertebrectomy
Bohlman triple-wire fusion
Boies forceps
Bollinger, posttraumatic apoplexy of
bolster
- abduction
- padded
- rubber
- Telfa

bolt (see also *pin*)
- Alvar condylar
- Barr
- Camino microventricular
- Camino ventricular

bolt *(cont.)*
- cannulated
- condylar
- Fenton
- fixation
- Harris
- Holt
- Moreira
- slotted
- subarachnoid
- tibial
- tibiofibular
- trochanteric
- Webb-Andreesen condylar
- Webb stove
- wire-fixation
- Zimmer tibia

bolt cutter
Boltzmann distribution
bolus, cotton
Bombelli-Mathys-Morscher hip prosthesis
Bond splint
bone
- AAA
- accessory
- autogenous
- Bethesda
- bicortical iliac
- bleeding
- Bonfiglio
- brittle
- Calcitite
- calvarial
- cancellous
- capitate
- chalky
- compact
- cortical
- cortical cancellous
- cuneiform
- displaced fragment of
- Durapatite
- eburnated

bone *(cont.)*
- electrical stimulation of
- endochondral
- flat
- fragment of
- fragmental
- freeze-dried
- freshening of
- frontal
- greater multangular (trapezium)
- hamate
- heterotopic
- hydroxyapatite
- infected
- Interpore
- ivory
- lamellar
- lamellated
- lesser multangular (trapezoid)
- long
- long axis of
- lunate
- lunocapitate
- luxated
- marble
- morcellized
- navicular
- necrotic
- Nicoll
- nonlamellated
- os trapezium
- os trapezoideum
- ossifying fibroma of long
- osteonal
- osteopenic
- osteoporotic
- pagetoid
- parietal
- perilesional
- petrous temporal
- Pirie
- pisiform
- primitive
- raw

bone *(cont.)*
- rider's
- rudimentary
- scaphoid
- semilunar
- sesamoid
- short
- split thickness cranial
- spongy
- subchondral
- subperiosteal new
- supernumerary sesamoid
- supracollicular spike of cortical
- temporal
- thick
- trabecular
- trapezium (greater multangular)
- trapezoid (lesser multangular)
- triangular wrist
- triquetrum
- tumor-bearing
- ulnar sesamoid
- Unilab Surgibone
- wing of sphenoid
- wormian
- woven
- wrist triquetrum

bone age according to Greulich and Pyle
bone age study as indicator of biologic age
bone allograft
bone bank
bone biopsy
bone block
bone-blocking procedure
bone borer
bone chip
bone core
bone cutter, Horsley
bone-cutting forceps
bone debris
bone density
bone dowel
bone dysplasia
bone ends
bone-forming tumor
bone fracture (see *fracture*)
bone fragment
bone graft (see *graft*)
Bone Grafter instrument
bone graft incorporation
bone graft substitute material, CHAG (coralline hydroxyapatite Goniopora)
bone growth stimulator
bone harvesting
bone holder
bone implant
bone infection
bonelet
bone marrow
bone marrow pressure (BMP)
bonemeal tablet
bone mineral content (BMC)
bone mineral density (BMD)
bone plate
bone powder
bone rasp
bone remodeling
bone replacement material
bone resurfacing
bone rongeur
bone scan
bone scintigraphy
bone screw
bone sequestrum
bone shaft
bone skid
bone sliver
bone spreader
bone spur
bone stock
bone substance
bone-tendon exposure
bone wax
Bonfiglio bone graft
Bonfiglio bone replacement material
Bonfiglio modification of Phemister technique

Bonney hallux valgus outcome scale
Bonney-Kessel dorsiflexionary tilt-up osteotomy
bony abnormality
bony ankylosis
bony bridging
bony callus
bony eburnation
bony encroachment
bony erosion
bony exostosis
bony fragment
bony island
bony landmark
bony necrosis and destruction
bony osteophyte
bony overgrowth
bony prominence (spur)
bony spurring
bony structures
bony tenderness
bony tufts of fingers
bony union
boom, overhead
boot, Boot
  Bunny
  cast
  gelatin compression
  Gibney
  Moon
  rocker
  Unna
  Unna paste
  Wilke
boot-top fracture
boot wrap, Unna
Booth test
Boplant surgibone
Bora operation
Borchardt olive-shaped bur
Borden-Spencer-Herman osteotomy
borer
  bone
  cork
Borg-Warner orthopedic bed
Borggreve-Hall technique
Bornholm disease
Borrelia burgdorferi antibody
Bose nail fold excision
boss, bossing
bosselated, bosselation
bossing
  frontal
  occipital
Boston Classification System
Boston Diagnostic Aphasia Examination
Boston LINAC (linear accelerator)
Boston Naming Test
Boston neurosurgical couch
Boston scoliosis brace
Boston soft body jacket
Boston thoracic brace
Boston thoracic splint
Bosworth femoroischial arthrodesis
Bosworth fracture
Bosworth lumbar spinal fusion
Bosworth procedure
Bosworth screw
Bosworth screwdriver
Bosworth shelf procedure
bottle sign
bottoming out of prosthetic component
Bouchard node
bouche de tapir (tapir's mouth, in muscular dystrophy)
Bouge needle
bouncing, ligamentous
bound, stimulus
boundary, tumor
Bourneville disease
Bourneville-Pringle disease
boutonnière deformity
Bovie electrocautery apparatus
bovine collagen graft
bovine cough
bow
  aiming
  Boehler extension
  extension

bow *(cont.)*
  finger extension
  Framer finger extension
  Kirschner wire traction
  posterior
  Schwarz finger extension
  traction
  wire traction
Bowden cable suspension system
bowed legs
bowel and bladder dysfunction
Bowen-Grover meniscotome
Bowers radial arthroplasty
bowing of forearm
bowing of tendons in arthritis
bowl, cement mixing
Bowlby splint
bowleg (genu varum)
bowler's thumb
Bowman angle
bowstringing
bowstring sign
bowstring tear
bow-tie sign
box
  anatomic snuffbox
  high-toe
  ligamentous
  snuff
  toe
box and block test of arm disability
boxcar effect
boxer's elbow
boxer's fracture
boxer's punch (fracture of the fifth metacarpal)
boxwood mallet
Boyd amputation
Boyd-Anderson biceps tendon repair
Boyd bone graft
Boyd-Bosworth procedure
Boyd-Griffin classification
Boyd-McLeod procedure
Boyd-Sisk posterior capsulorrhaphy
Boyd type II fracture
Boyes brachioradialis transfer
Boyes-Goodfellow hook
Bozzini light conductor
BPB (bone-patellar ligament-bone) autologous graft
BPB (bone-patellar tendon-bone) graft
BPS spinal angiographic catheter
brace, bracing (see also *bar*; *orthosis*; *splint*)
  Abbott
  accommodative
  adjustable
  Air-Stirrup Ankle Training Brace
  Aircast Air-Stirrup
  Aircast pneumatic air stirrup
  Aircast Swivel-Strap
  Aircast walking
  ankle
  Ankle Ligament Protector (ALP)
  Arnold lumbar
  athletic
  back
  bipivotal hinge knee
  Bledsoe
  Blount-Schmidt Milwaukee
  Boehler
  boot
  Boston scoliosis
  Boston thoracic
  bowleg
  cable twister
  caliper
  Callender derotational
  Cam Walker leg
  Can Am
  carpenter's
  cast
  Castaway leg
  Castiglia ankle
  cervical
  cervical collar
  chairback
  Charleston nighttime bending

brace *(cont.)*
Charleston scoliosis
Charnley
CHH cervical
Chopart
clam-shell
Cole hyperextension
contraflexion
controlled-motion
Cook walking
cowhorn
CRS (Counter Rotation System)
CTi (or C.Ti.)
CTi2 knee
custom-fitted
cutout patellar
D.A.C.O.
Dennyson cervical
derotational
dial-lock
DonJoy
DonJoy Gold Point knee
dorsiflexion stop
drop foot
drop-lock knee
dynamic abduction
eclipse ankle
Elite knee
English
felt
Florida cervical
Florida J-24
Florida J-35
Florida J-45
Florida J-55
foot-ankle
footdrop
49er knee
four-point cervical
four-poster cervical
Friedman
functional
gait lock splint (GLS)
Galveston metacarpal

brace *(cont.)*
Genutrain knee
GLS (gait lock splint)
Gold Point knee
Goldthwait
GII Unloader knee
Guilford cervical
Hennessy knee
Hi-Top foot/ankle
hinged knee
Hudson
hyperextension
I-Plus humeral
Ilfield
InCare ankle
Industrial Work
internal tibial torsion
ischial weightbearing
J-55 postfusion
Jewett
Jewett-Benjamin cervical
Jewett contraflexion
Jewett hyperextension
Jewett postfusion
Kalessy
King cervical
Klengall
Klenzak spring
knee
knee cage
knee MD
Knight back
Knight-Taylor thoracic
knock-knee
Korn Cage knee
Kydex
kyphosis
lace-on
lacing
lacing ankle
Lenox Hill
Lenox Hill derotational knee
long arm
long leg

brace *(cont.)*
- long leg hinged
- LSU reciprocation-gait orthosis
- lumbar
- lumbosacral
- Lyman-Smith
- MacCausland lumbar
- McClintoch
- McCollough internal tibial torsion
- MCL (medial collateral ligament)
- MD (Medical Design)
- Medipedic Multicentric knee
- Miami TLSO scoliosis
- Milwaukee
- Milwaukee scoliosis
- Moon Boot
- Mooney
- Multi-Lock knee
- Murphy
- neoprene support
- Newington
- Nextep knee
- night
- nonweightbearing
- Oppenheim
- OS-5/Plus 2 knee
- OS-5/Plus knee
- out-of-cast ankle
- P.C. Williams
- Palumbo knee
- Palumbo stabilizing
- pantaloon
- patellar
- patellar tendon-bearing (PTB)
- pelvic
- performer ultralight knee
- PFT (postop flexor tendon) traction
- Phelps
- Philadelphia Plastizote cervical
- piano-wire dorsiflexion
- postfusion
- Pro-8 ankle
- PTS knee
- range of motion

brace *(cont.)*
- reamer
- rigid postoperative
- Rolyan tibial fracture
- Saltiel
- SAS II (shoulder arm system)
- SAWA shoulder
- Schanz
- scoliosis
- Scottish Rite
- Seton hip
- short arm
- short leg caliper (single or double bar)
- short leg double upright
- six-point knee
- snap-lock
- SOMI (sternal occipital mandibular immobilizer)
- Sports
- Sports-Caster I and II knee
- stirrup
- stop action
- Stromgren ankle
- Swede-O
- Swede-O-Universal
- Swivel-Strap
- Taylor-Knight
- Teufel
- Thomas
- 3-D fracture walker
- TLSO (thoracolumbosacral orthosis)
- toe-drop
- Toronto
- Townsend knee
- Tracker knee
- Trinkle
- UBC (University of British Columbia)
- unilateral calcaneal (UCB)
- Varney acromioclavicular
- Victorian
- walking
- Warm Springs

brace *(cont.)*
  Watco
  weightbearing
  Wheaton
  Williams
  Wilmington scoliosis
  Yale
  Zimmer reamer
  Zinco CAM walker
brace/corset, Hoke lumbar
bracelet test
brachial neuritis
brachial plexus neuritis
brachialgia
brachiocephalic artery
brachiocephalic trunk of aorta
brachioradialis muscle
brachioradialis reflex
brachioradialis tendon
brachium (pl. brachia)
brachium conjunctivum
brachium of colliculus
brachycephalic head shape
brachycephaly
brachymetatarsia
brachytherapy
  ^{125}I
  ^{192}I
  interstitial
  remote afterloading (RAB)
  volumetric interstitial
Brackett-Osgood-Putti-Abbott
  technique
Brackett osteotomy
Braden flushing reservoir
Bradford fracture frame
Brady-Jewett technique
Brady leg splint
bradykinesia
bradykinin
bradyphemic
bradyphrenia
Bragard sign
Bragg ionization peak
Bragg peak photon beam therapy
Bragg peak radiosurgery
Brahms procedure
Braille TeleCaption system
brain
  architecture of
  atrophic lesion of the
  base of
  unicameral
  Virchow-Robin spaces of the
  water on the
  wet
brain abscess (see *abscess*)
brain biopsy
brain concussion
brain contusion
brain cyst
brain-dead patient
brain death syndrome
brain disease, organic (OBD)
brain dysfunction
  diffuse
  minimal
brain electrical activity map
  (or mapping) (BEAM)
brain function
brain-impaired person
brain laceration
brain lesion, atrophic
brain mantle
brain map
brain mass, posterior fossa
brain parenchyma, bleeding into
brain spatula
  Children's Hospital
  D'Errico
  Payton
  Scoville
brain spatula spoon, Ray
brain stem
brain stem auditory evoked potential
  (BAEP)
brain stem auditory evoked response
  (BAER)

brain stem compression
brain stem demyelination
brain stem disease
brain stem displacement
brain stem dysfunction
brain stem evoked potential
brain stem function
brain stem gaze mechanism
brain stem glioma tumor
brain stem hemorrhage
brain stem infarct
brain stem infarction
brain stem lesion
brain stem, motor nuclei in the lower
brain stem pyramidal tract
brain stem reflex
brain stem reticular formation
brain stem signs
brain stem stroke
brain stem symptom
brain stem syndrome
brain swelling
brain syndrome, organic (OBS)
brain tests
  BAEP (brain stem auditory evoked potential)
  BAER (brain stem auditory evoked response)
  EP (evoked potential)
  ER (evoked response)
  MEP (multimodality evoked potential)
  noninvasive
  SEP (somatosensory evoked potential)
  SER (somatosensory evoked response)
  VEP (visual evoked potential)
  VER (visual evoked response)
brain tumor (see *tumor*)
brain tumor forceps
Brain variation, hip arthroplasty
brain wave activity
branch
  digital
  distal
  feeding
  motor
  phalangeal
  proper digital nerve
branch of artery
Brand forceps
Brand palmaris tendon stripper
Brand plantaris stripper
Brand tendon-holding forceps
Brand tendon-passing forceps
Brand tendon transfer technique
Brand tendon-tunneling forceps
Brannock foot measuring device
Brannon-Wickstrom technique
Brant aluminum splint
Brantigan-Voshell procedure
brassiere, Jobst
Braun shoulder tenotomy
Braun skin graft
Braun-Yasargil right-ankle clip
Bravais-jacksonian epilepsy
bread-crumbling movement
breaker (see *cast breaker*)
breastbone
breaststroker's knee
breathholding spells
breathing
  apneustic
  ataxic
  labored
Breck pin
bregma, bregmatic
bregmatomastoid suture
Bremer AirFlo halo vest
Bremer halo crown traction (cervical spine)
Breschet sinus
Brett arthrodesis
Brett-Campbell tibial osteotomy
Breuerton x-ray view of hand

bridegroom's palsy
bridge
  interthalamic
  osseous
  skin
bridge autograft
bridge of meniscus
bridging, bony
bridging osteophytes
Brief Cognitive Rating Scale (BCRS)
Brief Neuropsychological Mental Status Examination (BNMSE)
Brigham brain tumor forceps
Brigham prosthesis
Brighton electrical stimulation system
brim sign
brisement therapy
Brissaud syndrome
Bristow-Helfet procedure
Bristow-May procedure
Bristow procedure
Bristow rasp
Bristow shoulder reconstruction
British test
Brittain ischiofemoral arthrodesis
brittle bones failure
broach
  barbed
  Charnley femoral
  drilling
  femoral
  femoral prosthesis
  Harris
  intramedullary
  Mittlemeir
  root canal
  smooth
  Swanson intramedullary
  Zimmer femoral canal
broached
Brobdingnagian disorder of visual perception in migraine
Broca aphasia
Broca area
Broca convolution
Broca diagonal band
Broca gyrus
Broca motor speech area of the brain
Broca region
Broca syndrome
Brockman-Nissen arthrodesis
Brockman procedure of foot
Broden view
Brodie abscess
Brodie disease
Brodie metaphyseal abscess
Brodmann area
Brodmann cytoarchitectonic fields
Brook wire
Brooker classification of heterotopic ossification
Brooker femoral nail
Brooker-Wills nail
Brookes-Jones tendon transfer
Brooks atlantoaxial arthrodesis
Brooks cervical fusion operation
Brooks-Gallie cervical fusion
Brooks-Jenkins atlantoaxial fusion
Brooks-Seddon tendon transfer
broom-stick cast
Broomhead approach
Brophy periosteal elevator
Broström-Gordon arthrography
Broström-Gould ankle instability operation
brown tumor (osteoclastoma)
Brown-Adson tissue forceps
Brown-Cushing forceps
Brown knee joint reconstruction
Brown rasp
Brown-Roberts-Wells (BRW) head ring halo
Brown-Roberts-Wells (BRW) stereotactic head frame
Brown-Séquard syndrome
Brown tissue forceps

Bruce protocol
Brucella arthritis
Brucella osteomyelitis
brucellosis, cerebral
Brudzinski sign
Brudzinski test
Bruening chisel
Bruening-Citelli rongeur
bruisability
bruise
bruit, bruits
  aneurysmal
  asymptomatic carotid (ACB)
  carotid
  cranial
  high-pitched
  loud
  subclavian
Brunhilde strain (type I poliomyelitis virus)
Brunner modified incision
Brunner palmar incision
Brunner rib shears
Brunnstrom-Fugl-Meyer (BFM) arm impairment assessment
Bruns ataxia
Bruns bone curet
Bruns gait apraxia
Bruns nystagmus
Bruns plaster shears
Bruns syndrome
Bruser skin incision (knee surgery)
brush, delta
bruxism
BRW (Brown-Roberts-Wells) stereotactic head ring
BRW-Mayfield head adapter
Bryan-Morrey elbow approach
Bryant sign
Bryant traction
BSSS (benign small sharp spike)
BTE (Baltimore Therapeutic Equipment)
BTE Assembly Tree
BTE Bolt Box
BTE Dynamic Lift
BTE Work Simulator
BTS (Back Therapy System), NordiCare
buccofacial apraxia
Buch-Gramcko gouge
Buchholz acetabular cup
Buchholz ankle prosthesis
Buchholz hip prosthesis
Buck bone curet
Buck cement restrictor insertor
Buck convoluted traction apparatus
Buck elevator
Buck-Gramcko pollicization
Buck neurological hammer
Buck percussion hammer
Buck periosteal elevator
Buck plug
Buck Redi-Traction apparatus
Buck splint
Buck traction
Buck traction stockinette
bucket, Denis Browne
bucket-handle tear
buckle fracture
buckle, wire-fixation
Buckley chisel
Bucky x-ray tray
Bucy cordotomy knife
Bucy-Frazier coagulation cannula
Bucy-Frazier suction cannula
Bucy laminectomy rongeur
Budde-Greenberg-Sugita stereotactic head frame
Budde retractor
buddy splint
buddy taping of fingers
Budge, ciliospinal center of
Budin-Chandler anteversion determination
Budin hammertoe splint
Budin toe splint
BUE strength

Buerger disease
Buerger symptom
Bugg-Boyd technique
buildup of seizure discharges
bulb
  baroreceptor in the carotid
  carotid
  high jugular (HJB)
  irrigation
  jugular
  olfactory
bulb dynamometer
bulb of internal jugular vein
bulb of occipital horn of lateral ventricle
bulb of posterior horn of lateral ventricle
bulb syringe
bulbar abnormality
bulbar palsy
bulbar reflex
bulbo cavernous reflex
bulbous stump
bulbus (n.), bulbous (adj.)
bulge of disk
bulging disk
bulk, muscle
bull's eye deformity
bulla (pl. bullae)
bulldog response (chewing reflex)
bullet
  hollow-point
  stabilizing
  tri-point
bullous
bump
  hip
  inion
  runner's
bumper fracture
Buncke technique
bundle
  Flechsig bundle in cerebellum
  Gowers bundle in cerebellum
  maculoneural

bundle *(cont.)*
  neurovascular
  Schultze
bundle function
bundle-nailing method
bundle of Vicq d'Azyr
Bunge amputation
bunion complex
bunionectomy
  Akin
  Austin
  base wedge osteotomy
  chevron
  closing wedge osteotomy
  crescentic base wedge osteotomy
  DuVries-Mann modified
  Hauser
  Joplin
  juvenile
  Kelikian modified Z osteotomy
  Keller
  Kreuscher
  Lapidus
  Mayo
  McBride
  Mitchell
  Mitchell osteotomy
  modified Mau
  modified McBride
  open base wedge osteotomy
  rotational scarf osteotomy
  scarf osteotomy
  Silver
  Stone
  supratubercular wedge osteotomy
  tailor's
  tricorrectional
  Wu
bunionette, excision of
bunionette-hallux valgus-splay foot complex
Bunker foot-piece
Bunnell active hand and finger splints
Bunnell anvil

Bunnell crisscross suture
Bunnell digital exertion measurer
Bunnell dissecting probe
Bunnell drill
Bunnell finger extension splint
Bunnell finger loop
Bunnell forwarding probe
Bunnell hand drill
Bunnell knuckle bender splint
Bunnell-Littler test
Bunnell modification of Steindler flexorplasty
Bunnell posterior tibial tendon transfer operation
Bunnell reverse knuckle bender splint
Bunnell safety-pin splint
Bunnell splint
Bunnell stitch
Bunnell suture
Bunnell tendon needle
Bunnell tendon passer
Bunnell tendon stripper
Bunnell tendon suturing technique
Bunnell tendon transfer
Bunnell wire pull-out suture
Bunny Boot splint
bur (also burr)
  Adson enlarging
  Adson perforating
  Adson-Rogers cranial
  air-driven
  Albee olive-shaped
  arthroplasty
  Bailey
  barrel
  bone
  Borchardt olive-shaped
  Burwell
  Caparosa
  carbide
  cone
  conical
  cranial
  craniotomy

bur *(cont.)*
  crosscut
  Cushing cranial
  cutting
  cylindrical
  D'Errico enlarging drill
  D'Errico perforating drill
  dental
  diamond
  Doyen cylindrical
  Doyen spherical
  Dyonics arthroplasty
  enlarging
  finish
  flame tip
  high-speed
  high-torque
  Hudson bone
  Lindermann
  McKenzie enlarging
  Midas Rex craniotomy
  motorized
  MTM 2
  olive-shaped
  Ossotome
  pear
  perforating
  power
  right-angle
  Rosen
  Rotablator rotating
  round
  Shannon
  spherical
  Stille
  water-cooled power
  Zimmer rotary
bur hole
bur hole cover
  Accu-Flo polyethylene
  Accu-Flo silicone rubber
bur surgery
Burch-Greenwood tendon tucker
Burford-Finochietto rib spreader

Burford rib spreader
Burgess below-knee amputation
Burke Bariatric bed
Burkhalter modification of Stiles-Bunnell technique
burned-out tabes
Burnham thumb and finger splint
burning-feet syndrome
Burns bench test
Burns plate
Burow skin flap operation
burr (see *bur*)
bursa (pl. bursae)
  adventitious
  calcaneal
  flexor
  intermediate
  intermetatarsophalangeal
  ischiogluteal
  Luschka
  olecranon
  prepatellar
  radial
  retrocalcaneal
  subacromial
  subdeltoid
  suprapatellar
  trochanteric
  ulnar
bursal adhesion
  subacromial
  subdeltoid
bursal flap
bursal fluid
bursal inflammation
bursal sac
bursectomy
bursitis (pl. bursitides)
  anserine
  chronic retrocalcaneal
  infracalcaneal
  intermetatarsophalangeal
  ischiogluteal
  olecranon

bursitis *(cont.)*
  patellar
  pigmented villonodular (PVB)
  postcalcaneal (posterior calcaneal bursitis)
  posterior calcaneal
  prepatellar
  retrocalcaneal
  septic
  subacromial
  subdeltoid
  Tornwaldt
bursocentesis
bursography
bursolith
bursopathy
bursotomy
burst
  asynchronous
  bilaterally synchronous
  bisynchronous
  epileptogenic
  onset
  positive
  rhythmic theta
  spindle
  synchronous
  synchronous paroxysmal
  theta wave
  unilateral
burst (compression) fracture of the atlas
bursting fracture
bursting, synchronous paroxysmal
burst of activity
burst of delta activity
burst of muscle potentials
burst of REM
burst of slow wave activity
burst of theta activity
burst phase
burst suppression on EEG
bursts between hemispheres on EEG
Burton sign
Burwell bur

Burwell-Charnley classification of
  fracture reduction
bushing, guide
Butler fifth toe operation
butterfly flap
butterfly fracture
buttock sign
button
  Biomet
  Charnley suture
  collared
  Drummond
  Hewson ligament
  padded
  patellar
  polyethylene
  Silastic
  subdural
  suture
  Wisconsin
buttonhole rupture
Button Spacer
button toe amputation
buttress plate
buttress, screws used to
buttressing
buzz bleeders
buzzing sensation
BVR (basal vein of Rosenthal)
B wave form on ICP monitor
B wave of cerebrospinal fluid (CSF)
bypass
  dorsal pedal
  EC-IC (extracranial-intracranial)
  extended tibial in situ
  femorodistal
  femoropopliteal
  intracranial arterial
  synthetic graft bypass to ankle

C, c

C.A. (chiropractic assistant)
cable
  braided
  chrome-cobalt
  Dall-Miles cerclage
  Dwyer scoliosis
  Gallie fusion-using
  Howmedica cerclage
  Songer spinal
  twister
cable and screws
cable telemetry EEG
cable twisters as treatment for internal tibial torsion
Cabot splint
Cacchione syndrome
cachexia, pituitary
CAD (computer-assisted design) femoral prosthesis
cadence of gait
Cadenza panty girdle
Cadwell 5200A somatosensory evoked potential unit
café au lait spot
Caffey disease
Caffey hyperostosis
Caffinière prosthesis
Cairns hemostatic forceps
caisson worker's disease (decompression sickness) (the bends)
Cajal interstitial nucleus
calamus scriptorius
Calandriello hip reduction
Calandruccio compression apparatus
Calandruccio fixation device
Calandruccio triangular compression fixation device
calcaneal apophysitis
calcaneal fracture, intra-articular
calcaneal gait
calcaneal pain
calcaneal spur
calcaneal spur cookie orthosis
calcaneal spur pad in shoe
calcanectomy
calcaneocavus (clubfoot)
  talipes calcaneus
  talipes cavus
calcaneocuboid arthrodesis
calcaneocuboid joint
calcaneocuboid ligament
calcaneofibular (CF) ligament
calcaneonavicular coalition
calcaneoplantar angle
calcaneotibial fusion
calcaneovalgus flatfoot
calcaneovalgus, pes
calcaneus
  excursion of the
  paralytic
  pes
  subtalar posterior displacement osteotomy of the
  sulcus
  talipes
  thalamic fracture of the
calcaneus altus
calcaneus deformity

calcar avis
calcar, pivot of
calcarine cortex
calcarine fissure
calcarine sulcus
calcification
  basal ganglia (on x-ray)
  dural
  dystrophic
  foci of
  gyriform
  intracranial
  periarticular
  periventricular
  pineal body
  sella turcica
  soft tissue
  tramline cortex
calcification of basal ganglia
calcification of dentate nuclei
calcification of falx
calcification of pineal gland
calcific tendinitis
calcified glial tumor
calcified pineal body, shift of
calcify
calcinosis circumscripta
calcinosis, tumoral
calcis, os
Calcitite bone replacement material
calcium alginate dressing
calcium hydroxyapatite
Caldwell-Coleman flatfoot technique
Caldwell-Durham tendon transfer
Caldwell hanging cast
calf circumference
calf muscle pump (anatomical)
calibration
  biological
  square wave
calibration pulse on EEG
calibration voltage for EEG
California viral encephalitis
calipers
  blunt
  body fat
  Harpenden
  Mitutoyo digital
  Thomas walking
  Townley femur
  vernier
  weight-relieving
Callahan extension of cervical injury
Callahan fusion technique
Callander amputation
Callaway test
Calleja exercises
Callender derotation brace
callosal area
callosal commissurotomy
callosal gyrus
callosal lesion
callosal sulcus
callosity, plantar
callosomarginal artery
callostomy, corpus
callosum, corpus
callous (adj.)
callus
  bony
  bridging
  florid
  fracture
callus formation
callus weld
Calman carotid clamp
Calnan-Nicolle metatarsophalangeal prosthesis
Calnan-Nicolle synthetic joint prosthesis
caloric requirements
  athletic
  basal
caloric stimulation test for vestibular function
calorics
  cold water
  ice water

Caltagirone chisel
calvarial bone
calvarium (pl. calvaria)
Calvé-Perthes disease
Cambridge test battery
camelback sign
camera
  DyoCam arthroscopic video
  gamma
Cameron-Haight periosteal elevator
CAM 5.2 antibody
Camino ICP monitor
Camino intracranial catheter
Camino microventricular bolt
Camino subdural transducer
Camino ventricular bolt
Camitz tendon transfer
Camp corset
Campbell-Akbarnia procedure
Campbell ankle operation
Campbell arthrodesis
Campbell-Goldthwait procedure
Campbell nerve root retractor
Campbell periosteal elevator
Campbell posterior bone block
Campbell root retractor
Campbell tibial osteotomy
Camper chiasma
camptocormia
camptodactyly
Cam Walker ankle walker
Cam Walker leg brace
Cam Walker leg walker
Can Am brace
Canadian crutches
Canadian Neurological Scale
Canakis pin
canal
  Alcock
  arachnoid
  Bichat
  carotid
  central spinal
  cervical

canal *(cont.)*
  Dorello
  ethmoidal
  femoral medullary
  Guyon
  haversian
  Hunter
  hydrops
  intramedullary
  lumbar
  medullary
  narrowing of spinal
  neural
  Richet tibio-astragalocalcaneal
  semicircular
  spinal
  spinal cord
  tarsal
  tibial medullary
  tibio-astragalocalcaneal of Richet
  tight spinal
  Volkmann
canal decompression
Canale-Kelly classification of talar neck fracture
Canale osteotomy
canaliculus, canaliculi
canal paresis
Canavan disease
Canavan leukodystrophy
Canavan-van Bogaert-Bertrand disease
cancellectomy
cancellous versus cortical bone
candelabra, sylvian
Candida albicans fungus
Candida albicans meningitis
Candida albicans invasion of the nervous system
candle wax appearance of bone
cane
  quad
  single-point
  small-base quad
  tripod

C angle
cannula
  Acufex double-lumen
  Adson brain exploring
  arthroscopic
  Bergstrom
  biopsy
  brain exploring
  Bucy-Frazier suction
  coagulating suction
  biopsy
  Dohrmann-Rubin
  Dorsey ventricular
  Dyonics
  Elsberg brain
  Elsberg ventricular
  Eriksson muscle biopsy
  exploring
  Fischer ventricular
  Ford Hospital ventricular
  Frazier brain exploring
  Frazier ventricular
  Haynes brain
  inflow
  intraventricular
  large-bore inflow
  large-egress
  McCain TMJ
  microirrigating
  Portnoy ventricular
  Ray ventricular
  Scott ventricular
  Sedan-Vallicioni
  small-egress
  suction
  suprapatellar
  ventricular
cannulated guided hip screw system
Cantelli sign
CAP (carotid Amytal procedure)
capacitor plate for electrical stimulation
Caparosa bur
Caparosa wire crimper
CAPE (Clifton Assessment Procedures for the Elderly)
CAPE (continuous anatomical passive exerciser)
Capello total hip replacement
Capener lateral rhachotomy
capillary filling time
capillary hemangioma
capital epiphysis (CE) angle
capital extension
capital flexor
capital fragment
capital mover
capitate bone of wrist
capitate, volar
capitellocondylar total elbow arthroplasty
capitellum
capitolunate joint
capitular epiphysis
capitulocondylar elbow arthroplasty
capitulum
Capner gouge
Capner splint
caps, Carnation corn
capsular imbrication
capsular incision
capsular plane
capsular reefing
capsular release
capsule
  articular
  dorsal
  external
  facet
  Gerota
  internal
  joint
  limb of anterior
  metatarsophalangeal joint
  MTP (metatarsophalangeal)
  plantar
  posterolateral
  redundant

capsule *(cont.)*
  rim of
  suprasellar
  talonavicular
  wrist
capsulectomy
  anterior
  circumferential
capsulitis, adhesive
capsulocaudate infarction
capsulodesis, Zancolli
capsulolabral complex
capsuloperiosteal envelope
capsuloplasty, Zancolli
capsuloputaminal infarction
capsuloputaminocaudate infarction
capsulorrhaphy (see *operation*)
  medial
  pants-over-vest
  staple
capsulotomy (see *operation*)
  Curtis PIP joint
  dorsal transverse
  dorsolateral and medial
  L-shaped
  medial V-Y
  stereotaxic anterior
  subtalar
  talonavicular
  transmetatarsal
  V
  vertical
car hand controls
car-sickness
carbide bur
carbohydrate loading
carbon dioxide intoxication
carbon monoxide intoxication
carbon tetrachloride poisoning
Carborundum grinding wheel
Carceau-Brahms ankle arthrodesis
carcinoma, medullary
carcinomatosis
carcinomatous meningitis
Cardan screwdriver
cardiac ganglion, Wrisberg
cardinal directions of gaze
Cardiopulmonary Paragon 8500 bed
cardiovascular seizure
Caregiver Strain Index (CSI)
Carl P. Jones traction splint
C-arm portable x-ray unit
Carnation corn caps
carnosinemia
Carolina rocker
caroticocavernous fistula
carotid angiography
carotid artery endarterectomy
carotid bruit
carotid bulb baroreceptor
carotid cavernous fistula occlusion
carotid distribution TIA (transient ischemic attack)
carotid endarterectomy
carotid occlusive disease
carotid plexus
carotid pulses
carotid sheath
carotid siphon
carotid stenosis
  bilateral
  unilateral
carpal arch
carpal coalition
carpal deviation
carpal row
carpal scaphoid bone fracture
carpal tunnel release (CTR)
carpal tunnel release system, Endotrac
carpal tunnel syndrome (CTS)
carpal tunnel view (x-ray)
carpal tunnel wrist syndrome
carpectomy
Carpenter syndrome
carphology
carpometacarpal (CMC) articulation
carpometacarpal (CMC) joint
carpopedal spasm

carpophalangeal joint
carporadial articulation
carpus
Carr-Purcell-Meiboom-Gill sequence
Carr-Purcell sequence
Carrell fibular substitution technique
Carrell-Girard screw
carrier
  Cave-Rowe ligature
  double-headed stereotactic ligature
  Yasargil ligature
Carroll and Taber arthroplasty
Carroll arthrodesis
Carroll-Bennett retractor
Carroll bone-holding forceps
Carroll dressing forceps
Carroll hand retractor
Carroll-Legg periosteal elevator
Carroll skin hook
Carroll-Smith-Petersen osteotome
Carroll tendon-pulling forceps
Carroll tissue forceps
Carrom orthopedic bed
carrying angle
Carter foam pillow
Carter immobilization cushion
Carter-Rowe view
Carter splint
Cartesian coordinate system for neurosurgery
cartilage
  articular
  cryopreserved
  degenerated
  free flap of
  nonossified tarsal navicular
  patellofemoral groove
  physeal
  quadrangle
  semilunar
  shelling off of
  triradial
  triradiate
cartilage degeneration, articular
cartilage joint space
cartilage reduction, Aston
cartilage shaver blade
cartilaginous anlage
cartilaginous cap of phalangeal head
cartilaginous lesion
cartilaginous navicular
cartwheel fracture
cascade, diagnostic
CASH (cruciform anterior spinal hyperextension)
CASH thoracolumbosacral orthosis
CASP (contoured anterior spinal plate)
Caspar alligator forceps
Caspar anterior cervical plating technique
Caspar blade
Caspar cervical plate
Caspar cervical screw
Caspar craniotome
Caspari arthroscopic portal
Caspari repair
cast, casting
  airplane
  arm cylinder
  banjo
  below-knee walking
  below-the-knee
  bent-knee
  Bermuda spica
  bivalved cylinder
  body
  body jacket
  Boston bivalve
  broom-stick
  Caldwell hanging
  corrective
  Cotrel
  Cotrel scoliosis
  cotton
  Cotton-Loader position
  cylinder walking
  Dehne

cast *(cont.)*
- double-hip spica
- double spica
- EDF scoliosis
- Equilizer short leg walking
- extension body
- fiberglass
- figure 8 (figure-of-8)
- flexion body
- Fractura Flex
- Frejka
- full-thumb spica
- Gaiter
- gauntlet
- gel
- Gelocast
- groin-to-ankle
- Gypsona
- halo
- hanging arm
- Hexcelite
- hinged cylinder
- hip spica
- inhibitive
- intermediate
- Kite clubfoot
- Kite metatarsal
- light
- long arm (LAC)
- long arm thumb spica
- long leg (LLC)
- long leg bent-knee
- long leg walking (LLWC)
- long leg weightbearing (LLWBC)
- Lorenz
- Lovell clubfoot
- MaxCast
- Minerva
- Moe modified Cotrel
- Mooney
- Neufeld
- nonwalking
- O'Donoghue cotton
- one and one-half spica

cast *(cont.)*
- one-half spica
- pantaloon
- patellar tendon-bearing (PTB)
- patellar tendon weightbearing
- petaling edges of
- Petrie spica
- plantar flexion
- plaster of Paris (POP)
- polyurethane
- Quengel
- Risser localizer scoliosis
- Risser turnbuckle
- Sarmiento short leg patellar tendon-bearing
- Sbarbaro spica
- Schmeisser spica
- scoliosis
- serial
- serial wedge
- short arm (SAC)
- short arm fiberglass
- short leg (SLC)
- short leg walking (SLWC)
- shoulder spica
- slipper
- spica
- sugar-tong
- three-finger spica
- 3M fiberglass
- thumb spica
- toe spica
- toe-to-groin
- toe-to-midthigh
- tone-inhibiting leg
- total contact
- turnbuckle
- univalve
- Unna boot
- Velpeau
- walking
- walking boot
- warm-and-form
- wedging

cast *(cont.)*
  well-leg
  windowed
cast application
Castaway ankle walker
Castaway leg brace
Castaway leg walker
castbelt, Posey below-the-knee
cast bender
cast boot
cast brace
cast breaker
cast cover
  AquaShield orthopedic
  Dryspell
cast cushion
cast cutter
Cast Gard cast protector
Castiglia ankle brace
cast immobilization
Castle procedure
cast padding, cotton
cast sock
cast spreader
  Beeson
  Henning
  Hoffer-Daimler
cast syndrome
cast table
cast tape
  Scotchcast 2
  TufStuf II
cast walker
  rubber sole
  Sabel
cast wedge
cast with dorsal (or volar) toe plate extension
Castroviejo bladebreaker knife
Castroviejo needle holder
CAT-CAM conversion
CAT (CT) scan
CAT (CT) scan cradle
CAT (CT) scan gantry
cataclysmic headache
catalepsy
cataleptic attack
catamenial migraine
cataplexy
cataract knife
cataract knife Beaver blade
catastrophic reaction (of a demented person)
catatonia
catecholamines
Categories, Functional Ambulation (FAC)
category, Westin-Turco
Cateye Ergociser
"cath'd" or "cathed" (slang for catheterized)
Cathcart Orthocentric hip prosthesis
catheter
  Abramson
  Accu-Flo ventricular
  angiographic
  BPS spinal angiographic
  Camino ICP (intracranial pressure)
  cardiac
  dummy seed
  epidural
  Fogarty embolectomy
  Foltz
  guide
  guiding
  Heplock
  high-pressure
  HNB angiographic
  hyperthermia
  ICP (intracranial pressure)
  indwelling
  interstitial
  intratumoral
  intraventricular
  ITC radiopaque balloon
  kinking of CNS
  low-pressure
  medium-pressure

catheter *(cont.)*
- peritoneal
- Phoenix ventriculostomy
- Portnoy ventricular
- Pudenz peritoneal
- Raimondi peritoneal
- Raimondi spring
- Raimondi ventricular
- Scott silicone ventricular
- Seletz nonrigid ventricular
- Shaw
- Simpson
- subarachnoid
- subcutaneous ventricular reservoir
- subdural drainage
- toposcopic
- Tracker-10
- Tracker-18
- ventricular

catheterization, superselective
Catlin amputating knife
Catterall classification
cauda corporis striati
caudad
cauda equina compression syndrome
caudally
caudalward
caudate nucleus
cauliflower ear
causalgia
- major
- minor
- trauma-related

causalgic pain
cautery
- Aesculap bipolar
- BICAP
- bipolar
- Bovie
- Concept hand-held
- Mira
- monopolar
- unipolar

cautery probe, McCain TMJ
Cavanaugh-Rogers classification of footprints
cave, Meckel
Cave-Rowe ligature carrier
Cave-Rowe shoulder dislocation technique
cavernous hemangioma
cavernous sinus lesion
cavernous sinus thrombosis
Cavin osteotome
cavitas medullaris
cavitation (in gunshot wounds)
Cavitron dissector
Cavitron ultrasonic aspirator (CUSA)
cavity
- absorption
- cotyloid
- epidural
- glenoid
- joint
- marrow
- Meckel
- popliteal
- saclike
- sigmoid cavity of radius
- sigmoid cavity of ulna
- subarachnoid
- subdural
- synovial
- syringomyelic
- syrinx
- trigeminal

cavity of septum pellucidum
cavovalgus
- pes
- talipes

cavovarus
- pes
- talipes

cavovarus deformity
cavovarus foot
cavum meckelii
cavum subdurale
cavum trigeminale

cavum vergae
cavus
  anterior
  forefoot
  global
  local
  midfoot
  pes
  posterior
  posttraumatic
  talipes
cavus deformity
cavus foot
CAWO (closing abductor wedge osteotomy)
CBF (cerebral blood flow)
CBI (convergent beam irradiation)
CBI stereotactic head holder
CBI stereotactic ring
CBS (chronic brain syndrome)
CBT (corticobulbar tract)
CBVH (Commission for the Blind and Visually Handicapped)
CBWO (closed base wedge osteotomy)
CCA (common carotid artery)
CCD (central collodiaphyseal) angle
CCF (carotid cavernous fistula)
CCS (Children's Coma Score)
CCTA (coronal computed tomographic arthrography)
CCTV/EEG (closed circuit TV and EEG recording)
CD (Cotrel-Dubousset) instruments
CD fixation device
CDH (congenital dislocation of hip)
CDH (congenital dysplasia of hip)
CE (capital epiphysis) angle of Wiberg
CEA (carcinoembryonic antigen)
CEA (carotid endarterectomy)
Cebotome drill
cecocentral scotoma (central cecal)
Cedell-Magnusson classification of arthritis on x-ray
C-EEG (computerized electro-encephalogram)
C electrode (central) (C_1-C_6)
cell, cells
  agranular chromophobe cell in adenohypophysis
  anterior horn
  Antoni A and B
  Betz
  Betz giant pyramidal
  cortical pyramidal
  degeneration of ganglion
  ependymal
  excitable
  foam
  germ
  giant pyramidal Betz
  glial
  gitter (microglia) (not glitter)
  globose
  granular cerebellar
  granular chromophil
  hemosiderin-laden
  injured
  intermediolateral horn
  lactotrophic
  motor horn
  multipotential
  myxomatous
  nests of tumor
  null
  oligodendroglial
  osteoclastic giant
  osteogenic
  plasma
  proliferation of
  Purkinje cerebellar
  Renshaw
  Sayk preparation of CSF
  Schwann
  shrinkage of ganglion
  specialized
  spindle
  stromal
  synovial lining
  thalamic pacemaker
cell leukodystrophy, globoid

cell sarcoma, reticulum
cell saver
cellulitis
CEM (central extensor mechanism)
cement (see also *adhesive*)
  acrylic
  bone
  centrifugation of
  CMW bone
  Implast bone
  Ketac
  low-viscosity
  methyl methacrylate
  orthopedic
  Palacos bone
  PMMA bone
  polymerized
  pressurization of
  pressurized
  Protoplast
  removal of excess
  residual
  Simplex
  surface
  Surgical Simplex P radiopaque
  Zimmer low-viscosity
cementation
cement compactor, acetabular
cemented total hip arthroplasty
Cement Eater
  Anspach
  Zimmer Cibatome
cementless technique
cement gun
cement line
cement mantle
cementome, Anspach
cementophyte
cement pump
cement removal
cement restrictor inserter
cement spacer inserter
cement spatula
cement technique
center
  ciliospinal center of Budge
  cortical
  emetic
  growth center of bones
  hearing
  motor
  pontine lateral gaze
  speech
  visual
  vomiting
center of gravity (CG)
center of joint
central cervical cord syndrome
central collodiaphyseal angle (CCD)
central-core disease
central facial paresis
central gray matter
central language deficit
central lesion
central motor pathways disease
central nervous system (CNS)
central nervous system, aspergillosis of the
central nervous system hemorrhage
central nervous system infection
central nervous system toxoplasmosis
central neurogenic hyperventilation
central nystagmus
central origin weakness
central rays
central retinal vein thrombosis
central scotoma (pl. scotomata)
central sensory deficit
central sensory loss
central slip of tendon
central stenosis
central sulcus
central tegmental tract
central thrombosis
Central European encephalitis
Centralign hip prosthesis
centralization procedure
centrally caused nystagmus

centrally uninhibited bladder
centrencephalic epilepsy
centrencephalic seizure
centrifugation of cement (in joint replacement)
centripetal wrapping, compressive
centroid on EEG
centronuclear myopathy
centroparietal head region
centrotemporal discharges on EEG
centrotemporal epilepsy
centrum semiovale
cephalad
cephalalgia (cephalgia)
cephalalgic (or cephalgic) attack
cephalgia (cephalalgia)
  cervical
  histamine
cephalgic attack
cephalgic seizure
cephalhematocele
cephalhematoma
cephalic angulation
cephalofacial proportionality
cephalohematoma, parietal
cephalometer, Bertillon
cephalometric analysis
cephalometrics
cephalostat
Ceramion prosthesis
cerclage
  cable
  Dall-Miles cable
  Howmedica
cerclage suture
cerclaged component
cerebellar ataxia
cerebellar degeneration
cerebellar disease
cerebellar dysarthria
cerebellar fibers
cerebellar fits (seizure)
cerebellar hemorrhage
cerebellar infarction
cerebellar malaria
cerebellar mass
cerebellar nystagmus
cerebellar pathway
cerebellar peduncle
cerebellar retractor
cerebellar signs
cerebellar syndrome
cerebellar tonsillar herniation
cerebellar tract
cerebellar tremor
cerebellar vermis
cerebellopontile angle (CP angle) tumor
cerebellopontine angle (CP angle) tumor
cerebellum
  basal ganglia of
  dentate nucleus of
  midline
  petrosal
  Purkinje cells of
  stimulation of the
  unilateral lesion of the
cerebellum tumor
cerebral abscess
cerebral amoebiasis (amebiasis)
cerebral angiography
cerebral anoxia
cerebral apotentiality
cerebral aqueduct
cerebral arteriography
cerebral Aspergillus abscess
cerebral atrophy
cerebral autoregulation
cerebral blood flow (CBF)
cerebral brain death
cerebral brucellosis
cerebral commissure
cerebral contusion (bruise)
cerebral cortex
cerebral death
cerebral disorder
cerebral dominance

cerebral dysfunction
cerebral dysrhythmia
cerebral edema
cerebral fat embolism
cerebral gigantism
cerebral hemidecortication
cerebral hemisphere
cerebral herniation
cerebral infarct, infarction
cerebral ischemic event
cerebral lesion
cerebral lipidosis
cerebral malaria, *Plasmodium falciparum*
cerebral mantle
cerebral metabolic rate of oxygen consumption ($CRMO_2$)
cerebral nocardiosis
cerebral palsy (CP)
  ataxic
  athetoid
  choreoathetoid
  dyskinetic
  dystonic
  extrapyramidal
  flaccid
  hypotonic
  pyramidal
  spastic
cerebral paraplegia
cerebral parenchyma
cerebral peduncle
cerebral perfusion pressure
cerebral poliodystrophy
cerebral potentials
cerebral revascularization
cerebral salt wasting
cerebral signs
cerebral steal syndrome
cerebral thrombophlebitis
cerebral trauma
cerebral vasospasm
cerebri (pl. of cerebrum)
  commotio
  contusio
cerebri *(cont.)*
  falx
  familial gliomatosis
  pseudotumor
cerebriform
cerebritis
  bacterial
  saturnine
Cerebrograph
cerebrohepatorenal syndrome
cerebromacular degeneration (CMD)
cerebroside lipidosis
cerebroside reticulocytosis
cerebroside sulfatase
cerebrospinal fluid (CSF)
  A wave of
  AFB (acid-fast bacilli) in
  anti-Borrelia antibody in
  antibody to herpes simplex in
  antibody to St. Louis encephalitis in
  antigen to *H. influenzae* in
  antigen to meningococci in
  antigen to Mycobacterium in
  antigen to pneumococci in
  B wave of
  blood in
  bloody
  C wave of
  C&S (culture and sensitivity)
  cellular pleocytosis in
  centrifuged sediment of
  clear
  cloudy
  coccidioidal complement fixation of
  counterimmune electrophoresis of
  cryptococcal antigen in
  cryptococcal antigen titer of
  CSF-serum HSV antibody ratio in
  culture and sensitivity (C&S) of
  cytology of
  dammed-up
  decreased absorption of
  elevated protein in
  ELISA test on

cerebrovascular circulation
cerebrovascular disease
cerebrovascular insufficiency
cerebrum, great vein of
certified disability examiner
Cerva Crane halter
cervical acceleration/deceleration
  syndrome (whiplash)
cervical AOA halo traction
cervical arthritis
cervical brace (see *brace*)
cervical cephalgia
cervical collar
cervical cord lesion
cervical corpectomy
cervical disk disease
cervical dorsal outlet syndrome
cervical extension
cervical fracture
cervical halter traction
cervical mover ligament
cervical movers
cervical musculature
cervical nerve root
cervical orthosis (see *orthosis*)
cervical pillow
cervical radiculitis
cervical retractor
cervical rib
cervical rongeur
cervical spine (C1 to C7)
cervical spine, dens view of
cervical spine injury
cervical spondylosis of the spinal cord
cervical spondylosis, washboard effect
  on myelography in
cervical spondylotic myelopathy
  (CMS)
cervical support
cervical sympathectomy
cervical tension myositis (CTM)
cervical traction
  AOA halo
  Bremer halo
cervical traction *(cont.)*
  Georgiade visor
  Houston halo
  Miami acute collar
  Miami J collar
  Philadelphia collar
cervical vertigo
cervical wire passer, Batzdorf
cervical wire twister, Batzdorf
cervico-occipital fusion
cervicomedullary junction
cervicothoracic level
cervicothoracic region
cervicothoracolumbosacral orthosis
cervicotrochanter
CES (cauda equina syndrome)
Céstan-Chenais syndrome
CFQ (Cognitive Failures
  Questionnaire)
CFQ-for-others assessment
CFS (contoured femoral stem) hip
  prosthesis
CG (center of gravity)
CGIC (Clinical Global Impression
  of Change)
Chaddock reflex
Chaddock sign
CHAG (coralline hydroxyapatite
  Goniopora) bone graft substitute
  material
Chagas disease
chain of electrodes
chain, sympathetic
chains, wheelchair
chair
  ergonomically correct
  Gardner
chairback brace
chairback orthosis
chalk bones
chamber, Pudenz flushing
Chamberlain line
chamfer cut
chamfer reamer

Champ elastic bandage
champagne-bottle legs in Charcot-Marie-Tooth disease
Champion Trauma Score (CTS)
Championnière bone drill
Chance spinal fracture
Chance vertebral fracture
Chandler arthrodesis
Chandler bone elevator
Chandler felt collar splint
Chandler knee retractor
Chandler procedure
Chandler retractor
Chandler spinal perforating forceps
Chandler tendon transfer
change, changes
 abulic mental
 age-related EEG
 arthritic talonavicular
 behavioral
 binocular acuity
 chondromalacial
 cystic
 dystrophic
 Fairbanks
 focal degenerative
 histological tendon
 mental
 monocular acuity
 osteoarthritic
 paroxysmal
 pre-slip (on x-ray)
 pupillary
 spondylitic
 subchondral
 trophic
 trophic skin
 ultrastructural (in wound healing)
 vasomotor
change in mentation
channel, EEG recording
channels, enlarged vascular (on x-ray)
Chapchal knee arthrodesis
Chaput tubercle
characteristics, stride
Charcot arthropathy
Charcot-Bouchard intracerebral aneurysm
Charcot-Bouchard microaneurysm
Charcot foot, diabetic
Charcot gait
Charcot joint
Charcot-Marie-Tooth (CMT) disease
Charcot-Marie-Tooth disease, stork's legs in
Charcot-Marie-Tooth syndrome
Charcot triad
Charest head frame
Charleston nighttime bending brace
Charleston scoliosis brace
charley horse
Charlie Chaplin type of gait
Charnley ankle arthrodesis
Charnley bone curet
Charnley brace
Charnley centering ring
Charnley compression apparatus
Charnley compression clamp
Charnley deepening reamer
Charnley drill
Charnley expanding reamer
Charnley external fixation apparatus
Charnley femoral broach
Charnley femoral condyle drill
Charnley femoral condyle radius gauge
Charnley femoral inlay aligner
Charnley femoral inlay guillotine
Charnley femoral prosthesis neck punch
Charnley femoral prosthesis pusher
Charnley foam suture pad
Charnley-Hastings prosthesis
Charnley hip arthroplasty
Charnley hip replacement
Charnley horizontal retractor
Charnley-Houston shoulder arthrodesis
Charnley initial incision retractor

Charnley introducer
Charnley knee retractor
Charnley-Merle D'Aubigné disability grading system
Charnley-Mueller hip prosthesis
Charnley pain and function grading scale
Charnley pin retractor
Charnley socket gauge
Charnley suction drain
Charnley suture button
Charnley taper reamer
Charnley template
Charnley tibial onlay jig
Charnley total hip system
Charnley trochanter holder
Charnley trochanter reamer
Charnley vertical retractor
Charnley wire-holding forceps
Charnley wire passer
Charriere amputation saw
Charriere bone saw
Chatfield-Girdlestone splint
Chatzidakis hinged Vitallium implant
chauffeur's fracture
Chaves muscle transfer
Chaves-Rapp muscle transfer technique
check, pupil
check socket
checking
Checklist
  McGill pain
  Low Back Pain Symptom
Chédiak-Higashi syndrome
cheek puffing, repetitive
cheese reaction headache (tyramine)
cheilectomy
  Garceau
  Mann-Coughlin-DuVries
cheilotomy
cheiralgia paresthetica
cheirarthritis
cheirobrachialgia
cheirognostic
cheiromegaly
cheiroplasty
cheiropodalgia
cheirospasm
chemical neurectomy
chemical rhizotomy
chemical shift
chemical sympathectomy
chemicals, stellate
chemoneurolysis
chemonucleolysis, double-needle
chemoreceptors
chemotherapy
  intracavitary
  intrathecal
  intratumoral
chemotic eyes in migraine
cherry-red macula of Tay-Sachs disease
Cherry-Austin drill
Cherry brain retractor
Cherry-Kerrison laminectomy forceps
Cherry-Kerrison laminectomy rongeur
Cherry laminectomy retractor
Cherry osteotome
Cherry traction tongs
chest expansion test
chest roll
chevaux de frise (migraine aura)
chevron laceration
chevron osteotomy
chewing automatism
chewing reflex (bulldog response)
Cheyne periosteal elevator
Cheyne-Stokes respirations
CHH cervical brace
CHI (closed head injury)
Chiari-Foix-Nicolesco syndrome
Chiari formation
Chiari innominate osteotomy
Chiari malformation
chiasm of digits of hand

chiasm
  optic
  tendinous
chiasma, Camper
chiasmal compression
chiasmal lesion
chiasmatic defect
Chick CLT operating table and frame
Chick-Foster orthopedic bed
Chick fracture table
Chiene test
chilblains
child, health-handicapped
Children's Coma Score (CCS)
Children's Hospital brain spatula
Children's Hospital hand drill
Children's Hospital scalp clips
Children's Hospital spatula
Childress ankle fixation technique
Childress duck waddle test
chin-occiput piece
Chinese flap
chip
  cancellous bone
  corticocancellous bone
Chippaux-Smirak arch index
Chiro-Manis chiropractic table
chiropodical
chiropodist
chiropody
chiropractic (noun)
  doctor of (D.C.)
  sports
  World Federation of (WFC)
chiropractic adjustment
chiropractic assistant (C.A.)
chiropractic joint manipulation
chiropractic laser nonsurgical face lift
chiropractic manual manipulation of the spine
chiropractic mattress
chiropractic spinal adjustments
chiropractic x-rays
chiropractor
chiropraxis
chisel (see also *gouge*)
  Adson
  Adson laminectomy
  Alexander
  ASIF
  Austin Moore
  Ballenger-Hajek
  beveled
  Bishop
  Blair
  bone
  Bowen
  box
  Brittain
  Bruening
  Buckley
  Caltagirone
  Cinelli-McIndoe
  Cloward cervical
  Cloward spinal fusion
  cold
  Converse
  Cottle
  D'Errico lamina
  Dautrey
  Fomon
  Freer
  Hajek
  Hibbs
  hollow
  Lambert-Lowman
  laminectomy
  Lexer
  Lowman-Hoglund
  Lucas
  Martin cartilage
  meniscotomy
  Metzenbaum
  Meyerding
  Miles bone
  mortising
  neurosurgical
  Partsch

chisel *(cont.)*
  Passow
  Pick
  Puka
  Schwartze
  seating
  Sheehan
  Simmons
  Smillie cartilage
  Smillie meniscotomy
  Smith-Petersen
  square hollow
  Stille bone
  straight
  swan-neck
  Trautmann
  U.S. Army bone
  West bone
chisel-tip wire
Cho cruciate ligament reconstruction
choked disk
cholelithiasis
cholesterol emboli
cholinergic crisis
cholinergic enzyme
chondral defect
chondral fragment
chondralgia
chondrectomy
chondrification
chondritis
chondroblastoma
chondrocalcinosis
chondrocytes, harvesting of
chondrodiastasis
chondrodysplasia
chondrodystrophia calcificans
chondrodystrophia fetalis
chondrodystrophy, myotonic
chondroepiphysitis
chondrofibroma
chondroitin (in osteoarthritis)
chondrolipoma
chondrolysis
chondroma, juxtacortical
chondromalacia of the patella
chondromalacia patellae
chondromalacial changes
chondromalacic changes
chondromatosis
  Henderson-Jones
  synovial
chondrometaplasia
chondromyofibroma
chondromyxofibroma
chondromyxoid fibroma (CMF)
chondromyxoma
chondromyxosarcoma
chondronecrosis
chondro-osteodystrophy
chondropathology
chondrophyte
chondroplastic
chondroplastic dwarfism
chondroplastic myotonia
chondroplasty blade
chondroporosis
chondrosarcoma
  clear cell
  differentiated
  extraskeletal
  mesenchymal
  myxoid
  parosteal
  periosteal
chondrosarcomatosis
chondrosteoma
chondrosternoplasty
chondrotomy
Chopart ankle dislocation
Chopart dislocation
Chopart hindfoot amputation
Chopart joint
Chopart partial foot prosthesis
Cho-Pat knee strap
Cho tendon technique
choppy sea sign
chorda magna

chorda tympani
chordae Willisii
chordoblastoma
chordocarcinoma
chordoepithelioma
chordoma
  cavern
  sacrococcygeal
chordosarcoma
chordotomy (see *cordotomy*)
chorea
  acute
  benign hereditary
  Bergeron
  chronic progressive hereditary
  dancing
  degenerative
  diaphragmatic
  Dubini
  electric
  fibrillary
  hemilateral
  Henoch
  hereditary
  Huntington
  hysterical
  juvenile
  kinesigenic
  limp
  malleatory
  methodic
  mimetic
  minor
  Morvan
  nocturnal
  one-sided
  oral contraceptive-induced
  paralytic
  phenytoin-induced
  posthemiplegic
  prehemiplegic
  rheumatic
  rhythmic
  saltatory

chorea *(cont.)*
  Schrötter (Schroetter)
  senile
  simple
  Sydenham
  thyrotoxicosis-induced
  unilateral
chorea gravidarum
chorea insaniens
chorea minor
chorea mollis
chorea nutans
choreic
choreic dyskinesia
choreic movement disorder
choreic movements
choreic syndrome
choreiform movement
choreoathetoid movement
choreoathetosis
  familial paroxysmal
  paroxysmal
  paroxysmal kinesigenic
  phenytoin-induced
  psychotic
  thyrotoxicosis-induced
choreoathetotic movements
choreoid
choreomania (dancing mania)
choriocarcinoma, pineal gland
choriomeningitis, benign lymphocytic
chorioretinitis
choroid plexus papilloma tumor
choroidal fissure
choroidal pericallosal artery
choroidectomy
Chrisman-Snook ankle technique
Chrisman-Snook reconstruction of ankle ligaments
Christensen interlocking nail
Christiansen hip prosthesis
Christmas hemophiliac disease
Christmas tree adapter
Christmas tree photopsias

Christmas tree reamer
chromatolysis
chromogranin, immunoreactive
chromophobe adenoma, pituitary tumor
chromophobe pituitary tumor
chronaxy (on EMG)
chrondroblastoma
chronic Achilles tendinitis
chronic ankle sprain
chronic basal meningitis with cranial nerve paralysis
chronic foot strain
chronic functional instability
chronic leg ulcer
chronic meningitis
chronic musculoskeletal pain syndrome (CMPS)
chronic pain syndrome
chronic paroxysmal hemicrania
chronic pyogenic osteomyelitis
chronic recurrent dislocation of ankle joint
chronic retrocalcaneal bursitis
chronic spinal epidural infection
  brucellosis
  coccidioidomycosis
  cryptococcosis
  syphilis
  tuberculous cold abscess
chronic spinal intradural infection
chronic sprain
chronic subtalar joint pain
chronic whiplash
chronologic age
chuck
  hand
  Jacobs
  pin
  universal
chuck key
Chuinard autogenous bone graft
Chuinard-Petersen ankle arthrodesis
Chvostek-Weiss sign
chymopapain injection
cicatrix
Cicherelli bone rongeur
CIDP (chronic inflammatory demyelinating polyradiculopathy)
CIDPN (chronic inflammatory demyelinating polyneuropathy)
ciliary ganglion
ciliary migraine
ciliary neuralgia
ciliospinal center of Budge
ciliospinal or pupillary-skin reflex
Cincinnati incision
cinefluoroscopy
Cinelli-McIndoe chisel
Cinelli osteotome
cinematographic vision disorder of visual perception in migraine
cinereum, tuber
cinesalgia
cingulate gyrus
cingulate herniation
cingulate sulcus
cingulectomy
cingulotomy
cingulum hemispherii
Cintor bone rongeur
Cintor knee prosthesis
CIP (chronic inflammatory poly-radiculoneuropathy)
circannual cycle
circannual rhythm
circle bed
circle of Weber
circle of Willis
  arterial
  forks of
CircOlectric bed
CircOlectric frame
circuit, Papez
circulation
  cerebrovascular
  collateral
  systemic

circulation *(cont.)*
spider-web (on angiography of glioblastomas)
circulation stroke
anterior
posterior
circulatory compromise
circulatory embarrassment
circumduction with spastic gait
circumference
calf
head
pelvic
circumferential fracture
circumferentially
circumlocution of speech
circumscripta, myositis ossificans
circumstantial migraine
circumstantial speech
cistern
ambient
arachnoiditis of the opticochiasmatic
basal
basal arachnoid
basilar
carotid
cerebellomedullary
cerebellopontine
chiasmatic
crural
effacement of
great
increased basilar
interpeduncular
mesencephalic
opticochiasmatic
parasellar
posterior
prepontine
puncture of
quadrigeminal
subarachnoidal
trigeminal
widening of crural
cisterna ambiens
cisterna basalis
cisterna cerebellomedullaris
cisterna chiasmatica
cisterna chiasmatis
cisternae subarachnoidales
cisterna fossae lateralis cerebri
cisterna fossae Sylvii
cisterna intercruralis profunda
cisterna interpeduncularis
cisternal puncture
cisterna magna
cisterna sulci lateralis
cisterna Sylvii
cisterna venae magnae cerebri
cistern of chiasma
cistern of fossa of Sylvius
cistern of lateral fossa of cerebrum
cistern of Pecquet
cistern of Sylvius
cisternogram, cisternography
indium
isotope
metrizamide CT (MCTC)
oxygen
radioisotope
radionuclide
cisternographic
Citelli angle
Citelli punch forceps
citrullinemia
CIVRA (continuous intravenous regional anesthesia)
CJD (Creutzfeldt-Jakob disease)
CKS (Continuum knee system) prosthesis
CKS knee implant
Claiborne external fixator
clamp
Acland
Adair breast
Allis
Böhler (Boehler)
Backhaus towel

clamp *(cont.)*
- Berens
- Berens muscle
- Bigelo calvarium
- Bircher bone/cartilage
- Bishop
- bone extension
- bone-holding
- Boyes muscle
- bulldog
- C
- Calman carotid
- calvarium
- carotid artery
- cartilage
- Charnley compression
- Crutchfield carotid artery
- Dandy
- Diethrich bulldog
- double
- Edna towel
- Fukushima C-clamp
- gallbladder
- Gardner neurosurgical skull
- Greenberg
- Halifax interlaminar
- Harrington hook
- Harrington rod
- Hoen
- hook
- infant skull
- interlaminar
- intracranial
- Jackson bone extension
- Jacobson bulldog
- Jacobson-Potts vascular
- Javid carotid
- Johns Hopkins bulldog
- Kartchner carotid
- Kelly
- Kern bone-holding
- Kindt carotid artery
- Kocher
- Lahey

clamp *(cont.)*
- Lambert-Lowman bone
- Lamis patella
- Lane bone
- Lane bone-holding
- Lewin bone-holding
- Locke
- Lowman bone-holding
- Lowman-Gerster bone
- Lowman-Hoglund bone-holding
- Martin cartilage
- Martin meniscus
- Martin muscle
- Mastin muscle
- Matthew cross-leg
- Mayfield neurosurgical skull
- Mayo
- meniscus
- microvascular
- mosquito
- Moynihan towel
- muscle biopsy
- Parham-Martin
- patellar
- Pean
- Pemberton spur-crushing
- pin
- Poppen-Blalock carotid
- Price muscle biopsy
- Rayport muscle biopsy
- rod
- saddle
- Salibi carotid artery
- Schlein
- Schwartz temporary intracranial artery
- self-retaining
- Selverstone carotid artery
- single
- skull
- Slocum meniscal
- Smith bone
- spur-crushing
- Steinhauser bone

clamp *(cont.)*
swivel
Thompson carotid
three-point skull
towel
trochanter-holding
Ulrich bone-holding
vascular
Verbrugge
VSF (Vermont spinal fixator)
Walton cartilage
Walton meniscus
wire-fixation
Yasargil carotid
clam-shell brace
Clancy-Andrews reconstruction
Clancy cruciate ligament reconstruction
clang associations
Clark transfer technique
Clarke arch angle
Clarke column
clasp-knife response
class, pyranocarboxylic acid
classic amnesic spell
dissociative state
fugue state
classical abdominal migraine
classic Kaposi sarcoma
classic migraine headache
classic-type spongiform encephalopathy
classification (see also *fracture*)
AAOS acetabular abnormalities
acromioclavicular injury
Aitken epiphyseal fracture
Allman acromioclavicular injury
American Rheumatism Association
American Spinal Cord Injury Association
Anderson-D'Alonzo odontoid fracture
Anderson tibial pseudarthrosis
Antoni-A neurinoma
AO ankle fracture
AO-Danis-Weber ankle fracture

classification *(cont.)*
Arthritis Impact Measurement Scales
Bayne radial agenesis
Benson-Geschwind aphasia
Berndt-Harty talar lesion staging
Bleck metatarsus adductus
Boston Classification System
Boyd-Griffin trochanteric fracture
Brooker
Burwell-Charnley fracture reduction
Canale-Kelly talar neck fracture
Carnesale-Stewart-Barnes hip dislocation
Catterall
Cavanaugh-Rogers footprint
Cedell-Magnusson arthritis (on x-ray)
Colonna hip fracture
Copeland-Kavat metatarso-phalangeal dislocation
D'Antonio acetabular
Danis-Weber ankle fracture
Daseler-Anson plantaris muscle anatomy
Delbert hip fracture
Denis seat belt injury
Denis spinal injury
Dickhaut-DeLee discoid meniscus
Dyck-Lambert
Eckert-Davis peroneal tendon subluxation
Engel postoperative seizure
Essex-Lopresti calcaneal fracture
Evans intertrochanteric fracture
Ficat femoral head osteonecrosis
Ficat stage of avascular necrosis
Fielding-Magliato subtrochanteric fracture
Fränkel spinal cord injury
Freeman calcaneal fracture
Fries score for rheumatoid arthritis
Frykman hand fracture
Frykman radial fracture

classification *(cont.)*
- Frykman wrist fracture
- Garden femoral neck fracture
- Gartland supracondylar fracture
- Gertzbein seat belt injury
- Grantham femur fracture
- Greenfield (spinocerebellar ataxia)
- Gumley seat belt injury
- Gustilo-Anderson tibial plafond fracture
- Gustilo puncture wound
- Gustilo tibial fracture
- Hahn-Steinthal capitellum fracture
- Hansen fracture
- Hardy-Clapham sesamoid
- Hawkins talar neck fracture
- Herbert-Fisher fracture system
- Herbert scaphoid bone fracture
- Hohl tibial condylar fracture
- Holdsworth spinal fracture
- Holdsworth spinal injury
- Hughston Clinic injury
- Hunt-Hess aneurysm
- Hunt-Hess neurological
- Hunt-Kosnik aneurysm
- Hunt-Kosnik nuchal stiffness
- Ingram-Bachynski hip fracture
- International OCu tetraplegia
- Jahss ankle dislocation
- Jahss metatarsophalangeal joint dislocation
- Jeffery radial fracture
- Johnson-Boseker scale
- Johnson-Jahss posterior tibial tendon tear
- Jones congenital tibial deficiency
- Jones diaphyseal fracture
- Kalamchi-Dawe congenital tibial deficiency
- Kelikian nail deformity
- Kernohan astrocytoma/glioblastoma
- Kernohan brain tumor
- Key-Conwell pelvic fracture
- Kilfoyle condylar fracture

classification *(cont.)*
- King classification of thoracic scoliosis
- Kistler subarachnoid hemorrhage
- Kocher-Lorenz capitellum fracture
- Kostuik-Errico spinal stability
- Kyle fracture
- Lauge-Hansen ankle fracture
- Leung thumb loss
- LSUMC motor and sensory function
- LSUMC nerve injury
- MacNichol-Voutsinas
- Mangled Extremity Severity Score (MESS)
- Mason radial fracture
- Mazur ankle evaluation
- McLain-Weinstein spinal tumor
- Medical Research Council (MRC) muscle function
- Merland perimedullary arterio-venous fistula
- Meyers-McKeever tibial fracture
- Milch elbow fracture
- Minaar coalition
- MRC muscle strength
- Mueller humerus fracture
- Neer femur fracture
- Neer-Horowitz humerus fracture
- Neer shoulder fracture (I, II, III)
- Nevaiser frozen shoulder
- New York diagnostic criteria
- Newman radial fracture
- Nurick spondylosis
- O'Brien radial fracture
- O'Rahilly limb deficiency
- Oden peroneal tendon subluxation
- Ogden epiphyseal fracture
- Ovadia-Beals tibial plafond fracture
- Paley complications
- Pauwels femoral neck fracture
- Pipkin femoral fracture
- Poland epiphyseal fracture
- Prosthetic Problem Inventory Scale
- Ratliff avascular necrosis

classification *(cont.)*
  Riordan club hand
  Riseborough-Radin intercondylar fracture
  Ritchie index
  Rockwood acromioclavicular injury
  Rome criteria
  Rosser Classification of Illness States
  Rowe calcaneal fracture
  Rowe-Lowell fracture-dislocation
  Ruedi-Allgower tibial plafond fracture
  Russell-Rubinstein cerebrovascular malformation
  Sage-Salvatore acromioclavicular joint injury
  Saha shoulder muscle
  Sakellarides calcaneal fracture
  Salter epiphyseal fracture
  Salter-Harris epiphyseal fracture
  Salter-Harris-Rang epiphyseal fracture
  Salter-Harris tibial-fibular injury
  Schatzker fracture
  Seddon nerve injury
  Seinsheimer femoral fracture
  Shelton femur fracture
  Smith sesamoid position
  Sorbie calcaneal fracture
  Steinbrocker rheumatoid arthritis
  Steinert epiphyseal fracture
  Steward-Milford fracture
  Sunderland nerve injury
  Sundt carotid ulceration
  talocalcaneal index
  Thompson-Epstein femoral fracture
  Tronzo intertrochanteric fracture
  Trunkey fracture
  Vostal radial fracture
  Wagner diabetic foot ulcer
  walking footprints
  Warren-Marshall
  Wassel thumb duplication

classification *(cont.)*
  Watanabe discoid meniscus
  Watson-Jones navicular fracture
  Watson-Jones spinal fracture
  Watson-Jones tibial fracture
  WHO (World Health Organization) astrocytoma
  Wiberg
  Wilkins radial fracture
  Winquist-Hansen femoral fracture
  Zickel fracture
  Zlotsky-Ballard acromioclavicular injury
Claude syndrome
claudication, neurogenic
clausa, rhinolalia
claustrum
clavicectomy
clavicle, condensing osteitis of
clavicotomy
clavicular head of sternocleidomastoid
clavipectoral fascia
clavus
  interdigital
  soft
clavus durus
clavus mollis
clawfoot deformity
  hollow foot
  pes arcuatus
  pes cavus
claw hand (main en griffe)
clawing of toes
clawtoe deformity
clay shoveler's fracture
Clayton forefoot arthroplasty
Clayton-Fowler technique
Clayton resection arthroplasty
CLBP (chronic low back pain)
CLCS (Comprehensive Level of Consciousness Scale)
clean wound
clear-cut cerebral dominance, lack of
Cleeman sign

cleft
  intergluteal
  interinnominoabdominal
  synaptic
  ventricular
clefting of meniscus
cleidocranial dysostosis
Cleland ligament in the hand
clenched fist attitude (of spastic hand)
clenched fist view
Cleveland bone-cutting forceps
Cleveland bone rongeur
Cleveland-Bosworth-Thompson
  technique
Cleveland rongeur
click, clicking
  hip
  Ortolani
click stimulus rate
Clifton Assessment Procedures for the
  Elderly (CAPE)
climbing up the legs (Gowers sign)
Clinical Dementia Rating (CDR) Scale
clinical EEG recording
Clinical Global Impression of Change
  (CGIC)
clinical seizure manifestation
Clinisert mattress
Clinitron air bed
clinodactyly
clinoid
clip (see also *clamp*)
  Acland
  Adson scalp
  aneurysm
  aneurysm window
  Biemer-Clip aneurysm
  brain
  Braun-Yasargil right-angle
  Children's Hospital scalp
  Codman aneurysm
  Cologne pattern scalp
  Drake aneurysm
  fenestrated Drake
clip *(cont.)*
  Heifitz
  hemostasis or hemostatic
  Housepan aneurysm
  Ingraham-Fowler tantalum
  Khodadad
  LeRoy-Raney scalp
  Ligaclip hemostatic
  ligating
  Mayfield aneurysm
  McFadden temporary aneurysm
  McKenzie brain
  McKenzie hemostasis
  McKenzie silver
  Michel
  Olivecrona aneurysm
  pin
  Raney hemostatic
  Raney scalp
  ring angled
  scalp
  Schwartz aneurysm
  silver
  skin
  sponge stopper
  Sugita aneurysm
  Sundt-Kees aneurysm window
  supracondylar medial
  surgical
  temporary vessel
  vari-angle aneurysm
  vessel
  Weck
  Yasargil vessel
clip applier (or applicator)
  Mayfield miniature
  Mayfield temporary aneurysm
clipping of aneurysm
clival region
clivus meningioma tumor
clivus tumor
clock, Deaf-Blind Alarm
Clodius dissector

clogs, Clogs
  Markell Mobility Health Clogs
  wooden postoperative
clonic movement
clonic phase spike and wave (on EEG)
clonic seizure
clonus
  ankle
  drawn ankle
  patellar
  persistent
  sustained ankle
  three-beat
  transient
  unsustained
closed circuit TV (CCTV)
closed disk-space infection
closed fracture
closed head injury
closed reduction and internal fixation
closed goggle-type eyeguards
closing abductor wedge osteotomy (CAWO)
closing base wedge osteotomy (CBWO)
closing pressure (on lumbar puncture)
closing wedge manipulation and reapplication of plaster
closing wedge osteotomy
Clostridium perfringens meningitis
Clostridium tetani (cause of tetanus)
closure (see also *suture*)
  delayed
  epiphyseal
  fascial
  incomplete
  myofascial
  partial
  physeal
  primary
  purse-string or pursestring
  secondary
  vein patch
closure tasks, sentence
clot
  blood
  evacuation of blood
  old blood
  subarachnoid
  subdural
clothespin graft
clouding of consciousness
Cloutier unconstrained knee prosthesis
cloverleaf Küntscher nail
Cloward anterior spinal fusion
Cloward blade retractor
Cloward bone graft impactor
Cloward brain retractor
Cloward cautery hook
Cloward cervical chisel
Cloward cervical retractor
Cloward cervical vertebrae spreader
Cloward-Cone ring curet
Cloward-Cushing vein retractor
Cloward depth gauge
Cloward disk rongeur
Cloward dowel cutter
Cloward dowel ejector
Cloward drill guide
Cloward drill tip
Cloward dural hook
Cloward dural retractor
Cloward elevator
Cloward-English laminectomy rongeur
Cloward hammer
Cloward-Harper laminectomy rongeur
Cloward-Hoen laminectomy retractor
Cloward intervertebral disk rongeur
Cloward lamina spreader
Cloward lumbar lamina retractor
Cloward nerve root retractor
Cloward osteophyte elevator
Cloward periosteal elevator
Cloward punch forceps
Cloward rongeur forceps
Cloward skin retractor
Cloward spinal fusion chisel
Cloward spinal fusion osteotome

Cloward tissue retractor
Cloward vertebrae spreader
clubbing of fingers and toes
clubfoot, clubfeet
clubfoot release
clubfoot splint, Denis Browne
clubhand deformity
clumsy gait
clumsy-hand dysarthria
clumsy-hand syndrome
cluneal nerve
cluster headache
Clyburn Colles fracture fixator
CMAP (compound motor action potential)
CMAP (compound muscle action potential)
CMC (carpometacarpal) fusion
CMD (cerebromacular degeneration)
CMF (chondromyxoid fibroma)
CMPS (chronic musculoskeletal pain syndrome)
CMRglu (regional cerebral glucose metabolism)
$CMRO_2$ (cerebral metabolic rate of oxygen consumption)
CMT (Charcot-Marie-Tooth) disease
CMV (cytomegalovirus) viral encephalitis
CMV meningitis
CMV myelopathy
CMW bone cement
CMW cement gun
CNAP (compound nerve action potential)
CNS (central nervous system)
CNS tumor
coagulase negative
coagulase positive
coagulator
  ASSI
  bipolar
  Concept bipolar
  Malis bipolar
coagulator *(cont.)*
  Malis CMC-II bipolar
  Polar-Mate
coalition
  bony
  calcaneonavicular
  carpal
  fibrous
  intercarpal
  lunate-triquetral
  Minaar classification of
  osseous
  talocalcaneal
  tarsal
coapt, coapted
coaptation, skin
coarse up-beat nystagmus
coating of aneurysm
Coballoy implant metal
Coballoy twist drill
cobalt-60 Gamma knife radiosurgical treatment
cobalt-chromium alloy
Coban elastic dressing
Cobb attachment for Albee-Compere fracture table
Cobb curet
Cobb elevator
Cobb gouge
Cobb method of measuring kyphosis
Cobb periosteal elevator
Cobb scoliosis angle
Cobb scoliosis measuring technique
Cobb spinal elevator
Cobb spinal gouge
Cobb syndrome
cobra retractor
Coccidioides immitis
coccidioidomycosis
coccygeal procedures
coccygeal spine (coccyx)
coccygectomy
coccygodynia
coccygotomy

coccyx (coccygeal spine)
cochlear nucleus
  dorsal
  ventral
cock-up deformity of toe
cock-up hand splint
Cockayne syndrome
cocking injury
Cocklin toe operation, modified
Co-Cr-Mo (cobalt-chromium-molybdenum) alloy implant metal
Co-Cr-W-Ni (cobalt-chromium-tungsten-nickel) alloy implant metal
codfish vertebrae
Codivilla tendon lengthening
Codman angle
Codman cranial blade
Codman curet
Codman drill
Codman exercises
Codman-Harper laminectomy rongeur
Codman-Kerrison laminectomy rongeur
Codman-Leksell laminectomy rongeur
Codman-Schlesinger laminectomy rongeur
Codman sign
Codman slit valve
Codman spinal curet
Codman surgical patties
  non-x-ray detectable
  x-ray detectable
Codman triangle, on x-ray
Codman tumor
Codman wire pass drill
Coe-pak paste
coefficient
  attenuation
  stiffness
coenesthesia
coenzyme Q
Cofield shoulder prosthesis
Cogan lid twitch sign
Cogan syndrome
cognition
cognitive deficit
cognitive dysfunction
Cognitive Failures Questionnaire (CFQ)
cognitive function, higher level
cogwheeling
cogwheel gait
cogwheel rigidity (in parkinsonism)
Cohen periosteal elevator
Cohen rongeur
coherence, coherent
coil
  crossed
  endovascular
  Golay
  gradient
  Helmholtz
  platinum
  radiofrequency (RF)
  receiver
  RF (radiofrequency)
  saddle
  shim
  solenoid
colchicine
Colclough-Scheicher laminectomy rongeur
Cole fracture frame
Cole osteotomy
Coleman flatfoot technique
collagen fibrils within tendon
collagen matrix
collagen, microcrystalline
Collagraft bone graft matrix
collapse of vertebral body
collar
  calcar
  cervical
  Exo-static cervical
  foam
  Forrester-Brown
  implant
  Lewin

collar *(cont.)*
  Mayo Thomas
  Miami Acute Care (MAC) cervical
  Miami J cervical
  myocervical rigid
  Nec Loc cervical
  periosteal bone
  Philadelphia cervical
  Philadelphia rigid
  pillow
  Plastizote cervical
  rigid
  Schanz
  serpentine foam
  soft cervical
  Thomas rigid
collar bone
collar-button abscess
collateral blood flow
collateral circulation
collateral ligaments of hand
collateral sprouting of neuron
collateral sulcus
collateral vessels
collection, intratendinous fluid
collectomy, shortening
Colles fascia
Colles fracture
Colles ligament
Colles splint
collet screwdriver adapter
Collet-Sicard syndrome
collicular fracture of medial malleolus
colliculus (pl. colliculi)
Collier sign
collimation
collimator helmet
Collimator, Multileaf
Collimator plugging pattern
Collin amputating knife
Collins dynamometer
Collins law of survival after brain tumor
Collins rib shears
Collis broken femoral stem technique
Collis-Taylor retractor
Collis TDR instruments
Collison drill
Collison plate
Collison screw
collodion dressing
colloid cyst of the third ventricle
colloid cyst tumor
colloid oncotic pressure (COP)
colloidal gold test (of CSF)
Collostat
Colonna-Ralston ankle approach
Colonna shelf procedure
color agnosia
color desaturation on vision test
color-flow Doppler
color-flow duplex imaging
Colorado tick fever viral encephalitis
Colpac
Coltart fracture technique
column
  anterior gray (of spinal cord)
  Clarke
  contrast
  demyelination of posterior
  displacement of spinal
  intermediolateral spinal gray
  medial (of calcaneus)
  posterior
  posterior gray, of cord
  vertebral
column of dye
coma
  adrenocortical
  agrypnodal
  alcoholic
  alpha
  alpha frequency
  apoplectic
  beta
  deep
  depth of
  diabetic

coma *(cont.)*
  evolution of
  hepatic
  hyperosmolar nonketotic
  hypopituitary
  incipient
  irreversible
  Kussmaul
  metabolic
  myxedema
  nonketotic hyperglycemic
    hyperosmolar
  pentobarbital
  postanoxic
  psychogenic
  spindle
  theta
  uremic
coma dépassé
comatose
coma vigil
comb rhythm on EEG
combative, combativeness
combined-flexion phenomenon
Comfeel Ulcus occlusive dressing
Comforfoam splint
commands
  inability to follow
  responds to verbal
  verbal
  unable to follow simple
commemorative sign
comminuted fracture
comminuted intra-articular fracture
Commission for the Blind and
  Visually Handicapped (CBVH)
commissural myelorrhaphy
commissure
  anterior (AC)
  cerebral
  gray commissure of spinal cord
  posterior (PC)
  white commissure of spinal cord
commissurotomy
  callosal
  central
commode, bedside
common migraine headache
common peroneal nerve palsy
commotio cerebri
communicating hydrocephalus
communication, asyndetic
communication/cognition treatment
communis, extensor digitorum
community rehabilitation
Comolli sign
compacter, acetabular cement
compartment
  anterior
  deep posterior
  extensor
  extradural
  fifth
  first
  fourth
  infratentorial
  lateral
  medial
  patellofemoral
  posterior
  posterolateral
  posteromedial
  second
  sixth
  superficial posterior
  third
Compartmental II knee prosthesis
compartment lesion, posterior
compartment syndrome
Compass hinge
Compass stereotactic system
compensable accident
Compensation, Workers'
"compensationitis"
compensatory wedge
Compere fixation wire

Compere-Thompson arthrodesis
Comperm tubular elastic bandage
complement-fixation studies for herpes
simplex
complete Achilles tendon rupture
complete elective mutism
complete nerve lesion
complete phocomelia
complete ptosis of third nerve paresis
complete ulnar nerve palsy
completed stroke
complex
AIDS dementia (ADC)
ankle joint (AJC)
anterior communicating artery
aperiodic
arcuate
atypical spike-and-wave
bunion
bunion–hallux valgus
bunionette–hallux valgus–splay foot
complex
capsulolabral
discoligamentous
Edinger-Westphal
fabellofibular
foot–ankle
gastrocnemius–soleus
Ghon-Sachs
hallux valgus–metatarsus primus
varus
hindfoot joint
hippocampal–amygdala
K
ligamentous
Lyme disease
morphology
multiple spike
OEIS
parkinsonism-dementia (of Guam)
periodic
polyspike
polyspike-and-slow-wave
quasi-periodic

complex *(cont.)*
sesamoid
sharp wave
slow spike-and-wave
spike-and-dome
spike-and-wave
subluxation
superior olivary
symptom
syndesmotic ligament
tibiocalcaneal joint
triangular fibrocartilage
triphasic wave
vertebrobasilar
complex multistep task
complications, neurologic
complications of antibiotics
complications of antipsychotic and
phenothiazine drugs
complications of griseofulvin
complications of stroke
complications of surgery
complications of tumor
component (see also *prosthesis*)
acetabular
AML trial hip
Amstutz femoral
Aufranc-Turner femoral
Bechtol acetabular
Bombelli-Morscher femoral
cerclaged
Charnley narrow stem
Charnley standard stem
cobra-design femoral
DePuy trispiked acetabular
glenoid
hallucinatory
Harris-Galante acetabular
head-neck
humeral
internal rotary component of force
(in gait)
metal-backed acetabular
Neer II humeral

component (cont.)
  Press-Fit
  prosthesis
  straight stem femoral
  Tri-Con
  trial femoral
component trial
composite graft
compound fracture
compound skull fracture
comprehension deficit
Comprehensive Level of
  Consciousness Scale (CLCS)
compression
  brain stem
  cervical cord
  chiasmal
  extradural spinal cord
  interfragmental
  intermittent pneumatic (IPC)
  lower lumbar root
  lumbar root
  mean maximal
  median nerve
  multiplanar
  nerve
  nerve root
  orbital mass
  radicular
  spinal cord
compression apparatus
compression arthrodesis
compression flexion injury
compression fracture (burst)
compression fracture of atlas
compression-plus-torque theory of
  cervical injury
compression syndrome, root
compression test
  ulnar nerve
  vasopneumatic
compression wrap dressing
compressive centripetal wrapping
compressive hyperextension injury
compressive neuropathy
compromise, spinal cord
Compton clavicle pin
computer-assisted design (CAD)
computer-assisted EEG signal analysis
computerized cranial tomography
computerized signal analysis of EEG
Conaxial total ankle prosthesis
concave-convex surface of first
  metacarpal bone
concavity
concealed straight leg raising test
concentrate, inability to
concentration (vigilance)
concentration
  lack of
  poor
concentric muscle training
Concept bipolar coagulator
Concept cannulated screw
Concept hand-held cautery
Concept shaver
concepts, time/money/number
conceptual ability
Conceptual Series Completion mental
  status test
concha of cranium
Conco elastic bandage
concrete thought processes
concretion
concurrent
concussion amnesia
concussion of brain (grades 1-3)
concussion of spinal cord
condensing osteitis of clavicle
conditions, triggering
conduction
  ephaptic
  motor nerve
  saltatory nerve
conduction aphasia
conduction studies, nerve
conductive jelly or paste for EEG

conductor
  Adson
  Bailey
  Davis
conduits, detour
condylar hypoplasia
condyle
  femoral
  flare of
  lateral femoral
  medial femoral
  occipital
  tibial
condylectomy, DuVries phalangeal
condyle resection
condylocephalic nailing
condylotomy
C1-C7 cervical vertebrae
C_1-C_5 segments of internal carotid artery
cone and socket bone
cone arthrodesis
cone biopsy cannula
cone biopsy needle
Cone-Grant technique
Cone laminectomy retractor
Cone ring curet
Cone scalp retractor
Cone skull punch forceps
Cone skull traction tongs
Cone suction biopsy curet
Cone suction tube
Cone ventricular needle
Cone wire-twisting forceps
coned-down x-ray view
confabulation of speech
configuration, horizontal dipole
configuration of wave
configuration, winged
confluent, superior
Conform dressing
conforming splint
confrontation naming test
confuse, confused
confusion
  episodic
  nocturnal
  postictal
  right-left
confusional episode
confusional state
congenita
  myotonia
  pseudohypertrophic musculature in myotonia
congenital arteriosclerotic aneurysm
congenital bars
congenital double athetosis
congenital dysplasia of the hip (CDH)
congenital flatfoot
congenital hippocampal sclerosis
congenital Horner syndrome
congenital idiopathic nystagmus
congenital insensitivity to pain
congenital intercalary limb absence
congenital latent nystagmus
congenital laxity of ligament
congenital myopathy
congenital nystagmus
congenital rubella
congenital syringomyelia
congenital terminal limb absence
congenital toxoplasmosis, Sabin-Feldman dye test for
congenital vertical talus
congenitally short limb
congestion, flap
congruence of mood and affect
congruent reduction
congruity, joint
congruous cup-shaped reamer
conical-point wire
conjugate deviation of the eyes
conjugate eye movements
conjugate fixed gaze
conjugate gaze
conjugate-horizontal gaze deviation
conjugate overshooting

conjugately, swing
Conley pin
connection
  corticocerebellar
  dendritic
  dentatorubrothalamic
  rostral
connective tissue disease
conoid ligament
Conrad-Bugg trapping of soft tissue in ankle fracture
Conray contrast medium
conscious, fully
consciousness
  change in level of
  clouding of
  crude
  declining
  depression of
  discrimination
  episodic changes of
  impaired
  impairment of
  level of
  loss of
  state of
conscious state, parasomniac
consensual constriction
consensual gaze
consensual light reflex
consensual pupillary response
conservative management
consolidation
constant touch perception
continuous performance test
constitution, migrainous
constitutional white finger (primary Raynaud phenomenon)
constriction
  absent consensual
  consensual
  direct (eyes)
  hourglass
  pupillary
constriction band syndrome
construct validity of rehabilitation testing
constructional ability
constructional apraxia
constructional impairment
constructional praxis
consumptive anoxia
contact, electrode
contaminated wound
content
  bone mineral (BMC)
  brain water (on MRI scan)
content validity of rehabilitation testing
contiguous articular surfaces
contiguous supramarginal gyrus
continua, epilepsia partialis
continuing absence seizure
continuing petit mal seizure
continuity
continuous passive motion (CPM) device
continuous performance test
continuous wave Doppler study
Continuum knee system (CKS)
contour, Wiberg type II patellar
Contour DF-80 total hip replacement
Contour internal prosthesis
Contour scalp retractor
contoured waveform
contract enhancement
contractile fibers
contraction
  agonist-antagonist
  nonepileptic myoclonic
  Rossolimo
  synergistic
contractor
  Bailey-Gibbon rib
  Bailey rib
  Lemmon rib
  rib
  Sellors rib
contracture
  Dupuytren
  elbow

contracture *(cont.)*
  fixed flexion
  flexion-adduction
  gastroc/soleus (gastrocnemius/ soleus)
  hip
  hip flexion
  ischemic
  joint
  knee
  knee flexion
  muscle
  myostatic
  postpoliomyelitic muscle
  scar
  secondary
  Skoog release of Dupuytren
  soft tissue
  Volkmann ischemic
  web
contralateral facial paralysis
contralateral foot
contralateral hemiparalysis
contralateral hemiplegia
contralateral homonymous inferior quadrantanopsia
contralateral homonymous superior quadrantanopsia
contralateral loss
contralateral sign
contrast arteriography
contrast baths (hot and cold)
contrast column
contrast enhancement
contrast medium (pl. media)
  Amipaque
  Angiovist 282
  Angiovist 292
  Angiovist 370
  Conray
  diatrizoate meglumine
  diatrizoate sodium
  Ethodian (iophendylate)
  Hexabrix

contrast medium *(cont.)*
  Hypaque-76
  iohexol
  iopamidol
  iothalamate meglumine
  ioversol
  ioxaglate meglumine
  ioxaglate sodium
  Isovue-200, Isovue-300, Isovue-370
  Isovue-M 200, Isovue-M 300
  Magnevist
  MD-60
  metrizamide
  Neurolite
  Neurotrast
  OctreoScan (indium-111 pentetreotide)
  Omnipaque
  Optiray 320
  radiopaque
  Renografin-60
  Reno-M-Dip
contrast myelography
contrecoup injury
control
  Dupaco knee
  exsanguination tourniquet
  image
  swing phase
controls
  car hand
  static reflex
  stato-kinetic reflex
contusio cerebri
contusion
  brain
  cerebral
  contrecoup
  frontal lobe
  hip
  occipital lobe
  parietal lobe
  pontine
  soft tissue

contusion *(cont.)*
  spinal cord
  temporal pole
contusion of brain or spinal cord
conus medullaris lesion
convergence
  ocular
  visual axis point of
convergence deficit
convergence of eyes
convergence paralysis
convergence-retraction nystagmus
convergence spasm
Converse chisel
Converse periosteal elevator
conversion, CAT-CAM
conversion reaction, hysterical
conversion symptom
Convery polyarticular disability index
convex
convexity, frontocentral
convexobasia
convoluted
convolution
  Broca
  cerebral
  Heschl
  occipitotemporal
  Zuckerkandl
convolutional
convulsant
convulsion
convulsion (see also *epilepsy*; *seizure*)
  central
  clonic
  coordinate
  epileptiform
  essential
  febrile
  generalized tonic/clonic (GTC)
  hysterical
  local
  mimetic
  mimic

convulsion *(cont.)*
  paroxysmal
  puerperal
  salaam
  spontaneous
  tetanic
  tonic/clonic
  uremic
convulsive disorder
Cook walking brace
cookie (pad)
  arch
  Gelfoam
  navicular shoe
  scaphoid shoe
  shoe
cookie cutter
Cooley-Baumgarten wire twisters
Cooley rib retractor
Cooley rib shears
Coonrad hinge prosthesis
Coonse-Adams technique
Coopernail sign
Coopervision irrigation/aspiration handpiece
coordination
COP (colloid oncotic pressure)
Copeland-Howard shoulder procedure
Copeland-Kavat classification of metatarsophalangeal dislocation
copolymer ankle-foot orthosis
copper wire effect
coprolalia
copropraxia
coracoacromial arch of scapula
coracoacromial ligament
coracoacromial process
coracoclavicular fixation device
coracohumeral ligament
coracoid process
coracoid tip avulsion
Corbett bone rongeur
cord
  anterior horns of spinal
  anterolateral white matter of

cord *(cont.)*
  cervical spinal
  cervical spondylosis of spinal
  compression of spinal
  encroachment on spinal
  fasciculi of
  heel cord advancement
  intramedullary spinal
  Lissauer tracts of spinal
  lumbar spinal
  neoplasm of spinal
  oblique elbow
  pretendinous
  rostral spinal
  sacral spinal
  severely compromised spinal
  spinal
  substantia gelatinosa of spinal
  tethered
  thoracic spinal
  tight heel
  Weitbrecht
cord compression
cord damage
  neoplastic
  traumatic
  vascular
cord embarrassment
Cordis implantable drug reservoir
Cordis multipurpose access port (MPAP)
Cordis Orbis Sigma shunt valve
cordlike structure
cordotomy, percutaneous
cord portion
corduroy cloth pattern on myelogram
core, bone
corencephalopathy
corkscrew dural hook
corkscrew esophagus (diffuse esophageal spasm)
corn
  apical
  end

corn *(cont.)*
  hard
  neurovascular
  plantar
  soft
  web
corneal reflex
corneal response
Cornelia de Lange syndrome
Cornell Scale for Depression, Dementia (CSDD)
corner of knee
corn-picker's pupil
corn removal plaster
corona radiata, in brain
coronal computed tomographic arthrography (CCTA)
coronal craniectomy
coronal orientation
coronal plane
coronal scalp incision
coronal suture
coronal synostosis
coronoid process
corpectomy
  anterior
  cervical
  subtotal
corporal agnosia (somatagnosia)
corpus, anterior
corpus callosum
  agenesis of
  central bands of
  splenium of
corpus callosum tumors
corpus Luysii (subthalamic nucleus in brain)
corpus striatum
corpuscle, Meissner
correction
  degree of
  subluxation
  V-Y plasty correction of varus toe
correction of scoliosis, Dwyer

corrective shoe
correlates, neuroanatomic
corset
  Camp
  elastic ankle
  Kampe
  leather ankle
  lumbosacral
cortectomy, parietal
cortex (pl. cortices)
  articular
  association, of parietal lobes
  bilateral orbital frontal
  calcarine
  cerebellar
  cerebral
  entorhinal
  excitomotor
  femoral
  homotypical
  insular
  limbic
  mesial-frontal
  motor
  nonolfactory
  opercular
  orbitofrontal
  parastriate
  parietal
  perirolandic parietal
  peristriate
  perisylvian
  postsensory
  premotor
  primary auditory
  primary visual
  pyriform
  rolandic
  sensorimotor
  striate
  visual
cortical atrophy
cortical blindness, total
cortical bone
cortical bone screw
cortical branch of middle cerebral
  artery
cortical cancellous bone
cortical cerebellar degeneration
cortical deafness
cortical deficit
cortical desmoid
cortical disease, advanced
cortical dysfunction, posttraumatic
cortical evoked potential
cortical function
cortical functioning, higher
cortical hinge axis
cortical infarcts, multiple
cortical ischemia
cortical lesion
cortical mapping
cortical margin
cortical neuronal dysfunction
cortical sensory loss
cortical testing
cortical thumb position
cortical transient ischemia
cortical-type eye deviation
cortical versus cancellous bone
corticectomy
corticifugal pathway
corticobulbar fibers
corticobulbar pathway
corticobulbar tract
corticocancellous bone graft
corticocancellous bone strip
corticocancellous strut
corticocerebellar connection
corticogram
corticography
corticoreticular theory
corticospinal disease
corticospinal fibers
corticospinal motor pathway
corticospinal motor system dysfunction
corticospinal pathway lesion
corticospinal tract fiber

corticosteroids
corticotomy
  Ilizarov
  percutaneous
  proximal tibia
  subperiosteal
Cor-Tech guidance to stereotactic head frame
Corti organ
Coryllos-Doyen periosteal elevator
Coryllos rasp
Coryllos rib shears
Cosman ICP Tele-Sensor
Cosman-Roberts-Wells (CRW) arc
Cosman-Roberts-Wells (CRW) stereotactic head frame
cosmesis
  poor
  subjective
cosmetically acceptable foot
cosmetically and functionally normal
Cosmolon closure for splint
costectomy
Costen syndrome
costocervical artery
costocervical trunk
costochondral junction of ribs
costochondral junction separation
costochondritis
costoclavicular maneuver
costoclavicular syndrome
costosternal angle
costotransversectomy technique
costovertebral angle (CVA) tenderness
costovertebral articulation
Cotrel cast
Cotrel-Dubousset derotation operation
Cotrel-Dubousset hook-rod
Cotrel-Dubousset spinal instrument
Cotrel scoliosis
Cotrel traction
Cottle chisel
Cottle-MacKenty elevator
Cottle-MacKenty rasp
Cottle mallet
Cottle osteotome
Cottle rasp
Cottle saw
Cotton ankle fracture
Cotton ankle instability test
Cotton Loader position cast
cotton (or cottonoid) patty (or pattie)
  moist
  saline-soaked
CO_2 laser (carbon dioxide)
cotyloid cavity
couch, neurosurgical
Couch-Derosa-Throop transfer technique
cough fracture of a rib
cough headache
count, white blood cell
counter
  extended medial shoe
  Geiger
  heel
Counter Rotation System (CRS)
counterbore, cloverleaf
countermovement
countersink, Synthes minifragment
countersunk
countertraction
counterweight
counting chamber, Fuchs-Rosenthal (for CSF cells)
counting-money tremor
Cournand-Grino arteriogram needle
course
  relapsing
  remitting
course of artery
course of nerve
Coventry femoral osteotomy
Coventry staple
cover
  Accu-Flo polyethylene bur hole
  Accu-Flo silicone rubber bur hole
  pedicle

Coverlet adhesive
Cover-Roll adhesive gauze
Cowdry type A intranuclear inclusion bodies in herpes simplex
Cowdry-type intranuclear inclusion body
COWS (cold opposite, warm same) caloric testing for vestibular function
coxa adducta
coxa brevis
coxa magna
coxa plana
coxa saltans
coxa senilis
coxa valga
coxa vara
coxa vara deformity
coxa vara luxans
coxarthria
coxarthritis
coxarthropathy
coxarthrosis
coxitis
Coxsackie A viral encephalitis
Coxsackie B viral encephalitis
Cozen-Brockway Z-plasty
Cozen test
CP (cerebral palsy)
CPAP, nasal (continuous positive airway pressure)
CP electrode (centroparietal) (CP_1-CP_6, CP_z)
CPM (continuous passive motion) device
CPM device for wrist, JACE W550
CPM exerciser machine
CPP (cranial perfusion pressure)
CPS (central pain syndrome)
CPS (complex partial seizure)
CPT (congenital pseudarthrosis of tibia)
crab gait
crabmeat-like appearance
Cracchiolo forefoot arthroplasty
Cracchiolo-Sculco implant arthroplasty
cracked pot sound
cracking of joint
cradle
  CT scan (computed tomography)
  head
  heel
Crafoord thoracic scissors
Craig splint
Craig vertebral body biopsy instrument
Cram test
Cramer wire splint
cramp
  benign nocturnal
  calf
  heat
  leg
  muscle
  night
  noctural muscle
  nocturnal leg
  writer's
Crane mallet
Crane osteotome
Crane shoulder exercise
cranial anomaly
cranial arteritis
cranial drill set
  Hudson
  Mira Mark III
cranial nerve abnormalities
cranial nerve deficit
cranial nerve I (olfactory)
cranial nerve II (optic)
cranial nerve III (oculomotor)
cranial nerve IV (trochlear)
cranial nerve V (trigeminal)
cranial nerve VI (abducens)
cranial nerve VII (facial)
cranial nerve VIII (auditory)
cranial nerve IX (glossopharyngeal)
cranial nerve X (vagus)
cranial nerve XI (spinal accessory)
cranial nerve XII (hypoglossal)

cranial nerve involvement
cranial nerve palsy
cranial nerves II-XII intact
cranial neuralgia
cranial neuropathy
cranial rongeur
cranial suture
craniectomy
  bilateral
  coronal
  decompressive
  metopic
  retromastoid
  suboccipital
cranioblade
  Acra-Cut
  Codman
craniocerebral penetrating wound
craniocerebral trauma
craniocervical junction
craniofacial dysjunction fracture
craniofacial microsomia
craniofacial reconstruction
craniofacial region
craniofacial remodeling
craniofacial resection
craniometric landmark
cranio-orbital deformity
craniopharyngioma tumor
cranioplastic powder
cranioplasty
craniorachischisis
craniostomy, twist drill
craniosynostosis, primary
craniotome
  Anspach
  B5 Midas Rex
  Caspar
  Freiberg
  Hall neurosurgical
  Mira Mark V
  Smith air
craniotome blade
craniotomy
  CT-assisted stereotactic
    (or stereotaxic)
  emergency
  emergent
  frontal
  frontotemporal
  frontotemporoparietal
  osteoplastic
  parietal
  parieto-occipital
  posterior fossa
  pterional
  retromastoid
  stereotaxic or stereotactic
  subfrontal
  supratentorial
  temporal-occipital
  trephine
craniotomy defect
cranium bifidum occultum
cranium, vertex of
crash induction of anesthesia
Crawford-Adams acetabular cup
  arthroplasty
Crawford dural elevator
Crawford low lithotomy crutches
Crawford small parts dexterity test
Crawler, Maddacrawler
CRDs (complex repetitive discharges)
C-reactive protein (CRP)
creaking
  alar
  back
  distal medial
  flexion
  infragluteal
  metatarsal-phalangeal
  palmar
  PIP flexion
  popliteal
  popliteal flexion
  skin
  thenar

creaking *(cont.)*
  ulnar
  wrist
Creed dissector
C_z reference montage on EEG
Crego elevator
Crego femoral osteotomy
Crego hip reduction
Crego-McCarroll traction
Crego retractor
cremasteric reflex
crepe bandage
crepitation, patellofemoral
crepitus, bony
crepuscular state
crescent-shaped fibrocartilaginous disk
crescentic osteotomy
crescentic rupture
crest
  gyral
  iliac
  tibial
Creutzfeldt-Jakob disease
Creutzfeldt-Jakob syndrome
cribriform plate, meningioma of the
cribriform plate of ethmoid bone
"crick" in the neck
cricopharyngeal achalasia
Crile artery forceps
Crile dissector
Crile forceps
Crile gasserian ganglion knife and dissector
Crile head traction
Crile knife
Crile needle holder
Crile nerve hook and dissector
Crile-Wood needle holder
crimper, washer
C ring
crisis
  cholinergic
  myasthenic
  oculogyric

crisis *(cont.)*
  parkinsonian
  spondylolisthetic
  tabetic
crispation
crista galli
criteria
  Insall
  Mulholland and Gunn
criterion-related validity of rehabilitation testing
CRN (cerebral radiation necrosis)
crossed leg/straight leg raising test
cross-irrigation of wounds
cross ligament
cross-pin, tensioned
crossed coil
crossed sciatica sign
crossed signs
crossed straight leg raising
Crosslink, TSRH (Texas Scottish Rite Hospital)
cross-union
Crouzon syndrome
Crowe pilot point
crown
  Adaptic
  halo
  Unitek steel
CRP (C-reactive protein)
CRS (Counter Rotation System)
CRS brace
cruciate fashion
cruciate ligament of fingers
cruciform screwdriver
crude consciousness
crural ataxia
crural fascia
crural monoplegia
crural paresis
cruris, fascia
crus (leg), crura (pl.)
crus phenomenon
crush injury

crushing osteochondritis
crutch walking, nonweightbearing
crutches
  Canadian
  Crawford low lithotomy
  Lofstrand
  platform
  weightbearing
Crutchfield carotid artery clamp
Crutchfield drill point
Crutchfield hand drill
Crutchfield-Raney skull traction tongs
Cruz trypanosomiasis
CRW (Cosman-Roberts-Wells) stereotactic head frame
crying, pathologic laughing and
Cryo/Cuff ankle dressing
Cryocup ice massager
cryohypophysectomy, transsphenoidal
cryolesion, brain
cryomagnet
cryostat
cryotherapy and compression
cryotherapy, liquid nitrogen
cryptococcal meningitis
Cryptococcus neoformans
cryptogenic drop attack
cryptotic medial border
crystal-induced arthroses
crystal-related arthropathy
crystal-related joint disease
crystalloid
crystals
  birefringent lipid
  oxalate
  sodium urate
  urate
  uric acid
CSC3 cervical support cushion
CSF (see *cerebrospinal fluid*)
CSF absorption and production
CSF cytologic study
CSF dissemination
CSF-induced peritonitis (via catheter)
CSF leak (otorrhea or rhinorrhea)
CSF pathway
CSF pleocytosis
CSF serology for lues
CSI (Caregiver Strain Index)
CSL (central sacral line)
CSM (cervical spondylotic myelopathy)
C-spine (cervical spine)
CSR (complete subtalar release) operation
CSSEP (cortical somatosensory evoked potential)
CST (corticospinal tract)
CSTi (cancellous-structured titanium)
CT (computed tomography) scan; scanning
CT-guided stereotactic surgery
CT reconstruction image of skull
CT scan with contrast
CT, thin-section
CTD (cumulative trauma disorder)
ctenoid spike on EEG (silent *c*)
CTi or C.Ti. brace
CTi2 knee brace
CTLSO (cervicothoracolumbosacral orthosis)
CTLV (cross-table lateral view) (x-ray)
CTM (cervical tension myositis)
CTR (carpal tunnel release)
CTS (carpal tunnel syndrome)
CTS (Champion Trauma Score)
CTT (central tegmental tract)
C-2 OsteoCap hip prosthesis
Cubbins screw
Cubbins shoulder dislocation technique
cubist disorder of visual perception in migraine
cubital fossa
cubital tunnel syndrome
cubitocarpal
cubitoradial
cubitus valgus
cubitus varus

cuboid squeeze technique
cuboid whip technique
cubonavicular joint
cucullaris muscle
cue, cueing (or cuing)
cuff
  arm
  musculotendinous
  pneumatic tourniquet
  rotator
  thigh
cuff of fascia
cuff of tissue
cul-de-sac, dural
Culler hook
Culley splint
cultures, fungal, on Sabouraud medium (in meningitis)
cumulative trauma disorder (CTD)
cuneatus, fasciculus
cuneiform fracture-dislocation
cuneiform joint
cuneiform mortise
cuneiform osteotomy
cuneus
cup (see also *prosthesis*)
  acetabular
  Arthopor
  Aufranc-Turner acetabular
  Aufranc-Turner hip
  Biomet acetabular
  bipolar acetabular
  bipolar prosthetic
  Buchholz acetabular
  ceramic acetabular
  Charnley acetabular
  Crawford-Adams acetabular
  custom-made acetabular
  DePuy bipolar
  Hallister heel
  Harris-Galante acetabular
  heel
  Integrity acetabular
  Laing concentric hip

cup *(cont.)*
  low-profile
  Luck hip
  Mueller-type
  McKee-Farrar acetabular
  metal-backed acetabular
  migration of acetabular
  New England Baptist acetabular
  oblong polyethylene acetabular
  Opti-Fix II acetabular
  Osteonics acetabular
  plastic heel
  Press-Fit
  prosthesis
  retroversion of acetabular
  Smith-Petersen
  Sorbuthane II heel
  SROM acetabular
  SROM super
  trial acetabular
  Tuli heel
cup arthroplasty
cup on cup arthroplasty of the hip
CUP (cancer of unknown primary)
Curdy blade
curet, curette
  Acufex
  angle-tipped
  angled Scoville
  bone
  bowl
  box
  Bruns bone
  Buck bone
  cement
  Charnley bone
  Cloward-Cone
  Cobb
  Codman spinal
  Cone ring
  Cone suction biopsy
  cup
  cupped
  curved

curet *(cont.)*
- Daubenspeck
- Dawson-Yuhl-Cone
- Epstein
- Faulkner
- fine
- fine-angled
- 45-degree
- forward-angled
- Halle bone
- Hardy hypophysial
- Hatfield
- hex handle
- Hibbs spinal
- Hibbs-Spratt spinal fusion
- horizontal ring
- Howard spinal
- hypophysial
- Innomed bone
- Jansen bone
- Kerpel bone
- Kerrison
- Kevorkian
- Lempert bone
- long
- loop
- Malis
- Marino transsphenoidal
- Martini bone
- mastoid
- Mayfield spinal
- McCain TMJ
- McElroy
- Meyhoeffer bone
- micro
- Moe bone
- oval curved cup
- pituitary
- Raney stirrup-loop
- Ray pituitary
- reverse-angled
- Rhoton loop
- Rhoton micro
- Rhoton pituitary

curet *(cont.)*
- Rhoton spoon
- Richards
- ring
- ruptured disk
- Schede bone
- Scoville ruptured disk
- Semmes spinal fusion
- short
- Simon
- spinal fusion
- spoon
- Spratt bone
- Spratt mastoid
- stirrup-loop
- T-handle
- transsphenoidal
- vertical ring
- Volkmann bone
- Walker ruptured disk
- Williger bone
- Yasargil micro

curettage
curetted (verb)
curettement
curettings
curls, towel (postoperative exercises)
current
- alternating
- direct
- pulsing

Curry hip nail
Curschmann-Steinert disease
curse, Ondine
cursiva, epilepsia (running seizures)
curtain pulled across visual field
Curtin plantar fibromatosis excision
Curtis-Fisher knee technique
Curtis PIP joint capsulotomy
curtsying pupil
curvature
- dorsal kyphotic
- humpbacked spinal
- kyphotic
- radius of

curve
  cervical spine
  fatigue
  flattening of normal cervical
  flattening of normal lumbar
  flattening of normal thoracic
  lumbar lordotic
  normal lordotic
  standardized growth
  superincumbent spinal
  thoracic spine
curvilinear distortion on EEG
curvilinear incision
CUSA (Cavitron ultrasonic aspirator)
CUSALap ultrasonic accessory for fragmentation, irrigation, and aspiration
Cushing basophilism
Cushing bipolar forceps
Cushing brain depressor
Cushing brain retractor
Cushing brain spatula spoons
Cushing bur
Cushing cranial bur
Cushing cranial perforator
Cushing cranial rongeur
Cushing decompression retractor
Cushing disk rongeur
Cushing dressing forceps
Cushing dural hook knife
Cushing elevator
Cushing flat drill
Cushing gasserian ganglion hook
Cushing-Gigli saw guide
Cushing-Hopkins periosteal elevator
Cushing intervertebral disk rongeur
Cushing-Landolt transsphenoidal speculum
Cushing Little Joker elevator
Cushing monopolar forceps
Cushing nerve hook
Cushing nerve retractor
Cushing perforator drill
Cushing periosteal elevator
Cushing pituitary elevator
Cushing pituitary scoop
Cushing pituitary spoon
Cushing response
Cushing retractor
Cushing rongeur forceps
Cushing saw guide
Cushing spatula spoon
Cushing staphylorrhaphy elevator
Cushing syndrome
Cushing tissue forceps
Cushing vein retractor
Cushing ventricular needle
cushion
  abduction
  Anti-Shox foot
  Back-Huggar lumbar support
  Carter immobilization
  cervical
  CSC3 cervical support
  Dry Flotation wheelchair
  FB cast
  foam
  foot
  immobilization
  Isch-Dish Plus
  lumbar
  lumbar support
  Posture Curve lumbar
  pressure
  pressure-relief
  Roho
  Sat-A-Lite seat
  Satalite cushion by Bodyline
  Sorbuthane heel
  Viscoheel K heel
  Viscoheel N
  Viscoheel SofSpot heel
  wheelchair
cut
  CT (cut or slice)
  homonymous field
  tomographic
  visual field

cutaneous adenoma
cutaneous angioma
cutaneous icing
cutoff, nerve root
cutter
  A-P
  bolt
  bone plug
  cast
  Cloward dowel
  cookie
  cushion-throat wire
  diamond wire
  dowel
  end
  femoral
  Howmedica Microfixation System plate
  Kalish Duredge wire
  Kirschner wire
  Kleinert-Kutz bone
  Leibinger Micro System plate
  Luhr Microfixation System plate
  Martin diamond wire
  meniscal
  milling
  motorized meniscus
  multiple action
  pin
  Rochester harvest bone
  Rochester recipient bone
  side
  Storz Microsystems plate
  Synthes Microsystem plate
  wire
  Wister wire/pin
Cutter cast
cutter guide
cutting jig for chevron osteotomy
cutting probe
cutting, water jet
CUWD (cold up, warm down) test
CVA (cerebrovascular accident) (stroke)
CVA (costovertebral angle)
CVM (cryptic vascular malformation)
C washer
C wave form on ICP monitor
C wave of cerebrospinal fluid
C wire inserter
cyanoacrylate (Superglue) adhesive
cyberphysiology
Cybex 340 isokinetic rehabilitation and testing system
Cybex back rehabilitation equipment
Cybex I (and II+) exercise system
Cybex II dynamometer
Cybex II (and II+) isokinetic exerciser
Cybex machine
Cybex test
Cybex Torso Rotation Testing and Rehabilitation Unit
Cybex Trunk Extension Flexion unit
cycle
  circannual
  disordered sleep
  gait
  phase shift of sleep-wake
  sleep
  sleep-wake
  sleep-wakefulness
  sleep-waking
  walking
cycles per second (c/sec)
cyclothymia
cyclothymic disorder
cyclotron
  helium
  proton
cyst
  aneurysmal bone
  arachnoid watery
  Baker
  bone
  brain
  central nervous system
  cerebral hydatid
  colloid cyst of the third ventricle

cyst *(cont.)*
  Dandy-Walker
  dermoid cyst of brain
  epidermoid cyst of brain
  foramen magnum
  ganglion
  glial
  inclusion
  interhemispheric
  intracranial
  intramedullary epidermoid
  intraneural ganglion
  intrasellar Rathke cleft
  meniscal
  mucous
  paraphyseal
  paraventricular
  pilonidal
  popliteal
  porencephalic
  Rathke cleft (RCC)
  rheumatoid
  sacral
  scalp inclusion
  subarticular
  subchondral bone
  suprasellar arachnoid
  suprasellar Rathke cleft
  synovial
  traumatic
  unicameral bone
  unifocal
  xanthomatous Rathke cleft
cystathioninuria
cystic brain tumor
cystic changes (in arthritis)
cystic hydroma
cystic hygroma (preferred)
cystic lysis of bone
cystic sac
cystic tumor
cystic wall
cysticercosis
  cerebral
  parenchymal brain
cysticercosis cerebri
cysto-atrial shunt
cyst wall
cytoarchitectonic abnormality
cytoarchitectonic field, Brodmann
cytokeratin immunostain
cytokeratin, low molecular weight
cytokeratins antibody
cytology, spinal fluid
cytomegalic inclusion disease
cytomegalovirus (CMV) viral
  encephalitis
cytoplasm, scanty
cytotoxic leukocyte test
Czerny suture

D, d

D.A.C.O. brace
Dacron graft
Dacron-impregnated silicone rod
Dacron suture
dacryocystic epilepsy
dactylitis, blistering distal (BDD)
DAF (dynamic axial fixator)
Dahlgren cranial rongeur
Dakin tubing
Dale abdominal binder
Dale first rib rongeur
Dall-Miles cable cerclage
Dall-Miles cable grip system
daltons of force (SI units)
DALYs (Disability Adjusted Life Years)
dam, rubber
damage
- anoxic
- brain
- cerebral
- epileptogenic cerebral
- focal
- hemisphere
- mesial frontal lobe
- myelin
- neoplastic cord
- physeal
- traumatic cord
- vascular cord

D'Ambrosia test
D'Antonio classification of acetabular abnormalities
dammed-up CSF
DANA shoulder prosthesis
dance, St. Vitus
dancing bear gait
dancing bear syndrome
dancing eyes (opsoclonus, or opsoclonia)
dancing-eyes dancing-feet syndrome
dancing mania (choreomania)
Dandy clamp
Dandy myocutaneous scalp flap
Dandy nerve hook
Dandy neurosurgical scissors
Dandy probe
Dandy scalp hemostatic forceps
Dandy trigeminal nerve scissors
Dandy ventricular needle
Dandy-Walker cyst
Dandy-Walker deformity
Dandy-Walker syndrome
Daniel iliac bone graft
Danis-Weber classification of ankle fractures
Danniflex CPM exerciser
Darco foot splint
Darco medical-surgical shoe and toe alignment splint
Darco moldable insole
Darco surgical shoe
Darier disease
Darkschewitsch, nucleus of (Darkshevich, Darkschevich)
Darrach-Hughston-Milch fracture
Darrach-McLaughlin shoulder technique
Darrach procedure
dart and dome EEG complexes

DAS (double-armed suture)
DASA (distal articular set angle)
Dasco Pro angle finder
Daseler-Anson classification of plantaris muscle anatomy
Das Gupta scapulectomy
Daubenspeck bone curet
Dautrey chisel
Dautrey osteotome
Davey-Rorabeck-Fowler decompression technique
Davidson-Sauerbruch-Doyen periosteal elevator
Davis brain retractor
Davis brain spatula
Davis coagulating forceps
Davis conductor
Davis dural dissector
Davis dural separator
Davis monopolar forceps
Davis muscle-pedicle graft
Davis nerve separator-spatula
Davis percussion hammer
Davis rib spreader
Davis saw guide
Davis scalp retractor
Davol drain
Dawbarn sign
Dawson encephalitis
Dawson inclusion body encephalitis
Dawson-Yuhl-Cone curet
Dawson-Yuhl gouge
Dawson-Yuhl impactor
Dawson-Yuhl-Kerrison rongeur forceps
Dawson-Yuhl-Key elevator
Dawson-Yuhl-Leksell rongeur forceps
Dawson-Yuhl osteotome
Dawson-Yuhl periosteal elevator
Dawson-Yuhl rongeur forceps
Dawson-Yuhl suction tube
Day fixation device
Day fixation pin
Day fixation staple
daze, patient in a
dazed patient
DB (Denis Browne) bar
DBM (demineralized bone matrix)
D.C. (doctor of chiropractic)
DC (dynamic compression) plate
DC-101 chiropractic table
DC-EEG (direct current electroencephalogram)
DCP (dynamic compression plate)
DCS (dorsal column stimulator)
DDH (developmental dysplasia of hip)
deaf, Deaf
  National Association for the
  National Technical Institute for the (NTID)
  Registry of Interpreters for the (RID)
  TeleCaption TV decoders for the
  telecommunication device for the (TDD)
Deaf-Blind Alarm Clock
deaf-blindness
deafferentation pain
deafness
  cortical
  midbrain
  pure word
de Andrade-MacNab occipitocervical arthrodesis
Dean bone rongeur
Dean scissors
Deane unconstrained knee prosthesis
death
  brain
  cerebral
  cerebral brain
  suspected cerebral
Deaver retractor
DeBakey endarterectomy scissors
DeBakey forceps
DeBakey rib spreader
DeBastiani distractor
DeBastiani external fixator
DeBastiani frame
Debeyre-Patte-Elmelik rotator cuff technique

Debré-Sémélaigne pseudomyotonia
debride
debridement
  Ahern trochanteric
  arthroscopic
  cortical
  hemidiaphyseal
  Magnuson
debris
  bone
  extra-articular
  intra-articular
  joint
  particulate
debulk
debulking of tumor
deburring
Decadron rash
decalcification
decalcified dorsum sellae
decancellation procedure
decarboxylase inhibitor
decarboxylation of levodopa
decerebrate attack
decerebrate posturing
decerebrate rigidity
decerebration, furious
dechondrification
deciduous
Decker alligator forceps
Decker alligator scissors
Decker microsurgical forceps
Decker microsurgical rongeurs
Decker microsurgical scissors
deckplate
decompression
  canal
  laser-assisted disk (LDD)
  microvascular (MVD)
  peripheral nerve
  suction
  surgical
decompression fasciotomy
decompression of tumor
decompression sickness (caisson disease; the bends)
decompression technique
decompressive craniectomy
decompressive laminectomy
decompressive osteotomy
deconditioned foot
decorticate and decerebrate
decorticate posturing
decorticate rigidity
decortication
decreased tonus
Decubinex pad/protector
decubitus ulcer
decussation
Dee elbow hinge
DEEG (depth EEG, electro-encephalogram)
deep arch
deep blade knife
deep massage
deep-seated lesion
deep-seated tumor
deep-shelled acetabulum
deep tendon reflexes (DTRs)
  hyperactive
  hypoactive
deep transverse metacarpal ligament
deep transverse palmar ligament
deep venous incompetence
deep venous insufficiency (DVI)
deep venous occlusion
deep venous thrombosis (DVT)
defect
  afferent pupillary
  arcuate visual field
  bony
  bar-like ventral (in myelography)
  bridging of
  centrocecal visual field
  chiasmatic
  chondral
  cortical
  craniotomy
  developmental

defect *(cont.)*
  extradural
  field
  focal plaquelike
  fusiform
  hemianopic visual field
  homonymous
  intercalary
  mapping of the
  neural tube
  nonhomonymous field
  nonsubperiosteal cortical
  optic nerve
  osseous
  osteochondral
  parietal field
  partial homonymous field
  postoperative skull
  protrusio
  radial ray
  segmental bone
  soft tissue
  subcortical
  subperiosteal cortical
  temporal field
  trochlear
  visual field
defervesce, defervesced
defervescence
deficiency
  Aitken femoral
  aminoaciduria
  arginase
  factor VIII
  factor IX
  hemispheral gaze
  mental
  myopathic carnitine
  phosphorylase
  protein S
  sulfite oxidase
deficit
  attentional
  central language

deficit *(cont.)*
  cognitive
  comprehension
  convergence
  cortical
  cranial nerve
  emotional
  fixed neurologic
  focal neurologic
  Fränkel classification of spinal cord injury
  gaze
  global cognitive
  gross neurologic
  language
  lateralizing
  march of sensory
  motor
  neural
  neurologic(al)
  peripheral nerve function
  peripheral neural
  posterior column
  postictal
  radicular neural
  resolving (or reversible) ischemic neurologic (RIND)
  saddle distribution of sensory
  sensory
  space
  spinal cord injury
  spinal neural
  thalamic
deficits of ideation and speech in migraine
deflection of EEG pen
deformans
  dystonia musculorum
  Paget osteitis
deformers, active (in arthritis)
deformity
  angular
  Arnold-Chiari
  back-knee

deformity *(cont.)*
- bifid thumb
- bony
- boutonnière
- bowing
- bull's eye
- bunion
- bunionette
- buttonhole
- calcaneus
- cavovarus
- cavus
- Charcot
- checkrein
- clawfoot
- clawhand
- clawtoe
- clubhand
- cock-up
- cock-up toe
- codfish
- compensatory
- congenital vertical talus foot
- cranio-orbital
- cubitus varus
- curly toe
- Dandy-Walker
- digitus flexus
- dinner-fork
- DISI (dorsal intercalary segment instability)
- equinovalgus
- equinovarus
- equinovarus hindfoot
- equinus
- eversion-external rotation
- femoral head
- flatfoot
- flexible spastic equinovarus
- forefoot abduction
- genu valgum
- genu varum
- gibbous
- gun stock

deformity *(cont.)*
- Haglund
- hallux abductovalgus
- hallux valgus
- hammer toe
- hatchet-head
- Hill-Sachs
- hindbrain
- hindfoot
- hourglass
- internal rotation
- intrinsic minus
- intrinsic plus
- joint
- Kirner
- lobster-claw
- Madelung
- mallet
- mallet finger
- Michel
- neuropathic midfoot
- pannus
- pes cavus
- pes planus
- planovalgus
- planovalgus deformity
- plantar flexion-inversion
- procurvature
- pseudo-Hurler
- rockerbottom foot
- rotational
- round shoulder
- sabre shin
- shepherd's crook
- silver-fork
- spastic equinovarus
- spastic hindfoot valgus
- splay foot
- split foot
- Sprengel
- static foot
- step-down shoulder
- supination
- swan-neck

deformity *(cont.)*
- swan-neck finger
- thumb-in-palm
- triphalangeal thumb
- turned-up pulp
- ulnar drift (motor)
- valgus
- valgus heel
- varus
- Velpeau
- VISI
- wasp-tail (in Duchenne dystrophy)
- windblown
- windswept

Defourmentel bone rongeur

degeneration
- Alzheimer neurofibrillary
- articular cartilage
- ascending
- axon
- axonal
- cartilaginous
- cerebellar
- cerebromacular (CMD)
- cobblestone
- cortical cerebellar
- corticobasal ganglionic
- corticostriatospinal
- descending
- familial cerebellar
- ganglion cells
- Gombault
- granulovacular
- gray
- great toe degeneration, Regnauld-type
- hepatocerebral
- hepatolenticular
- heterogeneous system
- Holmes cerebellar
- Holmes cortical cerebellar
- lattice
- Menzel olivopontocerebellar
- muscle fiber

degeneration *(cont.)*
- neurofibrillary
- Nissl
- olivopontocerebellar
- pallidal
- paraneoplastic cerebellar
- parenchymatous cerebellar
- paving stone
- pigmentary degeneration of the globus pallidus
- Ramsey Hunt type of inherited dentatorubral
- rim
- spinocerebellar
- spongy white matter
- striatal nigral
- subacute combined spinal cord
- Türck
- Terrien
- transneuronal
- wallerian
- wear and tear

degenerative arthritic change
degenerative disk disease
degenerative joint disease (DJD)
degenerative spine disease
degenerative spondylosis
degenerative spur
degloving injury
deglutition paralysis
degradable polyglycolide rods
degree of correction
dehiscence, wound
Dehne three-finger spica cast
Deiter nucleus of cerebellum
déjà entendu (already heard)
déjà éprouvé (already tested)
déjà fait (already done)
déjà pensé (already thought)
déjà raconté (already told)
déjà vécu (already lived)
déjà voulu (already desired)
déjà vu (already seen)
dejection

Dejerine aberrant pyramidal tract
Dejerine anterior bulbar syndrome
Dejerine-Davis percussion hammer
Dejerine disease
Dejerine-Klumpke palsy
Dejerine-Klumpke paralysis
Dejerine percussion hammer
Dejerine-Roussy syndrome
Dejerine sign
Dejerine-Sottas atrophy
Dejerine-Sottas disease
Dejerine-Sottas syndrome
Deknatel autotransfusion system
Deknatel orthopedic autotransfusion system
De La Caffinière trapeziometacarpal prosthesis
de Lange syndrome
delay
  developmental
  reflex relaxation
delayed apoplexy
delayed bone imaging
delayed onset muscle soreness (DOMS)
delayed union
Delbet splint for heel fracture
deliberant-dizziness therapy
deliriant
delirifacient
delirious
delirium
  acute
  alcohol withdrawal
  exhaustion
  febrile
  low
  senile
  toxic
  traumatic
delirium tremens (DTs)
deliriumlike state
Delitala T nail
DeLorme exercises
delta activity on EEG
delta band on EEG
delta brush pattern on EEG
delta electrode
delta frequency band on EEG
delta index on EEG
delta occipital pattern
delta pattern on EEG
delta rhythm on EEG
delta slowing on EEG
delta wave EEG activity
delta waveform
deltoid branch of posterior tibial artery
deltoid insertion over joint
deltoid ligament of ankle
deltoid ligament of foot
deltoid ligament of shoulder
deltopectoral interval
delusion
delusional
demarcate, demarcated
demarcation, level of (in sensory testing)
DeMarneffe meniscotomy knife
DeMartel neurosurgical scissors
DeMartel scalp flap forceps
DeMartel wire saw
Demel wire-tightening forceps
Demel wire-twisting forceps
demented
dementia
  Alzheimer
  atrophic
  Binswanger
  dialysis
  early
  epileptic
  familial
  frontal lobe
  global
  lacunar
  multi-infarct
  paralytic
  Pick

dementia *(cont.)*
  presenile
  primary degenerative
  senile
  subcortical
  toxic
  vascular
  Wernicke
Dementia Behavior Disturbance (DBD) Scale
Dementia Mood Assessment Scale (DMAS)
dementia praecox
dementia pugilistica
Demianoff sign
demineralization, bony
demineralization from disuse
demineralized bone matrix (DBM)
demodulator
DeMuth screw
demyelinating disease
demyelinating neuropathy
demyelination
  brain stem
  large-fiber
  postinfectious
  segmental
demyelination of posterior columns
demyelinative disorder
denatured alcohol
dendrite
dendritic connections
dendritic spine
denervated muscle fiber
denervation
  autonomic
  distal
  level of
  proximal
  somatic
  sympathetic
  zone of
denervation of muscle
dengue viral encephalitis
Denham external fixation
Denham pin
denial
  organic
  psychiatric
Denis Browne bar
Denis Browne clubfoot splint
Denis Browne talipes hobble splint
Denis Browne neuropathy
Denis Browne syndrome
Denis classification of seat belt injury
Denis classification of spinal injury (A-E)
Dennyson-Fulford arthrodesis
de novo
dens fracture
dens (odontoid) x-ray view of cervical spine
dense sensory loss
densitometry
  bone
  dual-photon
  photon
density
  bone mineral (BMD)
  periventricular
  spicular (on x-ray)
dental freer elevator
dentata
dentate fracture
dentate ligament
dentate nucleus of cerebellum
dentate suture of skull
dentato-olivary pathway
dentatorubral degeneration
dentatorubropallidoluysian atrophy
dentatorubrothalamic connections in upper brain stem
dentatothalamic
dentatum
denticulatum, ligamentum
dentinogenesis imperfecta

denude, denuded
denudation
Denver Developmental Screening Test
Denver hydrocephalus shunt
Deon hip prosthesis
deossification
DePalma modified patellar technique
Department of Vocational
  Rehabilitation (DVR)
dependence
  economic
  emotional
  physical
depersonalization, transient states of
  (in migraine)
depigmentation of the iris with
  neonatal Horner syndrome
depigmented spots in tuberous
  sclerosis
depolarization, nerve fiber membrane
depolarization of neuronal membrane
depolarize
deposit, calcium
deposition, monosodium urate crystal
  (in gout)
depressed and compound skull
  fracture
depression
  endogenous
  exogenous
  postictal
  spinal cord
depression of fragment
depression of tendon reflexes with
  cervical disk disease
depressor, Cushing brain
deprivation, sleep
depth EEG (DEEG)
depth gauge
depth-sense esthesiometry
depths of wound
DePuy acetabular liner
DePuy AML Porocoat stem prosthesis
DePuy nerve hook
DePuy orthopedic implant
de Quervain disease
de Quervain fracture
de Quervain stenosing tenosynovitis
derangement, mental
Derby nail
dermabrader
Dermacentor andersoni
Dermacentor variabilis
dermal electrodes (for EEG)
dermatoarthritis
dermatofibrosarcoma protuberans
dermatomal area
dermatomal diagram of pain
dermatomal distribution of pain
dermatomal pain
dermatomal pattern
dermatomal rash
dermatome
  Brown
  Reese
  sacral
  sensory
  Stryker
dermatome sensory changes with
  cervical disk disease
dermatomyositis
  heliotrope rash of
  intertriginous
dermodesis, resection
dermoid cyst of brain
dermoid tumor
dermometer
derotate, derotated
derotation
D'Errico-Adson retractor
D'Errico bayonet pituitary forceps
D'Errico brain spatula
D'Errico elevator
D'Errico enlarging bur
D'Errico hypophyseal forceps
D'Errico lamina chisel
D'Errico nerve root retractor
D'Errico perforating drill

D'Errico periosteal elevator
D'Errico pituitary forceps
D'Errico retractor
D'Errico skull trephine
D'Errico tissue forceps
D'Errico ventricular needle
desaturation of color on visual test
Desault sign
Desault wrist dislocation
descending tracts
desmalgia
desmectasis
desmitis
desmocytoma
desmodynia
desmoid, cortical
desmoma
desmopathy
desmoplasia
desmoplastic
desmorrhexis
desmosis
desmotomy
Desormaux endoscope
destructive lesion
desynchronized pattern on EEG
DeTakats-McKenzie brain clip forceps
detector
deterioration
  intellectual
  irradiation-induced mental
  mental
  neurologic(al)
  radiation-induced mental
  rostral-caudal
  uniformly progressive
deterioration of mental status
determinants of gait
  combined ankle and knee motion
  knee flexion during stance phase
  pelvic rotation
  pelvic shift
  pelvic tilt
determination, $TCPO_2$ (transcutaneous oxygen)
detour conduit
detritus
developmental delay
developmental dyslexia
developmental milestones of infants
deviation
  angular
  carpal
  conjugate eye
  cortical-type eye
  disconjugate eye (or dysconjugate)
  downward eye
  dysconjugate eye (or disconjugate)
  eye
  gait
  ipsilateral tonic
  radial
  rotary
  skew eye
  tongue
  tonic eye
  ulnar
deviation of eyes to one side
Devic disease
device (also *apparatus*; *orthosis*)
  Ace-Fischer external fixator
  Ace Unifix fixation
  activator table
  Acufex bioabsorbable fixation
  adjustable aiming
  Anderson fixation
  Anderson leg lengthening
  ankle disk
  anterior fixation
  antirotation
  antisiphon (ASD)
  AO compression
  AO contouring
  articular motion (AMD)
  assistive technology (ATD)
  Automator
  Axer compression
  Back Specialist chiropractic table
  Bassett electrical stimulation

device *(cont.)*
- biodegradable fixation
- Blanchard traction
- body fat calipers
- body-powered prosthetic
- Bovie electrocautery
- Brannock foot measuring
- Buck convoluted traction
- Buck Redi-Traction
- Cadwell 5200A somatosensory evoked potential unit
- Calandruccio triangular compression fixation
- Cameron fracture
- CD (Cotrel-Dubousset) fixation
- Charnley centering
- Charnley compression
- Charnley external fixation
- Chiro-Manis chiropractic table
- closed goggle-type eyeguards
- collapsible internal fixation
- compression screw-plate
- coracoclavicular fixation
- Cordis implantable drug reservoir
- Cordis MPAP system
- coring
- CPM (continuous passive motion)
- cranial
- Day fixation
- DC-101 chiropractic table
- Denham external fixation
- DeWald spinal
- Deyerle fixation
- DIGIT-grip
- driver tunnel locator
- Dunn fracture
- Dwyer-Wickham electrical
- dynamic external fixator
- EBI (Electro Biology, Inc.) bone healing system
- EBI SpF-2 implantable bone stimulator
- electrocautery
- Evershears surgical instrument

device *(cont.)*
- EX-FI-RE external fixation
- extensor (of fingers)
- external fixation
- external skeletal fixation
- eyeglass-type eyeguards
- fixating
- fixation
- four-bar external fixation
- Fox internal fixation
- fracture
- Gemini chiropractic table
- Georgiade fixation
- Giliberty
- Golgi
- halo fixation
- halo vest
- halo-pelvic distraction
- handgrip ergometer
- Hare
- Harrington fixation
- Harrington outrigger
- Harrington-Kostuik distraction
- Heyer-Schulte antisiphon
- Hirschhorn compression
- Hoffmann external fixation
- Hoffmann-Vidal external fixation
- ICLH
- Ikuta fixation
- Ilizarov
- internal fixation
- intramedullary fixation
- JACE-STIM electrotherapy stimulation
- JACE W550 CPM wrist
- Kaneda distraction
- Kin-Con
- kinesiologic testing
- Kinetron muscle strengthening
- Kirschner
- Kronner external fixation
- Kuhlman cervical traction
- Küntscher traction
- Leander chiropractic table

device *(cont.)*
leather lacer gauntlet
leg-holding
Leinbach
Lloyd chiropractic table
Luque fixation
McLaughlin osteosynthesis
Mobilimb CPM
Mueller compression (Müller)
nail-bending
nail-plate
Nauth traction
Neufeld
oculomotor
Ommaya reservoir
Omni-Flexor physical therapy
Orthofix
Oxford unicompartmental
Parham-Martin fracture
passive traction table
PGK (Panos G. Koutrouvelis, M.D.) stereotactic
plate-and-screw fixation
polycarbonate eyeguards
Polytechnic foot pressure measuring plate
Pro-Trac measurement
Quengel
Rancho anklet foot control
Ray TFC (threaded fusion cage)
Re-Lax-O chiropractic table
Redi-Trac traction
Reichert-Mundinger stereotactic
Rezinian external fixation
Rezinian interbody
Richards lag screw
RMC knee replacement
Rochester bone trephine
rod-mounted targeting
Roger Anderson compression
Roger Anderson external fixation
screen plate
screw fixation
Secor I (or II) drug pump

device *(cont.)*
Secor implantable drug reservoir
semirigid carbon fiber-reinforced plastic plate
Servox
shock-absorbent heel pad
Slot distraction
snap-fit
Sofamor spinal
Somanetics INVOS cerebral oximeter
SomaSensor
Southwick pin-holding
StairClimber assist
Statak
Sukhtian-Hughes fixation
Suretac bioabsorbable shoulder fixation
Sutter-CPM knee
Tekscan in-shoe monitoring
Telectronics electrical stimulation
telos radiographic stress
tensioning
Therex programmable drug pump
tilt board
toe-straight
trampoline
triangular compression fixation
TSRH pedicle fixation
unconstrained elbow
Unidose drug delivery system
Vidal-Adrey modified Hoffmann external fixation
visor halo fixation
Volkov-Oganesian external fixation
Wagner distraction
Wagner external fixation
Wagner leg-lengthening
Wagner-Schanz screw
Wasserstein fixation
Wrist Pro wrist support
Zenith chiropractic table
Zickel medullary
Zickel supracondylar fixation

device *(cont.)*
  Zielke distraction
  Zimmer electrical stimulation
DeVilbiss cranial rongeur
DeVilbiss rongeur forceps
DeVilbiss skull trephine
devitalized soft tissue
DeWald spinal appliance
Dewar-Barrington clavicular dislocation technique
Dewar cervical operation
Dewar-Harris shoulder technique
Dewar procedure
Dexon suture
Dexter hand evaluation
dexterity
  finger
  manual
dextrorotoscoliosis
dextroscoliosis
Deyerle II pin
Deyerle plate
Deyerle sciatic tension test
Deyerle sign
Deyerle technique
DF80 (Wilson-Burstein) hip internal prosthesis
DFA (hallux dorsiflexion angle)
DFI (dye fluorescence index)
DFS (distraction-flexion stage)
DGR cranial perforator
diabetes insipidus
diabetes mellitus
diabetic amyotrophy
diabetic Charcot foot
diabetic coma
diabetic encephalopathy
diabetic gangrene
diabetic neuropathy
diabetic neuroarthropathy of the foot and ankle
diabetic peripheral neuropathy
diabetic pseudotabes
diabetic third nerve mononeuropathy
diabetic third nerve palsy
Diabetic D-Sole foot orthosis
diacondylar fracture
diadochokinesia
diadochokinesis
diagnosis, gold standard of
Diagnostic and Statistical Manual III—Revised (DSM-III-R)
diagnostic arthroscopy and debridement
diagnostic cascade
dial-lock brace
Dial Away Pain 400 electrotherapy unit
dialysis dementia
diamagnetic
diameter
  midsagittal (MSD)
  spinal cord
diamond bur
Diamond-Gould syndactyly operation
diamond nail
diamond-point wire
diamond rasp
diapering, triple
diaphragma sellae
diaphyseal cortical mortise
diaphyseal fracture
diaphyseal nonunion
diaphysectomy
diaphysis (pl. diaphyses)
diaplasis
diarrhea, weekend
diarthrodial joint
diarthrosis
Dias-Giegerich fracture technique
diaschisis, cerebral
Diasonics
diastasis
  syndesmotic
  tibiofibular
diastasis of sutures
diastatic fracture
diastatic skull fracture
diastematomyelia
diastrophic dwarfism

diathermy
  microwave (MWD)
  shortwave (SWD)
diathesis
  epileptic
  migraine
DiChiara hand tray
Dickhaut-DeLee classification of discoid meniscus
Dickinson calcaneal bursitis technique
Dickinson-Coutts-Woodward-Handler osteotomy
Dickson-Diveley foot procedure
Dickson osteotomy
Dickson transplant technique
diencephalic herniation
diencephalic autonomic epilepsy
diencephalic seizure
diencephalon
diet
  Evers diet for multiple sclerosis
  gluten-free diet for multiple sclerosis
  gouty
  high manganese diet for multiple sclerosis
  low purine
  MacDougall diet for multiple sclerosis
  purine-free
  tea-and-toast
  tyramine
diet for athletes, American Dietetic Association
Diethrich bulldog clamp
differentially abled athlete
difficulty
  phrase-completion
  word-finding
diffuse axonal tearing (in head injury)
diffuse brain dysfunction
diffuse cerebral disease
diffuse delta slowing (on EEG)
diffuse encephalopathic process
diffuse encephalopathy
diffuse esophageal spasm (corkscrew esophagus)
diffuse idiopathic skeletal hyperostosis (DISH)
diffuse sclerosis
diffuse syphilitis meningitis
diffuse thalamic projection system
diffuse tract disease
diffusion
DiGeorge syndrome
Digi-Flex finger exerciser
Digikit finger tourniquet
digit, digits
  accessory
  arthrodesed
  flail
  replanted
  supernumerary
  syndactylization of
Digit-Aid fifth toe splint
digital branches
digital color (color of digit)
digital exertion measurer
digital flexor tendon quartet
digital grasp method
digital nerve block
digital opposers
digital paresthesia
digital plethysmography
digital replantation
digital signal analysis of EEG
digital subtraction angiography (DSA)
digital to analog converter
DIGIT-grip device
digit repetition test
digit reversal test
digit span test of recall after head injury
digit-symbol test
digitized spinography
digitorum
Dilantin loading
Dilantin rash

dilantinization
dilatation
  aneurysmal
  fusiform
  pupillary
  ventricular
dilatation of the sulcus
dilatation of the ventricle
dilated and fixed pupils
dilated pupil
dilator, Eder-Puestow metal olive
Dimension/C femoral stem
Dimension hip prosthesis
Dimon-Hughston fracture fixation
Dimon osteotomy
dimple, pilonidal
dimple sign
dimple the bone
DIMS (disorder of initiating and maintaining sleep)
Dingman bone-holding forceps
Dingman mouth gag
Dingman osteotome
dinner-fork deformity
DIP (distal interphalangeal)
DIP articulation
DIP joint
DiPalma shoe lift
diparesis, spastic
diphasic wave on EEG
diplegia, spastic
diplegia spinalis brachialis traumatica
diplopia
  central
  horizontal
  unequivocal
  vertical
diploscope
dipole
  corneoretinal
  horizontal
diect constriction (eye exam)
director, grooved
disability benefits
disability
  global measures of
  learning
  mobility
  neurologic
  partial permanent
  pedal
  percent of total
  permanent
  posttraumatic chronic
  progressive
  tapping tests of arm
  total
  Viscolas heel pain and
Disability Adjusted Life Years (DALYs)
Disability Division of the Social Services Administration
disabled for work
disarticulate
disarticulation
  Batch-Spittler-McFaddin knee
  Boyd hip
  elbow
  hip
  knee
  shoulder
  wrist
disc (see *disk*)
discectomy (see *diskectomy*)
discharge, discharges
  anteromesial temporal EEG
  bilateral independent periodic lateralizing
  epileptiform (BIPLED)
  bilaterally synchronous EEG
  biphasic
  centrotemporal (on EEG)
  complex repetitive (CRD)
  contralateral
  decrescendo
  dive-bomber
  epileptic
  epileptiform burst

discharge *(cont.)*
  focal epileptiform
  generalized epileptiform
  ictal focal epileptiform
  ictal generalized spike-and-wave
  interictal focal epileptiform
  interictal generalized spike-and-wave
  interictal spike
  irregular
  lateralizing
  local contralateral
  midtemporal
  multifocal spike
  myokymic
  myotonic
  neuromyotonic
  paroxysmal
  periodic lateralizing epileptiform (PLED)
  polyspike-and-wave
  regular
  rhythmical midtemporal (RMTD)
  rolandic epileptiform (on EEG)
  sharp-and-slow wave
  slow spike-and-wave
  spike
  spike-and-wave
  subclinical
  synchronous bilateral PLED
discharges of adults, subclinical rhythmical EEG (SREDA)
discission knife
discitis (diskitis)
discogenic
discogram (see *diskogram*)
discography (see *diskography*)
discoid lateral meniscus
discoligamentous complex
discoligamentous injury
disconjugate (or dysconjugate) gaze
disconjugate eye deviation
disconnection apraxia
disconnection syndrome
discopathy
discrepancy
  biomechanics of limb length
  leg-length
discrepant intellectual functioning
discreta, porokeratosis plantaris
discrete blood supply
discrimination consciousness
discrimination
  fine tactile
  sensory
  temperature
  two-point
  Sweet two-point
discus, disci
disease (also *disorder*; *syndrome*)
  advanced cortical
  Albers-Schönberg (Schoenberg)
  albuminocytologic dissociation in Guillain-Barré
  Alexander
  Alper
  Alzheimer (presenile dementia)
  amyotrophic lateral sclerosis (ALS)
  anterior horn cell
  Apert
  Atton
  Azorean-Joseph-Machado
  Baló
  basilar vertebral artery
  Bassen-Kornzweig
  Batten
  Bielschowsky-Jansky
  bilateral corticobulbar
  bilateral frontal lobe
  Binswanger
  Blount
  Bornholm
  Bourneville-Pringle
  brain stem
  brancher enzyme deficiency
  brittle bone
  Brodie

disease *(cont.)*
- Buerger
- bulky metastatic
- Caffey
- caisson worker's
- Calvé-Perthes
- Canavan
- Canavan-van Bogaert-Bertrand
- carnitine palmityltransferase (CPT) deficiency
- carotid artery
- carotid occlusive
- central core
- central motor pathways
- cerebellar
- cerebrovascular
- cervical disk
- Chagas
- champagne-bottle legs in Charcot-Marie-Tooth
- Charcot joint
- Charcot-Marie-Tooth (CMT)
- cherry-red macula of Tay-Sachs
- Christmas hemophiliac
- congenital disorder (skeletal hypoplasia)
- connective tissue
- cortical
- cortical gray-matter
- corticospinal
- Creutzfeldt-Jakob (CJD)
- crystal-related joint
- Curschmann-Steinert
- cytomegalic inclusion
- Darier
- de Quervain
- Debré-Sémélaigne
- degenerative
- degenerative disk
- degenerative disorder (osteoarthritis)
- degenerative joint (DJD)
- degenerative spinal
- Dejerine

disease *(cont.)*
- Dejerine-Sottas
- demyelinating
- developmental disorder (scoliosis)
- Devic
- diffuse cerebral
- diffuse tract
- disk
- diver's
- Dubini
- Duchenne
- Duplay
- Eales
- Ehrenfeld
- Emery-Dreifuss
- emotional lability following infectious neurologic
- end-organ
- Engelmann
- Erb-Goldflam
- Erb-Landouzy
- Erdheim-Chester
- Eulenburg
- extracranial carotid occlusive
- Fabry
- facioscapulohumeral muscle atrophy
- Fahr
- familial paroxysmal choreoathetosis
- Farber
- Fazio-Londe
- fibromuscular
- flareup of
- Flatau-Schilder
- Foix-Alajouanine
- Forbes
- Forbes-Cori
- Forestier
- Freiberg
- Freiberg-Kohler
- Friedreich
- frontal lobe
- Fukuyama
- Garré

disease *(cont.)*
- Gaucher
- Gilbert
- glial
- Goldflam
- Gorham
- Gowers
- Greenfield
- Haglund
- Hallervorden-Spatz
- Hand-Schüller-Christian
- Hartnup
- hereditary striatopallidal
- heterogeneous system
- histiocytosis X group
- Holmes cerebellar degeneration
- Hunt
- Huntington
- Hurler
- Hurst
- Iceland (or Icelandic)
- intractable
- intraneuronal inclusion
- intrauterine cytomegalic inclusion
- Jaffe
- Jakob-Creutzfeldt
- Jansky-Bielschowsky
- jeep driver's
- Joseph
- Kearns-Sayre
- Kienböck (Kienboeck)
- Kimura
- Kinnier-Wilson
- knee knob of Osgood-Schlatter
- Köhler (Koehler)
- König (Koenig)
- Kümmell (Kuemmell)
- Krabbe
- Kufs
- Kugelberg-Welander
- Lafora body
- Landouzy-Dejerine
- large-vessel disease of the diabetic foot

disease *(cont.)*
- Leber
- Legg
- Legg-Calvé-Perthes
- Legg-Perthes
- Leigh
- leptomeningeal
- Letterer-Siwe
- Lhermitte-Duclos
- Lichtheim
- lipid storage
- Little
- long tract
- Lou Gehrig
- lower motor neuron
- Lyme
- maple syrup urine (MSUD)
- Machado-Joseph
- Marchiafava-Bignami
- Marie-Bamberger
- Marie-Charcot-Tooth
- Marie-Foix-Alajouanine
- Marie-Strümpell (Struempell)
- McArdle
- Menkes
- metabolic bone
- milk-alkali
- milk leg
- Milroy
- minicore
- mixed connective tissue (MCTD)
- Morquio
- Morvan
- motor neuron (MND)
- moyamoya
- multicore
- multisystem
- neoplastic disorder
- neurodegenerative
- neurologic
- neuromuscular
- neurotraumatic evolution of Charcot joint
- Niemann-Pick

disease *(cont.)*
- oasthouse urine
- oculocraniosomatic
- Ollier
- Oppenheim
- organic brain (OBD)
- Osgood-Schlatter
- Paget
- Panner
- parietal lobe
- Parkinson
- Parsonage-Turner
- Pelizaeus-Merzbacher
- Pellegrini-Stieda
- Perthes
- Peyronie
- phytanic acid storage
- Pick
- Pompe
- posterior column
- posterolateral sclerosis
- Pott
- Prieser
- pseudomyotonia
- pulseless
- Quervain
- Rabot
- Raynaud
- Refsum
- retinal pathways
- Roussy-Lévy
- Santavuori-Haltia
- Santavuori-Haltia-Hagberg
- scapuloperoneal muscle atrophy
- Scheuermann
- Schilder
- Schmitt
- Seitelberger
- Sever
- Sinding Larsen–Johansson (SLJD)
- small-vessel disease of diabetic foot
- Spielmeyer-Vogt
- Spielmeyer-Vogt-Sjögren
- spinocerebellar

disease *(cont.)*
- Steele-Richardson-Olszewski
- Still
- Strümpell-Lorrain
- Sudeck
- Takayasu
- Tangier
- Tay-Sachs
- Thiemann
- Thomsen
- traumatic disorder
- Trevor
- unilateral supranuclear
- Unverricht
- Unverricht-Lafora
- Unverricht-Lundborg
- upper motor neuron
- vertebrobasilar
- Vogt
- von Economo
- von Eulenberg
- von Gierke
- von Hippel-Landau
- von Recklinghausen
- Voorhoeve
- VTED (venous thromboembolic)
- Welander
- Werdnig-Hoffmann
- Whipple
- white matter
- Wilson
- wing-beating tremor of Wilson
- Wolman

disease-modifying antirheumatic drugs (DMARDs)
disease of the retinal pathways
disease of motor units
disease-specific measures of impairment
disequilibrium (or dysequilibrium)
disequilibrium state
DISH (diffuse idiopathic sclerosing [or skeletal] hyperostosis)
disheveled appearance

DISI (dorsal intercalary segment
  instability) deformity
disimpaction
disinhibitions of a frontal lobe
  syndrome
disinsertion of tendon
disinterest
disjointing
disk (also *disc*)
  articular
  Bardeen
  bulge of
  bulging
  choked
  crescent-shaped
  epiphyseal
  fibrocartilaginous
  fibrous ring of
  fixation
  frayed
  hard
  herniated
  herniated cervical
  herniated intervertebral (HID)
  herniation of lumbosacral
    intervertebral
  herniation of thoracic intervertebral
  hydrodynamic potential of
  interarticular
  intervertebral
  locking
  massive herniated
  midline herniation of
  pale
  pallid swelling of (in eye)
  protruding
  ruptured
  Schiefferdecker
  sequestered
  slipped
  soft
  tactile
Diskard head halter
Disk-Criminator sensory tester
disk disease
diskectomy (also *discectomy*)
  automated percutaneous lumbar
    (APLD)
  cervical
  Cloward fusion
  microlumbar
  microsurgical
  percutaneous automated
  percutaneous lumbar
  Smith-Robinson
  Williams
disk extrusion
diskiform
disk interspace
diskitis
disk margin
disk material
disk matrix proteoglycans
diskogenic pain
diskogram, diskography (discography)
  cervical
  intranuclear
disk plication
disk protrusion
disk rongeur
disk space, height of
disk space infection
disk space narrowing
disk water signal (on MRI)
dislocate, dislocated
dislocation
  anterior hip
  anterior-inferior
  Bankart shoulder
  bayonet
  Bell-Dally
  Bell-Dally cervical
  Bennett
  Bennett basic hand
  boutonnière hand
  bursting
  carpometacarpal
  central
  Chopart ankle
  chronic recurrent ankle joint

dislocation *(cont.)*
  closed
  complete
  compound
  congenital dislocation of hip (CDH)
  congenital dysplasia of hip (CDH)
  consecutive
  Desault wrist
  divergent elbow
  facet
  fracture
  frank
  gamekeeper's
  habitual
  Hill-Sachs shoulder
  hip
  incomplete
  interphalangeal
  isolated
  Jahss classification of ankle
  joint
  Kienböck (Kienboeck)
  knee
  Lisfranc
  lunate
  luxatio erecta shoulder
  metacarpophalangeal
  milkmaid's elbow
  Monteggia
  Nélaton ankle
  nontraumatic
  old
  open
  Otto pelvis
  partial
  patellar
  pathologic fracture
  perilunate carpal
  peroneal tendon
  posterior hip
  primitive
  radial head
  recent
  recurrent

dislocation *(cont.)*
  simple
  Smith
  subastragalar
  subcoracoid shoulder
  subglenoid shoulder
  subspinous
  swivel, of midfoot
  talar
  tarsal
  tarsometatarsal
  tendon
  transscaphoid perilunate
  traumatic
  triquetrolunate
  volar semilunar wrist
dislocations of time and space perception in migraine
disorder
  acute labyrinthine
  apperceptive
  apraxic
  attention deficit (ADD)
  attention-deficit hyperactivity (ADHD)
  cerebral
  choreic movement
  convulsive
  cubist disorder of visual perception in migraine
  cumulative trauma (CTD)
  cyclothymic
  demyelinative
  end-stage
  extrapyramidal
  functional
  gait
  hyperkinetic motor
  labyrinthine
  lilliputian disorder of visual perception, in migraine
  median nerve
  motor
  movement

disorder *(cont.)*
multifocal seizure
neurogenic
perseverative
personality
pointilliste disorder of visual perception in migraine
potential cumulative trauma
seizure
sleep
sleep arousal
somatization
supranuclear disorder of ocular movement
syntactical
target
thalamic
vestibular nerve
zoom disorder of visual perception in migraine
disorder of initiating and maintaining sleep (DIMS)
disorder of visual perception in migraine
disorganization, spatial
disorganized pattern on EEG
disorientation
geographic
right-left
spatial
visuospatial
disoriented patient
displaced intra-articular fracture of the tarsal navicular
displacement
brain stem
Ellis Jones peroneal
midbrain
radial epiphyseal
vertebral body
displacement of fracture fragment
displacement of interhemispheric fissure
displacement of spinal column
displacement of the midbrain
disproportion, fiber-type
disrupted syndesmosis
disruption
facet capsule
joint
ligamentous
traumatic
dissecans, osteochondritis (OD)
dissected out
dissecting intracranial aneurysm
dissection
blunt
bone
cranial nerve
extracapsular
field of
finger
microsurgical
sharp
spontaneous arterial
subperiosteal
vertebral artery
dissector
aneurysm neck
Angell James
angled
ball
bunion
Cavitron
Clodius
Creed
Crile
Crile gasserian ganglion knife and
Crile nerve hook and
Davis dura
dura
Effler-Groves
endarterectomy
Fager pituitary
Feild suction (not Field)
golf-stick
grooved
Hajek-Ballenger

dissector *(cont.)*
  hand
  Hardy pituitary
  hockey-stick
  Holinger endarterectomy
  Jannetta aneurysm neck
  Kennerdell-Maroon
  Kocher
  Lewin bunion
  MacDonald
  Malis
  Marino transsphenoidal
  Maroon-Jannetta
  micro
  Milligan
  nerve root
  Oldberg
  Olivecrona dura
  Penfield (No. 1, 2, 3, 4, 5)
  pituitary
  Rayport dural and knife
  Rhoton ball
  Rhoton spatula
  Rochester lamina
  round
  Schmieden-Taylor
  Scoville
  sesamoidectomy
  Smithwick
  spatula
  suction
  teardrop
  Toennis-Adson
  Toennis dura
  transsphenoidal
  West hand
  Woodson
  Yasargil micro
disseminated sclerosis
disseminated-type pigmented villonodular synovitis
dissipate
dissociated (ataxic) nystagmus
dissociated sensory loss
dissociation
  albumino-cytologic (in Guillain-Barré)
  scapholunate
  segmental sensory
dissociative state
distal Akin phalangeal osteotomy
distal articular set angle (DASA)
distal branches
distal denervation
distal L osteotomy
distal medial crease (of hand)
distal phocomelia
distal third of shaft
distal tibial physes
distalward, distally
distance
  intercaudate
  interelectrode
  interlaminar
  interorbital
  interpediculate
  interspinous
disto-occlusal
distorted synaptic input (in epilepsy)
distortion
  EEG curvilinear
  spatial
  visual-spatial
distortion trauma
distract, distracting
distractibility
  easy
  heightened
distractible
distraction
  callus
  physeal
  segment
  small-step
  soft tissue
distraction-flexion stage (DFS)
distraction gap
distraction hyperflexion injury

distraction lengthening for the congenitally short metatarsal
distraction of fracture
distraction of joint
distraction osteogenesis
distraction phase
distractor
  Acufex ankle
  Anderson
  Bliskunov implantable femoral
  DeBastiani
  femoral
  Ilizarov
  Kessler metacarpal
  Monticelli-Spinelli
  Orthofix M-100
  Pinto
  Santa Casa
  turnbuckle
  Wagner
distribution
  field of
  glovelike
  lateral
  lateralized
  myotomal
  onion skin (of sensation)
  regional
  stocking
  stocking-glove
  stocking-like
distribution of activity on EEG
disturbance
  articulation
  focal neurologic
  gait
  high level perceptual
  oculomotor
  sphincter
  visual
  visual field
disturbed orientation
disuse
  demineralization from
  lesser atrophy of
disuse atrophy
disuse osteoporosis
dive-bomber discharges on electromyogram
dive-bomber sound on electromyography
divergence, ocular
diving reflex
divisionary line (in a bipartite sesamoid)
divopontocerebellar atrophy
divot
Divry-van Bogaert familial corticomeningeal angiomatosis
Dix-Hallpike maneuver
dizziness
DJD (degenerative joint disease)
DMA (distal metatarsal angle)
DMARDs (disease-modifying antirheumatic drugs)
DMD (Duchenne muscular dystrophy)
DMD gene
DMD phenotype
DMI orthopedic bed
DNA flow cytometry
D.O. (doctor of osteopathy)
DOA (diagnostic and operative arthroscopy)
Doane knee retractor
docility
doctor of chiropractic (D.C.)
doctor of osteopathy (D.O.)
doctor of podiatric medicine (D.P.M.)
doctor of podiatry (D.P.)
Doctor's First Report of Injury
doctrine, Monro-Kellie
DOES (disorders of excessive sleep)
doffing prosthesis (taking it off)
dog-ear
Dohn-Carton brain retractor
Dohrmann-Rubin cannula
dolichoectasia, vertebrobasilar
dolichostenomelia
Doll trochanteric reattachment technique

doll's eye (head) phenomenon
doll's eye reaction
doll's eye reflex
doll's eyes
doll's eye sign
doll's head maneuver
dolorimeter
dome
  anterior talar
  shoulder
  talar
  weightbearing acetabular
dome of aneurysm
dome osteotomy
Domen laminoplasty
domiciliary setting (evaluation for rehabilitation)
dominance
  cerebral
  lack of clear-cut cerebral
  left hemisphere
  left/right hemisphere
  mixed cerebral
  right hemisphere
dominant hemisphere lesion
dominant waking frequency (on EEG)
DOMS (delayed-onset muscle soreness)
Donaghy angled suture needle holder
Donati suture
DonJoy Gold Point knee brace
DonJoy knee splint
DonJoy wrist splint
donning prosthesis (putting it on)
donor team
Dooley nail
door-bell sign
dopa-decarboxylase
dopamine
dopamine agonist
dopamine levels in corpus striatum
dopaminergic-cholinergic balance
dopaminergic receptor
Doppler
  color-flow
  continuous wave
  duplex
  duplex B-mode
  range-gated pulsed
  range-gated transcranial
  transcranial
Doppler ankle systolic pressure
Doppler calf systolic pressure
Doppler flowmetry
Doppler insonation
Doppler study
Doppler thigh systolic pressure
Doppler ultrasound segmental blood pressure testing
Dorello canal
Dorrance hand prosthesis
dorsal aponeurotic expansion hood
dorsal closing wedge metatarsal osteotomy
dorsal cochlear nucleus
dorsal column stimulator (DCS)
dorsal interosseous
dorsal medial nucleus of the thalamus
dorsal metacarpal ligament
dorsal nucleus of vagus
dorsal pedal bypass
dorsal root entry zone (DREZ) lesion
dorsal root ganglia (DRG)
dorsal root rhizotomy
dorsal spine (D1 to D12)
dorsal spinocerebellar tracts
dorsal subaponeurotic space
dorsal subcutaneous space
dorsal wing fracture
dorsal wrist ligament
dorsalis pedis
dorsalis pedis myofascial flap
dorsalis pedis pulse
dorsalis tabes
dorsalward
Dorsey dural separator

Dorsey separator
Dorsey ventricular cannulas
dorsiflexed
dorsiflexion, neutral
dorsiflexors
dorsiflexion stop brace
dorsolateral and medial capsulotomy
dorsomedial incision
dorsoplantar talonavicular angle
dorsoplantar view
dorsoradial
dorsorostral
dorsum of hand
dorsum sellae
double athetosis
double bubble flushing reservoir
double camelback sign (knee)
double consecutive coma of epidural hematoma
double-contrast arthrography
double-contrast laryngography
double drape
double hemiplegia
double-jointed (patient with hyper-extensible joints)
double leg raise test
double-leg stance phase of gait
double simultaneous sensory stimulation
double simultaneous stimulation
  tactile
  visual
double-stem silicone lesser MP implant
double-threaded Herbert screw
doughnut, foam
Douglas skin graft
douloureux, tic (trigeminal neuralgia)
Dow Corning Wright prosthesis
dowager's hump
dowel, doweling
  bone
  bone bank
  calf bone
  cylindrical

dowel *(cont.)*
  graft
  iliac
  iliac crest
dowel arthrodesis
dowel cutters, Cloward
dowel graft technique
doweling spondylolisthesis technique
dowel spinal fusion
Dowling intracranial cyst removal technique
down-beat (down-beating) nystagmus
Down epiphyseal knife
Down syndrome
downbeating nystagmus
Downey hemilaminectomy retractor
downgoing toes
Downing cartilage knife
Downing retractor
Doyen bone mallet
Doyen costal rasp
Doyen cylindrical drill
Doyen rib elevator
Doyen rib rasp
Doyen spherical bur
DRA (distal reference axis)
draggy, feeling
Dragstedt skin graft
drain
  Becker external
  Charnley suction
  Davol
  external ventricular (EVD)
  Hemovac
  Hemovac Hydrocoat
  Heyer-Schulte wound
  Jackson-Pratt
  lumbar
  monofilament nylon
  Nélaton rubber tube
  nylon threads as
  Penrose
  rubber
  Shirley
  Silastic

drain *(cont.)*
    spinal
    suction
    Surgivac
    ventriculoperitoneal
    ventriculostomy
    wound
    Wound-Evac
drainage
    fish-mouth
    mucopurulent
    purulent
    ventricular
Drake aneurysm clip
DRAM (deepithelialized rectus
    abdominis muscle) flap
drape
    adhesive
    double
    fenestrated
    foot
    head
    impervious
    isolation
    lint-free
    Loban adhesive
    NeuroDrape surgical
    Opmi microscope
    Opraflex incise
    plastic
    povidone-iodine (Betadine)
        impregnated
    3M skin
draped out
drawer sign (at ankle or knee)
drawn ankle clonus
dream, dreaming
dreamless sleep
dreamy state
Drennan metaphyseal-epiphyseal angle
Dressinet netting bandage
dressing (see also *bandage*; *packing*)
    ABD
    ABD pad
    ACU-derm wound

dressing *(cont.)*
    Adaptic
    Aeroplast
    Allevyn
    Aquaphor
    Betadine
    Bioclusive transparent
    bulky
    Bunnell
    calcium alginate
    Coban
    collodion
    Comfeel Ulcus occlusive
    compression wrap
    compressive
    Conform
    corrective soft
    cotton
    Coverlet adhesive surgical
    Cover-Roll adhesive gauze
    Cryo/Cuff ankle
    dry
    DuoDerm
    elastic salve
    elasticized gauze
    Elastikon
    Elastomull
    Elastoplast
    Esmarch
    Fabco gauze bandage
    felt
    figure-of-8 (or figure 8)
    Flexinet
    fluff
    foam gauze
    4 x 4 gauze
    Fuller shield
    Furacin gauze
    gauze
    Glasscock ear
    Inerpan flexible burn
    iodoform gauze
    Jones
    Kaltostat
    Kerlix

dressing *(cont.)*
- Kling adhesive
- Koch-Mason
- Lyofoam
- Microfoam
- Mills
- modified Robert Jones
- moleskin
- moleskin strips
- Mother Jones (modified Robert Jones)
- nonadherent gauze
- Nu Gauze
- O'Donoghue
- occlusive
- Op-Site
- Owen gauze
- palm-to-axilla
- patch
- pledget
- polyurethane foam (PFD)
- pressure
- Reston
- rigid
- Robert Jones
- Schanz
- silk mesh gauze
- Sof-Rol
- Sof-Wick
- soft bulky
- stent
- sterile
- Stimson
- T strap in single-bar ankle brace
- Tegaderm
- Telfa gauze
- toe-to-groin modified Jones
- Tubex gauze
- Tubigrip
- Velpeau
- Vigilon
- Webril
- wet-to-dry
- wide-mesh petroleum gauze
- Xeroform gauze

dressing and bathing ability

dressing apraxia

Dreyer formula

Dreyer test

DREZ (dorsal root entry zone) lesion

DREZ modification of Eriksson technique

DREZ-otomy, microsurgical

DREZ procedure

DRG (dorsal root ganglia)

Driessen hinged plate

drift, drifting
- arm
- eye
- finger pursuit
- finger-to-nose exam
- leg
- medial metatarsal
- pronator

drill
- Acra-Cut wire pass
- Adson twist
- air
- air-powered cutting
- Anspach power
- archimedean hand
- battery-driven hand
- biflanged
- Black and Decker
- bone
- Bosworth
- brace
- Bunnell hand
- cannulated
- Cebotome
- Cement Eater
- centering
- cervical
- Championnière bone
- Charnley centering
- Charnley femoral condyle
- Cherry-Austin
- Children's Hospital hand
- chuck
- Cloward

drill *(cont.)*
- Coballoy twist
- Codman wire pass
- Collison
- cortex
- cortical
- cranial
- Crutchfield hand
- Cushing flat
- Cushing perforator
- D'Errico perforating
- dental
- Elan-E power
- femoral condyle
- fingernail
- flat
- flex
- Gray
- Hall air
- Hall large bore
- Hall Micro E
- Hall Surgairtome
- Hall Versipower
- hand
- hand-operated
- high-speed twist
- Hudson brace
- Hudson cranial
- Kirschner hand
- Kirschner wire
- Küntscher (Kuentscher)
- Mathews hand
- McKenzie perforating twist
- Micro-Aire
- microsurgery
- Mira Mark III cranial
- Moore hand
- Osteone air
- otologic
- patellar
- Pease bone
- penetrating
- Penn fingernail

drill *(cont.)*
- perforating twist
- Phoenix cranial
- pilot
- pneumatic
- Ralk hand
- Raney cranial
- Raney perforator
- right-angle dental
- Shea
- Smedberg hand
- Smedberg twist
- Smith automatic perforator
- Smith cranial
- spiral
- step
- Stille bone
- Stille cranial
- Stille hand
- Stille-Sherman bone
- Stryker microsurgery
- Toti trephine
- Treace
- trephine
- Trinkle
- twist
- wire
- wire pass
- Xomed
- Zimmer hand

drill bit
- cannulated
- Howmedica Microfixation System
- Leibinger Micro System
- Luhr Microfixation System
- Storz Microsystems
- Synthes Microsystem

drill bushing

drill flat

drill guide
- ACL (anterior cruciate ligament)
- Adson

drill hole

drill point
  cannulated
  carbon steel
  Crutchfield
  Raney-Crutchfield
  Stille
drill points, burs, and trephine
drill/reamer, Micro-Aire
drill set, Hudson cranial
drive
  Jacobs chuck
  worm
driver
  blade plate
  bullet
  Flatt
  Hall
  Harrington hook
  Jewett
  K-wire
  Küntscher nail (Kuentscher)
  Linvatec
  Lloyd nail
  Massie
  Micro Series wire
  nail
  Orthoairtome wire
  Paramax angled
  plate
  power
  prosthesis
  staple
  supine position
  Sven-Johansson
  Teflon-coated
driver-bender-extractor, Rush
driver-extractor
  Hansen-Street
  Ken
  McReynolds
  Sage
  Schneider
  Zimmer
driving, photic (on EEG)
driving response (on EEG)
dromedary gait
drooling
droop, facial
droopy shoulder thoracic outlet syndrome
drop-arm test
drop
  foot
  wrist
drop attack, akinetic
dropfoot
dropfoot gait
drop Lasègue sign
droplets, lipid (within muscle fibers)
dropout, neuronal
drowsiness
  excessive daytime
  postictal
  state of
  transition to
drowsy
drug delivery pump system (see *pump*)
drug delivery system, DUPEL iontophoretic
drug holiday, therapeutic
drug-induced nystagmus
drug-induced parkinsonism
drugs (see also *medications*)
  absorption of
  acetaminophen
  addictive potential of
  administration of
  adrenergic
  aerosolized
  alternate-day steroids
  aminoglycoside
  amphetamine
  analgesic
  anaphylactic
  anesthetic
  antianxiety
  antibiotic

drugs *(cont.)*
anticholinergic
anticonvulsant
antidepressant
antidote for drug overdose
antiemetic
antifungal
anti-infective
anti-inflammatory
antimetabolite
antineoplastic
antiparkinsonian
antipruritic
antipsychotic
antipyretic
antiseizure
antiseptic
antispasmodic
antitussive
antiviral
antiyeast
anxiolytic
azaspirodecanedione (ASD)
bactericidal
bacteriostatic
barbiturate
barbiturate hypnotic
benzodiazepine
beta blocking
blood screen for
branched chain amino acids (BCAA)
broad-spectrum antibiotic
calcium channel blocking
CNS-stimulating (central nervous system)
cephalosporin
chemotherapy
cholinergic
combination
corticosteroid
CR (controlled release)
curare-like
dextrorotatory

drugs *(cont.)*
disease-modifying antirheumatic (DMARDs)
disinfectant
diuretic
emergency
epidural anesthetic
fibrinolytic agents
fractionalized fish oil
general anesthetic
gold salts
half-life of
heterocyclic antidepressant
high-dose
hydantoin
hypnotic
ICV (intracerebroventricular) administration of
illicit
inhalation of
insomnia
intolerance of
intracavitary chemotherapy
intradiscal
intramuscular (IM)
intranasal
intrathecal
intratumoral chemotherapy
intravenous (IV)
investigational
isomer
LA (long-acting)
levorotatory
loading dose of
local anesthetic
maintenance dose of
MAO (monoamine oxidase) inhibitor
monocyclic antidepressant
monoclonal antibody
muscle relaxant
musculoskeletal relaxant
naphthylalkalone
narcotic

drugs *(cont.)*
  narcotic agonist
  narcotic analgesic
  narcotic antagonist
  neuroleptic
  neurological
  neuromuscular blocking
  neuroprotector
  nonbarbiturate hypnotic
  non-narcotic analgesic
  nonsteroidal anti-inflammatory (NSAIDs)
  nootropics
  oral
  over-the-counter
  peak level of
  peak and trough levels of
  peripheral vasodilating
  phenothiazine
  placebo
  prescription
  prophylactic
  psychiatric
  psychotic
  SA (sustained action)
  salicylate
  sedative
  sedative/hypnotic
  skeletal muscle relaxant
  SL (sublingual)
  slow-release (SR)
  spinal anesthetic
  SR (slow release, sustained release)
  stepwise increase in dosage of
  steroid
  succinimide
  sulfa
  sulfonamide (sulfa)
  sustained release (SR)
  systemic
  tapering doses of
  tetracyclic antidepressant
  tetracycline
  therapeutic effects of

drugs *(cont.)*
  therapeutic index of
  titrated dose of
  tolerance of
  topical
  topical antiviral
  toxic effects of
  tranquilizer
  tricyclic antidepressant
  trough level of
  vasoconstrictor
  vasodilating
  vasopressor
drug-withdrawal seizure
Drummond button
Drummond hook holder
Drummond wire technique
drunken sailor gait
Dry Flotation wheelchair cushion
dry gangrene
Dryspell cast cover
DTICH (delayed traumatic intracerebral hemorrhage)
DTRs (deep tendon reflexes)
DTs (delirium tremens)
DTT (dynamic transverse traction) screw
DuVries phalangeal condylectomy
dual-lock hip prosthesis
dual-lock total hip replacement system
dual-photon densitometry test for osteoporosis
Duane retraction syndrome
Dubini chorea
Dubini disease
Duchenne-Aran spinal muscular atrophy
Duchenne muscular dystrophy
  duck's waddle gait in
  wasp-tail deformity in
Duchenne-Erb palsy
Duchenne muscular dystrophy (DMD)
Duchenne sign
duck gait

duck waddle gait in Duchenne dystrophy
duck waddle test
Dudley Morton syndrome
Dugas test
Dumbach cranial titanium mesh
dumbbell neurofibroma tumor
dumbbell type neuroblastoma
Duncan prone rectus test
Dunlop-Shands view
Dunlop traction
Dunn-Brittain foot stabilization technique
Dunn fracture device
Dunn-Hess trochanteric osteotomy
Dunn procedure (of hip)
Duo-Cline bed wedge
DuoDerm dressing
Duo-Driv screw
Duo-Lock
Duopress guide
Dupaco knee control
DUPEL iontophoretic drug delivery system
Duplay disease
duplex imaging, color-flow
DuPont CRONEX x-ray film
DuPont Rare Earth Imaging System
Dupuytren contracture release
Dupuytren fasciitis
dura
  attenuated
  bulging
  freeze-dried
dura mater of the brain
dura mater of the spinal cord
Duracon prosthesis
Dura-Kold wrap
dural arteriovenous fistula
dural arteriovenous malformation
dural attachment
dural dissector and knife
dural elevator
dural guard
dural hook
dural hook knife
Duraloc acetabular liner
dural puncture
dural retractor
dural ring
dural root pouches
dural sac
dural scar
dural scissors
dural separator
dural separator-spatula
dural sheath
dural sinus thrombosis
dural tear
dural venous sinus
Duran-Houser wrist splint
Durapatite bone replacement material
duraplasty, decompressive
Duray-Read gouge
Duret hemorrhage
Duret lesion
Durham flatfoot
durus, clavus
duToit-Roux staple capsulorrhaphy
Duval elevator
Duverney fracture
DuVries arthroplasty
DuVries condylectomy
DuVries deltoid ligament reconstruction technique
DuVries hammer toe repair
DuVries-Mann bunionectomy
DuVries modified McBride hallux valgus operation
DuVries technique for overlapping toe
DVI (deep venous insufficiency)
DVR (Department of Vocational Rehabilitation)
DVT (deep venous thrombosis)
dwarfism
  achondroplastic
  chondroplastic
  diastrophic

Dwyer cable and screw
Dwyer cable for correction of scoliosis
Dwyer clawfoot operation
Dwyer correction of scoliosis
Dwyer osteotomy
Dwyer-Wickham electrical stimulation
Dycal base
Dyck-Lambert classification
dye fluorescence index (DFI)
dye, methylene blue
Dyke-Davidoff-Masson syndrome
Dynagrip blade handle
Dyna knee splint
dynamic ambulatory balance
dynamic aphasias
dynamic compression-plating
dynamic entrapment of vertebral
  artery
dynamic external fixation
dynamic friction
dynamic pedobarography
dynamic splint
dynamic standing balance
dynamics, foot
dynamometer
  ballistic
  Biodex
  bulb
  Collins
  Cybex II
  hand
  isokinetic
  Jamar hand
Dynaplex knee prosthesis
DyoCam 550 arthroscopic video camera
Dyonics arthroplasty bur
Dyonics arthroscopic blade
Dyonics arthroscopic instruments
Dyonics cannula
Dyonics Golden Retriever magnet
Dyonics rod-lens endoscope
Dyonics shaver
Dyonics shaving system
DyoVac suction punch

dysarthria
  apraxic
  cerebellar
  clumsy-hand
  hypophonic
  labial
  laryngeal
  lingual
  moderate
  pharyngeal
  severe
dysarthria literalis
dysarthria syllabaris spasmodica vagal
dysarthric speech
dysautonomia, familial
dysbasia lordotica
dysbaric
dyscalculia, developmental
dyschondroplasia
dyscollagenosis
dysconjugate eye movement (also
  disconjugate)
dyscrasia, dyscratic
dysdiadochokinesia
dysdiadochokinesis
dysdiadochokinetic
dysequilibrium syndrome
dyserethesia
dyserethism
dysergia
dysesthesia
  burning
  painful
dysesthesic sensation
dysesthetic sensation
dysfluency (stammering or stuttering)
dysfunction
  autonomic
  bilateral cerebral
  bilateral hemisphere
  bilateral upper motor neuron
  bowel and bladder
  brain
  brain stem

dysfunction *(cont.)*
  cerebral
  cognitive
  cortical neuronal
  corticospinal motor system
  diffuse brain
  eighth nerve
  fiber tract
  frontal lobe
  hemispheral
  higher cerebral (HCD)
  higher cortical
  language
  lingual airway
  lumbopelvic
  midbrain
  minimal brain
  neurologic
  neuromotor
  oculomotor
  parietal lobe
  posttraumatic cortical
  premotor areas of cerebral cortex
  progressive rostral-caudal brain stem
  severe diffuse brain
  subcortical neuronal
  supranuclear (bilateral upper motor neuron)
  swallowing
  sympathetic
dysgenesis
  alar
  epiphyseal
dysgnosia
dysgraphia with dyslexia
dysinhibition, emotional
dysjunctive eye movement
dysjunctive gaze
dyskinesia
  choreic
  facial
  faciobuccolingual
  L-dopa-induced

dyskinesia *(cont.)*
  neuroleptic-induced
  oral-buccal-lingual
  orofacial
  tardive
  tardive oromandibular
  withdrawal-emergent
dyskinesia intermittens
dyskinetic
dyskoimesis
dyslalia
dyslexia
  developmental
  dyseidetic
  dysphonetic
  mixed dysphonetic-dyseidetic
dyslexia with dysgraphia
dyslexia without dysgraphia
dyslexic
dyslogia
dysmaturity of EEG
dysmemory
dysmetria
  cerebellar
  lower limb
  ocular
  truncal
dysmetric overshoot of eye movement
dysmimia
dysmnesia
dysmnesic
dysmorphophobia
dysmyelinatus, status
dysmyotonia
dysnomia
  amnestic
  literal paraphasic
  paraphasic
  verbal paraphasic
dysosteogenesis
dysostosis
  cleidocranial
  craniofacial
  metaphyseal

dysostosis multiplex
dysphasia
  concomitant
  global
  motor
  sensory
dysphasic
dysphonia
dysplasia
  acropectorovertebral
  bone
  cleidocranial
  congenital dysplasia of hip (CDH)
  congenital hip
  cranioskeletal
  developmental
  diaphyseal
  epiarticular osteochondromatous
  fibromuscular (FMD)
  fibrous
  foot
  mesomelic
  Mondini
  monostotic fibrous
  multiple epiphyseal
  Namaqualand hip
  oculoauriculovertebral (OAV)
  odontoid
  osseous
  polyostotic fibrous
  progressive diaphyseal
  Sponastrine
  spondyloepiphyseal
  Streeter
dysplasia of the hip, congenital
dyspractic movement
dyspraxia
  ideational
  ideomotor
  innervatory
  limb-kinetic
  sympathetic
  vocal
dysprosody
dysraphism
  closed spinal
  occult spinal
  spinal
dysreflexia, autonomic
dysrhythmia
  anterior slow
  cerebral
  slow anterior
dysrhythmic movement
dysrhythmic, scattered, slow activity (on EEG)
dysrhythmic speech
dyssynergia (jerky incoordinate movement)
dyssynergia cerebellaris myoclonica syndrome
dyssynergia, Ramsay Hunt cerebellar myoclonic
dystasia, hereditary areflexic
dystonia
  body
  facial
  focal
  focal appendicular
  kinesogenic
  nonkinesogenic
  spasmodic
  tardive
  torsion
dystonia musculorum deformans
dystonic posture
dystonic posturing
dystrophia myotonica
dystrophic calcification
dystrophic changes
dystrophic gait
dystrophin
dystrophy
  adiposogenital
  Becker-Kiener
  Becker muscular (BMD)
  Becker type of muscular
  Becker variant of Duchenne

dystrophy *(cont.)*
benign X-linked muscular
benign X-linked recessive muscular
cerebromacular
congenital muscular
congenital myotonic
distal muscle
Duchenne muscular (DMD)
Emery-Dreifuss
Erb muscular
faciohumeral muscular
facioscapulohumeral (FSH) muscular
Fröhlich adiposogenital (Froehlich)
Gowers muscular
humeroperoneal muscular
infantile neuroaxonal
juvenile muscular
juvenile neuroaxonal
Kiloh-Nevin ocular form of
progressive muscular

dystrophy *(cont.)*
Landouzy-Dejerine
limb-girdle muscular
minor reflex
muscular
myopathic
myotonic muscular
ocular muscular
oculopharyngeal muscular
postinjection reflex sympathetic
pseudohypertrophic muscular
reflex sympathetic (RSD)
scapuloperoneal
sympathetic reflex
Thomsen
Welander muscular
X-linked recessive muscular

E, e

EADL (extended activities of daily living)
Eagle arthroscope
Eagle straight-ahead arthroscope
Eales disease
ear
  cauliflower
  scrum (in rugby players)
  swimmer's
  wrestler's
early dementia
early traumatic epilepsy
early ulnar nerve paresis
ear reference montage on EEG
EAST (external rotation abduction stress test)
eastern equine viral encephalitis
East-West retractor
Eater, Anspach Cement
Eaton-Lambert syndrome
Eaton-Littler technique
Eaton-Malerich fracture-dislocation technique
Eaton prosthesis
Eberle contracture release technique
EBI (Electro-Biology, Inc.) bone healing system
EBI SpF-T bone stimulator
EBI SpF-2 implantable bone stimulator
EBI spinal fusion (SpF) stimulator
EBL (estimated blood loss)
eburnated area
eburnated bone
eburnation, bony
ECA (external carotid artery)
eccentric axis of rotation of the ankle
eccentric muscle training
ecchondroma
ecchondrotome
ecchymosis
  periorbital (raccoon eye sign)
  postauricular (Battle sign)
eccrine angiomatous hamartoma
Echlin duckbill rongeur
Echlin laminectomy rongeur
Echlin-Luer rongeur
echo, echoes
ECHO (enteric cytopathic human orphan) virus
echo planar imaging
echo time (TE)
encephalitis (pl. encephalitides)
echoencephalogram
echoencephalography
echolalia
Echols retractor
echopraxia
ECI (electrocerebral inactivity)
ECIC (extracranial-intracranial) arterial bypass
Ecker-Lotke-Glazer tendon reconstruction technique
Eckert-Davis classification of peroneal tendon subluxation
Eclipse ankle brace
Eclipse TENS unit
ECoG (electrocorticogram)
ecological validity of rehabilitation testing
economic dependence

E-cotton bandage
ECR (evoked cortical response)
ECRB (extensor carpi radialis brevis) muscle
ECRB (extensor carpi radialis brevis) tendon
ECRL (extensor carpi radialis longus) muscle
ECRL (extensor carpi radialis longus) tendon
ECS (electrocerebral silence)
ECT (European compression technique) bone screw
ECT internal fracture fixation
ectasia, basilar artery
ectoderm, embryonic neural
ectopic foci of seizures
Ectra carpal tunnel instruments
Ectra system
ECU (extensor carpi ulnaris) muscle
ECU (extensor carpi ulnaris) tendon
EDAMS (encephaloduroarterio-myosynangiosis)
EDAS (encephaloduroarterio–synangiosis)
EDB (extensor digitorum brevis) muscle
EDB (extensor digitorum brevis) tendon
EDC (extensor digitorum communis) muscle
EDC (extensor digitorum communis) tendon
EDCP (eccentric dynamic compression plate)
eddy currents; eddies
edema
  brain
  cerebral
  dependent
  intracompartmental
  malignant brain
  mushy
  nerve root
edema *(cont.)*
  nonpitting
  papilledema
  peritumoral
  pitting
  plerocephalic
  pretibial
  scalp
edematous brain tissue
edematous stump
Eden-Hybbinette arthroplasty
Eden-Lange procedure
Eden test
Eder-Puestow metal olive dilator
EDF scoliosis cast
Edgarton-Grand thumb adduction
edge
  rough
  tentorial
EDH (epidural hematoma)
Edinburgh-2 Coma Scale (E-2CS)
Edinburgh Rehabilitation Status Scale (ERSS)
Edinger-Westphal complex
Edinger-Westphal nucleus
EDiT (electric differential therapy)
EDL (extensor digitorum longus) muscle
EDL (extensor digitorum longus) tendon
Edna towel clamp
EDQ (extensor digiti quinti) muscle
EDQ (extensor digiti quinti) tendon
edrophonium (Tensilon) test
Education, Foundation for Chiropractic (FCE)
educed EEG electrode array
Edwards D-L modular fixator
Edwards D-L modular screw-rod
Edwards hook
Edwards-Levine hook
Edwards-Levine rod
Edwards-Levine sleeve
Edwards procedure
Edwards syndrome
EEA stapler (end-to-end anastomosis)

EEG (see *electroencephalogram*)
EEG focus
EEG frequency
 alpha
 beta
 delta
 theta
EEG leads, nasopharyngeal
EEG telemetry
EFA (Epilepsy Foundation of Amercia)
EFF (electromagnetic focusing field) probe
effacement of cistern
effacement of dural sac
effacement of nerve root sheath
effacement of sulcus
effacement of ventricle
effect
 boxcar (with arterial emboli to the retinal vessels)
 copper wire (in arteriosclerosis of the retina)
 doorstopper
 extrapyramidal side
 fetal alcohol (FAE)
 halo effect on x-ray
 hemispheral mass
 lag
 mass
 on-off effect of L-dopa in parkinsonism
 side
 washboard effect on myelography in cervical spondylosis
 wearing off effect of drugs
efferent digital nerve
Effler-Groves dissector
Effler-Groves hook
effleurage massage
effusion
 bloody
 inflammatory joint
 joint
 noninflammatory joint
effusion *(cont.)*
 recurrent
 subdural
Eftekhar broken femoral stem technique
Egawa sign
egg-crate mattress
Eggers plate
Eggers screw
Eggers splint
Eggers tendon transfer technique
égoïsme à deux
egress of arthroscopic fluid
EHL (extensor hallucis longus) muscle
EHL (extensor hallucis longus) tendon
Ehlers-Danlos syndrome
Ehrenfeld disease
Eicher femoral prosthesis
eighth cranial nerve (auditory and vestibular divisions)
eighth nerve dysfunction
eighth nerve tumor
EIP (extensor indicis proprius) muscle
EIP (extensor indicis proprius) tendon
ejector, Cloward dowel
Ekbom restless leg syndrome
Elan-E power drill
elastic bandage
elastic stable intramedullary nailing (ESIN)
Elastic Foam bandage
elasticity, modulus of
elasticum, pseudoxanthoma
Elastikon elastic tape for pressure dressings
elastin
Elasto-Gel shoulder therapy wrap
elastofibroma dorsi
elastomer, thermoplastic (TPE)
Elastomull elastic gauze bandage
Elastomull splint
elbow
 baseball pitcher's
 boxer's
 floating

elbow *(cont.)*
  golfer's
  javelin thrower's
  Little Leaguer's
  milkmaid's
  reverse tennis
  tennis
  thrower's
  wrestler's
elbow prosthesis (see *prosthesis*)
elbow replacement
elbow-wrist-hand orthosis
elective mutism
  complete
  relative
elective surgery
electric differential therapy (EDiT)
Electri-Cool cold therapy system
electric wheelchair
electrical impedance
electrical potential
electrical stimulation of bone
electrical stimulation therapy
electro-oculogram (EOG)
electro-oculographic analysis
Electro-Link joint wrap
electrocautery apparatus
electrocautery, Aspen
electrocerebral activity
electrocerebral inactivity (ECI)
electrocerebral silence (ECS)
electrocoagulation, radiofrequency (RFE)
electrocorticogram (ECoG)
electrocorticographic electrode
electrode, electrodes
  A (auricular)
  A_1
  A_2
  active recording
  AF (anterior frontal)
  AF_3
  AF_4
  AF_7

electrode *(cont.)*
  AF_8
  AF_z
  Ag-AgCl (silver-silver chloride)
  anterior temporal surface
  Aspen laparoscopy
  auricular (A)
  average potential reference of
  average reference
  ball
  bar
  basal
  bipolar
  bipolar depth
  C (central)
  C_1-C_6
  C_z
  chains of
  chlorided silver
  clip
  coaxial
  common reference
  concentric
  cortical
  CP (centroparietal)
  CP_1-CP_6
  CP_z
  DBS (deep-brain-stimulating)
  delta
  depolarizing
  depth
  dermal
  diamond-shaped
  disc
  disposable
  earlobe
  EEG
  electrocorticographic
  electroencephalogram (EEG)
  electromyogram (EMG)
  epidural
  epidural peg
  equipotential
  exploring

electrode *(cont.)*
F (frontal)
F_1-F_{10}
F_z
FC (frontocentral)
FC_1-FC_6
FC_z
FF (frontopolar-frontal)
4-contact strip
Fp (frontopolar)
Fp_1-Fp_2
Fp_z
FpF (frontopolar-frontal)
frontal (F)
frontocentral (FC)
frontopolar (Fp)
frontotemporal (FT)
FT (frontotemporal)
FT_7-FT_{10}
G_1
G_2
gold
gold bulb
gold-coated
Goldmann-Offner reference of
grid of
ground
grounding
impedance of
inactive
indifferent
interhemispheric
intracerebral
I_z
International 10-20
Levin thermocouple cordotomy
loop
M_1 (mastoid)
M_2 (mastoid)
mandibular angle
mastoid (M)
metal cup
metal surface
monopolar

electrode *(cont.)*
multipolar
Nashold TC
nasopharyngeal
neck muscle
needle
neighboring
neutral
Nichrome cylindrical
noncephalic reference
nonpolarizable
N_z
O (occipital)
O_1
O_2
O_z
P (parietal)
P_1-P_{10}
P_z
pad
peak N20
peak N22
peak N9
peak P14
peak P38
peg
pipe-cleaner
placement of EEG
platinum
platinum-coated
PO (parieto-occipital)
PO_3
PO_4
PO_7
PO_8
PO_z
prefrontal
recording
reference recording
resistance of
ring
rod
scalp
scalpel

electrode *(cont.)*
  silver chloride-coated
  silver-silver chloride
  silver-ball
  Silverman placement of
  Sluyter-Mehta thermocouple
  sphenoid
  sphenoidal
  stainless steel
  Stephenson-Gibbs reference
  stereotactic or stereotaxic
  sternospinal reference
  stick-on
  stigmatic
  stimulating
  subdural
  suction
  surface
  T (temporal)
  T_7-T_{10}
  temporal (T)
  10-20 System of
  tin-coated
  TP (temporal-posterior)
  TP_7-TP_{10}
  true anterior temporal
  21 recording
  unchlorided silver
  uninsulated tip of
  VPL (ventroposterolateral) thalamic
  watchband
  zero potential reference
electrode grid
electrode headband
electrode insertion point
electrode paste
electrode placement
electrode polarization
electrodecremental seizure
electrodesiccated bleeding points
electrodiagnostic studies
electrodynography
electroencephalogram (or -graph) (EEG) (see also *montage*, *potential*, *wave*)
  absolute band frequency on
  absolute band value on
  absolute peak frequency on
  after-discharge on
  age-related changes on
  alerting maneuver during
  aliasing on
  all-night sleep recording with
  alpha activity on
  alpha blocking on
  alpha coma pattern on
  alpha frequency range on
  alpha rhythm on
  alpha spindles on
  alpha variant rhythm on
  alphoid rhythm on
  ambulatory recording of
  amplifier drift on
  anachronism on
  anterior slow dysrhythmia on
  aperiodic waves (or complexes) on
  apiculate waveform on
  arceau rhythm on
  arch-shaped waves on
  arrhythmic delta activity on
  arrhythmical repetitive
  arrhythmical waves on
  artifact-free
  artifact on
  asymmetric waveforms on
  asynchronous bursts of activity on
  asynchronous delta waves on
  asynchronous epileptiform activity on
  asynchronous sleep spindles on
  asynchronous slow waves on
  asynchronous spindles on
  asynchronous waves on
  attack-specific potential on
  attenuation of alpha rhythm on
  attenuation of background rhythm on
  atypical spike-and-wave complexes

electroencephalogram *(cont.)*
audiovisual (AVEEG)
auditory stimulation during
augmenting response on
autoregressive signal analysis of
background disorganization on
BAERs during
Bancaud phenomenon on
barbiturate-induced activity on
baseline distortion on
baseline on
baseline waking
benign epileptiform pattern on
benign epileptiform transients of sleep (BETS) on
beta activity on
beta coma pattern on
beta rhythm on
beta spindles on
BETS (benign epileptiform transients of sleep) on
bilateral activity on
bilateral synchrony on
bilaterally synchronous bursts on
bilaterally synchronous discharges
bilaterally synchronous slow waves
bilaterally synchronous waves on
biparietal hump on
biphasic discharges on
biphasic wave on
biphasic waveforms on
BIPLEDs (bihemispheric PLEDs) on
bipolar montage on
bipolar recording of
bisynchronous bursts on
bisynchronous delta waves on
bisynchronous slow waves on
bisynchronous waves on
blink artifact on
blood oxygen saturation during
blood pressure monitoring during
brain stem auditory evoked potentials during

electroencephalogram *(cont.)*
burst phase on
burst-suppression pattern on
bursts between hemispheres on
bursts of delta waves on
bursts of REM on
bursts of theta waves on
bursts on
cable telemetry
calibration pulse on
cardiac pacemaker artifact on
cassette recording of
C-EEG (computerized)
centroid on
centromidtemporal spikes on
centroparietal slow waves on
centrotemporal spikes on
cerebral activity on
cerebral blood flow measurement during
cerebral death on
cerebral potentials on
channels on
Ciganek rhythms on
circumferential bipolar
clinical
clipping of waves on
clonic phase-spike and wave on
closed circuit TV (CCTV) recording during
comb rhythm on
common average reference montage
common reference montage on
complex of waves on
compressed spectral array
computer-assisted analysis of
computer-assisted signal analysis of
computerized (C-EEG)
computerized signal analysis of
conductive jelly for
cone waves on
continuous
continuous slow wave pattern on

electroencephalogram (*cont.*)
contoured waveform on
contralateral discharges on
coronal bipolar montage on
cortical spikes on
ctenoids on (silent *c*)
curvilinear distortion on
C_z reference montage on
delta activity on
delta brush pattern on
delta focus on
delta index on
delta occipital pattern on
depth (DEEG)
desynchronization of
desynchronized pattern on
diagnostic
diffuse delta pattern on
diffuse distribution of activity on
diffusely low-voltage
digital
digital signal analysis of
diphasic spikes on
diphasic wave on
direct current (DC-EEG)
discontinuous activity on
disorganized electrical activity on
disorganized pattern on
double-banana montage on
driving response on
drowsiness during
dysmaturity on
dysrhythmia on
dysrhythmic delta activity on
dysrhythmic pattern on
ear reference montage on
ear reference recording during
electrocardiogram during
electrocerebral inactivity (ECI) on
electrocerebral silence (ECS) on
electrodecremental seizure on
electrode-popping artifact on
electrographic maturation seen on

electroencephalogram (*cont.*)
electrolyte gel for
electrolyte jelly for
electrolyte paste for
electro-oculogram (EOG) during
electroretinogram and
EMG by submental monitor during
encoches frontales on
epileptiform activity on
epileptiform burst discharges on
epileptiform event on
epileptiform pattern on
epileptiform spike on
epileptiform waveform on
epileptogenic burst on
epileptogenic focus on
epochs on
evoked potential (EP) mapping of
extracerebral activity on
eye blinks on
eye closing on
eye movement (EM) monitor on
eye opening and closing maneuver
eye opening on
eye position monitoring on
eyelid flutter on
fast alpha variant rhythm on
fast alpha variants on
fast Fourier transform (FFT) analysis
fast waves on
FIRDA (frontal intermittent rhythmic delta activity)
flash stimulation on
flat
flatline
flattening of tracing on
focal activity on
focal epileptiform discharges on
focal interictal epileptiform activity
focal parietal theta rhythm on
focal periodic pattern on
focal sharp waves on
focal slow waves on

electroencephalogram (*cont.*)
focal slowing on
frequency domain mapping of
frontal beta rhythm on
frontal rhythmic theta activity on
frontal sharp transient
frontal sharp waves on
frontocentral slow waves on
fused alpha wave morphology on
galvanic skin response during
gamma rhythm on
generalization on
generalized asynchronous slow waves on
generalized background slowing on
generalized distribution of activity on
generalized epileptiform activity on
generalized epileptiform discharges
generalized fast waves on
generalized flattening on
generalized paroxysmal fast activity
generalized periodic pattern on
generalized slow
generalized spike-and-wave discharges on
generalized spikes
glissando photic stimulation during
glossokinetic artifact on
grape juice for hypoglycemia during
hand movement monitoring during
high-amplitude
high-amplitude transients on
high-filter frequency (HFF) on
high-voltage complexes on
high-voltage pattern on
high-voltage slow pattern on
horizontal dipoles on
hypersynchronous
hyperventilation during
hypnagogic hypersynchrony during
hypoglycemic changes on
hypsarrhythmia on

electroencephalogram (*cont.*)
hypsarrhythmia pattern on
ictal epileptiform activity on
ictal focal epileptiform discharges on
ictal focal slow waves on
ictal pattern on
impedance pneumogram used during
in-phase waves on
independent waves on
indeterminate sleep during
infantile pattern of spikes on
instrumental phase reversal on
interburst interval measurement on
interference on
interhemispheric synchrony on
interictal continuous spikes on
interictal epileptiform activity on
interictal focal epileptiform discharges on
interictal focal slow waves on
interictal generalized epileptiform waves on
interictal spike
interictal temporal lobe spikes on
intermittent focal spikes on
intermittent rhythmical delta activity
intermittent slowing on
intermittent temporal slow waves on
intermixed spike pattern on
intracerebral
intracranial
invariant pattern on
ipsilateral reference montage on
IRDA (intermittent rhythmic delta activity) on
isoelectric pattern on
isopotential line on
Janz response on
jaw jerks on
juvenile pattern of spikes on
K complex on
kappa rhythm on

electroencephalogram (*cont.*)
lambda waves on
Laplacian montage on
larval spike-and-slow waves on
lateral rectus spike on
lateralized activity on
lateralized distribution on
lateralized epileptiform activity on
lateralized slowing on
lateralizing epileptiform discharges
left-sided lead on
lid flutter on
linear
linked ear reference montage on
local slow waves on
localized evoked potentials on
longitudinal bipolar (LB) montage
low-amplitude spikes on
low-filter frequency (LFF) on
low-voltage activity on
low-voltage pattern on
low-voltage slow waves on
M-type (minimal) alpha rhythm on
mean peak frequency on
medium-voltage slow waves on
methohexital given during
MFD (monorhythmic frontal delta) waves on
midline focus of
midline theta rhythm on
midtemporal discharges on
miniblinks on
mirror foci on
monomorphic waves on
monophasic sharp waves on
monorhythmic activity on
monorhythmic frontal delta (MFD) waves on
monorhythmic frontal slowing
monorhythmic pattern on
monorhythmic sinusoidal delta activity on
monorhythmic waves on

electroencephalogram (*cont.*)
MSTs (multifocal sharp transients)
multichannel
multifocal independent spikes on
multifocal sharp transients (MSTs)
multifocal spike discharges on
multifocal spikes on
multiple sleep latency test (MSLT) with
multiple spike-and-slow wave complexes on
multiple spike complexes on
mu rhythm on
nasal thermistor used during
negative vertex spike on
neonatal
non-REM sleep periods on
noncephalic reference montage on
noncerebral activity on
nonepileptiform activity on
nonphysiologic artifact on
nonspecific diffuse slowing on
nonspecific reaction to stimuli on
normalization of
notched rhythmic theta activity on
NREM (nonrapid eye movement) sleep on
O waves on
occasional periodic discharges on
occipital negative
occipital rhythm on
occipital spikes of blind person on
occipital spikes on
occipital waveforms on
OIRDA (occipital intermittent rhythmic delta activity) on
Omni Prep electrolyte gel for
on and off response on
onset bursts on
opposite polarity of signals on
oral thermistor used during
out-of-phase waves on
overreading of

electroencephalogram (*cont.*)
oversampling on
P-type (persistent) alpha rhythm on
paper stop artifact on
paradoxical alpha rhythm on
paradoxical μ (mu) rhythm on
paroxysmal activity on
paroxysmal alpha activity on
paroxysmal beta activity on
paroxysmal delta activity on
paroxysmal discharges on
paroxysmal hypnagogic hyper-synchrony on
paroxysmal pattern on
paroxysmal rhythmical waves on
paroxysmal theta activity on
paste for
pattern sensitivity on
PDA (polymorphic delta activity) on
peak of wave on
pentylene tetrazol given during
period between complexes on
periodic complexes on
periodic discharges on
periodic generalized sharp waves on
periodic lateralizing epileptiform discharges (PLEDs)
periodic slow waves on
persistent alpha rhythm slowing on
perspiration artifact on
phantom spike-and-wave pattern on
phase angle on
phase lag on
phase reversal on
photic driving with
photic stimulation during
photoconvulsive response on
photometrazol test during
photomyoclonic jerking on
photomyoclonic response on
photoparoxysmal response on
photosensitivity during
physiologic artifact on

electroencephalogram (*cont.*)
PLEDs (periodic lateralized epileptiform discharges) on
plotting field of potentials on
polymorphic delta activity on
polymorphic slow activity on
polymorphic waves on
polyphasic sharp wave on
polyphasic spike on
polyphasic transients on
polyphasic waves on
polyrhythmic waves on
polyspike-and-slow-wave complexes
polyspike-and-wave complexes on
polyspike-and-wave discharges on
polyspike complexes on
positive bursts on
positive occipitital spike-like sleep waves on
positive sharp waves on
positive spikes on
posterior beta rhythm on
posterior dominant activity on
posterior slow waves of youth on
posterior theta rhythm on
postictal alpha rhythm slowing on
postictal bisynchronous slow waves
POSTS (positive occipital sharp transients) on
potentials on
projected rhythms on
prominent flash evoked response during
propagation of activity on
pseudoepileptiform activity on
pseudoepileptiform pattern on
pulse wave artifact on
quadrant on
quadriphasic waves on
quantitative analysis of
quantitative (QEEG)
quasi-periodic waves on
quiet sleep during

electroencephalogram (*cont.*)
quiet wakefulness during
R-type (reactive) alpha rhythm on
radiotelemetry
rapid eye movements (REM) during sleep on
recruiting response on
reduction of amplitude on
referential alternating montage on
referential block montage on
referential montage on
referential recording of
relative band frequency on
relative band value on
REM sleep periods on
repetitive flashes of light used on
repetitive spikes on
repetitive waves on
respiratory monitoring during
resting wakefulness during
reversal of polarity on
rhythmic activity on
rhythmic artifacts on
rhythmic temporal theta waves on
rhythmic theta burst of drowsiness
rhythmic theta pattern on
rhythmical midtemporal discharges
rhythmical repetitive
rhythmical slow waves on
rhythmical waves on
rhythmicity of
right-sided lead on
RMTDs (rhythmical midtemporal discharges) on
rolandic dip on
rolandic sharp transient on
rolandic sharp waves on
rolandic spike on
runs of sharp theta activity on
saccadic eye movements on
salt bridges connecting electrodes during
sampling rate on

electroencephalogram (*cont.*)
sawtooth waves on
scalp (SEEG)
scalp-scalp montage on
SDEEG (stereotaxic depth)
seizure focus on
seizure pattern on
SEMs (slow lateral eye movements)
serial recording of
sharp-and-slow-wave discharges on
sharp transients on
sharp wave complexes on
sharp wave focus on
sharp waves on
sharply contoured waveform on
shut eye waves on
sigma rhythm on
signal analysis of
simultaneous opposite polarities on
simultaneous video monitoring during
simultaneous waves on
sinusoidal appearing sleep spindles
sinusoidal waves on
sleep
sleep-deprived
sleep onset REM period (SOREMP) on
sleep spindle on
slow alpha variant on
slow alpha variant rhythm on
slow anterior dysrhythmia on
slow lateral eye movements (SLEMs) on
slow-spike-and-wave complex on
slow spike-and-wave discharges on
slow wave sleep during
slow waves on
small sharp spikes (SSS) on
somatosensory stimulation during
SOREMP (sleep onset REM period)
spatial resolution on
spectral analysis of

electroencephalogram (*cont.*)
spectral averaging on
spectral edge frequency on
spicules on
spike-and-dome complexes on
spike-and-wave complex on
spike-and-wave discharges on
spike averaging on
spike focus on
spike-like artifact on
spike-wave discharges on
spikes on
spiking activity on
spiky transients on
spindle bursts on
spindle coma pattern on
spindle-like activity on
spindle-shaped activity on
spindles on
sporadic generalized slow waves on
sporadic waves on
squeak phenomenon on
SREDA (subclinical rhythmic epi– leptiform discharges of adults) on
SSS (small sharp spike) on
stage I (drowsiness) sleep on
stage II (light sleep) sleep on
stage III (deep sleep) sleep on
stage IV (very deep sleep) sleep on
stage W (wakefulness) sleep on
startling noise used during
startling stimulus used during
stepwise photic stimulation during
stereotactic (SEEG) (or stereotaxic)
stereotactic depth (SDEEG)
stereotyped spikes on
stimulus artifact on
stroboscopic flashes of light used on
subclinical rhythmical discharge on
subclinical seizure
submental EMG activity monitor used during
superimposed on

electroencephalogram (*cont.*)
suppression-burst pattern on
surface electromyogram (EMG) during
synchronous bursts of
synchronous waveforms on
synchronous waves on
tactile stimulation during
TB (transverse or triangular bipolar) montage on
telephone transmission of
temporal μ (mu) rhythm on
temporal negative sharp transient
temporal positive sharp transient on
temporal sawtooth pattern on
temporal spikes on
theta activity on
theta bursts on
theta coma pattern on
theta rhythm on
thoracic strain gauge monitor
time domain mapping
topographic mapping of
trains of mu (μ) rhythm on
trains of waves on
transient on
transitional sleep during
transverse bipolar (TB) montage on
triangular bipolar (TB) montage on
triangular waves on
triphasic wave pattern on
triphasic waves on
trough of wave on
true phase reversal on
unilateral bursts on
unilateral epileptiform activity on
unilateral focus of activity on
unilateral sleep spindles on
unilateral spikes on
unilateral waveforms on
unipolar montage on
V (vertex) waves on
VEPs (visual evoked potentials)

electroencephalogram *(cont.)*
- VERs (visual evoked responses) during
- vertex sharp
- vertex sharp transients on
- vertex waves on
- very low voltage
- video
- visual evoked potentials (VEPs) on
- visual evoked responses (VERs) on
- visual stimulation during
- voltage calibration on
- voltage suppression on
- wakefulness during
- waking
- waking portion of sleep
- wave-and-spike phantoms on
- waveform superimposed on wave form on
- wicket rhythm on
- wicket spike on
- wickets on
- widespread beta
- widespread distribution of activity on
- zero line on

electroencephalograph, -graphy
electroencephalographer
electrogalvanic stimulation
electrogoniometer, biaxial
electrographic maturation on EEG
electrographic seizure activity
electrolyte gel for EEG
electromyogram, electromyography (EMG)
- antidromic conduction velocity on
- antidromic sensory response on
- belly-tendon method on
- biphasic waves on
- brachial plexus motor study on
- CMAP (compound motor action potential) on
- CNAP (compound nerve action potential) on
- complex repetitive discharges on
- conduction velocity on
- cortical
- CRDs (complex repetitive discharges) on
- decline in latency on
- decreased motor amplitude on
- decreased sensory amplitude on
- decrement at rest on
- decrescendo discharges on
- distal motor latency on
- dive-bomber discharges on
- dynamic gait
- endplate spikes (or noise) on
- Erb point stimulation on
- F wave latency on
- F wave on
- F wave persistence on
- F wave study during
- fasciculation potential on
- femoral nerve motor study on
- fiber density on
- fibrillation potential on
- fibrillations on
- G1 (active recording electrode) on
- G2 (reference recording electrode)
- H reflex latency on
- H reflex study during
- high-frequency discharges on
- high-frequency repetitive discharges
- increased recruitment on
- jitter on
- lumbosacral root motor study on
- M wave latency on
- M wave study on
- mean consecutive difference (MCD)
- median mixed nerve action potential
- median motor response on

electromyogram *(cont.)*
median sensory response on
mixed nerve conduction study on
motor latency on
motor response amplitude on
motor unit recruitment on
MUAP (motor unit action potential) on
muscle belly-tendon method for
muscle interference pattern on
musculocutaneous nerve sensory study during
myokymic discharges on
myopathic interference pattern on
myotonic discharges on
needle
nerve conduction time on
neuromuscular transmission time on
neuromyotonic discharges on
neuropathic interference pattern on
Nomad
onset conduction velocity on
onset latency of potential on
onset of stimulus on
orthodromic conduction velocity on
orthodromic sensory response on
pattern of firing on
peak conduction velocity on
peak latency of potential on
peak-to-peak amplitude on
peroneal nerve motor study on
polyphasic potentials on
positive sharp waves on
postactivation exhaustion on
postactivation facilitation on
postactivation increment on
postexercise facilitation on
posttetanic facilitation on
prolonged distal latency on
prolonged latency on
pseudofacilitation
radial nerve motor/sensory

electromyogram *(cont.)*
recruitment ratio on
reduced conduction velocity on
repetitive discharges on
right-left latency difference on
rise time on
S (stimulating electrode) on
S1 (distal stimulation site) on
S1/H-reflex latency on
S2 (proximal stimulation site) on
saltatory nerve conduction on
saphenous nerve sensory study on
satellite potential on
sciatic nerve motor study on
sensory conduction latencies on
sensory latency on
sensory nerve conduction study during
serrated potential on
short potentials on
single-fiber (SFEMG)
small amplitude polyphasic motor units on
SNAP (sensory nerve action potential) on
spikes without baseline crossings on
SSR (sympathetic skin response) on
superficial peroneal nerve sensory study on
surface
sural nerve sensory study on
terminal latencies on
tibial nerve motor/sensory study on
triphasic wave on
turns on
ulnar nerve motor/sensory
electromyographic feedback
electromyographic incomplete interference pattern
electromyographic insertion study
electromyographic potentials
electromyographic recording

electromyographic study
electromyography (EMG)
electron beam therapy
electroneuromyography
electronystagmogram
electronystagmography (ENG)
electrophysiologic integrity (of nerve impulse)
electrophysiologic test
electrophysiological localization of nerve lesions
electrophysiology nerve study
electroretinogram (ERG)
  flash
  pattern
electrostimulation for nonunion of fracture
electrotherapy unit, Dial Away Pain 400
Elekta stereotactic head frame (*not* Elektra)
elements, neoplastic destruction of spinal
elephantiasis neurofibromatosa
elevate on pillows
elevation, head
elevation of extremity
elevator
  Adson
  Adson periosteal
  angular
  Aufranc periosteal
  Bennett
  Bennett bone
  Bethune periosteal
  Blair
  blunt
  bone
  Bowen periosteal
  Bristow periosteal
  Brophy periosteal
  Buck
  Buck periosteal
  Cameron-Haight periosteal

elevator *(cont.)*
  Campbell periosteal
  Carroll-Legg periosteal
  Chandler bone
  Cheyne periosteal
  chisel
  chisel-edge
  Cloward osteophyte
  Cloward periosteal
  Cobb periosteal
  Cobb spinal
  Cohen periosteal
  Converse periosteal
  Coryllos-Doyen periosteal
  Cottle-MacKenty
  Crawford dural
  Crego
  curved periosteal
  Cushing-Hopkins periosteal
  Cushing Little Joker
  Cushing periosteal
  Cushing pituitary
  Cushing staphylorrhaphy
  D'Errico periosteal
  Darrach
  Davidson-Sauerbruch-Doyen periosteal
  Dawson-Yuhl-Key
  Dawson-Yuhl periosteal
  Doyen rib
  duckbill
  dural
  Duval
  Farabeuf periosteal
  Fomon periosteal
  fracture reducing
  Frazier dural
  Freer periosteal
  Freer septal
  Gardner
  Hajek-Ballenger septal
  hand
  Harrington spinal

elevator (cont.)
- Henahan
- Herczel rib
- Hibbs chisel
- Hoen periosteal
- Iowa University periosteal
- J-periosteal
- Jannetta duckbill
- joker periosteal
- Joseph periosteal
- Kahre-Williger periosteal
- Kennerdell-Maroon
- Key periosteal
- Kirmission periosteal
- Kocher
- Lambotte
- lamina
- Lane periosteal
- Langenbeck periosteal
- Lempert periosteal
- Lewis periosteal
- Locke
- Love-Adson periosteal
- lumbosacral fusion
- MacKenty periosteal
- Malis
- Matson-Alexander
- Matson rib
- McGlamry
- Mead periosteal
- Molt periosteal
- Moore bone
- nasal
- OSI Extremity
- osteophyte
- Penfield
- periosteal
- Phemister
- Presbyterian Hospital staphylorrhaphy
- Ray-Parsons-Sunday staphylorrhaphy
- Rhoton
- rib

elevator *(cont.)*
- Roberts-Gill periosteal
- Rochester lamina
- Rochester spinal
- Rosen
- round-tapped periosteal
- Sauerbruch rib
- Sayre periosteal
- Scott-McCracken periosteal
- Sebileau periosteal
- Sedillot periosteal
- septal
- Sheffield hand
- Sisson fracture reducing
- spinal
- staphylorrhaphy
- straight periosteal
- Sunday staphylorrhaphy
- Swanson
- T handle
- Tegtmeier
- Tenzel
- Tronzo
- von Langenbeck periosteal
- Ward periosteal
- Wiberg periosteal
- wide periosteal
- Willauer-Gibbon periosteal
- Williger periosteal
- Woodson
- Yankauer periosteal
- Yasargil

elevator-dissector

elevator-periosteotome

elevatus
- iatrogenic
- metatarsus
- metatarsus primus

eleventh cranial nerve (spinal accessory nerve)

Elihorn Maze Test

ELISA (enzyme-linked immunosorbent assay) test

Elite Farley retractor for spinal
  surgery
Elite knee brace
Elizabethtown method osteotomy
Elliott femoral condyle blade plate
Elliott plate
ellipsoid joint
elliptical
Ellis Jones peroneal tendon technique
Ellis technique for Barton fracture
Ellison lateral knee reconstruction
Elmslie-Cholmeley foot procedure
Elmslie peroneal tendon operation
Elmslie-Trillat patellar procedure
elongata, plica alaris
elongation derotation flexion
eloquent areas of the brain
ELP broach
ELP femoral prosthesis
ELP stem for hip arthroplasty
Elsberg brain cannula
Elsberg ventricular cannula
Ely heel-to-buttock test
EM (eye movement) monitor used
  during EEG
EMA (epithelial membrane antigen)
  antibody
EMA immunostain
embarrassment
  circulatory
  cord
  nerve root
  respiratory
embarrassment of midbrain function
embolectomy
embolic cerebral infarction
embolic material, nidus of
embolic stroke
embolism
  air
  cerebral fat
  cholesterol
  fat
  intracranial
  polyurethane foam

embolism *(cont.)*
  pulmonary (PE)
  retinal
  silent cerebral
embolization
  balloon
  flow-directed
  microvascular
  super selective
embolus (pl. emboli)
embouchure
embryonal tumor
embryonic neural ectoderm
EMC (encephalomyocarditis)
  encephalitis
Emed-F foot force measurement system
emergency closed manipulative measure
emergency department
emergency room area, minor (MERA)
emergent, emergently
Emery-Dreifuss disease
Emery-Dreifuss dystrophy
emetic center
EMG (electromyogram, electro-
  myography)
eminence
  hypothenar
  medial
  thenar
  tibial
  wasting of hypothenar
  wasting of thenar
Emmon osteotomy
emotional deficits
emotional dependence
emotional dysinhibition
emotional lability
emotional lability following infectious
  neurologic disease
empirical
empty sella syndrome
empyema
  spinal
  subdural
EMS (encephalomyosynangiosis)

EMS (eosinophilia-myalgia syndrome)
emulsified
en bloc resection
en bloc turning in parkinsonism
en face
en plaque, meningioma
ENA (extractable nuclear antigen) test
encapsulated brain abscess
encephalalgia
encephalatrophy
encephalauxe
encephalic
encephalitic
encephalitis (pl. encephalitides) (see also *encephalitis, viral*)
  acute disseminated
  acute necrotizing
  benign myalgic
  bulbar
  California
  Central European
  chronic subcortical
  CMV (cytomegalovirus)
  Colorado tick fever
  cortical
  Coxsackie A
  Coxsackie B
  cytomegalovirus (CMV)
  Dawson inclusion body
  dengue
  diffuse necrotizing
  eastern equine
  EMC (encephalomyocarditis)
  epidemic
  Epstein-Barr virus
  focal
  fulminant
  Hayem
  hemorrhagic
  herpes simplex virus (HSV)
  herpes zoster
  herpetic
  HSV (herpes simplex virus) type II
  Ilheus

encephalitis *(cont.)*
  infantile
  infectious hepatitis
  infectious mononucleosis
  influenza
  influenzal
  Japanese
  Japanese B
  LaCrosse virus
  lead
  Leichtenstern
  limbic
  louping ill
  lymphogranuloma venereum
  measles
  mumps
  Murray Valley (Australian X)
  Mycoplasma pneumoniae
  necrotizing
  poliomyelitis
  postinfectious
  postvaccinal
  psittacosis
  purulent
  pyogenic
  rabies
  Rasmussen
  rubella
  rubeola
  Schilder
  St. Louis
  Strümpell-Leichtenstern
  subacute inclusion body
  suppurative
  tick-borne
  toxoplasmic
  vaccinal
  van Bogaert
  varicella-zoster
  Venezuelan equine
  viral
  West Nile
  western equine
  yellow fever

encephalitis, viral (see also *encephalitis*)
  Australian X
  California
  Colorado tick fever
  Coxsackie A
  Coxsackie B
  Creutzfeldt-Jakob
  cytomegalovirus (CMV)
  dengue
  eastern equine
  ECHO (enteric cytopathic human orphan)
  encephalomyocarditis (EMC)
  herpes simplex (HSV)
  herpes zoster
  Ilheus
  infectious hepatitis
  infectious mononucleosis
  influenza
  Jakob-Creutzfeldt
  Japanese B
  kuru
  louping ill
  lymphocytic choriomeningitis
  measles
  mumps
  Murray Valley
  poliomyelitis
  progressive multifocal leuko-
  J encephalopathy (PML)
  rabies
  slow virus
  St. Louis
  subacute sclerosing panencephalitis (SSPE)
  tick-borne
  Venezuelan equine
  West Nile
  western equine
  yellow fever
encephaloarteriography
encephalocele
  anterior fontanelle
  cranial vault
encephalocele *(cont.)*
  ethmoidal
  frontoethmoidal
  frontosphenoidal
  interfrontal
  interparietal
  intranasal
  middle fossa
  nasoethmoidal
  nasofrontal
  naso-orbital
  occipital
  posterior fontanel
  sphenoethmoidal
  sphenomaxillary
  spheno-orbital
  suboccipital
  temporal
  transethmoidal
  transsphenoidal
encephalocele with cranium bifidum
encephaloclastic lesion
encephalocystocele
encephalodialysis
encephaloduroarteriosynangiosis (EDAS)
encephalodysplasia
encephalogram
encephalography
encephaloid
encephalolith
encephaloma
encephalomalacia, macrocystic
encephalomeningitis
encephalomeningocele
encephalomeningopathy
encephalometer
encephalomyelitis
  acute disseminated (ADEM)
  acute hemorrhagic
  ascending
  benign myalgic
  disseminated
  granulomatous

encephalomyelitis *(cont.)*
- Leigh subacute necrotizing
- postinfectious
- postmeasles
- postvaccinal
- rabies postvaccinal
- toxoplasmic
- varicella zoster
- viral

encephalomyeloneuropathy
encephalomyelopathy
- postinfection
- postvaccinial
- subacute necrotizing

encephalomyeloradiculitis
encephalomyeloradiculopathy
encephalomyeloradiculoneuritis
encephalomyocarditis (EMC)
- encephalitis

encephalomyocarditis (EMC) viral
- encephalitis

encephalomyopathy, mitochondrial
encephalomyosynangiosis (EMS)
encephalon
encephalonarcosis
encephalopathic parkinsonism
encephalopathic process, diffuse
encephalopathy
- AIDS
- allergic
- amyotrophic type of spongiform
- anoxic
- biliary
- bilirubin
- childhood
- demyelinating
- diabetic
- dialysis
- diffuse
- Heidenhain type of spongiform
- hepatic (HE)
- hypernatremic
- hypertensive
- hypoglycemic

encephalopathy *(cont.)*
- hyponatremic
- hypoparathyroid
- hypoxic-ischemic (HIE)
- idiopathic
- ischemic-hypoxic
- lead
- Leigh necrotizing
- limbic
- metabolic
- myoclonic
- Nevin-Jones subacute spongiform
- painter's
- pancreatic
- portal-systemic (PSE)
- postanoxic
- postinfectious
- postshunt
- posttraumatic
- postvaccinal
- progressive subcortical
- progressive traumatic
- punch-drunk
- renal
- saturnine
- spongiform
- static
- subacute arteriosclerotic
- subacute necrotizing
- subacute spongiform
- thiamine deficiency (TDE)
- toxic
- transmissible spongiform viral
- traumatic
- uremic
- viral
- Wernicke
- Wernicke-Korsakoff

encephalopuncture
encephalopyosis
encephalorachidian
encephaloradiculitis
encephalorrhagia
encephalosclerosis

encephaloscope
encephaloscopy
encephalosepsis
encephalosis
encephalospinal
encephalothlipsis
encephalotome
encephalotomy
encephalotrigeminal angiomatosis
encerclage
enchondral ossification
enchondroma
enchondromatosis
encoches frontales on EEG
encopresis
encroachment
  bony
  foraminal
encroachment on the spinal cord
endarterectomized vessel
endarterectomy
  carotid (CEA)
  carotid artery
  carotid bifurcation
  eversion
  vertebral
  vertebral artery
Ender femoral fracture technique
Ender nail
Ender rod fixation
Endo-Model rotating knee joint prosthesis
endochondral ossification
endocranium
endocrine myopathy
endocrinopathy
endogenous depression
endolymphatic hydrops
endomysium
endoneural
endoneurial
endoneuritis
endoneurium
endoneurolysis
endoperineuritis
endoprosthesis (see *prosthesis*)
end organs, proprioceptive
endoscope
  Desormaux
  Dyonics rod-lens
endoscopy, stereotaxic
endoskeleton
endosteal revascularization
endosteal surface
endosteum
endotenon
endothelial cell chemotactic factor
endotheliomatous meningioma
Endotrac carpal tunnel release system
endotracheal intubation
endovascular coil
endplate
  hyaline-cartilage (of intervertebral disk)
  vertebral
end point of orthopedic tests
end point (physiologic) nystagmus
end post
end-range limitation of motion
end-stage disorder
end-to-end anastomosis (EEA) stapler
endurance
Enduron acetabular liner
energy, strain
enervation
ENG (electronystagmography)
engagement levels
Engel classification of postoperative seizures
Engelhardt femoral prosthesis
Engelmann disease
Engelmann splint
Engel-May nail
Engel plaster saw
Engen palmar finger orthosis
Engen palmar wrist splint
Engh total hip replacement
engineering, rehabilitation (RE)

English brace
enhanced scan
enhancement with contrast medium
enhancing mass (on CT or MRI scan)
Enker brain retractor
enlarged frontal horns
enlarged vascular channels
enlargement, ventricular
Enlon-Plus
Enneking staging of malignant soft tissue tumor
enophthalmos, unilateral (in migraine)
ensemble of epochs
enteric cytopathic human orphan (ECHO) viral encephalitis
enthesitis
enthesopathy
entrapment
  lateral
  nerve
  patellar
  PIN (posterior interosseous nerve)
  popliteal
  posterior tibial nerve
  soft tissue
  suprascapular nerve
  ulnar nerve (at the elbow)
entrapment mononeuropathy
entrapment myopathy
entrapment neuropathy
entrapment of nerve
entrapment syndrome
entrapped plantar sesamoid
enucleate
enucleation
enucleator
  Hardy
  Hardy micro
  Marino transsphenoidal
  Rhoton
  transsphenoidal
envelope
  soft tissue
  stem
environmental assessment
enzyme
  cholinergic
  lysosomal (in rheumatoid arthritis)
  proteolytic (in rheumatoid arthritis)
EOG (electro-oculogram)
eosinophilia-myalgia syndrome (EMS)
eosinophilic adenoma
eosinophilic granuloma
epaulet
EPB (extensor pollicis brevis) muscle
EPB (extensor pollicis brevis) tendon
ependymal cells
ependymitis
  granular
  purulent
ependymoblastoma
ependymoma
  malignant
  myxopapillary
ependymoma tumor
ephaptic conduction
epicondylar fracture
epicondyle
epicondylitis, lateral
epicortical lesion
epicritic
epicritic function
epidemic Kaposi sarcoma
epidermoid cyst of brain
epidermoid tumor
epidondyle
epicondylitis, medial
epidural abscess
epidural block anesthesia
epidural blood patch
epidural cavity
epidural electrode
epidural hematoma
epidural hemorrhage
epidural implant
epidural mass
epidural space
epidural spinal abscess

epidural steroid block
epidural venography
epidurography
epigastric sensation (prior to seizure)
epilemmal
epilepsia cursiva
epilepsia gravior
epilepsia major
epilepsia minor
epilepsia mitior
epilepsia nutans
epilepsia partialis continua
epilepsia partialis continua seizure
epilepsia tarda
epilepsy (see also *seizure*)
  abdominal
  absence
  acquired
  activated
  alcohol-precipitated
  alcoholic
  amygdalar
  anterior polar-amygdalar
  arithmetical
  automatic
  benign childhood
  benign familial myoclonic
  benign focal
  benign rolandic
  Bravais-jacksonian
  centrencephalic
  centrotemporal (rolandic)
  childhood
  chronic
  cingulate
  clouded state
  communicating
  cortical
  cryptogenic myoclonic
  cursive
  dacryocystic
  Dark Warrior
  dementia in
  deterioration

epilepsy *(cont.)*
  diencephalic autonomic
  diurnal
  dorsolateral
  early traumatic
  essential
  extrinsic
  familial progressive myoclonic
  focal
  focal cerebral
  focal motor with march
  frontal lobe
  gelastic (laughing seizures)
  generalized
  genetic
  glassy stare of petit mal
  grand mal
  GTC (generalized tonic-clonic)
  haut mal
  hippocampal
  hysterical
  idiopathic generalized
  impulsive petit mal
  insular
  intractable
  intrinsic
  Jackson
  jacksonian
  juvenile
  juvenile myoclonic
  Koshevnikoff
  Lafora inclusion body
  larval
  laryngeal
  late traumatic
  latent
  Lundborg myoclonic
  major
  matutinal
  menstrual
  mesiobasal limbic
  minor
  motor cortex
  musicogenic

epilepsy *(cont.)*
myoclonic
myoclonic-astatic
myoclonus
Nintendo
nocturnal
occipital
occipital paroxysms with
opercular
orbitofrontal
organic
paroxysmal patterns of
pattern-induced
perceptive
petit mal
photic
photogenic
photosensitive
physiologic
postanoxic
posttraumatic
precipitation of
primary reading
primary rhinencephalic psychomotor
procursive
progressive familial myoclonic
progressive myoclonic
provocative tests for
psychic
psychomotor
psychomotor variant of
quiritarian
reading
reflex
rolandic
running
secondary reading
sensorial
sensory
serial
situation-related
spinal
supplementary motor
symptomatic

epilepsy *(cont.)*
tardy
television-induced
temporal lobe (TLE)
temporolimbic
thalamic
tonic
tornado
traumatic
uncinate
Unverricht-Lundborg myoclonus
Unverricht myoclonic
versive
vestibulogenic
visual
xanthine derivatives-induced
epilepsy-causing brain tumors
Epilepsy Foundation of America (EFA)
epileptic
epileptic attack
epileptic automatism
epileptic diathesis
epileptic discharge on EEG
epileptic equivalent
epileptic foci
epileptic fugue state
epileptic mania
epileptic march
epileptic neuron
epileptic neuronal aggregate
epileptic prodrome
epileptic syndrome
epilepticus
focal status
furor
globus
status
epileptiform abnormalities on EEG
epileptiform activity on EEG
epileptiform event
epileptiform pattern on EEG
epileptiform response
epileptiform spike on EEG

epileptiform wave form
epileptiform waves on
epileptogenesis
epileptogenic burst
epileptogenic focus
epileptogenic lesion
epileptogenic stimulation
epileptogenic temporal lesion
epileptogenic zone
epileptogenicity, hemispheral
epileptogenous
epileptoid
epileptologist
epileptology
epimysium
epineural covering
epineural repair
epineurial neurorrhaphy
epineurium
epineurolysis, volar
epineurosis
epiphora, in migraine
epiphyseal or epiphysial
epiphyseal disk
epiphyseal fracture (see *fracture*)
epiphyseal growth
epiphyseal hyperplasia
epiphysealis
epiphyseal plate
epiphysial or epiphyseal
epiphysiodesis
  Blount
  bone peg
  percutaneous
epiphysiolysis, distraction
epiphysis (pl. epiphyses)
  capital femoral
  capitular
  Perthes
  slipped
  slipped capital femoral (SCFE)
  stippled
  tibial
epiphysitis
episode
  confusional
  gray-out
  sleep onset
episodic confusion
episodic vertigo
epistaxis (nosebleed)
epitendineum
epitenon
epithelial membrane antigen (EMA)
  antibody
epithelialization, creeping
epithelioid sarcoma
Epitrain elbow support
Epitrain knitted elbow support
epitrochlea, epitrochlear
EPL (extensor pollicis longus) muscle
EPL (extensor pollicis longus) tendon
E plane
epoch length on EEG
epochs
  averaged
  ensemble of
epochs of wakefulness
eponychium
Eppright dial osteotomy
EPSP (excitatory postsynaptic potential)
Epstein bone rasp
Epstein curet
Epstein neurological hammer
EQP (extensor quinti proprius) muscle
EQP (extensor quinti proprius) tendon
equilibratory ataxia
equilibrium reactions
Equilizer short leg walking cast
equine encephalitis
  eastern
  Venezuelan
  western
equine gait
equinocavovarus
equinovalgus
  pes
  spastic

equinovarus hindfoot deformity
equinovarus of spastic paralysis
equinovarus, talipes
equinus
  calcaneal
  metatarsus
  talipes
equinus deformity
equipment, adaptive
equipotential line
equivalent
  epileptic
  migraine
equivocal plantar reflex
ER (evoked response)
Erb-Duchenne-Klumpke injury to brachial plexus
Erb-Duchenne palsy
Erb-Duchenne paralysis
Erb-Goldflam disease
Erb injury to brachial plexus
Erb-Landouzy disease
Erb muscular dystrophy
Erb palsy
Erb paralysis
Erb point
Erb sign
Erb spastic paraplegia
Erdheim-Chester disease
ERE (external rotation in extension)
erector spinae
ERF (external rotation in flexion)
ERG (electroretinogram)
ergometer, handgrip
ergometry, bicycle
ergonomically correct chair
ergonomically designed transducer
ergonomics
Erich splint
Erichsen sign
Erickson-Leider-Brown technique
Eriksson cruciate ligament reconstruction
Eriksson knee prosthesis
Eriksson ligament technique
Eriksson muscle biopsy cannula
erosion
  articular
  bony
  osteoclastic
  pedicle (on x-ray)
erosion of articular surface
erosion of the dorsum sellae on x-ray
erosive osteoarthritis
errors
  aphasic
  paralexic
ERSS (Edinburgh Rehabilitation Status Scale)
erysipelas
erythema of joint
erythematous
erythrasma (from *Corynebacterium minutissimum*)
erythrocyte sedimentation rate (ESR)
erythroprosopalgia
eschar
escharotic
escharotomy
escharotomy and fasciotomy
ESCS (epidural spinal cord stimulator)
ESIN (elastic stable intramedullary nailing)
Esmarch bandage
Esmarch plaster knife
Esmarch plaster scissors
Esmarch plaster shears
Esmarch tourniquet
esophagus, corkscrew (diffuse esophageal spasm)
esophoria
ESR (erythrocyte sedimentation rate) test
essential cerebellar tremor
essential myoclonus
essential tremor
essential ultra trace elements (in nutrition)

Esser skin graft
Essex-Lopresti axial fixation technique
Essex-Lopresti calcaneal fracture classification
Essex-Lopresti fixation of calcaneal fracture
esthesia
esthesiometer
  Semmes-Weinstein
  Weber
esthesiometry, depth-sense
esthesioneuroblastoma
estimated blood loss (EBL)
Estridge biopsy needle
état criblé (atrophy of cerebral tissue)
état lacunaire (multiple small strokes)
état marbré (marble state)
Ethibond suture
Ethiflex suture
Ethilon suture
ethmoidal canal
ethmoidal foramen
ethmoidal meningoencephalocele
ethmoidal nerve
ethylene vinyl alcohol (EVAL)
E-2CS (Edinburgh-2 Coma Scale)
Eulenburg disease
euphoria
Euroglide MKII slide board
evacuation of blood clot
evacuation of hematoma
evacuator
  hematoma
  Hemo-Drain
  Reichert-Mundinger hematoma
EVAL (ethylene vinyl alcohol)
evaluation
  home
  Hughston knee
  neurosurgical
  noninvasive soft tissue
  orthopedic
  orthoptic
  postneurosurgical

evaluation *(cont.)*
  posttreatment neuropsychologic
  preneurosurgical
  pretreatment neuropsychologic
  rehabilitation
  Smith physical capacities (PCE)
  strain gauge
  vocational (VE)
Evans ankle joint instability operation
Evans ankle reconstruction technique
Evans calcaneal lengthening procedure
Evans fracture classification system
Evans tenodesis
EVD (external ventricular drain)
eventration
events, recall of
Evers diet for multiple sclerosis
Evershears surgical instrument
eversion of rearfoot
eversion sprain of the ankle
evert, everted
everyday memory questionnaire
evoked potential recording
evoked potentials
evoked response (ER)
evolution, stroke in
Evolution hip prosthesis
evolving hematoma
evolving stroke
Ewald total elbow replacement
Ewald-Walker kinematic knee arthroplasty
EWHO (elbow-wrist-hand orthosis)
Ewing's sarcoma, estraosseous
ex vacuo, hydrocephalus
EX-FI-RE external fixation device
exacerbate, exacerbated
exacerbation of pain
exam (examination)
examination, Examination (see also *test*)
  Boston Diagnostic Aphasia
  Folstein Mini-Mental Status
  intact neurologic

examination *(cont.)*
  mental status
  Neurobehavioral Cognitive Status
  neurological
  nonfocal neurologic
  ophthalmoscopic
  physiologic neurologic
  visual field
examiner, certified disability
Examining for Aphasia test
exarticulation
excessive diffuse low and medium wave beta activity (on EEG)
excessive joint play
excision (see *operation*)
  split-thickness skin (STSE)
  wedge
excision arthroplasty
excision of intervertebral disk
excision of osteochondroma
excitation
  TCR rebound
  wave of
excitatory lesion
excitatory postsynaptic potential (EPSP)
excitatory synapse
excitomotor cortex
excoriation
excrescence, bony
excretion, SIADH (syndrome of inappropriate antidiuretic hormone)
excursion
  calcaneus
  hindfoot
  range of
Exer-Cor exerciser
exercise, exercises
  active assisted range of motion
  active range of motion (AROM)
  ankle pump
  aquatic
  AROM (active range of motion)
  Calleja

exercise *(cont.)*
  chain reaction
  chin tuck
  closed-chain kinetic
  Codman
  contract/relax
  Crane shoulder
  DeLorme
  external rotation
  gastroc-resistive (gastrocnemius)
  graded
  hamstring-setting
  heel cord stretching
  heel raises
  heel rocks
  hip abductor strengthening
  hook-lying pectoral stretch
  horizontal shoulder abduction
  internal rotation
  inversion-eversion
  isokinetic passive mode
  isometric
  isotonic
  knee extension
  knee pump
  lower abdominal pelvic tilt
  MacKenzie
  muscle-setting
  muscle-strengthening
  myofascial stretching
  passive assistive
  passive range of motion (PROM)
  passive stretch
  pelvic tilt
  pendulum
  plyometric
  PNF (proprioceptive neuromuscular facilitation)
  progressive resistive
  PROM (passive range of motion)
  prone scapular retraction
  pulley
  quad-set (quadriceps-setting)
  quad-strengthening

exercise *(cont.)*
- range of motion
- Regen flexion
- resistive strengthening
- seated scapular retraction
- self-monitored
- straight leg raising
- strengthening
- strenuous
- supported extension
- Tai Chi Chuan
- tendon stretching
- therapeutic
- toe gripping
- toe raises
- translation
- Williams flexion
- wrist stretch

exercise-induced amenorrhea
exercise-induced myokymia
exercise intolerance
exerciser
- continuous anatomical passive (CAPE)
- CPM (continuous passive motion)
- Cybex II isokinetic
- Cybex II+ isokinetic
- Danniflex CPM
- Digi-Flex finger
- Exer-Cor
- ExtendaFLEX
- finger
- JACE shoulder
- jaw
- KineTec clubfoot CPM
- Nelson finger
- NordiCare Enabler
- NordiCare Strider
- Omni-Flexor wrist
- Orthotron
- Powerflex CPM
- Preston Traveler CPM
- strengthening
- Stryker CPM

exerciser *(cont.)*
- Stryker leg
- Therabite jaw
- Toronto Medical CPM
- Wilco ankle
- Zimmer continuous anatomical passive

Exeter bone lavage
Exeter hip prosthesis
exit wound
Exner area
Exner writing center (in brain, middle frontal convolution)
Exo-static cervical collar
exogenous depression
exogenous reaction, acute
exophthalmos
- bilateral
- unilateral

exostectomy
exostosis, exostoses
- blocker's
- bony
- epiphyseal
- hereditary multiple
- hypertrophic
- impingement
- marginal
- retrocalcaneal
- tackler's
- traction
- turret

exotoxin tetanospasmin
expander
- acetabular
- Mentor tissue
- tissue

expanding intracranial mass
expenditure, resting energy (REE)
exploration and debridement
exploration and revision
exploration, posterior fossa
explosivity of behavior
exposure, bone-tendon

expressive aphasia
expressive aphasic disorder
exsanguinate
exsanguinated
exsanguination
exstrophy
ExtendaFLEX CPM exerciser
extended activities of daily living (EADLs)
extended ADLs
extended tibial in situ bypass
extender
  nail
  stem
extension
  capital
  cervical
  flexion and
  headrest
  Hittenberger halo
  outward
  range of
  sitting knee
  suprasellar (of tumor)
  toe plate
extensor, extensors
  apparatus (of fingers and toes)
  mechanism (of hand and foot)
  radial
  ulnar
  wrist
extensor brevis arthroplasty
extensor carpi radialis brevis (ECRB) muscle
extensor carpi radialis brevis (ECRB) tendon
extensor carpi radialis longus (ECRL) muscle
extensor carpi radialis longus (ECRL) tendon
extensor digitorum communis (EDC) muscle
extensor digitorum communis (EDC) tendon
extensor digitorum longus (EDL) muscle
extensor digitorum longus (EDL) tendon
extensor hallucis longus (EHL) muscle
extensor hallucis longus (EHL) tendon
extensor indicis proprius (EIP) muscle
extensor indicis proprius (EIP) tendon
extensor pollicis brevis (EPB) muscle
extensor pollicis brevis (EPB) tendon
extensor pollicis longus (EPL) muscle
extensor pollicis longus (EPL) tendon
extensor quinti proprius (EQP) muscle
extensor quinti proprius (EQP) tendon
extensor retinaculum
extensor wad of three
extensus, hallux
external fixation
external immobilization
external rotation in extension (ERE)
external rotation in flexion (ERF)
external rotation recurvatum test
external ventricular drain (EVD)
external wire fixation
extinction of stimulus
extinction phenomenon
extirpation
  microsurgical
  tumor
extra-articular resection
extracapsular dissection
extracerebral activity on EEG
extracerebral potential on EEG
extracranial carotid occlusive disease
extracranial-intracranial bypass (ECIC)
extractor
  Austin Moore
  bone
  Cherry
  cloverleaf pin
  corkscrew femoral head
  femoral head
  FIN
  Jewett
  Küntscher
  Kalish Duredge wire

extractor *(cont.)*
  Massie
  metatarsal head
  Moore prosthesis
  Nicoll
  Rousek
  staple
  Sven-Johansson
extractor-driver, Schneider
extractor-impactor, Fox
extradural abscess
extradural anastomosis
extradural artery
extradural compartment
extradural defect
extradural hematoma
extradural space
extradural spinal metastasis
extradural tumor
extrafusal fibers
extramedullary hemangioma
extramedullary plasmacytoma
extraneous material
extraocular motility
extraocular muscle palsy
extraocular muscle paresis
extrapyramidal disorder
extrapyramidal side effects
extrapyramidal structures
extrapyramidal system
extrathecal nerve roots
extravasation
extremity, extremities
  lower (LEs)
  upper (UEs)
extrinsic-dominant runners
extrinsic foot muscles
extrinsically powered splint
extrinsics, finger or toe
extrusion, disk
exuberant granulation tissue
exuberant synovium
exudate
  fibrinoid
  perivascular
exude
eye, eyes
  affected
  black
  chemotic (in migraine)
  dancing
  doll's
  downward deviation of
  drifting of
  fixed
  immobile
  lazy (amblyopia ex anopsia)
  raccoon's
  saccadic movements of
  skew deviation of
  sunset
eye blink artifact on EEG
eye blinking, repeated
eye blinks, repetitive
eye closing on EEG
eye deviation, cortical-type
eyeglass-type eyeguards
eyeguards
  closed goggle-type
  eyeglass-type
  polycarbonate
eyelet, rod
eyelid flutter on EEG
eyelid, ptosis of
eye movements
  roving
  smooth pursuit
eye opening on EEG
eye rolling
eyes and head, deviation of
eye swinging conjugately back and forth
Eyler flexorplasty
E-Z Flap cranial bone plate

F, f

Fabco gauze bandage dressing
fabella
fabellofibular complex
fabere (flexion, abduction, external rotation, extension)
fabere sign
fabere test
Fabry's disease
FAC (Functional Ambulation Categories)
face-hand test
facet (also facette)
 inferior medial
 lunate
 scaphoid
facetal imbrication
facet capsule disruption
facetious
facet joint
facet of patella
facet surface of vertebra
facet syndrome
facet tropism
facetectomy, O'Donoghue
face validity of rehabilitation testing
facial dystonia
facial fracture
facial grimaces, repetitive
facial movement weakness
facial myoclonia
facial myokymia
facial nerve (seventh cranial nerve)
facial nucleus
facial palsy, persistent
facial paralysis
 contralateral
 ipsilateral
facial paresthesia
facial reflexes
facial spasm, medial (of Meige)
facies (pl. facies)
 birdlike
 hatchet
 mask (of parkinsonism)
 masklike
 moon
 myasthenic
 myopathic
 myotonic
 parkinsonian
 swan-neck
facilitation, proprioceptive neuromuscular (PNF)
Facilities, Health-Related (HRF)
facility, skilled nursing (SNF)
facing of metacarpal heads: radial, ulnar
facioauriculovertebral (FAV) syndrome
faciobuccolingual dyskinesia
faciohumeral dystrophy
facioplegic migraine
facioscapulohumeral (FSH) muscular dystrophy
faciostenosis
factitious attack
factor
 basal endothelium-derived relaxing
 endothelial cell chemotactic

factor *(cont.)*
  fibroblast growth
  growth hormone releasing (GRF)
  nerve growth (NGF)
  RA (rheumatoid arthritis)
  rheumatoid (RF)
  skeletal growth
factor I, insulin-like growth
factor VIII deficiency
factor IX deficiency
facultative pacemaker theory
fad therapy
fadir (flexion, adduction, internal rotation)
fadir sign
fadir test
FAE (fetal alcohol effects)
Fager pituitary dissector
Fahey-Compere pin
Fahey-O'Brien procedure
Fahey retractor
Fahr disease
FAI (Frenchay Activities Index)
failed back surgery syndrome (FBSS)
failure of conservative management
fainting
Fairbanks changes on x-rays
Fairbanks-Sever procedure
Fajersztajn crossed sciatic sign
falciparum, Plasmodium
falcotentorial meningioma
falling attack
false localizing sign
false negative result (in rehabilitation testing)
false positive result (in rehabilitation testing)
falx
  calcification of
  cerebral
falx cerebri
falx meningioma
familial amyotrophic lateral sclerosis
familial dysautonomia
familial gliomatosis cerebri
familial paroxysmal choreoathetosis
familial sensory radicular neuropathy
familial spastic ataxia
familial spastic paraplegia
familial tremor
fan, macular
fan sign
Fanconi syndrome
fanning of toes
Farabeuf bone-holding forceps
Farabeuf bone rasp
Farabeuf-Collin rasp
Farabeuf-Lambotte bone-holding forceps
Farabeuf-Lambotte raspatory
Farabeuf periosteal elevator
Farabeuf rasp
Faraday shield
faradic (electrical) stimulation
faradic current stimulation
Farber disease
Farber syndrome
Farmer operation
Farrior wire-crimping forceps
FAS (fetal alcohol syndrome)
fascia
  antebrachial
  clavipectoral
  Colles
  crural
  deep
  deltoid
  infraspinous
  investing
  lumbar
  medial geniculate
  palmar
  plantar
  quadratus femoris
  Sibson
  superficial temporalis
  superficial temporoparietal
fascia cruris

fascia lata (but tensor fasciae latae)
fascial arthroplasty
fascial release
fasciaplasty (also fascioplasty)
fasciatome
  Masson
  Moseley
fascicle, nerve
fascicular repair, grouped
fasciculations, muscle-wasting
fasciculi of the cord
fasciculus (pl. fasciculi)
  arcuate (AF)
  fibrous palmar
  palmar fibrous
  lenticular
  longitudinal
  longitudinalis medialis
  medial longitudinal (MLF)
fasciculus cuneatus
fasciculus gracilis
fasciculus lenticularis
fasciectomy, partial
fasciitis
  Dupuytren
  necrotizing
  nodular
  plantar
fasciocutaneous island flap
fasciodesis
fasciogram
fasciola cinerea
fasciorrhaphy
fasciotomy
  compartment
  decompression
  plantar
  subcutaneous palmar
fast component of nystagmus
fast Fourier transform (FFT) analysis of EEG
fastigial pressor response (FPR)
FAST (Frenchay Aphasia Screening Test)
Fas-Trac strips
fast-twitch fibers
fat
  Siri formula for percentage of body
  subcutaneous
FAT (Frenchay Arm Test)
fat embolism, cerebral
fat-free [body] mass (FFM)
fatigability, muscular
fatigue curve
fatigue fracture
fatigue strength
fatigue stress
fat pad
  foveal
  heel
  Hoffa
  infrapatellar
  scalene
fat pad sign (on x-ray)
fatty streak
fatty tumor
faucial sensation
Faulkner curet
faults, sagittal plane
Favoloro-Morse sternal spreader
favor the injured part
Fazio-Londe disease
Fazio-Londe syndrome
FB cast cushion
FBS (failed back syndrome)
FBSS (failed back surgery syndrome)
FC electrode (frontocentral) (FC_1-FC_6, FC_z)
FCE (Foundation for Chiropractic Education)
FCR (flexor carpi radialis) muscle
FCR (flexor carpi radialis) tendon
FCS (full cervical spine) series of x-rays
FCU (flexor carpi ulnaris) muscle
FCU (flexor carpi ulnaris) tendon
FDC (flexor digitorum communis) muscle

FDC (flexor digitorum communis) tendon
FDI (first digital interosseous) muscle
FDI (first digital interosseous) tendon
FDL (flexor digitorum longus) muscle
FDL (flexor digitorum longus) tendon
FDP (flexor digitorum profundus) muscle
FDP (flexor digitorum profundus) tendon
FDQ (flexor digiti quinti) muscle
FDQ (flexor digiti quinti) tendon
FDQB (flexor digiti quinti brevis) muscle
FDQB (flexor digiti quinti brevis) tendon
FDS (flexor digitorum sublimis) muscle
FDS (flexor digitorum sublimis) tendon
FDS (flexor digitorum superficialis) muscle
FDS (flexor digitorum superficialis) tendon
fecal incontinence
febrile convulsion
febrile seizure
Fédération International de Chiropractic Sportif (FICS)
feebleminded
feeblemindedness
feedback, electromyographic (EMG)
feeder arteries
feeders, arterial
feeding artery to aneurysm
feeding branch of artery
feeding vessel
feet
  burning
  calcaneocavus
  flail
  rockerbottom
Feild blade (not Field)
Feild-Lee brain biopsy needle
Feild suction dissector
Feingold diet
Feiss line
F (frontal) electrode
F_1-F_{10} electrode
felon infection
felt
  orthopedic
  rolled
felt collar splint
felt dressing
felt patch
Felty syndrome
femoral aligner
femoral anteversion
femoral canal restrictor (in hip replacement)
femoral condyle, medial
femoral cutter
femoral head amputation
femoral head and neck
femoral head deformity
femoral head, Matroc
femoral jig
femoral nerve stretch test
femoral nerve traction test
femoral prosthesis
femoral pusher
femorocrural graft
femorodistal bypass procedure
femorodistal PTFE graft (polytetrafluoroethylene)
femoroiliac thrombophlebitis
femoropopliteal bypass
femorotibial angle (FTA)
femur (pl. femora)
  apex of head of
  head and neck of
fender fracture
fenestrated Drake clip
fenestrated drape
fenestration saw
Fenton bolt
Ferciot-Thomson excision

Ferguson bone-holding forceps
Ferguson brain suction tip
Ferguson-Frazier suction tube
Ferguson hip reduction
Ferguson-Thompson-King two-stage osteotomy
Fergusson method for measuring scoliosis
Ferkel torticollis technique
Fernandez osteotomy
Ferris Smith bone-biting forceps
Ferris Smith intervertebral disk rongeur
Ferris Smith-Kerrison disk rongeur
Ferris Smith-Kerrison laminectomy rongeur
Ferris Smith rongeur forceps
Ferris Smith-Spurling disk rongeur
Ferris Smith tissue forceps
ferrocalcinosis, familial cerebral
ferromagnetic
festinant quality in parkinsonian speech
festinating gait
festination
fetal alcohol effects (FAE)
fetal alcohol syndrome (FAS)
fetal substantia nigra implants
Fett carpal prosthesis
FF (frontopolar-frontal) electrode
FFC (fixed flexion contracture)
FFM (fat-free [body] mass)
FFT (fast-Fourier transform) analysis of EEG
FHB (flexor hallucis brevis) muscle
FHB (flexor hallucis brevis) tendon
FHL (flexor hallucis longus) muscle
FHL (flexor hallucis longus) tendon
fiber, fibers
  anchoring (of hand)
  annular
  annulospiral
  cerebellar
  collagen

fiber *(cont.)*
  commissural
  contractile
  corticobulbar
  corticospinal
  degeneration of muscle
  demyelinated nerve
  denervated muscle
  extrafusal
  fast-twitch
  frontopontine
  general somatic efferent (motor)
  ghost muscle
  intrafusal (spindle system)
  mossy
  motor (general somatic efferent)
  muscle
  myelinated nerve
  nerve
  nerve root
  parasympathetic pupillary constrictor
  pontocerebellar
  postganglionic gray
  pupillomotor
  ragged-red
  regenerating peripheral
  regeneration of muscle
  retinacular
  secretomotor (parasympathetic)
  Sharpey
  slow C
  somatesthetic
  somatic alpha
  somatic nerve
  spinal sympathetic
  tendinous
  thalamofrontal
  trihelical collagen
  type I muscle
  type II muscle
  unmyelinated nerve
  white
fiber formation, Rosenthal (in leukodystrophy)

fiberglass cast
Fiberlase flexible system for CO_2
  surgical laser
fiberoptic light source
fiber tract dysfunction
fibrillary matrix
fibrillation
fibrillogenesis
fibrils of connective tissue
fibrin glue
fibrin mass
fibrinoid exudate
fibrinolytic agents
fibroarthrosis
fibroblast growth factor
fibroblastic meningioma
fibroblastoma, perineurial
fibrocartilage, triangular
fibrocartilaginous plate
fibrocartilaginous tissue
fibrocollagenous connective tissue
fibroma
  aponeurotic
  chondromyxoid (CMF)
  desmoplastic
  meningeal
  nonossifying
  nonosteogenic
  osteogenic
  periosteal
  subcutaneous
fibroma molle
fibroma molluscum
fibromatosis
  fascial
  infantile dermal
  irradiation
fibromatosis colli
fibromuscular disease
fibromyalgia joint pain
fibromyositis
fibro-osseous tunnel
fibrosarcoma
fibrosed muscles
fibrosis
  meningeal
  periarticular
  posttraumatic
fibrositis, periarticular
fibrous dysplasia ossificans progressiva
fibrous histiocytoma
fibrous palmar fasciculi
fibrous union
fibroxanthoma
fibroxanthosarcoma
fibula, apex of head of
fibular collateral ligament
fibular ostectomy
fibular physes
fibulocalcaneal
fibulotalar ligament
fibulotalocalcaneal (FTC) ligament
Ficat classification of femoral head
  osteonecrosis
Ficat-Marcus grading system
Ficat operation
Ficat stage of avascular necrosis
FICS (Fédération International de
  Chiropractic Sportif)
FID (free induction decay)
fiducial localization system attached to
  stereotactic frame
field, fields
  altitudinal loss of visual
  blind spot in visual
  bloodless
  Brodmann cytoarchitectonic
  central visual
  chiasmal visual
  concentric visual
  confrontation visual
  curtain pulled across visual
  EEG potentials plotting
  irregular loss of visual
  nasal retinal visual
  peripheral (of vision)
  pulsating electromagnetic (PEMF)
  temporal visual

field *(cont.)*
  vertical meridian of visual
  visual
  window shade pulled down on visual
field defect
field gradient
field H of Forel
Fielding-Magliato classification of subtrochanteric fracture
field lock
field of dissection
field of distribution on EEG
field stretcher
fifth compartment
fifth cranial nerve (trigeminal nerve)
  mandibular division
  maxillary division
  ophthalmic division
fighter's fracture
figure 4 position
figure 8 cast
figure 8 dressing
figure 8 interscapular bandage
figure 8 ring harness
fila of nerve roots
file
  bone
  McCain TMJ
filed
filiform
Fillauer bar
Fillauer night splint
filler, shoe
filling factor
filling, venous
film
  Accu-Flo dura
  DuPont Cronex x-ray
  scout
  stress
filter, Greenfield
filtered-back projection
Filtzer interbody rasp
filum terminale
FIM (Functional Independence Measure)
fin of prosthetic stem, lateral
FIN pin extractor
FIN pin guide
final handicap
finder
  angle
  Dasco Pro angle
  gravity-driven angle
  pedicle
finding
  angiographic
  focal
  lateralizing
  specious
fine-angled curet
fine tactile discrimination
fine tactile sensations
finger, fingers
  angle
  baseball
  Dasco Pro angle
  football
  gravity-driven angle
  index
  jammed
  jersey
  little
  long
  mallet
  middle
  pedicle
  pulp of
  pulley of
  replantation of
  replanted
  ring
  sausage (in syringomyelia)
  spider
  stoved
  trigger
finger agnosia

finger agnosis
finger count test
fingerbreadth
finger dexterity
fingerdrop
finger extrinsics
finger fracture
finger intrinsics
fingernail
  base of
  circumferential
finger of tumor
finger opposition
finger pad
finger pursuit drift
finger splint
  malleable metal
  Joint-Jack
fingertip
fingertip amputation
fingertip pad
finger-to-finger test
finger-to-nose test (F to N)
fingertrap
  Chinese
  Japanese
fingertrap suspension
finisher
  Küntscher
  Sven-Johansson
Finkelstein sign for synovitis
Finkelstein test
Finochietto laminectomy retractor
Finochietto rib spreader
FIRDA (frontal intermittent rhythmic delta activity)
firing of neuron
FirmFlex custom orthotic
first compartment
first cranial nerve (olfactory nerve)
first dorsal interosseous
FIRST knee prosthesis
first metatarsal angle
first ray instability
first ray stabilizers (muscles)
first rib resection
first temporal gyrus
first-toe Jones repair
FIRST total knee instrumentation
Fisch bone rongeur
Fisch dural hook
Fisch micro hook
Fisch rongeur
Fischer frame
Fischer ring
Fischer tendon stripper
Fischer ventricular cannula
Fish cuneiform osteotomy technique
Fisher guide
Fisher rasp
Fisher syndrome
fish-mouth drainage
fish-mouth incision
fissura petro-occipitalis
fissura petrosquamosa
fissura spheno-occipitalis
fissuration
fissure
  anterior median (of cord)
  calcarine
  cerebellopontine or cerebellopontile
  choroidal
  displacement of interhemispheric
  hippocampal
  inflammatory process of the superior orbital
  interhemispheric
  lateral
  longitudinal
  neoplastic process of the superior orbital
  rolandic
  superior orbital
  supraorbital
  sylvian
fisticuffs
Fist-Palm-Side Test
Fist-Ring Test

fistula
  arteriovenous (AVF)
  carotid-cavernous sinus
  congential
  CSF (cerebrospinal fluid)
  dural arteriovenous (AVF)
  durocutaneous
  iatrogenic
  intradural arteriovenous
  intradural retromedullary
    arteriovenous
  premedullary arteriovenous
  tangle of
  transdural
fit (see *seizure*)
Fitnet joint testing system
Fitron
fitting
  immediate postsurgical (IPSF)
  prosthetic
  Velcro
five-in-one knee repair
fix and focus attention
fixateur (see *fixator*)
Fixateur Interne fixation system
Fixateur Interne rod
Fixateur Interne screw
fixation (see also *fixator*; *operation*)
  Ace-Fischer
  Ace Unifix
  atlantoaxial
  atlantoaxial rotatory
  Barbour cervical
  Biofix absorbable
  bolt
  bone-ingrowth
  Calandruccio triangular compression
  cementless
  circumferential wire loop
  Cole tendon
  contoured loop
  dynamic
  dynamic external
  ECT (European compression
    technique) internal fracture

fixation *(cont.)*
  Ender nail
  Ender rod
  EX-FI-RE external
  external wire
  four-bar external
  four-point
  fracture
  Galveston sacral
  Georgiade visor halo
  greenstick
  Hammer external
  Herbert bone screw
  Hoffmann external
  hook-pin
  hook-plate
  hydroxyapatite
  internal
  internal fracture
  intrapedicular
  K wire (Kirschner)
  LPPS hydroxyapatite
  Luque loop
  Luque rod
  Luque segmental
  Magerl hook-plate
  Magerl transarticular screw
  Minerva
  minifragment plate
  monofilament wire
  Monticelli-Spinelli leg
  nail
  Olerud transpedicular
  open reduction and internal (ORIF)
  Orthofix
  OrthoSorb pin
  pedicle screw
  Pennig dynamic wrist fixator
  pin
  postural
  Precision Osteolock
  primary metallic
  primary rigid
  Rezinian external
  rigid internal

fixation *(cont.)*
  Rogozinski spinal
  screw
  screw-and-plate
  screw-and-wire
  screw-plate
  segmental spinal
  Seidel intramedullary
  spinal pedicle
  spring
  staple
  static
  suprasyndesmotic
  Suretac shoulder
  tension band
  TiMesh implantable hardware
  transarticular screw
  transpedicular
  transsyndesmotic screw
  triangular external ankle
  variable screw plate (VSP)
  Versa-Fx femoral
  Vidal-Adrey modified Hoffmann
  wire
  Wolvek sternal approximation
  Zickel nail
  ZMS intramedullary
fixation device
fixation nystagmus
fixation of a scoliosis
fixation peg
fixation reflexes
fixation system
fixation wire
fixator
  Ace-Colles external
  Ace-Fischer external
  AO internal
  articulated
  circular external
  Claiborne external
  Clyburn Colles fracture
  D-L internal
  DeBastiani external
  dynamic axial (DAF)

fixator *(cont.)*
  Edwards D-L modular
  external
  external spinal skeletal (ESSF)
  hinged articulated
  Hoffmann external
  Ilizarov
  Ilizarov external
  Kessler external
  mini-Hoffmann external
  mini-Orthofix
  Monofixateur external
  Monticelli-Spinelli
  Olerud internal
  Orthofix external
  Orthofix miniature
  Oxford
  Pennig dynamic wrist
  ReFix stereotactic head
  ring external
  thin-wire Ilizarov
  Thomas
  Vermont spinal (VSF)
  Wagner external
  Wiltse
fixed pupils
fixer, Wagner
flaccid
flaccidity
flaccid paralysis
flaccid weakness
flail digit
flail foot
flail joint
flail shoulder
flake fracture of the hamate
flaking of cartilage in osteoarthritis
Flanagan-Burem apposing
  hemicylindric graft
Flanagan spinal fusion gouge
flange
flap, flaps
  abdominal
  advancement
  Atasoy-Kleinert

flap *(cont.)*
- Atasoy palmar
- Atasoy triangular advancement
- axial pattern
- bilobed
- bipedicle
- bone
- bursal
- butterfly
- Chinese
- cross-finger
- cross-leg
- Dandy myocutaneous scalp
- digital
- dorsalis pedis myofascial
- DRAM (de-epithelialized rectus abdominis) muscle
- extended
- extensor carpi radialis longus
- fascial
- fasciocutaneous island
- free
- free fasciocutaneous
- free latissimus dorsi
- free temporal
- galeal
- gastrocnemius sliding
- gracilis muscle
- groin
- hemipulp
- horseshoe-shaped
- iliofemoral pedicle
- island pedicle
- Kutler digital
- latissimus dorsi musculocutaneous free
- microsurgical free
- modified dorsalis pedis myofascial
- muscle
- musculocutaneous free flap
- musculotendinous
- myocutaneous
- myofascial
- neurovascular island pedicle

flap *(cont.)*
- nutrient
- osteocutaneous free
- palmar
- pectoralis major
- pedicle
- pedicled muscle-tendon
- plantaris longus
- pulp
- radial-based
- radial forearm
- rectus abdominis
- rectus abdominis musculocutaneous free
- rectus muscle
- remote pedicle
- rotational
- rotator
- scalp
- scapular
- segmented
- skin
- Tait
- thenar
- transposition
- triangular
- tumbler
- turned-down tendon
- V-Y advancement
- vascularized
- wraparound

flap congestion

flap graft, Kutler V-Y

flapping tremor

flap tear

flare
- axon
- metaphyseal
- tibial

flare of condyle

flare of trochanter

flareup of disease

flareup of pain

flashback

flashes per second of photic stimulation
flash stimulation on EEG
flash visual evoked response
flat affect
flat EEG recording
flat (isoelectric) EEG record
flat nasolabial fold
Flatau-Schilder disease
flatfoot
  acquired
  adult
  calcaneovalgus
  congenital
  Durham procedure for
  hypermobile
  Kidner
  neonatal
  peroneal spastic
  pronated straight
  rigid
  rockerbottom
  spastic
flatfoot deformity
flatfootedness
flatfoot pathomechanics, juvenile
flatline EEG
Flatt finger/thumb prosthesis
flattened longitudinal arch of foot
flattening, generalized
flattening of EEG tracing
flattening of normal lumbar curve
flaval ligament
flavum, pleating of ligamentum
Flechsig bundle (in cerebellum)
Fleck sign
flesh
  live
  proud
flex against gravity
flexer (see flexor)
Flex-Foam bandage
Flexfoot foot prosthesis
flexibility, waxy
flexible spastic equinovarus deformity
Flexicair bed
Flexilite conforming elastic bandage
flexion
  dorsiflexion
  elongation-derotation
  forced plantar
  neutral
  plantar
  range of
  resisted active
  Riordan finger
  spasmodic
  toe
  uninhibited
flexion against resistance
flexion and extension
flexion contracture
flexion-distraction injury
flexion maneuver on cervical spine
  x-ray
flexion reflex
flexion-rotation-compression
  maneuvers
flexion test
Flexisplint flexed arm board
Flex-Master bandage
flexometer, Moeltgen
flexor, flexors
  capital
  hallux
  snapping thumb
  toe
  X-TEND-O knee
flexor carpi ulnaris (FCU) muscle
flexor carpi ulnaris (FCU) tendon
flexor digitorum profundus (FDP)
  muscle
flexor digitorum profundus (FDP)
  tendon
flexor digitorum superficialis (FDS)
  muscle
flexor digitorum superficialis (FDS)
  tendon
flexor hallucis longus (FHL) muscle

flexor hallucis longus (FHL) tendon
flexor palmar plates
flexor pollicis longus (FPL) muscle
flexor pollicis longus (FPL) tendon
flexor retinaculum
flexor wad of five
flexorplasty
  Bunnell modification of Steindler
  Eyler
  Steindler
flexors and extensors
flip angle
flipper hand
floating traction
floating time (in gait)
floccillation
flocculent foci of calcification
flocculonodular lobe of cerebellum
flocculonodular tumors
flocculus of cerebellum
floor effect in rehabilitation testing
floor of the acetabulum
floor of ventricle
floor, sellar
floppy infant
floppy infant syndrome
florid reactive periostitis
Florida cervical brace
Florida J-24 brace
Florida J-35 brace
Florida J-45 brace
Florida J-55 brace
Flotan thumb
flottant, pouce (floating thumb)
flow
  axoplasmic
  cerebral blood
  cerebrospinal fluid
  collateral blood
  regional cerebral blood (rCBF)
  total cerebral blood (TCBF)
flow images
flowmetry
  Doppler
  laser-Doppler (LDF)
flow of cerebrospinal fluid
flow scan, radionuclide
flow void
FLP (Functional Limitation Profile)
fludeoxyglucose F 18 PET
fluent aphasic speech
fluent paraphasic speech
fluffy rarefaction of Paget's disease (on x-ray)
fluid
  bursal
  cerebrospinal (CSF)
  egress of arthroscopic
  high-signal (on MRI) intratendinous collection of
  joint
  leakage of cerebrospinal
  serous
  subgaleal cerebrospinal
  synovial
FluidAir bed
fluorescein perfusion monitoring
fluorescence, laser-induced
fluorescent treponemal antibody (FTA) test
fluorometry
  fiberoptic
  image intensification
  portable C-arm image intensifier
  two-plane
  video (of swallowing mechanism)
flurry of myoclonic jerks
flush
  heparinized saline
  peroxide
flutes of cannulated screw
flutter
  eyelid
  lid
  ocular
fly-catching movements of the tongue
Flynn technique
FMA cephalometric measurement
FMH (first metatarsal head)
FO (foot orthosis)

foam cell
foam, velvet
foaming at the mouth during seizure
focal activity on EEG
focal cerebral epilepsy
focal damage
focal deficit
focal degenerative change
focal delta slow wave activity (EEG)
focal finding
focal motor seizure
focal neurologic sign
focal plaque-like defect
focal sensory seizure
focal sign
focal status epilepticus
focal weakness
foci of abnormal epileptic neurons
foci of calcification
focus (pl. foci)
  anaplastic
  asynchronous
  bilateral
  centrotemporal paroxysmal
  ectopic seizure
  EEG
  epileptic
  epileptogenic
  hemorrhagic
  mesial frontal
  midline parasagittal
  mirror
  multiple
  occipital
  resection of epileptogenic
  rolandic paroxysmal
  seizure
  sharp wave
  shifting
  spike
  stationary
  unilateral
focus of activity
  midline
  unilateral
Foerster forceps
Fogarty embolectomy catheter
Foix-Alajouanine disease
Foix syndrome
fold
  asymmetric thigh
  flat nasolabial
folia cerebelli
following abililty (of eyes)
following movements
Folstein Mini-Mental Status
  Examination
Foltz catheter
Foltz flushing reservoir
fomentation therapy
Fomon chisel
Fomon periosteal elevator
Fomon periosteotome
Fomon rasp
fontanel, fontanelle
  anterior
  bulging
  closed
  fused
  open
  overriding sutures of
  posterior
  tense
foot
  anesthetic
  architecture of the
  athlete's
  axial compression of the
  ball of
  calcaneocavus
  calcaneovalgus
  cavovarus
  cavus
  Charcot
  clawfoot
  contralateral

foot *(cont.)*
- cosmetically acceptable
- deconditioned
- diabetic Charcot
- drop
- flail
- flatfoot
- flat calcaneovalgus
- flat flexible
- flat neonatal
- flat pronated straight
- flat rigid
- Friedreich
- functional disability of the
- hollow (pes cavus, pes arcuatus, clawfoot)
- hypoflexibility of
- insensate
- ischemic
- Kidner flatfoot
- lateral wedges for sole of heel of
- lift-off of the foot (in gait)
- lobster-claw
- longitudinal arch of
- march
- monodactylous cleft
- Morton
- neuroarthropathic
- peroneal spastic flatfoot
- planovalgus
- plantigrade
- polydactylous cleft
- pronated
- propulsive
- push-off of the foot (in gait)
- Quantum
- revascularization of
- rigid
- rocker (rockerbottom flatfoot)
- rockerbottom
- SACH (solid-ankle, cushioned heel)
- SAFE (stationary attachment flexible endoskeletal)
- serpentine

foot *(cont.)*
- single-axis
- skew
- sole of
- splay
- supporting
- Syme prosthetic
- tabetic
- valgus
- venous pump of the

foot-ankle assembly
foot-ankle complex
football finger
footballer's ankle
footdrop
- paralytic peroneal
- postpartum
- steppage gait due to

footdrop of central origin
footdrop of peripheral origin
footdrop splint
foot dynamics
foot dysplasia
foot intrinsic muscle strength
foot ischemia
Foot Levelers orthotics
foot orthosis (FO)
foot piece
- Bunker
- traction

footplate, metal
foot pound
footprint
- dynamic
- static

footprint analysis
foot progression angle (FPA)
foot prosthesis
foot slap
foot strain
foot strike phase of gait
footwear
forage procedure

foramen (pl. foramina)
  ethmoidal
  intertransverse
  interventricular
  intervertebral
foramen interventriculare
foramen lacerum
foramen magnum herniation
foramen magnum of skull
foramen magnum pressure coning
foramen of Froesch
foramen of Luschka
foramen of Magendie
foramen of Monro
foramen ovale
foramen rotundum
foramen spinosum
foramen, stylomastoid
foraminal encroachment
foraminal space
foraminiferous
foraminotomy, keyhole
foraminulum
Forbes-Cori disease
Forbes disease
Forbes modification of Phemister graft technique
force, forces
  axial compression (loads on spine)
  daltons of (SI units)
  ground reaction
  impact
  lateral translation
  linear translation
  Newton
  pascals of (SI units)
  propulsive
  rotational
  shearing (on sacroiliac joints in runners)
  tension
  torque
  torsional impaction
  transverse plane
forced plantar flexion
forceps
  Acland clamp-applying
  Acufex curved basket
  Acufex rotary biting basket
  Adson bipolar
  Adson-Brown tissue
  Adson clip-introducing
  Adson dressing
  Adson dura protecting
  Adson hemostatic
  Adson hypophyseal
  Adson-Mixter neurosurgical
  Adson rongeur
  Adson tissue
  adventitial
  Aesculap bipolar cautery
  alligator
  alligator grasping
  Allis tissue
  Angell James hypophysectomy
  Angell James reverse-action hypophysectomy
  angled-down
  angled-up
  anterior
  AO reduction
  arthroscopy basket
  arthroscopy grasping
  Asch
  Backhaus towel
  Bacon rongeur
  Baer bone cutting
  Bane rongeur
  Bangerter muscle
  Bardeleben bone-holding
  basket
  bayonet
  bayonet-shaped
  Berens muscle
  Beyer rongeur
  biopsy
  bipolar cautery
  Bircher-Ganske cartilage

forceps *(cont.)*
- blunt
- Boies
- bone-biting
- bone-breaking
- bone-cutting
- bone-grasping
- bone-holding
- bone punch
- bone-splitting
- brain
- brain clip
- brain spatula
- brain tumor
- Brand tendon-holding
- Brand tendon-passing
- Brand tendon-tunneling
- Brigham brain tumor
- Brown-Adson tissue
- Brown-Cushing
- Cairns hemostatic
- Carroll bone-holding
- Carroll dressing
- Carroll tendon-pulling
- Carroll tissue
- cartilage
- Caspar alligator
- cervical punch
- Chandler spinal
- Chandler spinal perforating
- Charnley wire-holding
- Cherry-Kerrison laminectomy
- Citelli punch
- clamp-applying
- Cleveland bone-cutting
- clip-applying
- clip-bending
- clip-cutting
- clip-introducing
- Cloward punch
- Cloward rongeur
- coagulating
- Cone skull punch
- Cone wire-twisting

forceps *(cont.)*
- cranial rongeur
- Crile artery
- cup
- cupped-jaw
- curved
- Cushing bipolar
- Cushing dressing
- Cushing monopolar
- Cushing rongeur
- Cushing tissue
- cutting
- D'Errico bayonet pituitary
- D'Errico hypophyseal
- D'Errico pituitary
- D'Errico tissue
- Dandy scalp hemostatic
- Davis coagulating
- Davis monopolar
- Dawson-Yuhl-Kerrison rongeur
- Dawson-Yuhl-Leksell rongeur
- DeBakey
- Decker alligator
- Decker microsurgical
- DeMartel scalp
- DeMartel scalp flap
- Demel wire-tightening
- Demel wire-twisting
- DeTakats-McKenzie brain clip
- DeVilbiss rongeur
- Dingman bone-holding
- disk
- dissecting
- dressing
- dura protecting
- ear
- Echlin rongeur
- ethmoid
- extracting
- Farabeuf bone-holding
- Farabeuf-Lambotte bone-holding
- Farrior wire-crimping
- Ferguson bone-holding
- Fergusson

forceps *(cont.)*
Ferris Smith-Kerrison
Ferris Smith rongeur
Ferris Smith tissue
fine-tip
Foerster
Fox bipolar
Friedman rongeur
gall duct
Gardner bone
Gerald bipolar
Gerald dressing
Gerald tissue
Gildenberg biopsy
glenoid-reaming
grasping
Greene
Greenwood bipolar and suction
Gruenwald ear
Gruppe wire-crimping
Gunderson bone
Gunderson muscle
Hajek-Koffler bone punch
Halsted artery
Halsted mosquito
Hardy bipolar
Hardy dressing
Hardy microbipolar
Hardy sella punch
Harrison bone-holding
Hartmann mosquito
Heermann alligator
hemostatic
Hibbs bone-cutting
Hinderer cartilage
Hirsch hypophysis punch
Hoen angular
Hoen scalp hemostatic
Horsley bone-cutting
Horsley-Stille bone-cutting
Housepan clip-applying
Howmedica Microfixation System
Hudson
Hunt tumor

forceps *(cont.)*
Hunt-Yasargil pituitary
Hurd bone-cutting
hypophyseal
hypophysectomy
hypophysis punch
Ingraham skull punch
intervertebral disk
Jackson tendon-seizing
Jacobson dressing
Jacobson mosquito
Jannetta alligator
Jannetta bayonet
Jansen-Middleton septal
Jansen monopolar
Jarell
Jarit brain
Jarit tendon-pulling
jeweler's
Johnson brain tumor
Johnson tumor
Juers-Lempert rongeur
Kelly artery
Kern bone-holding
Kern-Lane bone
Kleinert-Kutz rongeur
Kleinert-Kutz tendon
Knight bone-cutting
knotting
Kocher
Lalonde hook
Lambotte bone-holding
laminectomy punch
Landolt spreading
Lane bone-holding
Lane screw-holding
Lane self-retaining bone-holding
Langenbeck bone-holding
Larsen tendon-holding
Leibinger Micro System plate-holding
Leksell rongeur
Lempert rongeur
LeRoy clip-applying

forceps *(cont.)*
LeRoy scalp clip-applying
Lester muscle
Lewin bone-holding
Lewin spinal-perforating
ligamentum flavum
lion
lion-jaw
Liston bone-cutting
Liston-Key bone-cutting
Liston-Littauer bone-cutting
Liston-Stille bone-cutting
Littauer-Liston bone-cutting
Llorente dissecting
Lore suction tube and tip-holding
Love-Gruenwald alligator
Love-Gruenwald intervertebral disk
Love-Gruenwald pituitary
Love-Kerrison rongeur
Lowman bone-holding
Luer rongeur
Luer-Whiting rongeur
Luhr Microfixation System plate-holding
Malis angled-up bipolar
Malis bipolar cautery
Malis bipolar coagulation
Malis irrigation
Malis-Jensen microbipolar
Malis jeweler bipolar
Markwalder rib
Martin cartilage
Mayfield
McCain TMJ
McGee-Priest wire
McGee wire-crimping
McIndoe rongeur
McKenzie brain clip
McKenzie clip-applying
McKenzie clip-bending
McKenzie clip-introducing
meniscus
microartery
microbipolar

forceps *(cont.)*
Micro-One dissecting
microsurgery
Micro-Two
microvascular
Mixter
mosquito
Moynihan
nail-pulling
Nicola
Niro bone-cutting
Niro wire-twisting
Oldberg pituitary
Olivecrona clip-applying and removing
Olivecrona-Toennis clip-applying
Overholt clip-applying
Pean
peapod intervertebral disk
perforating
Perman cartilage
pick-up
pituitary
plain tissue
plate-holding
Poppen
Potts-Smith dressing
Preston ligamentum flavum
punch
Raimondi hemostatic
Raimondi infant scalp hemostatic
Raimondi scalp
Raney coagulating
Raney rongeur
Raney scalp clip-applying
Rhoton bipolar
Rhoton cup
Rhoton-Cushing
Rhoton dissecting
Rhoton-Tew bipolar
rib
Riches artery
Richter laminectomy punch
ring

forceps *(cont.)*
- Rochester-Carmalt
- Rochester-Ochsner
- Rochester-Pean
- rongeur
- Rowe disimpaction
- Rowe glenoid-reaming
- Rowe-Harrison bone-holding
- Rowe modified-Harrison
- Ruskin bone-splitting
- Ruskin-Liston bone-cutting
- Ruskin rongeur
- Ruskin-Rowland bone-cutting
- Russian
- Samuels
- Sauerbruch rib
- scalp
- scalp clip
- scalp flap
- Scharff microbipolar and suction
- Scheicker laminectomy punch
- Schlesinger cervical punch
- Schlesinger rongeur
- Schwartz clip-applying
- Schwartz temporary clamp-applying
- Scoville brain clip-applying
- Scoville brain spatula
- screw-holding
- seizing
- sella punch
- Selverstone rongeur
- Semb bone
- Semb rib
- Semkin tissue
- septal
- sequestrum
- Sewall brain clip
- Sewall clip-applying
- Shutt Mantis retrograde
- skull punch
- Smithwick clip-applying
- smooth-tipped jeweler's
- spatula
- Spence rongeur

forceps *(cont.)*
- spinal perforating
- sponge-holding
- spreading
- Spurling-Kerrison rongeur
- Steinmann tendon
- Stevenson alligator
- Stevenson grasping
- Stille-Horsley bone
- Stille-Liston bone-cutting
- Stille-Luer rongeur
- Stiwer bone-holding
- Storz Microsystems plate-holding
- straight
- Synthes Microsystems plate-holding
- Takahashi
- Take-apart
- taper-jaw
- tenaculum-reducing
- tendon
- tendon-holding
- tendon-passing
- tendon-pulling
- tendon-retrieving
- tendon-seizing
- tendon-tunneling
- three-edge cutting
- thumb
- tissue
- titanium microsurgical bipolar
- Toennis tumor
- tonsil
- toothed tissue
- transsphenoidal bipolar
- Tudor-Edwards bone-cutting
- tumor-grasping
- tying
- Ulrich bone-holding
- Ulrich-St. Gallen
- Van Buren sequestrum
- vascular
- Verbrugge bone-holding
- Walter-Liston
- Walton-Ruskin

forceps *(cont.)*
  Walton wire-pulling
  Weller cartilage
  Wiet cup
  Wilde
  Wilde ethmoid
  Wilde rongeur
  wire
  wire-crimping
  wire-cutting
  wire-extracting
  wire-holding
  wire-pulling
  wire-tightening
  wire-twisting
  Yasargil artery
  Yasargil bayonet
  Yasargil clip-applying
  Yasargil hypophyseal
  Yasargil knotting
  Yasargil micro
  Yasargil tumor
forceps major
forceps minor
forceps occipitalis
forceps posterior
forceps speculum
Ford Hospital ventricular cannula
forearm
forearm lift-assist on prosthesis
forebrain
forefinger
forefoot
  angulation of the
  narrowing of
  splaying of
forefoot adductovarus
forefoot adduction correction test
forefoot adductus
forefoot angulation
forefoot cavus
forefoot digital amputation
forefoot splaying
forefoot striker
forehead
  free-floating
  prominence of
foreign body, retained
Forel, field H of
Forestier bowstring sign
Forestier disease
forgetful
forgetfulness, benign senescent
fork
  carotid
  double-prong
  Gardiner-Brown tuning
  Hardy three-prong
  implant application
  Jannetta
  Rhoton
  three-prong
  tuning
forking of sylvian aqueduct
forks of the circle of Willis
fork strap prosthetic support
formalin, 10% neutral buffered
formation
  brain stem reticular
  bunion
  callus
  Chiari
  gray reticular
  hippocampal
  lateral reticular
  mesencephalic reticular
  midbrain reticular (MRF)
  new bone
  osteophyte
  palisade
  paramedian pontine reticular
  periosteal bone
  pontine parareticular (PPRF)
  reticular
  rouleaux
  villus (in rheumatoid arthritis)
  white reticular
forme fruste

- formication
- formula
  - Abercrombie neuronal cell count
  - Dreyer
  - Siri (for percentage of body fat)
- fornix
- Forrester-Brown head halter
- Forrester splint
- Forte harness
- fortification scotomata
- fortification spectrum during migraine
- forward-head posture
- fossa (pl. fossae)
  - cranial
  - cubital
  - glenoid
  - infratemporal
  - intercondylar
  - interpeduncular
  - lateral cerebral
  - middle cerebral
  - middle cranial
  - pituitary
  - popliteal
  - posterior
  - pterygopalatine
  - rhomboid
  - sphenoidal
  - temporal
- fossae lateralis cerebri
- fossa of Rosenmüller
- fossa of Sylvius
- fossa ovalis
- Foster bed
- Foster frame
- Foster-Kennedy maneuver
- Foster-Kennedy syndrome
- Foster splint
- Foundation, Epilepsy F. of America (EFA)
- Foundation for Chiropractic Education (FCE)
- four-bar fixation device
- four-flanged nail
- four-flap Z-plasty
- four-in-one arthroplasty
- four-point walker
- four-poster cervical orthosis
- four-vessel cerebral angiography
- Fourier pulsatility index
- Fourier transform
- Fournier test for ataxic gait
- fourth compartment
- fourth cranial nerve (trochlear nerve)
- fourth ventricle tumor
- fovea
- foveal fat pad
- foveal vision
- Foville fasciculus
- Foville syndrome
- Fowler maneuver
- Fowles dislocation technique
- Fox bipolar forceps
- Fox-Blazina knee procedure
- Fox extractor-impactor
- Fox splint
- FP artery (frontopolar)
- FP electrode (frontopolar) (FP_1, FP_2, F_z)
- FPA (foot progression angle)
  - forefoot
  - hindfoot
- FPB (flexor pollicis brevis) muscle
- FPB (flexor pollicis brevis) tendon
- FpF (frontopolar-frontal) electrode
- FPL (flexor pollicis longus) muscle
- FPL (flexor pollicis longus) tendon
- FPR (fastigial pressor response)
- Frac-Sur splint
- fraction
  - ejection
  - linear
  - S-phase
  - transchondral
- Fractura Flex
- Fractura Flex bandage

Fractura Flex cast
fracture
  abduction
  acute avulsion
  adduction
  agenetic
  Aitken classification of epiphyseal
  alveolar bone
  anatomic
  angulated
  ankle mortise
  AO classification of ankle
  apophyseal
  articular
  atrophic
  avulsion
  avulsion chip
  axial compression
  backfire
  Barton
  basal neck
  basal skull
  baseball finger
  basilar femoral neck
  basilar skull
  basocervical
  bending
  Bennett basic hand
  Berndt-Harty classification of transchondral
  bicondylar
  bimalleolar ankle
  bipartite
  birth
  blow-in
  blow-out
  boot-top
  Bosworth
  both-bone
  boxer's
  Boyd type II
  bucket-handle
  buckle
  bumper

fracture *(cont.)*
  bunk bed
  burst (compression) (of the atlas)
  bursting
  butterfly
  buttonhole
  Canale-Kelly talar neck
  carpal navicular
  carpal scaphoid bone
  cartwheel
  cemental
  cementum
  cervical
  cervicotrochanteric
  Chance
  Chance spinal
  chauffeur's
  chip
  chisel
  circumferential
  clay shoveler's
  cleavage
  closed
  closed break
  Colles
  collicular
  comminuted
  complete
  complex
  complicated
  composite
  compound
  compound skull
  compression (burst) (of the atlas)
  condylar
  congenital
  Conrad-Bugg trapping of soft tissue in ankle
  contrecoup
  cortical
  Cotton ankle
  cough (of a rib)
  crack
  craniofacial dysjunction

fracture *(cont.)*
- crush
- cuboid
- cuneiform
- Danis-Weber classification of ankle
- Darrach-Hughston-Milch
- dashboard
- Denis (A, B, C, D, or E) spinal
- dens
- dentate
- depressed
- depressed and compound skull
- depressed skull
- diacondylar
- diaphyseal
- diastatic
- displaced
- displaced intra-articular (of the tarsal navicular)
- dogleg
- dome
- dorsal wing
- double
- Dupuytren
- Duverney
- dyscrasic
- epicondylar
- epiphyseal slip
- Essex-Lopresti calcaneal
- extracapsular
- facial
- fatigue
- femoral neck
- fender
- fighter's
- finger
- fissure
- flake
- flake (of the hamate)
- flexion-burst
- flexion-compression
- flexion-distraction
- floating arch
- Freiberg

fracture *(cont.)*
- Frykman radial
- fulcrum
- Galeazzi f. of radius
- Garden femoral neck
- Gosselin
- greenstick
- grenade-thrower's
- gross
- Guérin
- gutter
- Hahn-Steinthal capitellum
- Hansen
- hairline
- hamate tail
- hangman's
- Hawkins talar neck
- Hawkins II talar neck
- healed
- heat
- hemicondylar
- Herbert scaphoid bone
- Hermodsson
- hickory-stick
- hockey-stick
- horizontal
- humeral head-splitting
- hyperflexion
- idiopathic
- impacted
- incomplete
- indirect
- inflammatory
- infraction
- internally fixed
- interperiosteal
- intertrochanteric
- intra-articular
- intra-articular calcaneal
- intracapsular
- intraperiosteal
- intrauterine
- irreducible
- Jefferson

fracture *(cont.)*
- joint depression
- Jones
- juvenile Tillaux
- juxta-articular
- Kocher
- Kocher-Lorenz classification of capitellum
- lateral column calcaneal
- laterally displaced
- Lauge-Hansen classification of ankle
- Lauge-Hansen stage II supination-eversion
- lead pipe
- LeFort I, II, III
- linear and depressed skull
- Lisfranc
- long bone
- longitudinal
- loose
- lorry driver's
- low T humerus
- lunate
- Maisonneuve fibular
- malar
- Malgaigne pelvic
- mallet
- malunited
- mandibular
- march
- maxillary
- medial column calcaneal
- medial malleolar
- midfacial
- midshaft
- monomalleolar ankle
- Monteggia
- Montercaux
- Moore
- Müller classification of humerus
- multangular ridge
- multipartite
- nasal

fracture *(cont.)*
- navicular body
- naviculocapitate
- neck
- neoplastic
- neurogenic
- neuropathic
- neurotrophic
- nightstick
- nondisplaced
- oblique
- occult
- odontoid
- Ogden classification of epiphyseal
- old
- olecranon tip
- open
- open-break
- osteochondral fractures of the dome of the talus
- Pais
- panfacial
- paratrooper
- parry
- patellar
- pathologic
- Pauwels
- perforating
- pedicle
- periarticular
- pertrochanteric
- physeal
- Piedmont
- pillion
- pillow
- pilon
- ping-pong
- plafond
- pond
- posterior element
- postmortem
- Pott ankle
- pressure
- puncture

fracture *(cont.)*
- pyramidal
- Quervain (de Quervain)
- radial head
- radial styloid process
- resecting
- retrodisplaced
- reverse Barton
- reverse Colles
- rib
- ring
- Rolando
- rotation-burst
- Ruedi-Allgower tibial plafond
- Salter-Harris-Rang classification of epiphyseal
- Salter I-VI
- sandbagging (of long bones)
- scaphoid
- seat belt
- secondary
- segmental
- Segond
- SER-IV
- shaft
- Shepherd
- sideswipe elbow
- silver-fork
- simple
- simple skull
- skier's
- Skillern
- sleeve
- slice
- small
- Smith
- Sneppen talar
- spiral
- splintered
- spontaneous
- sprain
- Springer
- sprinter's
- stable

fracture *(cont.)*
- stairstep
- Steinert classification of epiphyseal
- stellate
- stellate undepressed
- step-off of
- Stieda
- straddle
- strain
- stress
- stress-type
- subcapital
- subcutaneous
- subperiosteal
- subtrochanteric
- supination-adduction
- supination-eversion
- supination, external rotation-type IV (SER-IV)
- supracondylar
- surgical neck
- T
- T condylar
- talar osteochondral
- teardrop
- teardrop-shaped flexion-compression
- temporal bone
- thalamic (of the calcaneal)
- through-and-through
- tibial plafond
- tibial plateau
- tibiofibular
- Tillaux
- Tillaux-Kleiger
- tongue
- tongue-type
- torsion
- torus
- transcapitate
- transcervical femoral
- transchondral talar
- transcondylar
- transhamate
- transscaphoid

fracture *(cont.)*
- transtriquetral
- transverse
- traversing the
- trimalleolar
- trimalleolar ankle
- triplane
- triquetral
- trophic
- tuft
- undisplaced
- unstable
- ununited
- vertebra plana
- vertebral wedge compression
- vertical shear
- wagon wheel
- Wagstaffe
- Watson-Jones navicular
- Watson-Jones spinal
- Weber C
- wedge
- wedge-compression
- wedge flexion-compression
- willow
- Y
- Y-T
- Zickel
- zygomatic-malar complex (ZMC)

fracture blister
fracture by contrecoup
fracture circumferential
fracture classification
fracture-dislocation
fracture en coin
fracture en rave
fracture frame
fracture in close apposition
fracture line
fracture nonunion
- elephant-foot
- horse-hoof
- oligotrophic
- torsion wedge

fracture reduction system, Agee-WristJack
fracture trauma
fragilitas ossium congenita
Fragmatome tip
fragment, fragments
- alignment of fracture
- articular
- avulsed fracture
- avulsion
- bony
- butterfly bone
- capital
- chondral
- cortical
- disk
- displacement of fracture
- free
- free-floating cartilaginous
- loose
- osteochondral
- overriding of fracture
- retrolisthesed
- retropulsed bony

fragmentation of the apophysis
frame
- Ace-Colles fracture
- Ace-Fischer fracture
- Ace-Fischer ring
- Alexian Brothers overhead
- Andrews spinal
- Andrews spinal surgery
- Boehler-Braun leg
- Boehler fracture
- Boehler reducing
- Balkan fracture
- Bradford fracture
- Braun
- Brooker
- Brown-Roberts-Wells stereotactic head
- Budde-Greenberg-Sugita stereotactic head
- Charest head

frame *(cont.)*
- Chick CLT operating
- CircOlectric
- claw-type basic
- Cole fracture
- Cole hyperextension
- Cosman-Roberts-Wells (CRW)
- stereotactic head
- Crawford head
- DeBastiani
- DePuy rainbow
- DePuy reducing
- double-ring
- Elekta stereotactic head
- Fischer
- fixation
- Foster turning
- four-poster
- fusion
- Gardner-Wells fixation
- gNomos head (lowercase g, capital N)
- Goldthwait
- Granberry
- Hastings
- head
- Heffington lumbar seat spinal
- surgery
- Herzmark
- Hibbs
- Hitchcock stereotactic head
- Hoffmann-Vidal double
- Ilizarov
- ISAH stereotactic immobilization
- Jones abduction
- Kessler traction
- Komai stereotactic head
- Laitinen stereotactic head
- laminectomy
- Leksell D-shaped stereotactic
- Leksell-Elekta stereotactic
- Leksell gamma stereotactic
- Leksell Model G stereotactic
- Leksell stereotactic coordinate

frame *(cont.)*
- Lex-Ton spinal
- Malcolm-Lynn C-RXF cervical retractor
- Mayfield fixation
- Monticelli-Spinelli
- Mundinger-Reichert stereotactic
- OBT stereotactic
- Olivier-Bertrand-Talairach stereotactic head
- Patil stereotactic head frame
- Pearson attachment to Thomas
- Pelourus stereotactic
- phantom
- Pittsburgh pelvic
- Radionics CRW stereotactic head
- Radionics stereotactic
- Reichert-Mundinger-Fischer stereotactic head
- Relton-Hall
- scoliosis operating
- Slatis pelvic fracture
- spine
- stereotactic coordinate
- stereotactic head
- stereotaxic head
- Stryker fracture
- Stryker turning
- Sugita head
- Talairach stereotactic
- Taylor spinal
- Thomas
- Thompson
- Todd-Wells stereotactic
- triangular ankle fusion
- Wagner
- Whitman
- Wilson
- Wilson convex
- Wingfield
- Wolfson
- Zimmer laminectomy

Framer finger extension bow

Framer splint

Framer tendon passer
Framer tendon-passing needle
frank dislocation
Fränkel classification of spinal cord injury (Fraenkel)
Fränkel sign
Fränkel white line
fray, frayed, fraying
fraying of meniscus
Frazier brain-exploring cannula
Frazier brain trocar
Frazier cordotomy knife
Frazier dural elevator
Frazier dural hook
Frazier dural scissors
Frazier dural separator
Frazier laminectomy retractor
Frazier lighted brain retractor
Frazier nerve hook
Frazier pituitary knife
Frazier retractor
Frazier scissors
Frazier separator
Frazier suction tip
Frazier suction tube
Frazier ventricular cannula
Frazier ventricular needle
free flap
free flap of cartilage
free flap transfer
free-floating osteotomy
free fragments
free induction decay (FID)
free induction signal
free latissimus dorsi flap
free phalangeal base autograft for hallux limitus
free revascularized autograft
free toe transfer
Freedom arthritis support for hand
Freeman modular total hip prosthesis
Freeman-Swanson knee prosthesis
Freer chisel
Freer elevator-dissector
Freer periosteal elevator
Freer septal elevator
Freer-Swanson ganglion knife
freeze-drying
freezing of movement
freezing phenomena
Freiberg cartilage knife
Freiberg craniotome
Freiberg disease
Freiberg infraction
Freiberg-Kohler disease
Freiberg meniscectomy knife
Frejka cast
Frejka jacket
Frejka pillow
fremitus
French brain retractor
French fracture technique
French scale for sizing catheters
Frenchay Activities Index (FAI)
Frenchay Aphasia Screening Test (FAST)
Frenchay Arm Test (FAT)
frenectomy
frenulum
Frenzel lens
frequency
  absolute peak (on EEG)
  alpha
  dominant waking (on EEG)
  EEG spectral edge
  high filter (HFF)
  low filter (LFF)
  mean peak (on EEG)
  treatment
frequency measured in cycles per second
frequency measured in hertz (Hz)
frequency range
freshen the surface
freshened surfaces
freshening of bone
Fresnel prism
F response

FRIA (Friends and Relatives of the Institutionalized Aged)
friable
friable feeder arteries
friction, dynamic
friction rub in knee
friction syndrome, iliotibial band
Fried-Green foot procedure
Fried-Hendel tendon technique
Friedman bone rongeur
Friedman brace
Friedman elbow support
Friedreich ataxia
Friedreich disease
Friedreich sign
Friends and Relatives of the Institutionalized Aged (FRIA)
Fries score for rheumatoid arthritis
fringe, synovial
frog splint
Fröhlich adiposogenital dystrophy
Frohse ligamentous arcade
Froimson-Oh arm procedure
Froin syndrome
FROM (full range of motion)
Froment paper sign
frond, synovial
frontal ataxia
frontal gyrus
frontal horn of lateral ventricle
frontal horns, enlarged
frontal lobe contusion
frontal lobe damage, mesial-
frontal lobe disease
frontal lobe dysfunction
frontal lobe lesion
frontal lobe personality
frontal lobe reflex
frontal lobe sign
frontal lobe syndrome
frontal lobe tumor
frontal neoplasm
frontal plane growth abnormalities
frontal release sign
frontocentral (FC) electrode
frontocentral convexity
frontocentral head region
frontoethmoidal encephalocele
fronto-orbital advancement
frontoparietal suture
frontopontine fiber
frontopontine tract
frontopontocerebellar pathway
frontosphenoid suture
frontosphenoidal encephalocele
frontotemporal (FT)
frontotemporal atrophy
frontotemporal craniotomy
frontotemporal electrode
frontotemporal region
frontotemporoparietal craniotomy
frontozygomatic region
frost, synovial
Frost posterior tibialis tendon lengthe ning
Frost foot procedure
Frost stitch
frostbite injury
frozen section diagnosis
frozen shoulder
F.R. Thompson femoral prosthesis
Fruehevald splint
Frykholm bone rongeur
Frykman classification of hand fractures
Frykman classification of wrist fractures
FSCAN pressure-sensitive insole sensor
FSH (facioscapulohumeral) dystrophy
FSI (Functional Status Index)
FSQ (Functional Status Questionnaire)
FTA (femorotibial angle)
FTA (fluorescent treponemal antibody) test
FTC (fibulotalocalcaneal) ligament
FT electrode (frontotemporal) (FT_9-FT_{10})
F to N (finger-to-nose) test

FTSG (full-thickness skin graft)
Fuchs-Rosenthal counting chamber for CSF cells
fugax, amaurosis
fugue state
  epileptic
  hysterical
Fujita snake retractor
Fujita suction retractor
Fukushima C-clamp
Fukuyama disease
fulcrum fracture
fulcrum, joint
fulgurate, fulgurated
full-circle goniometer
full recruitment pattern
full-thickness skin graft (FTSG)
fully jacketed (handgun) missiles
fulminant encephalitis
fulminant hydrocephalus
fulminate
Fulton laminectomy rongeur
Fulton rongeur
fumigatus, Aspergillus
function, functions, functioning
  brain stem
  bundle
  caloric test for vestibular
  cognitive
  cortical
  discrepant intellectual
  embarrassment of midbrain
  epicritic
  higher cerebral
  higher cortical
  higher integrative
  higher level cognitive
  independent
  neuro-ophthalmologic
  position of
  verbally mediated
Functional Ambulation Categories (FAC)
Functional Assessment Staging (FAST)
functional aphonia
functional disability of the foot
functional disorder
functional grip
functional hyperlordosis
functional inattention
Functional Independence Measure (FIM)
Functional Limitation Profile (FLP)
functional loss
functional movements
functional outcome
functional overlay
functional recovery
functional splint
Functional Status Index (FSI)
Functional Status Questionnaire (FSQ)
functional units of spine
fund of information
fund of information test
fund of knowledge
fundamental aspects of mobility
fundus, ocular
fundus of aneursym
funduscopically
fungal cultures on Sabouraud medium in meningitis
fungal meningitis
funiculus (pl. funiculi)
Funsten splint
Funston syndrome
Furlong tendon stripper
Furnas bayonet osteotome
Furnas-Haq-Somers technique
furor epilepticus
fused ankle
fused physis
fusiform aneurysm
fusiform dilatation
fusiform swelling
fusiformis

fusion (see also *operation*)
  Albee lumbar spinal
  ankle
  anterior cervical (ACF)
  anterior cervical body
  anterior spinal
  atlanto-occipital
  Blair ankle
  Blair talar body
  Bohlman triple-wire
  Bosworth lumbar spinal
  Brooks-Gallie cervical
  Brooks-Jenkins cervical
  calcaneotibial
  carpal-metacarpal (CMC)
  (also carpometacarpal)
  cervical interbody
  chevron
  Cloward back
  diaphyseal-epiphyseal
  diskectomy with Cloward
  dowel spinal
  extra-articular hip
  facet
  Gallie atlantoaxial
  Gallie cervical
  Gallie wire
  Hatcher-Smith cervical
  Horwitz ankle
  hyperostotic bony
  interbody
  interphalangeal
  interspinous process
  intra-articular knee
  McKeever metatarsophalangeal
  metatarsocuneiform joint
  metatarsophalangeal joint
  multilevel

fusion *(cont.)*
  occipitocervical
  pantalar
  posterior cervical
  posterior lumbar interbody (PLIF)
  posterior spinal
  posterolateral
  Robinson-Riley spinal
  Rowe
  screw
  Smith-Robinson interbody
  spinal
  subaxial posterior cervical spinal
  symmetric vertebral
  talocrural
  tibiocalcaneal
  tibiotalar
  tibiotalocalcaneal
  transfibular
  triple-wire
  two-stage
fusion defect
fusion of bone
fusion of joint
fusion of two or more vertebral
  segments
fusion frame
Futura cock-up splint
Futura wrist splint
fuzziness, mental
F wave
F wave measurements
F wave on electromyogram
F wave response
F wave on motor nerve conduction
  velocity study
fx (fracture)

G,g

GABA (gamma-aminobutyric acid)
GABA-T (GABA-transaminase)
gadolinium enhancement of MRI
Gaeltec catheter-tip pressure transducer
Gaenslen sign
Gaenslen split heel incision
Gaffney ankle prosthesis
Gaffney joint
gag reflex
Gage sign
Gagnon splint
gain (as a result of illness)
  primary
  secondary
gait
  abductor lurch
  antalgic
  apraxic
  astasia-abasia
  ataxic
  batrachian (frog)
  broad-based
  cadence of
  calcaneal
  calcaneous
  cerebellar
  Charcot
  Charlie Chaplin type of
  choreatic
  clumsy
  cogwheel
  crab
  cross-leg
  cross-legged

gait *(cont.)*
  dancing
  dancing bear
  double-leg stance phase of
  double-step
  double-tap
  drag-to
  dromedary
  drop-foot
  drunken sailor
  duck's waddle
  dystrophic
  equine
  festinating
  floating
  foot strike phase of
  four-point
  free-swinging knee
  glue-footed
  gluteal
  gluteus maximus
  gluteus medius
  heel
  heel-and-toe
  heel contact phase of
  heel-off phase of
  heel strike phase of
  heel-to-toe
  heel-toe
  helicopod
  hemiplegic
  high steppage
  hobbling
  hysterical

gait *(cont.)*
- instability
- intermittent double-step
- intoeing
- jerky
- listing
- lurching
- marche à petits pas
- narrow-base
- Oppenheim
- opposite foot strike phase of
- opposite toe-off phase of
- parkinsonian
- Petren
- pigeon toeing
- propulsion
- propulsion of
- push-off phase of
- quality of
- reeling
- retropulsion of
- reversal of fore-aft shear phase of
- rigid
- scissor
- scissor-leg
- scraping toe
- shuffling
- slap foot
- slapping
- spastic
- speed of
- stable
- staggering
- stance phase of
- steppage
- stiff
- stiff-legged
- stride length of
- strike phase of
- stuttering (in parkinsonism)
- swaying
- swing phase of
- swing-through
- swing-to
- tabetic

gait *(cont.)*
- tandem
- Thorazine shuffle
- three-point
- tiptoe
- toe-off phase of
- toe-walking
- toeing-in
- toeing-out
- tottering
- Trendelenburg
- two-point
- uncoordinated
- unsteadiness of
- unsteady
- waddling
- wide-based

Gait Abnormality Rating Scale (GARS)

gait analysis

gait and mobility

gait and station, unsteadiness of

gait apraxia

gait ataxia

gait biomechanics

gait cycle
- stance phase of
- swing phase of

gait determinants
- combined ankle and knee motion
- knee flexion during stance phase
- pelvic rotation
- pelvic shift
- pelvic tilt

gait deviations

gait disturbance

Gaiter cast

gait initiation

gait instability

gait lock splint (GLS) brace

gait pathomechanics

gait plate

GAIT (great toe arthroplasty implant technique) spacer

gait training for the pronated foot

Galant sign
Galante hip prosthesis
galea aponeurotica
galeal extension of tumor
Galeazzi fracture-dislocation
Galeazzi fracture of radius
Galeazzi patellar operation
Galeazzi sign
Galen, great cerebral vein of
Gallagher rasp
Gallannaugh bone plate
Gallie ankle arthrodesis
Gallie atlantoaxial arthrodesis
Gallie atlantoaxial fusion technique
Gallie cervical fusion
Gallie fusion-using cable
Gallie H-graft
Gallie wire fixation technique
gallium-67 bone scan
gallium scanning, with ^{67}Ga
Gallo traction
Galt hand trephine
Galt skull trephine
galvanic skin response (GSR) on EEG
galvanometer, EEG pen
Galveston metacarpal brace
Galveston Orientation and Awareness
  Test (GOAT)
Galveston sacral fixation
gambiense, Trypanosoma
game knee
game leg
gamekeeper's thumb
gamma-aminobutyric acid (GABA)
gamma camera
gamma efferent system
gamma globulin elevated in CSF
gamma irradiation
Gamma knife for radiosurgery
gamma locking nail
gamma loop nervous system
gamma motor neurons
gamma rhythm on EEG
gamma unit
gammopathy, monoclonal
ganglioglioma
gangliolysis, radiofrequency
ganglion (pl. ganglia)
  Acrel
  basal
  calcification of the basal
  cervical
  ciliary
  dorsal root (DRG)
  gasserian
  marbled appearance of basal
  otic
  palmar
  petrosal
  posterior root
  radiocapitellar joint
  Scarpa
  sensory
  sphenopalatine
  submandibular
  trigeminal
  Wrisberg
ganglion cells
  degeneration of
  shrinkage of
  vacuolation of
ganglioneuroma
ganglion hook, Cushing gasserian
ganglionic cyst in synovial tendon
  sheath
ganglion scissors, Adson
ganglioradiculitis
gangliosidosis, GM_1 and GM_2
gangrene
  dry
  gas
  ischemic
  Meleney synergistic
  peripheral
  wet
Ganley modification of Keller
  arthroplasty
GANS (granulomatous angiitis of the
  nervous system)
Ganser syndrome

Gant hip arthrodesis
Gant osteotomy
gantry of CT scanner
Garceau-Brahms arthrodesis
Garceau cheilectomy
Garceau tendon technique
Garcin syndrome
Garden angle
Garden femoral neck fracture
Gardiner-Brown tuning fork
Gardner bone forceps
Gardner chair
Gardner elevator
Gardner neurosurgical skull clamp
Gardner skull clamp pin
Gardner-Wells fixation frame
Gardner-Wells headrest
Gardner-Wells skull traction tongs
Garré, sclerosing osteomyelitis of
GARS (Gait Abnormality Rating Scale)
Gartland classification of supracondylar fracture
gas, subcutaneous tissue
gasserian ganglion tumor
gate clamp
gate clip
gastroc (gastrocnemius muscle)
gastroc-resistive exercises
gastroc/soleus contractures
gastrocnemius reflex
gastrocnemius-soleus complex
gastrocnemius-soleus muscle group
Gatch bed
gatched bed
gate control pain treatment
Gatellier-Chastang ankle approach
Gaucher disease
gauge
  acetabular
  B&L pinch
  bone screw ruler
  Charnley femoral condyle radius
  Charnley socket

gauge *(cont.)*
  Cloward depth
  Cobb
  depth
  elasticized
  foam
  isometric strain
  measuring
  Philips toe force
  pinch
  screw depth
  socket
  strain
gauge of wire
gauntlet
  Jobst
  leather lacer
gauntlet splint
gauze (see also *dressing*)
  Aquaphor
  elasticized
  foam
  Nu Gauze
  Owen
  tantalum
Gaynor-Hart position
gaze
  cardinal directions of
  conjugate
  conjugate fixed
  conjugate horizontal
  consensual
  disconjugate (or dysconjugate)
  down
  dysjunctive
  field of
  fixed
  following
  horizontal
  ipsilateral tonic conjugate
  lateral
  paresis of
  pontine center for
  preference of

gaze *(cont.)*
  refixational shift of
  up
  vertical
gaze center in brain (pontine)
gaze coordinating aggregate
gaze deficit
gaze impairment
gaze mechanism in brain stem
gaze palsy
gaze paralysis
gaze paresis
gaze-paretic nystagmus
gaze preference
GBM (glioblastoma multiforme)
GBS (Guillain-Barré syndrome)
GCS (Glasgow Coma Scale)
GCT (germ-cell tumor)
GCTSPS (germ-cell tumor with synchronous lesions in pineal and suprasellar regions)
Gd-DTPA contrast medium used in MRI scan
GDF-1 (growth differentiation factor-1)
Geckler screw
gegenhalten
Geiger counter
Geiger rongeur
gel
  electrolyte EEG
  Lectron II electrode
  Omni Prep electrolyte EEG
gelastic epilepsy
gelatin foam, thrombin-soaked
gelatinosa, substantia
gelatinous hematoma
gel cast
Gelfoam
  thrombin-soaked
  wafer of
Gelfoam cookie
Gelfoam pack
Gelfoam stam
Gelman foot procedure
Gelocast
Gelpi retractor
gemellus (pl. gemelli) muscle
Gemini chiropractic table
Gemini hip system
general endotracheal anesthesia
general paresis
general somatic efferent (motor) fibers
General Health Questionnaire (GHQ)
General Well-Being Schedule
generalization on EEG
generalized convulsive seizure with focal onset
generalized convulsive seizure without focal onset
generalized delta activity (on EEG)
generalized nonconvulsive seizure
generalized osteoarthritis
generalized slowing (on EEG)
generalized theta activity (on EEG)
generalized tonic-clonic seizure
Genesis knee prosthesis
Genesis total knee system
genetic epilepsy
genicular position, medial
geniculate body
geniculate herpes zoster
geniculate neuralgia
geniculate nucleus
geniculocalcarine region
geniculocalvarium
geniculocortical pathway
geniculum
Gennari
  band of
  line of
  stripe of (in brain)
genu recurvatum
genu valgum (knock-knee) deformity
genu varum (bowleg) deformity
Genucom ACL laxity analysis system
Genucom arthrometer
Genucom knee flexion analysis system
Genutrain P3 knee brace

Genutrain PE patellar realignment
geographic disorientation
Geomedic total knee prosthesis
Geometric total knee prosthesis
Georgiade fixation apparatus
Georgiade visor halo fixation apparatus
Gerald bipolar forceps
Gerald dressing forceps
Gerald tissue forceps
Gerard prosthesis
Gerard resurfacing procedure
Gerbode-Burford rib spreader
Gerdy tubercle in knee
Gerdy ligament
geriatric
Geriatric Depression Scale (GDS)
germ-cell tumor (GCT), intracranial
germinal matrix
germinoma
  basal ganglia
  medulla oblongata
  neurohypophyseal
  pineal
  suprasellar
Gerontological Society
gerontologist
Gerota capsule
Gerster traction bar
Gerstmann-Straussler syndrome
Gertzbein classification of seat belt injury
Gerzog bone mallet
gestalt
gestural automatism
Getty decompression technique
GFAP (glial fibrillary acidic protein) antibody
GFAP immunostain
Ghajar guide
Ghon-Sachs complex
Ghormley arthrodesis
Ghormley shelf procedure
ghost muscle fibers
GHQ (General Health Questionnaire)
Giannestras modification of Lapidus technique
Giannestras step-down modified osteotomy
giant cell arteritis, Horton
giant cell malignant tumor of soft tissue
giant cell reparative granuloma
giant neurons
giant pyramidal Betz cells
Gianturco prosthesis
gibberish
gibbous deformity
gibbus (hump)
Gibney bandage
Gibson approach
Gibson bandage
Gibson-Piggott osteotomy
Gibson splint
giddy headache (preceded by vertigo)
Giebel blade plate
Giertz rib shears
Giertz-Shoemaker rib shears
Giertz-Stille scissors
Gifford mastoid retractor
gigantism, cerebral
Gigli saw blade
Gigli saw guide
Gigli wire saw
Gilbert-Tamai-Weiland technique
Gilchrest test
Gildenberg biopsy forceps
Giliberty bipolar femoral head
Giliberty device
Giliberty femoral prosthesis
Gilles de la Tourette syndrome
Gillespie syndrome
Gillette joint orthosis
Gillette joint prosthesis
Gillette modification of ankle-foot orthosis
Gilliat-Summer nerve-damaged hand
Gillies bone hook
Gillies-Dingman hook
Gillies graft

Gillies-Millard cocked-hat technique
Gillies pollicization
Gillies suture
Gillis test
Gill-Manning-White spondylolisthesis technique
Gill modification of Campbell ankle operation
Gillquist joint instruments
Gill shelf procedure
Gill sliding graft technique
Gill-Stein arthrodesis
Gilmer splint
gimpy
gimpy leg
gingival hyperplasia
girdle
  limb
  pelvic
  shoulder
Girdlestone arthroplasty
Girdlestone pseudarthrosis
Girdlestone resection arthroplasty
Girdlestone-Taylor procedure
Girdlestone tendon transfer
Gissane angle
Gissane spike
gitter cells in cerebral degenerative processes
give-way phenomena
giving way of ankle
giving way of knee
glabella
glabella reflex
glabellar tap
glabellar tapping
gladiatorum, herpes
gland
  calcification of pineal
  haversian
  pineal
  pituitary
  von Ebner
glandular toxoplasmosis
Glaser automatic laminectomy retractor
Glaser laminectomy retractor
Glasflex material
Glasgow Assessment Schedule
Glasgow Coma Scale (GCS)
Glasgow Outcome Scale (GOS)
Glasgow screw
Glass-Bessen transfixion screw
glassy-eyed stare
glassy stare of petit mal epilepsy
G-lengthening of semitendinosus tendon
glenohumeral glide
glenohumeral joint subluxation
glenohumeral ligament
glenoid cavity
glenoid component, keel of
glenoid fossa
glenoid labrum
glenoplasty
Gliadel implant
glial cell
glial disease
glial fibrillary acidic protein (GFAP) antibody
glial nodule
glial reaction
glial scarring
glial tumor
glide, glenohumeral
glide hole
glioblast
glioblastoma multiforme (GBM)
glioma
  anaplastic
  anaplastic cerebral
  brain stem
  butterfly-type
  cerebral
  high-grade
  intracranial
  low-grade
  malignant

glioma *(cont.)*
  non-anaplastic
  optic
  optic nerve
  pontine
  rolandoparietal
  supratentorial
glioma tumor
gliomatosis cerebri, familial
gliomatosis, meningeal
gliosarcoma
gliosis
  astrocytic
  progressive subcortical
  reactive
gliosis of sylvian aqueduct
Glisson sling
global amnesia
global aphasia
global assessment of sensory disturbance
global cerebral ischemia
Global Deterioration Scale (GDS)
global measures of disability
Global total shoulder arthroplasty system
globoid cell leukodystrophy
globose cell
globulin, gamma (elevated in CSF)
globus epilepticus
globus hystericus
globus pallidus
glomerular basement membrane
glomeruloid formation
glomi of choroid plexus
glomus arteriovenous malformation
glomus jugulare tumor
glomus of choroid plexus
glomus (subungual) tumor
glomus-type arteriovenous malformation (AVM)
glossokinetic artifact on EEG
glossokinetic potential
glossopharyngeal nerve (ninth cranial nerve)
glossopharyngeal neuralgia
glove, gloves
  Biobrane
  Handeze fingerless
glove-and-stocking anesthesia distribution
glovelike distribution
GLS (gait lock splint) brace
Gluck rib shears
glue
  biomedical
  cyanoacrylate
  fibrin
  skin
glue-footed gait
"glued-to-the-floor" phenomenon in parkinsonism
gluteal bonnet
gluteal lines
gluteal lurch
gluteal maximus tensing test
gluteal punch test
gluten-free diet for multiple sclerosis
Gluterex
glutethimide intoxication
gluteus maximus muscle
gluteus maximus tensing test
gluteus medius gait
gluteus medius muscle
gluteus minimus muscle
glycogen supersaturation, muscle
Glynn-Neibauer technique
GM_1 gangliosidosis
GM_2 gangliosidosis
gNomos head frame (lowercase *g*, capital *N*)
GOAT (Galveston Orientation and Awareness Test)
Golaski graft
Golay coil
gold salts therapy for rheumatoid arthritis
gold standard of diagnosis
Gold Point knee brace

Golden Period for primary closure in infected wounds
Goldenhar syndrome
Goldflam disease
Goldmann-Offner reference of electrode
Goldmar opponensplasty
Goldner-Clippinger technique
Goldstein spinal fusion technique
Goldthwait brace
Goldthwait-Hauser procedure
Goldthwait sign
golfer's elbow
Golgi apparatus
Golgi reflex
Golgi system
Gombault degeneration
Gomori stain
gonarthrosis, unicompartmental
Golda reflex
gondii, Toxoplasma
G1 (grid 1) on EEG
goniometer
  electronic (for rheumatology testing)
  finger
  full-circle
  Polk finger
  Scerratti
  Sedan
gonion-gnathion plane
gonococcal arthritis
Gooch splint
Good rasp
Goodman orthopedic bed
Gordon-Broström technique
Gordon knee phenomenon
Gordon reflex
Gordon sign
Gordon splint
Gordon-Taylor technique
Gore bit
Gore Smoother Crucial Tool
Gore-Tex cast liner
Gore-Tex knee prosthesis
Gore-Tex graft
Gore-Tex nonabsorbable surgical suture
Gorham disease
GOS (Glasgow Outcome Scale)
Gosselin fracture
Gosset, spiral band of
Gouffon hip pin fixation
gouge (see also *chisel*)
  Abbott
  Acufex
  Alexander
  Andrews
  Army bone
  arthroplasty
  Aufranc
  Bishop
  bone
  Buch-Gramcko
  Campbell
  Capner
  Cobb spinal
  curved
  Dawson-Yuhl
  Duray-Read
  Flanagan spinal fusion
  gooseneck
  Guy
  Hibbs spinal fusion
  Hoen
  Hoen lamina
  Jewett
  Killian
  Lexer
  Lucas
  Metzenbaum
  Meyerding curved
  mini-Lexer
  Moe
  motorized
  Murphy
  oscillating
  Partsch
  Read

gouge *(cont.)*
  Ruben
  Sheehan
  Smith-Petersen curved
  Smith-Petersen straight
  spinal fusion
  Stille bone
  straight
  swan-neck
  tendon
  U.S. Army
  Watson-Jones bone
  West
  West bone
  Zielke
  Zimmer
Goulet retractor
gout
  acute
  overhanging edges or margins in
  pseudogout
  tophaceous (of the hand)
gouty arthritis
gouty diet
Gowers bundle (in cerebellum)
Gowers column
Gowers fasciculus
Gowers maneuver
Gowers muscular dystrophy
Gowers phenomenon
Gowers sign
Gowers syndrome
Gowers tract
grab bars
grabber, disk
Graber-Devernay hip procedure
Grace method of ratio of metatarsal length
gracilis muscle flap
Gradenigo syndrome
gradient
  amplitude
  anterior-posterior amplitude
  frequency-amplitude
  posterior dominant amplitude
gradient coil
gradient magnetic field
grading scale
grading system
Graflex material
graft
  ACL
  adrenal medulla
  advancement flap
  Albee bone
  allogeneic bone
  allogenous bone
  anterior iliac crest
  anterior sliding tibial
  autochthonous
  autogenous bone
  autogenous inlay
  autologous crest bone
  autologous reverse
  Banks bone
  bicortical iliac bone
  bicortical ilial strip
  BioPolyMeric
  bone
  bone chip
  bone peg
  bone-tendon-bone
  Bonfiglio bone
  bovine collagen
  Boyd dual onlay bone
  BPB (bone-patellar ligament-bone) autologous
  BPB (bone-patellar tendon-bone) autologous
  Braun skin
  bridge
  Calcitite
  Campbell onlay
  cancellous and cortical bone
  cancellous chip bone
  carbon fiber
  cartilage
  chip
  Chuinard autogenous bone
  clothespin spinal fusion

graft *(cont.)*
- Codivilla bone
- Collagraft bone graft matrix
- composite
- consolidated
- cortical strut
- corticocancellous bone
- corticocancellous chip
- cranial bone
- cutaneous
- Dacron
- Daniel iliac bone
- Davis muscle-pedicle
- demineralized bone
- devitalized bone
- diamond inlay
- Douglas skin
- dowel
- Dragstedt skin
- dual onlay bone
- dural
- Esser skin
- extra-articular
- fascia lata
- femorocrural
- femorodistal PTFE
- fetal substantia nigra
- fillet local flap
- Flanagan-Burem apposing hemicylindric
- free
- free fat
- free skin
- freeze-dried
- freeze-dried bone
- fresh frozen
- full-thickness skin
- fusion
- Gillies bone
- Golaski
- Gore-Tex vascular
- gracilis muscle
- Haldeman bone
- Harris superior acetabular

graft *(cont.)*
- harvesting of
- Hemashield enhanced
- hemicylindrical bone
- Henderson onlay bone
- Henry bone
- heterogeneous (heterogenous)
- Hey-Groves-Kirk bone
- Hoaglund bone
- homogeneous (homogenous)
- homologous
- H-shaped
- Huntington bone
- iliac bone
- iliac crest bone
- iliotibial band
- Inclan bone
- inlay bone
- in situ vein
- intercalary
- interfascicular nerve
- interposition bone
- intramedullary
- Isotec patellar tendon
- Judet
- jump
- keystone
- Krause-Wolfe skin
- Kutler V-Y flap
- Langenskiöld bone
- Lee bone
- lyophilized bone
- Massie sliding
- matchstick
- McFarland bone
- McMaster bone
- medullary bone
- morcelized bone
- nerve
- neurovascular island
- Nicoll cancellous bone
- nontubed closed distant flap
- nontubed open distant flap
- Ollier thick split free

graft *(cont.)*
- Ollier-Thiersch skin
- onlay
- onlay cancellous iliac
- osteoarticular
- osteocartilaginous
- osteochondral
- osteoperiosteal
- Overton dowel
- Papineau
- patellar tendon
- pedicle
- pedicle bone
- peg
- percutaneous autogenous dowel bone
- peroneus brevis
- Phemister onlay bone
- porous polyethylene
- postage stamp
- powdered bone
- prosthetic femorodistal
- PTFE (polytetrafluoroethylene)
- Reverdin epidermal free
- Russe bone
- Ryerson bone
- sandwiched iliac bone
- segmental
- semitendinosus
- single onlay cortical bone
- skin
- skull bone
- sliding inlay
- Soto-Hall bone
- split calvarial bone
- split-thickness skin
- strut bone
- subclavian-external carotid artery
- Tait
- temporal fascia
- Thiersch medium split free
- Thiersch thin split free
- Thomas extrapolated bar
- tricortical bone

graft *(cont.)*
- tricortical ilial strip
- tube flap
- tumbler
- vein
- Wilson bone
- Wolfe full-thickness free
- Wolfe-Kawamoto bone
- wraparound flap bone
- Z-plasty local flap

graft enhanced with collagen
Graham nerve hook
Granberry frame
Granberry splint
Granberry traction
grand mal seizure (tonic-clonic)
Grantham classification of femur fracture
granular chromophobe cell
granulation tissue
granulations, pacchionian
granules, pigment
granuloma
- eosinophilic
- giant cell reparative
- swimming pool

granulomatous giant cell angiitis
granulous fibrous tissue in rheumatoid arthritis
granulovacuolar change in hippocampus
granulovacuolar degeneration
graph, Moseley straight line
graphanesthesia
graphesthesia
graphic impairment
Grashey aphasia
grasp reflex
graspers, pituitary
grasping power
grate, grating
Gratiolet, optic radiation of
gravidarum, chorea
gravis, myasthenia

gravity
  center of (CG)
  flex against
gray commissure (of spinal cord)
gray horns in the spinal canal, posterior
gray matter of central nervous system
gray-out episode
gray-white differentiation on CT
gray-white matter junction
Gray drill
Gray Panthers
graying of vision in multiple sclerosis
Grayson ligament in hand
great toe push-off
great vein of cerebrum
greater multangular bone
Green-Anderson growth table
Green-Banks technique
Green-Joynt sign
Green-Laird modification of the Reverdin osteotomy
Green muscle hook
Green procedure
Green transfer
Greenberg clamp
Greenberg hand rest
Greenberg Universal retractor
Greene forceps
Greenfield classification of spinocerebellar ataxia
Greenfield disease
Greenfield filter
Greenfield osteotomy
greenstick fracture
Greenwood bipolar and suction forceps
grenade thrower's fracture
Grenoble-Paris-Rennes (GPR) robot neurosurgical microscope
Grenoble stereotactic robot
Greulich and Pyle, bone age according to
Grice-Green extra-articular subtalar arthrodesis
grid
  AdTech electrode
  epidural electrode
  subdural electrode
grid lead
grid of electrodes
grid 1 (G1) on EEG
grid 2 (G2) on EEG
Grierson tendon stripper
Griesinger sign
grimace, facial
grimace test
grimacing
Grimelius stain
grind, grinding
grinder, DePuy calcar
grip
  functional
  handle lift
  key
  pistol (of hand)
  power (of hand)
  precision (of hand)
Gripper acetabular cup prosthesis
grip pinch testing
grip strength
grip test, Jamar
Grisel syndrome
Gristina-Webb total shoulder arthroplasty
Gritti-Stokes distal thigh amputation
Gritti-Stokes knee prosthesis
grommet, titanium
groove
  annular
  biceps
  bicipital
  deltopectoral
  femoral
  fibular
  flexor
  intercollicular
  intercondylar
  meningioma of the olfactory

groove *(cont.)*
  neural
  olfactory
  parasagittal
  patellar
  patellofemoral
  peroneal
  Ranvier
  sagittal
  spiral
  spiral humeral
  trochlear
  ulnar
grooving of articular surface
groping reaction
Grosse-Kempf interlocking medullary nailing
Grosse-Kempf nail
ground-reaction forces
ground substance (of connective tissue)
group b arboviruses (causing encephalitis)
group, muscle
Grover meniscotome
Grover meniscus knife
Groves-Goldner technique
Groves opponensplasty
growth
  abnormal epiphyseal
  anchorage-dependent
growth arrest line
growth center of bones
growth curves, standardized
growth factor I, insulin-like
growth hormone antibody
growth hormone releasing factor (GRF)
growth plate arrest
growth plate, cartilaginous
growth plate injury
growth plate widening
growth spurt
Gruber suture
Gruca lower leg procedure
Gruenwald forceps
Gruenwald neurosurgical rongeur
grumous tissue
grunts, repetitive
Gruppe wire-crimping forceps
GSB (Gschwind-Scheier-Bahler) elbow prosthesis
GSR (galvanic skin response) on EEG
G suit
GSW (gunshot wound)
GSWH (gunshot wound to head)
GTC (generalized tonic-clonic) convulsions
GTC epilepsy
GTC seizures
G2 (grid 2) on EEG
G-II Unloader knee brace
guard
  ankle
  dural
  eye
  knee
  McDavid ankle
  McDavid hinged knee
guarding, muscle
Gudden atrophy
Gudden, nucleus of
Gudden tract
Gude tunneler
Guérin fracture
Guepar hinge-knee prosthesis
guide
  Accu-Line
  acetabular
  ACL drill
  Acufex tibial
  adjustable angle
  Adson drill
  Adson dural protector
  Adson saw
  alignment
  Bailey-Gigli saw
  ball-tipped Küntscher (Kuentscher)
  barrel

guide *(cont.)*
- Blair saw
- calibrated pin
- Cloward drill
- Cushing-Gigli saw
- Cushing saw
- Davis saw
- DePuy femoral acetabular overlay drill
- Duopress
- eccentric drill
- femoral intermedullary
- FIN pin
- Fisher
- Ghajar
- Gigli saw
- Hall-Dundar drill
- Hewson cruciate
- Hewson drill
- Hoffmann pin
- intercondylar drill
- intermedullary
- Lebsche saw
- ligature
- long axial alignment
- nail rotational
- neutral drill
- patellar drill
- PCA cutting
- PCA medullary
- picket fence
- Poppen Gigli saw
- Raney saw
- Richards angle
- saw
- stationary angle
- Synthes wire
- T-bar
- telescopic wire
- tibial cutter
- tibial cutting
- Todd-Wells
- tube
- tunnel drill

guide *(cont.)*
- wire
- XMB tibial reaming
- Yasargil ligature

guide bushing

guide pin
- ball-point
- ball-tip
- calibrated

guide sleeve

guideline
- Hartel
- Böhler (Boehler)
- Letournel

guidewire introducer

guidewire, steerable

Guild Memory Test

Guilford cervical brace

Guillain and Mollaret, triangle of

Guillain-Barré-Strohl syndrome

Guillain-Barré syndrome (GBS)

Guillain-Garcin syndrome

Guillain-Mollaret triangle

Guilland sign

guillotine, Charnley femoral inlay

Guleke bone rongeur

Guleke-Stookey approach

Guller resection

Gumley classification of seat belt injury

gumma (granulomatous lesion of neurosyphilis)

gun
- cement
- CMW cement
- Harris cement
- Lidge cement
- power-driven staple
- staple

Gunderson bone forceps

Gunderson muscle forceps

Gunn jaw winking

Gunning splint

gunshot wound (GSW)

gunshot wound to head (GSWH)
GunSlinger shoulder orthosis
Gunston-Hult knee prosthesis
Guppe forceps
gurney
gustatory aura
gustatory seizure
gustatory symptom
Gustilo-Anderson classification of tibial plafond fracture
Gustilo classification of puncture wounds
Gustilo classification of tibial fractures
Gustilo-Kyle cementless total hip arthroplasty
Gustilo knee prosthesis
Guthrie bacterial inhibition test
gutter
  lateral
  sacral
gutter fracture
guttering
Guttmann subtalar arthrodesis
guy suture
Guy gouge
Guyon tunnel release
Guyon canal
G/W Heel Lift
Gymnic ball
gymnast's wrist
Gypsona cast material
gyral crest
gyri cerebri
gyromagnetic ratio
gyrus (pl. gyri)
  angular (AG)
  annectant
  ascending parietal
  Broca
  callosal
  central
  cingulate
  contiguous supramarginal
  dentate

gyrus *(cont.)*
  first temporal
  flattening of
  frontal
  fusiform
  Heschl transverse
  hippocampal
  inferior frontal
  inferior temporal
  infracalcarine
  insular
  lamination of
  lateral occipitotemporal
  lingual
  marginal
  medial occipitotemporal
  middle frontal
  occipital
  occipitotemporal
  olfactory
  orbital
  paracentral
  parahippocampal
  paraterminal
  parietal
  postcentral
  posterior central
  precentral
  preinsular
  quadrate
  short insular
  subcallosal
  subcollateral
  superior frontal
  superior parietal lobule
  superior temporal
  supracallosal
  supramarginal
  temporal
  transverse temporal
  Turner marginal
  uncal
  uncinate
gyrus callosus

gyrus cerebelli
gyrus cingulatus
gyrus cinguli
gyrus isthmus fornicatus
gyrus rectus

H, h

Haacker sling
Haas osteotomy
Haas paralysis
habenula
habenular nucleus
habitus, spondylolisthetic
Hachinski Ischemic Score for Dementia
hacksaw
Haddad-Riordan arthrodesis
Hadfield hand board
Haemonetics Cell Saver
Haemophilus influenzae meningitis
Hagie pin
Hagie sliding nail plate
Haglund deformity
Haglund disease
Haglund-Stille plaster spreader
Haglund syndrome
Hahn bone nail
Hahn screw
Hahn-Steinthal classification of capitellum fracture
Haid cervical plate
Haid UBP (universal bone plate) system
Haight-Finochietto rib spreader
Haight rib spreader
Haines-McDougall medial sesamoid ligament
hairline fracture
Hajek-Ballenger dissector
Hajek-Ballenger septal elevator
Hajek chisel
Hajek-Koffler bone punch forceps
Hajek-Koffler laminectomy rongeur
Hajek mallet
Hakansson bone rongeur
Hakim-Cortis ventriculoperitoneal shunt
Haldeman bone graft
half and half nails
half base syndrome
half ring
Halifax interlaminar clamp
Hall air-driven oscillating saw
Hall driver
Hall-Dundar drill guide
Halle bone curet
Halle dura knife
Halle nasal speculum
Halle speculum
Hallermann-Streiff-François syndrome
Hallervorden-Spatz disease
Hallister heel cup
Hall large bore drill
Hall Micro E drill
Hall Micro E oscillating saw
Hall Micro E reciprocating saw
Hall Micro E sagittal saw
Hall Micro E wiredriver
Hall neurosurgical craniotome
Hall rod
Hall Surgairtome drill
hallucal pronation
hallucination
  auditory
  gustatory
  hypnagogic

hallucination *(cont.)*
  hypnopompic
  nocturnal
  olfactory
  simple
  structured
  tactile
  visual
hallucinatory component
hallucinosis
  alcoholic
  organic
  peduncular
hallux abductovalgus
hallux elevatus
hallux extensus
hallux flexus
hallux interphalangeal (IP) joint
  arthrodesis
hallux interphalangeal joint
hallux interphalangeus angle
hallux limitus (HL)
hallux limitus/rigidus
hallux malleus
hallux migrati
hallux migration
hallux nail
hallux rigidus
hallux valgus (HV)
  bilateral
  unilateral
hallux valgus angle (HVA)
hallux valgus interphalangeus angle
hallux valgus-metatarsus primus varus
  complex
hallux varus correction, Johnson-
  Spiegl
Hall Versipower drill
Hall Versipower oscillating saw
Hall Versipower reamer
Hall Versipower reciprocating saw
halo
  Bremer
  Brown-Roberts-Wells head ring

halo *(cont.)*
  Houston
  Philadelphia
  pulsating visual
  Twin Cities Lo-Profile
halo cast
halo crown system, Bremer
halo immobilization
halo ring
halo traction
halo vest
Halsey nail scissors
Halsey needle holder
Halstead-Reitan Battery
Halstead-Wepman Aphasia Screening
  Test
Halsted artery forceps
Halsted mosquito forceps
halter
  Cerva Crane
  DePuy
  Diskard head
  flannel head
  foam head
  Forrester-Brown head
  head
  Redi head
  Repro head
  Upper 7 head
  Zimfoam head
  Zimmer head
halter traction, cervical
hamartoma
  cartilaginous
  eccrine angiomatous
  subependymal
  vascular
  ventromedial hypothalamic
hamartomatous lesion
Hamas prosthesis
hamate bone, hook of
hamate, capitate
Hamilton bandage
Hamilton Rating Scale for Depression

- Hamilton ruler test
- Hamilton screw
- Hamilton test
- Hamilton traction
- Hamman sign
- hammer
  - Babinski percussion
  - Berliner percussion
  - Buck neurological
  - Buck percussion
  - Cloward
  - Davis percussion
  - Dejerine-Davis percussion
  - Dejerine percussion
  - Epstein neurological
  - Küntscher
  - neurological
  - percussion
  - Rabiner neurological
  - slotted
  - Taylor percussion
  - Traube neurological percussion
  - Trömner percussion (Troemner)
- hammer-marked skull secondary to thinning
- Hammer external fixation
- hammer toe (or hammertoe)
  - dynamic
  - fixed
- hammer toe repair
- hammocking of conventional mattresses
- Hammond foot procedure
- Hammond splint
- hamstring lengthening operation
- hamstring muscle
- hamstring release operation
- hamstring spasm
- hamstring stain
- hamstring strain
- hamstring tendon
- hamstring, tight
- hand
  - all-ulnar
  - ape
- hand *(cont.)*
  - apelike
  - bear's paw
  - claw
  - cleft
  - dorsum of
  - flipper
  - Gilliat-Summer nerve-damaged
  - hemiplegic
  - lobster-claw
  - mirror
  - Myobock artificial
  - oath
  - obstetrician's
  - opera-glass
  - preferential use of right/left
  - prosthetic
  - psychoextended
  - psychoflexed
  - spastic
  - web-area of
  - web-border of
- handbreadth
- hand-carpal unit
- hand drill, Children's Hospital
- handedness, right/left
- Handeze fingerless gloves
- hand-foot syndrome
- hand-foot-uterus syndrome
- handgrip ergometer
- hand-held assist
- hand-held weights (HHW)
- Hand Helper
- handicap
  - final
  - mobility
- handle
  - Bard-Parker
  - Beaver blade
  - cup holder
  - Dynagrip blade
  - multisided blade
  - surgical knife
- handlebar palsy

handle lift grip
hand preference
hand prosthesis
Hand-Schüller-Christian disease
hand sign, alien
hand-wringing, repetitive
Handy-Buck traction
hanging arm cast
hangman's fracture
hang-up
Hanna night splint
Hannover Polytrauma score
Hansen classification of fractures
Hansen-Street driver-extractor
Hansen-Street nail
Hansen-Street pin
Hansen-Street plate
Hapad (shoe insert)
Hapad heel pad
Hapad medial arch pad
Hapad metatarsal arch
Hapad metatarsal insole
Hapad scaphoid arch
HAQ (Health Assessment Questionnaire)
Harada, syndrome of
hard disk herniation
Hardinge femoral approach
Hardinge vastus lateralis operation
Hardt-Delima osteotome
hardware, orthopedic
Hardy bipolar forceps
Hardy-Clapham sesamoid classification
Hardy curet
Hardy dissector
Hardy dressing forceps
Hardy enucleator
Hardy hypophysectomy instruments
Hardy-Joyce triangle
Hardy micro bipolar forceps
Hardy micro dissector
Hardy micro enucleator
Hardy pituitary dissector
Hardy pituitary spoon
Hardy sellar punch forceps
Hardy speculum
Hardy suction tube
Hardy three-prong fork
Hare device
"hare's eye" (lagophthalmos)
Hare pin
Hare traction splint
Hark foot procedure
Harken rib spreader
Harlow plate
Harm posterior cervical plate
Harmon transfer technique
harmonics of waveform
harness
  acromioclavicular
  EEG head
  figure 8 ring
  immobilizer
  Pavlik
  weight-relieving Forte
Harpenden calipers
Harrington compression rod
Harrington distraction outrigger
Harrington distraction rod
Harrington fixation device
Harrington hook
Harrington-Kostuik distraction device
Harrington-Luque
Harrington rod clamp
Harrington rod to correct scoliosis
Harrington spinal elevator
Harrington spreader
Harris-Beath arthrodesis
Harris-Beath axial hindfoot x-ray
Harris-Beath footprint mat
Harris broach
Harris-CDH hip prosthesis
Harris Design 1 (or 2) femoral prosthesis
Harris footprint mat
Harris-Galante acetabular component
Harris-Galante hip prosthesis
Harris HD (or HD-2) hip prosthesis

Harris hip line
Harris hip nail
Harris hip scale
Harris hip score
Harris-Smith cervical fusion
Harrison bone-holding forceps
Harrison-Nicolle polypropylene peg
Hartel guideline
Hartmann bone rongeur
Hartmann mosquito forceps
Hartnup disease
Hart sign
Hart splint
harvesting of bone
harvesting of grafts
Harvey wire-cutting scissors
HA 65101 implant metal
Hass procedure
Hassmann-Brunn-Neer elbow technique
Hastings bipolar hemiarthroplasty
Hastings frame
Hastings prosthesis
Hatcher pin
Hatcher-Smith cervical fusion
hatchet-head deformity
Hatfield bone curet
Hauser ambulation index
Hauser bunionectomy
Hauser heel cord procedure
Hauser patellar tendon procedure
Hausted orthopedic bed
Haverfield-Scoville hemilaminectomy retractor
haversian canal
haversian gland
Hawiva test
Hawkeye suture needle for arthroscopy
Hawkins classification of talar neck fractures
Hawkins II talar neck fracture
Hawkins impingement sign
Hawkins line
Hay-Groves shelf procedure
Hayem encephalitis
Hayes retractor
Haygarth node
Haynes brain cannula
Haynes-Stellite 21 (HS-21) implant metal
Hays hand retractor
HCD (higher cerebral dysfunction)
HD II (or HD-2) total hip prosthesis
HE (hepatic encephalopathy)
head, heads
  Biolox ceramic ball for hip replacement
  cartilaginous cap of phalangeal
  clavicular head of the sternocleidomastoid
  doll's
  first metatarsal (FMH)
  forward positioning of
  metatarsal
  nerve
  Series-II humeral
  terminal
  tower
  transillumination of
  ulnar
  Zirconia orthopedic prosthetic
headache, headaches
  alarm-clock
  band-like
  benign exertional
  bifrontal
  bilateral
  bioccipital
  blind
  blood patch for post-LP
  cataclysmic
  chronic
  cheese reaction
  cluster
  combination
  conditions that precipitate a
  cough

headache *(cont.)*
- disabling
- dull
- duration of
- essential
- evening
- exertional
- frequency of
- frontal
- generalized
- giddy
- histamine
- Horton
- hot dog
- ice cream
- ice pick
- ipsilateral
- leakage (of CSF)
- matutinal (morning)
- migraine
- migrainelike
- mixed
- morning
- muscle contraction
- nitrite
- nonpulsating
- persistent
- post-LP (lumbar puncture)
- postconcussion
- postictal migrainous
- posttraumatic
- psychogenic
- pulsating
- recurrent
- recurring
- seasonal
- severity of
- sex
- sinus
- suboccipital
- sudden-onset
- Symonds
- temporal
- tension

headache *(cont.)*
- tension-type
- tension-vascular
- throbbing
- thunderclap
- traumatic
- unilateral
- vacuum
- vascular
- vasodilator
- vasomotor
- weekend
- whole cranial
- Willis
- Wolff

headache-free interval
headache syndrome
head and neck, femoral
headband, electrode
head bobbing
head circumference size
head cradle
head dislocation, radial
head elevation
head fracture, radial
headframe
- Kannon
- Sugita
- thousand-hands Kannon universal

head halter
head holder
head-injured patient
head injury (HI)
head injury instructions
head lag
head nodding
head of caudate nucleus
head of femur
headrest
- Gardner-Wells
- horseshoe
- Light-Veley
- Mayfield horseshoe
- Mayfield-Kees

headframe *(cont.)*
  Mayfield neurosurgical
  Multipoise
  pediatric
  pin
  pin fixation
  Reston foam-padded
  three-point
  Veley
headrest extension
head sheet
head subluxation, radial
head trauma
healing by primary intention
healing by secondary intention
healing, therapeutic ultrasound for tendon
health-handicapped child
Health Assessment Questionnaire (HAQ)
Health-Related Facilities (HRF)
heat
  application of
  moist
heat fracture
Heath mallet
heave, parasternal
heavy-metal neuritis
heavy-particle irradiation
Heberden node
hebosteotomy
hebotomy
Hebra blade
Hector, tendon of
Hedblom rib retractor
Hedley-Hungerford hip prosthesis
heel
  anterior
  black-dot
  cucumber
  high-prow
  painful
  prominent
  reverse Thomas

heel *(cont.)*
  rubber walking
  SACH (solid ankle, cushioned heel) orthopedic
  Thomas
  valgus
  varus
  walking
Heelbo decubitus heel/elbow protector
heel contact phase of gait
heel cord advancement
heel cord stretching exercise
heel cradle
heel cup
heel height
heel lift in shoe
heel-off phase of gait
heel pad thickness
heel pads ("cookies")
heel-strike phase of gait
heel-to-knee test
heel-to-shin test
heel-toe gait
heel-toe runners
heel-walking
Heerfort syndrome
Heermann alligator forceps
Heffington lumbar seat spinal surgery frame
Heidenhain-type of spongiform encephalopathy
Heifetz cranial perforator
Heifetz procedure
Heifitz clip
height, heel
heightened attention, state of
heightened awareness, state of
Hein rongeur
Heiss soft tissue retractor
Helal osteotomy
Helbing sign
Helenca bandage
Helfet test
helicopod gait

Heliodorus bandage
heliotrope rash in polymyositis or
  dermatomyositis
helmet, Sheffield collimator
Helmholtz coil
helminthic infection of the nervous
  system
heloma durum
heloma (pl. helomata)
heloma molle
hemangioblastoma, cerebellar
hemangioblastoma tumor
hemangioendothelioma, Masson
  vegetant intravascular
hemangioma
  capillary
  cavernous
  extramedullary
  leptomeningeal
  trigeminal
hemangiomatosis
hemangiopericytoma
hemarthrosis
Hemashield enhanced graft
hematogenous osteomyelitis
hematogenous spread of metastases to
  brain
hematogenous spread of tumor
hematoma
  balancing subdural
  carotid plaque
  dural
  epidural (EDH)
  evacuation of
  evolving
  extracerebral
  extradural
  gelatinous
  hemispheral
  hypertensive
  intracerebral
  intracranial
  intraparenchymal
  intraventricular
hematoma *(cont.)*
  nasal septum
  posterior fossa
  retromembranous
  scalp
  spinal epidural
  subdural
  subgaleal
  subungual
  traumatic
hematoma evacuator
hematomyelia
hematopoietic reticulum of marrow
hemeralopia (blurred vision in bright
  light)
hemianesthesia, contralateral
hemianopia
  altitudinal
  bilateral homonymous
  bitemporal
  congruous
  contralateral
  dense
  homonymous
  ipsilateral
  macular
  paracentral
  partial
  quandrantic
hemianopsia
  bitemporal
  dense
  homonymous
hemiarthroplasty
  Bateman
  I-Beam hip
  Austin Moore
  I-beam
  Neer
hemiataxia
hemiballism
hemiballismus
hemibasal syndrome
hemichondrodiasthesis

hemichorea-hemiballism syndrome
hemichorea, vascular
hemichoreic
hemiconvulsions, hemiplegia, and epilepsy (HHE syndrome)
hemicorpora
hemicorporectomy
hemicrania, chronic paroxysmal
hemicraniectomy
hemicraniotomy
hemicranium
hemidecortication, cerebral
hemidepot form of triamcinolone for joint injections
hemidiaphyseal debridement
hemidystonia
hemiepiphyseodesis
hemifacial microsomia
hemifacial spasm
hemifacial weakness
hemifield of vision
hemifield loss
hemihypesthesia
hemi-inattention
  auditory
  tactile
  visual
hemijoint arthroplasty
hemiknee, Savastano
hemilaminectomy
  partial
  segment
  unilateral
hemilaminectomy retractor, Scoville-Haverfield
hemimelia, paraxial (complete and incomplete)
hemiparalysis, contralateral
hemiparesis
  ataxic (AH)
  contralateral
  dense
  hemiparetic
  paradoxical ipsilateral

hemiparesis *(cont.)*
  pure motor (PMH)
  residual
  spastic
hemiparesthesia
hemiparetic hemiparesis
hemiparkinsonism
hemipelvectomy
hemipelvis
hemiphalangectomy, Johnson
hemiplegia
  acutely acquired
  alternating
  contralateral
  dense
  double
  hysterical
  infantile
  left
  motor
  pure motor
  right
  spinal
  Wernicke-Mann spastic
hemiplegia alternans
hemiplegic gait
hemiplegic hand
hemiplegic migraine headache
hemisection of spinal cord
hemisensory loss
hemisensory syndrome
hemisoma
hemisomatognosia
hemispheral dysfunction
hemispheral gaze deficiency
hemispheral mass
hemispheral mass effect
hemisphere
  cerebellar
  cerebral
  dominant
  mesial
  nondominant
hemisphere atrophy

hemispherectomy
hemisphere damage
hemisphere dominance, left/right
hemisphere lesion, dominant
hemisphere stroke
hemispherical contact probe
hemivertebra
  balanced
  unbalanced
Hemo-Drain evacuator
Hemo-Drain needle
hemoclamp
hemodynamics
  limb
  microvascular
hemogenesis
hemophilia A
hemophilia B
hemophilia, classic
hemophiliac
hemorrhage
  aneurysmal
  brain stem
  central nervous system
  cerebellar
  delayed traumatic intracerebral (DTICH)
  Duret
  eight-ball
  epidural
  flame-shaped
  focus of
  hypertensive
  hypothalamic
  intertrabecular
  intracerebral (ICH)
  intracranial
  intraparenchymal
  intraventricular (IVH)
  lobar intracerebral
  nondominant putaminal
  old
  parenchymal
  parenchymatous

hemorrhage *(cont.)*
  periaqueductal
  petechial
  pontine
  putaminal
  retrobulbar
  slit
  spinal epidural (SEH)
  spinal subarachnoid
  spinal subdural (SSH)
  splinter
  striate
  subacute
  subarachnoid (SAH)
  subdural (SDH)
  subependymal
  subhyaloid preretinal
  subhyaloid retinal
  thalamic
  traumatic meningeal
hemorrhagic infarct
hemorrhagic necrosis
hemorrhagic stroke
hemorrheology
hemostasis
hemostat (see also *forceps*)
  curved
  Hoen scalp
  Kelly
  Mixter
  mosquito
  tonsil
hemotympanum
Hemovac Hydrocoat drain
Hemovac suction tube
Henahan elevator
Hendel guided osteotome
Henderson-Jones chondromatosis
Henderson lag screw
Henderson onlay graft
Henle, ligament of
Henley carotid retractor
Hennessy knee brace
Henning cast spreader

Henning mallet
Henning meniscal retractor
Henning plaster spreader
Henoch chorea
Henoch-Schönlein purpura (Schoenlein)
Henry
  master knot of
  vertebral artery by
Henry acromioclavicular technique
Henry and Wrisberg, ligaments of
Henry-Geist spinal fusion technique
Henschke-Mauch SNS knee prosthesis
heparinized Ringer lactate solution
hepatic coma
hepatic encephalopathy
hepatic encephalopathy tremor
hepatolenticular degeneration
Heplock catheter
Herbert bone screw fixation
Herbert-Fisher fracture classification system
Herbert knee prosthesis
Herbert saw
Herbert screw fixation
Herbert-Whipple bone screw
Hercules plaster shears
Herczel rib elevator
Herczel rib rasp
hereditary areflexic dystasia
hereditary progressive arthro-ophthalmology
hereditary sensory radicular neuropathy
hereditary spastic ataxia
hereditary spastic paraplegia
heredoataxia
heredofamilial tremor
Hermodsson fracture
Hermodsson internal rotation technique
Hernandez-Ros bone staple
Herndon-Heyman foot procedure
herniated cerebellar tonsil
herniated cervical disk
herniated disk
herniated intervertebral disk (HID)
herniated nucleus pulposus (HNP)
herniation
  brain
  central
  cerebellar tonsil
  cerebral
  cingulate
  concentric
  foramen magnum
  frank disk
  hard disk
  hippocampal
  impending
  internal disk
  intraspongy nuclear disk
  phalangeal
  soft disk
  subfalcine (subfalcial)
  temporal lobe
  tentorial notch
  tonsillar
  transtentorial
  uncal
herniation of brain tissue
herniation of lumbosacral intervertebral disk
herniation of thoracic intervertebral disk
herniorrhaphy
herpes encephalitis
herpes gladiatorum
herpes simplex encephalitis
herpes simplex myelitis
herpes zoster
herpes zoster encephalitis
herpes zoster viral encephalitis
herpes zoster virus
herpetic whitlow
hersage (Fr. "combing")
hertz (Hz) (cycles per second)
Hertzler rib retractor
Herzmark frame
Heschl convolution

Heschl transverse gyrus
hesitation test
Hessel-Nystrom pin
heterogeneous (or heterogenous)
heterogeneous system degeneration
heterogeneous system disease
heterogenesis
heterografts, porcine
heterotopic ossification
Heubner, recurrent artery of
Heubner syphilitis endarteritis
Heuter-Volkmann law
Hewson cruciate guide
Hewson ligament button
Hewson suture passer
hex nut
hex screw
Hexcel total condylar knee system
Hexcelite cast
Heyer-Schulte antisiphon device (ASD)
Heyer-Schulte bur hole valve
Heyer-Schulte neurosurgical shunt
Heyer-Schulte wound drain
Hey-Groves-Kirk bone graft
Hey-Groves ligament reconstruction
Heyman-Herndon clubfoot operation
Heyman-Herndon procedure
Heyman-Herndon-Strong technique
HFF (high filter frequency) on EEG
HG Multilock hip prosthesis
HHA (homonymous hemianopia)
HHE syndrome (hemiconvulsions, hemiplegia, and epilepsy)
HHW (hand-held weights)
HI (head injury)
HIAD (high-impact aerobic dance)
hiatus, popliteal
Hibbs blade
Hibbs bone-cutting forceps
Hibbs chisel elevator
Hibbs curet
Hibbs gouge
Hibbs-Jones spinal fusion procedure
Hibbs mallet
Hibbs metatarsocalcaneal angle
Hibbs osteotome
Hibbs retractor
Hibbs spinal curet
Hibbs spinal fusion gouge
Hibbs-Spratt spinal fusion curet
Hibbs test
Hibiclens scrub
Hibiclens solution
hickory-stick fracture
Hicks lugged plate
HID (herniated intervertebral disk)
HIE (hypoxic-ischemic encephalopathy)
hierarchical scales of ADLs
HIF (higher integrative functions)
high-air-loss bed
high-caliber, low-velocity handgun injury
high-energy gunshot wound
high-energy trauma
high-grade astrocytoma tumor
high-impact activities
high-impact aerobic dance (HIAD)
high level motor problem
high level perceptual disturbance
high manganese diet for multiple sclerosis
high muscular resistance bed
high-pitched bruit
high pontine lesion
high-power athlete
high-resolution infrared (HRI) imaging
high-resolution, low-speed radiography
high-resolution ultrasound scanning for foreign bodies
high-signal (on MRI) intratendinous collection of fluid
high steppage gait
high-torque bur
high-velocity gunshot wound
high-volt biphasic stimulator
high-volt inferential stimulator
high voltage slow and sharp activity

higher cerebral dysfunction (HCD)
higher cognitive functions
higher cortical dysfunction
higher cortical functioning
higher integrative functions (HIF)
higher integrative language processing
higher level cognitive functions
Hilgenreiner angle
Hilgenreiner horizontal Y line
Hilgenreiner line
Hilgenreiner-Pauwels line
Hilgenreiner-Perkins line
Hilger facial nerve stimulator
Hill-Nahai-Vasconez-Mathes technique
Hill-Rom orthopedic bed
Hill-Sachs deformity
Hill-Sachs shoulder lesion
hillock, axon
Hillock arch
hilum, hilar
hindbrain deformity
Hinderer cartilage forceps
hindfoot arthrodesis
hindfoot excursion
hindfoot instability
hindfoot joint complex
hindfoot kinematics
hindfoot motion
hindfoot valgus
hinge
  Arizona Health Sciences Center-Volz
  Bahler
  Compass
  Dee elbow
  flail-elbow
  implant
  Kinematic rotating
  Kudo
  Lacey
  Noiles
  Quengel
  Rancho swivel
  stabilizing
hinged implant
hinge joint, stable
hip
  congenital dislocation of (CDH)
  congenital dysplasia of (CDH)
  developmental dysplasia (DDH)
  dislocated
  hanging
  pillow orthosis for
  Precision total
  snapping
  Senegas approach to
hip abduction stress test
hip arthroplasty, Mark II Sorrells
hip bump
hip dislocation
hip-knee-ankle-foot orthosis (HKAFO)
hip pointer
hip prosthesis
hip replacement
hip skid
hip spica cast
hippocampal-amygdala complex
hippocampal formation
hippocampal gyrus
hippocampal herniation
hippocampal infarction
hippocampal region
hippocampal seizure
hippocampus
  CA1, CA2, CA3 subfields of
  dentate granule subfield of
  granulovacuolar change in
  hilar subfield of
  hippocampal
  Sommer sector of
Hippocrates bandage
Hippocrates manipulation
hippotherapy
hippus
Hirano bodies
HiRider motorized/lift wheelchair
Hirsch hypophyseal punch
Hirsch hypophysis punch forceps

Hirschberg sign
Hirschhorn compression approach
Hirschtick splint
His-Haas muscle transfer
Hi Speed Pulse Lavage
hissing respiration in uremic coma
histamine cephalalgia
histamine headache
histinemia
histiocytoma
  angiomatoid
  fibrous
  low-grade malignant
  malignant fibrous
histiocytosis X group of diseases
Histoacryl glue
histological tendon changes
histolytica, Torula (earlier name for *Cryptococcus neoformans)*
Histoplasma capsulatum meningitis
history of seizures
hitch, ankle
Hitchcock arm procedure
Hitchcock stereotactic head frame
Hitchcock tendon technique
Hi-Top foot/ankle brace
Hi-Top foot/ankle walker
Hittenberger halo extension
Hittenberger prosthesis
HIV viral antigen
HJB (high jugular bulb)
HKAFO (hip-knee-ankle-foot orthosis)
HL (hallux limitus)
HLA-B27
HMPAO (hexamethyl propylene amine oxime) for SPECT scan
HMSN (hereditary motor and sensory neuropathy)
HMT (Hodkinson Mental Test)
HNA (hypothalamoneurohypophyseal axis)
HNB angiographic catheter
HNP (herniated nucleus pulposus)
Hoaglund bone graft
Hobb view
hobble, hobbling
hockey-stick incision
Hodes, surface method of
Hodgen splint
Hodgkin lymphoma, intracranial
Hodgkin tumor
Hodkinson Mental Test (HMT)
Hoek-Bowen cement removal system
Hoen angular forceps
Hoen clamp
Hoen dural separator
Hoen hemilaminectomy retractor
Hoen intervertebral disk rongeur
Hoen lamina gouge
Hoen laminectomy rongeur
Hoen nerve hook
Hoen periosteal elevator
Hoen scalp hemostat
Hoen scalp retractor
Hoen skull plate
Hoen ventricular needle
Hoffa fat pad
Hoffa tendon shortening
Hoffa test
Hoffer-Daimler cast spreader
Hoffer ankle procedure
Hoffmann-Clayton operation
Hoffmann external fixation device
Hoffmann metatarsal operation
Hoffmann monosynaptic reflex (H reflex)
Hoffmann reflex
Hoffmann sign
Hoffmann syndrome
Hoffmann-Vidal double frame
Hogg chair
Hohl tibia condylar fracture classification
Hohmann bone retractor
Hohmann osteotomy
Hoke Achilles tendon lengthening operation
Hoke lumbar brace/corset

Hoke-Martin traction
Hoke osteotome
Hoke procedure for tibial palsy
Hold-and-Hold positioner
Holdaway ratio
holder
  acetabular cup
  Adson dural needle
  Adson needle
  Aesculap head
  Alvarado knee
  Alvarado leg
  arm
  arthroscopic leg
  Ayers needle
  Barraquer needle
  Böhler-Steinmann pin (Boehler)
  bone
  Castroviejo needle
  CBI stereotactic head
  Charnley trochanter
  Crile-Wood needle
  cup
  Donaghy angled suture needle
  Drummond
  Drummond hook
  Ferguson bone
  Halsey needle
  head
  Jacobson needle
  knee
  leg
  lithotomy leg
  Low Profile leg
  Malis needle
  Mayfield skull-pin head
  Mayo-Hegar needle
  microneedle
  microsurgery needle
  Micro-Two needle
  needle
  neurosurgical needle
  operative leg
  OSI Arthroscopic Leg

holder *(cont.)*
  Patil stereotactic head
  pin
  Prep-Assist leg
  ReFix stereotactic head
  Rhoton needle
  Ryder needle
  Schmidt rod
  shell
  skull-pin head
  staple
  Surbaugh leg
  Surg-Assist leg
  tibial track
  trochanter
  Wangensteen
  Webster needle
  well-leg
  Yasargil needle
  Zollinger leg
Holdsworth classification of spinal injury
hole
  acetabular seating
  anchor
  anchoring
  bur (or burr)
  centering
  drill
  glide
  guide
  offset drill
  pullout
hole cutter
holiday, drug (therapeutic)
Holinger endarterectomy dissector
holistic approach
hollow foot
hollow mill Asnis cannulated screw
hollow-point bullet
Hollywood bed extension hook set
Holmes-Adie pupil
Holmes cerebellar degeneration
Holmes cortical cerebellar degeneration

Holmes degeneration
holocrania
holoprosencephaly
Holscher nerve root retractor
Holt bolt
Holt nail
Holt-Oran syndrome
Holt plate
Holzheimer retractor
Homans sign
home assessment
home evaluation
homeostatic balance
homocystinuria
homogeneity
homogeneous graft
homograft
homologous graft
homonymous defect
homonymous hemianopsia (HHA)
homonymous scintillating scotomata
honeymoon palsy
hood
  dorsal aponeurotic expansion
  extensor
  retinacular
hook
  Acufex nerve
  Adson dissecting
  Adson dural
  Adson nerve
  André
  APRL (Army Prosthetics Research Laboratory)
  Austin Moore
  Barr
  bifid
  blunt
  blunt nerve
  Bobechko
  bone
  Boyes-Goodfellow
  button
  buttressed

hook *(cont.)*
  C-D
  Carroll skin
  caudal
  cautery
  clawed pedicle
  Cloward cautery
  Cloward dural
  compression
  cordotomy
  corkscrew dural
  Cotrel-Dubousset
  Crile nerve
  Culler
  Cushing dural
  Cushing gasserian ganglion
  Cushing nerve
  Dandy nerve
  DePuy nerve
  dissecting
  distraction
  double
  Drummond
  DTT (dynamic transverse traction)
  dura
  dural
  Edwards
  Edwards-Levine
  Effler-Groves
  Fisch dural
  Fisch micro
  Frazier dural
  Frazier nerve
  ganglion
  garment
  Gillies
  Gillies bone
  Gillies-Dingman
  Graham muscle
  Graham nerve
  Green muscle
  Harrington
  Hoen nerve
  Isola

hook *(cont.)*
- Jameson muscle
- Jannetta
- Joseph
- Küntscher nail extracting
- Keene compression
- Kennerdell-Maroon
- Kilner
- Kirby muscle
- Knodt
- Krayenbuehl (Krayenbühl)
- Lahey Clinic dural
- Lahey Clinic nerve
- Lambotte bone
- laminar
- Leatherman
- Love nerve root
- Lucae nerve
- Malis nerve
- Marino transsphenoidal
- meniscus
- micro
- micro dural
- Micro-One
- Moe spinal
- Moe square-ended
- Moss
- muscle
- nail-extracting
- nerve
- O'Brien rib
- pedicle
- prosthetic
- Rhoton
- rib
- right-angle
- Rogozinski
- Rosser crypt
- Sachs dural
- Scoville nerve
- Scoville nerve root
- Selby II
- Selverstone cordotomy
- sharp
- shoe of the
- side opening
- skin
- sliding barrel
- Smithwick button
- Smithwick nerve
- Smithwick sympathectomy
- Speare dural
- spring
- straight dura
- Strully dural
- sympathectomy
- T-handled
- tendon
- Toennis dura
- traction
- transsphenoidal
- transverse
- transverse process
- Trautman Locktite prosthetic
- TSRH (Texas Scottish Rite Hospital)
- twist
- Tyrell
- vessel
- Volkmann bone
- Weary nerve
- Yasargil spring
- Zielke
- Zimmer caudal
- Zuelzer

Hook hemi-harness shoulder immobilizer

hooklike osteophyte formation

hook of hamate bone

hook-plate fixation

hook-rod
- Cotrel-Dubousset
- Isola
- TSRH (Texas Scottish Rite Hospital)

Hoover sign

Hoover test

Hopkins plaster knife
Hoppenfeld-Deboer technique
horizontal gaze
horizontal shoulder abduction exercises
hormone
  growth
  luteinizing
  prolactin
  thyrotropin
horn
  Ammon
  anterior
  central
  dorsal spinal cord
  enlarged frontal
  frontal
  occipital
  posterior
  posterior gray (of spinal cord)
  spinal cord
  spinal dorsal
  splaying of frontal
  temporal
Horner syndrome
  congenital
  neonatal
horn of ventricle
horse, charley
horse's tail (cauda equina)
horseshoe abscess of hand
horseshoe appearance
Horsley bone-cutting forceps
Horsley bone rongeur
Horsley dural separator
Horsley saw
Horsley separator
Horsley-Stille bone-cutting forceps
Horsley-Stille rib shears
Horton cephalalgia
Horton giant cell arteritis
Horton headache
Horton histamine cephalalgia
Horwitz-Adams arthrodesis
Horwitz ankle fusion
hose, TED (thromboembolic disease) (see also *stockings*)
Hospital Anxiety and Depression Scale
hot and cold contrast baths
hot cross bun skull
hot fomentation therapy
hot packs
hot shot cervical or brachial plexus injury
hot spot on isotope bone scan
hot sulfur baths
Hot/Ice System III
Houghton-Akroyd fracture technique
Hounsfield unit
hourglass deformity on myelogram
hourglass tumors of the cord
hourglass-type of neurilemmoma
House-Dieter malleus nipper
House-Fisch dural retractor
House-Fisch dural spatula
housemaid's knee
Housepan aneurysm clips
Housepan clip-applying forceps
House suction-irrigator
Houston halo cervical support
Houston halo traction
Hovanian procedure
Howard bone block
Howard spinal curet
Howmedica cerclage cable
Howmedica ICS screw
Howmedica Kinematic II knee prosthesis
Howmedica Microfixation cranial plate
Howmedica Microfixation System drill bit
Howmedica Microfixation System plate cutters
Howmedica Microfixation System plate-holding forceps
Howmedica Microfixation System pliers
Howmedica Vitallium staple
Howmedica VSF fixation system
Howorth-Keillor procedure

Howse total hip replacement
Hoyer lift
HPS II hip prosthesis
HRF (Health-Related Facilities)
HRI (high-resolution infrared) imaging
HS (Haynes-Stellite) implant metal
HSE (herpes simplex encephalitis)
HSMN (hereditary sensorimotor neuropathy)
HSMN III (hereditary sensorimotor neuropathy, type III)
HSN (hereditary sensory neuropathy)
HSS (Hospital for Special Surgery)
HSS knee prosthesis
HSS knee score
HSS ligament rating scale
HSV particles on brain biopsy
Hubbard physical therapy tank
Hubbard plate
Huber needle
Huber transfer of abductor digiti quinti
Huck towel
Huckstep nail
Hudson bone bur
Hudson brace drill
Hudson bur
Hudson cerebellar attachment
Hudson chuck adapter
Hudson cranial drill set
Hudson cranial rongeur
Hudson forceps
Hueter bandage
Hueter fracture sign
Hueter line
Hueter sign
Hughston Clinic classification of injury
Hughston-Degenhardt reconstruction technique
Hughston external rotation recurvatum test
Hughston-Hauser procedure
Hughston-Jacobson technique
Hughston knee evaluation
Hughston knee score
Hughston-Losee jerk test
Hughston view
humeroperoneal muscular dystrophy
humeroradial articulation
humeroulnar articulation
humerus, humeral
hump
  buffalo
  dowager's
  hip
humpback
hung-up (sustained) knee jerk
Hungerford-Krackow-Kenna knee arthroplasty
Hunt disease
Hunt-Hess aneurysm grading system
Hunt-Hess neurological classification
Hunt-Hess subarachnoid hemorrhage scale
Hunt-Kosnik classification of aneurysms
Hunt-Kosnik classification of nuchal stiffness
Hunt neuralgia
Hunt tumor forceps
Hunt-Yasargil pituitary forceps
Hunter canal
Hunter dural separator
Hunter open cord tendon implant
Hunter Silastic rod
Hunter syndrome
Hunter tendon prosthesis
Hunter tendon rod
hunterian ligation of aneurysm
Huntington bone graft
Huntington chorea
Huntington disease
Huntington sign
Hurd bone-cutting forceps
Hurler disease
Hurler syndrome
Hurst disease
Hurteau skull plate anvil
Husk bone rongeur

Hutchinson pupil
Hutchinson type of neuroblastoma
HV (hallux valgus)
HVA (hallux valgus angle)
HVO forefoot splint (hallux valgus orthosis)
hyaline-cartilage endplate of the intervertebral disk
hyaluronidase, synovial
hybrid seizure
Hydra-Cadence gait control unit
hydranencephaly (hydrocephalus)
hydrated proteoglycan gel of annulus fibrosus
hydrencephalomeningocele
hydrencephaly
hydrocephalic patient
hydrocephalocele
hydrocephalus
  acquired
  acute
  asymptomatic
  bilateral
  chronic
  communicating
  congenital
  delayed
  fulminant
  idiopathic
  infantile
  noncommunicating
  normal-pressure (NPH)
  normotensive
  obstructive
  occult
  otitis
  posthemorrhagic
  postinfectious
  posttraumatic
  primary
  secondary
  symptomatic
  unilateral
  unshunted
hydrocephalus ex vacuo
hydrocephaly
hydrocollation
Hydrocollator pad
Hydrocollator steam pack
hydrodipsomania
hydrodynamic potential of disk
hydroencephalocele
hydroencephaly
hydrogen peroxide
hydroma (see *hygroma*)
hydromyelia
Hydron Burn Bandage
hydrophobia (rabies)
hydropneumogony
hydrops
  endolymphatic
  labyrinthine
hydrops of the semicircular canals
Hydro-Splint II
hydrosyringomyelia
hydrotherapy pool
Hydroxial hip prosthesis
hydroxyapatite
  APS (air plasma spray)
  calcium
  LPPS (low-pressure plasma spray)
hydroxyapatite adhesive
hydroxyapatite bone replacement material
hydroxyisovaleric aminoaciduria
hygroma
  cystic
  subdural
Hylamer acetabular liner
Hylin rasp
hypalgesia (hypoalgesia)
Hypaque contrast medium
Hypaque myelography
hyper-ß-alaninemia
hyperactive behavior
hyperactive deep tendon reflexes
hyperactive reflexes
hyperactive syndrome

hyperactivity
  autonomic
  sudomotor (not pseudomotor)
    autonomic
hyperacusis
hyperalgesia
hyperalgesic
hyperbaric oxygen for osteomyelitis
hyperbradykininism
hypercalcemia
hypercholesterolemia
hyperdopaminergic state
hyperdynamic abductor hallucis
hyperemia test
hyperemic
hyperesthesia, stocking-glove
hyperesthetic
hyperexcitability, neuronal
hyperexplexia
hyperextensibility of joints
hyperextension injury
hyperextension stress
hyperextension test
hyperflexion/hyperextension cervical injury
hyperflexion injury
hyperglycemia
  ketotic
  nonketotic
hyperhidrosis
hyperintense marrow space
hyperkeratosis
hyperkeratotic plantar lesion
hyperkinesia
hyperkinesis
hyperkinetic motor disorder
hyperkinetic movement
hyperlaxity
hyperlisenemia
hyperlordosis, functional
hyperlysinemia
hypermetria
hypermobile first ray
hypermobility
hypermyelination
hypernephroma, cerebral
hyperostosis
  ankylosing spinal
  Caffey
  diffuse idiopathic sclerosis (DISH)
  diffuse idiopathic skeletal (DISH)
  idiopathic cortical (ICH)
  infantile cortical
  skull
hyperparathyroidism, brown tumor of
hyperpathia, thalamic
hyperpigmented lesion
hyperpituitary state
hyperplasia
  epiphyseal
  gingival
hyperplastic
hyperpolarization
hyperpolarize
hyperprolactinemia
hyperprolinemia
hyperpronation
hyperreflexia
  asymmetric
  autonomic
  bilateral
  pathologic
  spastic
  unilateral
hyperreflexic
hypersarcosinemia
hypersensitivity reaction to anticonvulsants
hypersomnia
hypersomnolence
hypersynchrony, paroxysmal hypnagogic (on EEG)
hypertelorism
hypertension
  benign intracranial (BIH)
  intracranial
  striate hemorrhage in intracranial
hypertension injury

hypertensive encephalopathy
hypertensive hemorrhage
hypertensive stroke
hyperthermia
  volumetric interstitial
  whole body
hypertonia
hypertonicity
hypertrichosis
hypertrophic infiltrating tenosynovitis
hypertrophica, pachymeningitis
  cervicalis
hypertrophy
  ligamentous-muscular
  muscular
  olivary
hyperuricemia
hypervalinemia
hyperventilation
  autonomic
  central neurogenic
  forced
  neurogenic
  psychogenic
  stertorous
hyperventilation as activating
  technique during EEG
hypervigilance
hypesthesia (hypoesthesia)
hypnagogic hallucinations
hypnagogic hypersynchrony on EEG
hypnagogic state
hypnalgia
hypnic jerks
hypnolepsy
hypnopedia
hypnopompic hallucinations
hypoactive deep tendon reflexes
hypoalgesia (hypalgesia)
hypocalcemia
hypochondriac region
hypochondriasis
hypocycloidal ankle tomography
hypoesthesia (hypesthesia)
hypoesthesic
hypoflexibility of foot
hypogeusia
hypoglossal nerve (twelfth cranial
  nerve)
hypoglossal neuralgia
hypoglycemia
hypoglycorrhachia
hypokinesia, parkinsonian
hypokinesis
hypomelanosis, Ito
hypometria
hypomyelination neuropathy
hyponychium
hypo-osmolar glucose solution
hypoparathyroidism
hypophyseal (or hypophysial)
hypophysectomy
  transcranial
  transsphenoidal
hypophysectomy kit, Zervas
hypophysial (or hypophyseal)
hypophysis cerebri
hypophysis, infundibulum
hypopituitarism
hypopituitary coma
hypoplasia
  cartilage-hair
  skeletal
hyporeflexia
hyporeflexic
hypothalamic lesion
hypothalamic-pituitary-adrenal axis
hypothalamic-pituitary axis
hypothalamus
  anterior
  rostral
hypothalamus tumor
hypothenar eminence
hypothenar muscle groups of hand
hypothermia
hypotonia
  benign congenital
  cerebral
  congenital
hypotonic

hypotonic patient
hypoxia
  anemic
  anoxic
  cerebral
  hypoxic
  ischemic
  toxic
hypoxic brain damage
hypoxic encephalopathy
hypsarrhythmia
  asymmetrical
  unilateral
hypsarrhythmia pattern on EEG
hypsokinesis
hysteric coma-like state
hysterical aphonia
hysterical blindness
hysterical conversion reaction
hysterical fugue state
hysterical gait
hysterical hemiplegia
hysterical mutism
hysterical pseudodementia
hysterical seizure
hysterical trance
hysterical tremor
hysterical visual loss
hysterical overbreathing, voluntary
hystericus, globus
hysteroepilepsy
Hz (hertz or cycles per second)

I, i

IADL (instrumental activities of daily living)
IADSA (intra-arterial digital subtraction angiography)
I&D (incision and drainage)
IAP (intracranial amobarbital procedure)
IAS (intra-articular shaver)
IAT (intraoperative autologous transfusion)
iatrogenic dural tear
iatrogenic elevatus
IBCA (n-isobutyl-cyanoacrylate) glue
I-beam, Jergesen
IBF (Insall-Burstein-Freeman) knee instruments
IBM (inclusion body myositis)
IC (intermittent catheterization)
ICA (internal carotid artery)
ice, application of
ice massage
ice water caloric response
ice water irrigation
ICEDP (intracranial epidural pressure)
Iceland (or Icelandic) disease
ICF (Intermediate Care Facilities)
ICH (idiopathic cortical hyperostosis)
ICH (intracerebral hemorrhage)
ichthyosis in Refsum disease
ICIDH (International Classification of Impairments, Disabilities, Handicaps)
ICIDH model of the World Health Organization
icing, cutaneous
ICLH (Imperial College, London Hospital)
ICLH ankle prosthesis
ICLH apparatus
ICLH double-cup arthroplasty
ICP (intracranial pressure)
ICP catheter
ICP monitor
ICP wave form
ICS (intercostal space)
ICST (isolated cold stress test)
ictal amnesia
ictal automatism
ictal confusional seizure
ictal epileptiform activity
ictal epileptiform pattern
ictal focal epileptiform discharge
ictal pattern on EEG
ictal period
ictus
ICV (internal cerebral vein)
ideational apraxia
ideational dyspraxia
ideomotor apraxia
ideomotor dyspraxia
idiocy, mongolian
idioglossia
idiopathic cortical hyperostosis (ICH)
idiopathic encephalopathy
idiopathic epilepsy
idiopathic facial nerve palsy
idiopathic fracture
idiopathic generalized epilepsy

idiopathic polymyositis myopathy
idiopathic polyneuropathy
idiopathic scoliosis
idiopathic seizure
idiot-savant
IDK (internal derangement of knee)
I_z electrode
Ikuta fixation device
ileus as response to spinal injury
Ilfeld-Gustafson splint
Ilheus encephalitis
Ilheus viral encephalitis
iliac apophysitis
iliac compression test
iliac dowel
iliac wing
ilioinguinal syndrome
iliopsoas test
iliotibial band augmentation
iliotibial band friction syndrome
ilium
Ilizarov ankle arthrodesis
Ilizarov corticotomy
Ilizarov distractor
Ilizarov external fixator
Ilizarov fixator
Ilizarov frame
Ilizarov leg lengthening technique
Ilizarov limb lengthening procedure
Ilizarov ring
Ilizarov screw
Ilizarov system
Ilizarov technique
Ilizarov wire
illicit drug, blood levels of
illness behaviors
illness, progressive dementing
illusion
illusory strabismus
IM (intermetatarsal) joint
IM (intramedullary) rod, rodding
IMA (intermetatarsal angle)
image acquisition time
image control
image intensification
image intensifier
image, persistence of visual
images, flow
imaging
  blood pool
  color-flow duplex
  delayed bone
  magnetic resonance (MRI)
  neurodiagnostic
imbalance
  biomechanical
  muscle
imbecility
imbibition
imbricate
imbrication
  capsular
  facetal
imbrication of facets
immediate memory; recall (short-term memory)
immediate postsurgical fitting (IPSF)
immitis, Coccidioides
immobilization after spinal injury
immobilization
  cast
  external
  halo
  joint
  postoperative
  Rowe-Zarin shoulder
  sling
  Velcro
immobilization jacket
immobilizer
  Hook hemi-harness shoulder
  knee
  long leg
  OEC knee
  Raymond shoulder
  sateen knee
  shoulder
  shoulder abduction

immobilizer *(cont.)*
  sterno-occipitomanubrial
  Tab-Strap knee
  Trimline knee
  Velcro
  Velpeau shoulder
  Watco 2001 knee
  Westfield acromioclavicular
  Y-strap knee
  Zimmer knee
  Zinco thumb-wrist
immunization, tetanus
immunocytochemistry
immunoglobulin, tetanus
immunoreactive chromogranin
immunostain
  chromogranin
  cytokeratin
  epithelial membrane antigen (EMA)
  GFAP (glial fibrillary acidic protein)
  pancytokeratin
  proliferating cell nuclear antigen
  S-100 protein
  vimentin
immunostaining
IMPA cephalometric measurement
IMP Surgical Leg Pedestal
IMP-Turnstile Casting Stand
impact force
Impact total hip prosthesis
impactor
  Austin Moore
  Cloward bone graft
  Dawson-Yuhl
  Küntscher
  Moe
  shell
  Smith-Petersen
  vertebral body
impactor-extractor, Fox
impactor rod
impaired consciousness
impairment
  anterior horn cell motor
  constructional

impairment *(cont.)*
  disease-specific measure of
  gaze
  graphic
  intellectual
  memory
  motor
  objective symptoms of
  perceptual-motor
  peripheral nerve level motor
  reading comprehension
  root level motor
  spinal nerve level motor
  subjective symptoms of
  upper motor neuron
  visual
impairment-based measures
impairment of consciousness
impairment of coordination
impedance
  electrical
  electrode
  interelectrode
  ohms
impedance meter
imperfect regeneration
impinge
impinged upon
impingement
  dural
  lateral
  ligamentous (ankle)
  talar
  talofibular
impingement on nerve root
impingement syndrome
impingement tendinitis
impingement exostosis
implant (see also *prosthesis*)
  AO-ASIF
  Arenberg-Denver inner-ear valve
  Biocoral
  Biodel
  Biofix biodegradable
  Biomatrix ocular

implant *(cont.)*
cochlear
Custodis
DePuy orthopedic
double-stem silicone lesser MP
Durapatite
epidural
gentamicin
Gliadel
Global total shoulder
hinged
Hunter open cord tendon
hydroxyapatite
IMEX scleral
Insall-Burstein total knee
Interpore
islet cell
LaPorta great toe
McCutchen
methyl methacrylate beads
Miragel
Nexus
PMMA (poly-methyl methacrylate)
polyglycolide
polylactide
ProOsteon synthetic bone
Septacin
Ship hammertoe
silicone
silicone elastomer rubber ball
Sinterlock
Sutter double-stem silicone
Swanson metacarpophalangeal
Techmedica
TheraSeed
tobramycin-impregnated PMMA
vagal nerve
vagus stimulator
Zielke VDS (ventral derotating spinal)
implantable bone growth stimulator, Osteo Stim
implant collar
implant hinge
implant metal
Implast bone cement
impulse, simultaneous nerve
impulsive petit mal
impulsiveness
impulsivity
in-a-chair test
in extremis
in phase
in situ pinning
in situ vein graft
in situ vein graft to ankle
in-toeing
in toto
inability to attend
inactivity, electrocerebral (ECI)
inappropriate ADH (antidiuretic hormone) secretion
inappropriate affect
inappropriate words (paraphrasia)
inattention
functional
organic
inattentiveness, momentary
InCare ankle brace
incarnatus, unguis
incise
incision
anteromedial
battledore (racquet-shaped)
bifrontal
bikini skin
Brunner modified
Brunner palmar
Bruser skin (knee)
capsular
Charnley
chevron
Cincinnati
circumscribing
coronal
coronal scalp
Cubbins
Curtin

incision *(cont.)*
- curved
- curvilinear
- deltoid-splitting
- dorsal linear
- dorsomedial
- double
- DuVries
- elliptical
- exploratory
- fascial-splitting
- fiber-splitting
- fish-mouth
- Gaenslen split heel
- H-shaped capsular
- Henderson skin
- Henry
- hockey-stick
- J-shaped skin
- Kocher
- Kocher collar
- L-curved
- L-shaped
- lateral
- lateral utility
- lazy-S
- longitudinal
- Ludloff
- Mayfield
- medial
- medial parapatellar
- median parapatellar
- midaxillary line
- muscle-splitting
- oblique
- Ollier
- palmar
- paramedial
- parapatellar
- posterior
- racquet-shaped
- relaxing
- relieving
- S

incision *(cont.)*
- S-flap
- S-shaped
- saber-cut
- serpentine
- skin
- split
- stab
- standard
- straight
- T-shaped
- tangential
- transverse
- U-shaped
- V-shaped
- volar
- Wagner skin
- Watson-Jones
- webspace
- Y
- Y-shaped
- Z-plasty
- zigzag finger

incision and drainage (I&D)
incisional scar
Incisor arthroscopic blade
incisura of tentorium
incisura, tentorial
incisural sclerosis
Inclan modification of Campbell ankle operation
Inclan-Ober procedure
inclinometer
inclusion
- retinal
- intracytoplasmic hyaline

inclusion bodies
inclusion cyst
Income, Supplemental Security (SSI)
incompetence
- deep venous
- sphincter

incomplete closure
incomplete stroke

incongruity, angle of
incontinence
  bowel
  bowel and bladder
  emotional
  fecal
  urinary
incontinent after seizure
incontinentia pigmenti
incontinent of feces/stool
incontinent of urine
incoordination, motor
incorporation (new-bone formation)
increased basilar cisterns
increased intracranial pressure
increased tonus
increment
indentation of the myelography dye with incomplete tumors
independent in bed mobility
independent in bed transfers
Independent Living movement
index, Index (pl. indices)
  ADL (activities of daily living)
  alpha
  ambulation
  ankle/arm
  ankle/brachial (ABI)
  ankle-brachial blood pressures
  arch
  arch length
  Arthritis Helplessness (AHI)
  Barthel ADL
  Benink tarsal
  beta
  Caregiver Strain (CSI)
  Chippaux-Smirak arch
  Convery polyarticular disability
  CSF immunoglobulin
  delta
  dye fluorescence (DFI)
  footprint
  Fourier pulsatility
  Frenchay Activities (FAI)
index *(cont.)*
  Functional Status (FSI)
  Garden alignment
  Hauser ambulation
  ischemic
  Jette Functional Status
  Katz ADL Index
  Keitel
  Kenny ADL
  laxity
  Life Satisfaction (LSI)
  Lucas and Drucker Motor
  maturation
  McDowell Impairment (MII)
  McMurtry kinematic
  Motricity
  multi-item
  Northwick Park Index of Independence in ADL
  Nottingham Extended ADL
  pipe stemming of ankle-brachial
  Porch Index of Communicative Ability (PICA)
  poststress ankle/arm Doppler
  pulsatility
  QL
  Reintegration to Normal Living
  resting ankle/arm Doppler
  Ritchie
  Rivermead ADL (RAI)
  Rivermead Mobility (RMI)
  Roland i. of low back pain
  Singh osteoporosis
  Spinal Cord Motor Index and Sensory Indices
  systolic toe/brachial
  talocalcaneal
  theta
  toe
  truncated arch
  valgus
  Waddell Chronic Back Pain Disability
Index of Well-Being (IWB)

Indiana conservative prosthesis
Indiana reamer
indices (pl. of index)
indifférence, la belle
indirect fracture
indium-111-labeled leukocyte bone scan
indium scintigraphy with ^{111}In oxine white blood cells
Indong Oh hip prosthesis
inductance
indurated, induration
indusium griseum
Industrial Work Brace, by Bodyline
indwelling catheter
inequality, limb-length
Inerpan flexible burn dressing
inertia, polar moment of
infancy, pre-walking treatment of pronated feet in
infantile hemiplegia
infantile hydrocephalus
infantile polymyoclonus syndrome
infantile seizure
infantile spasms
infarct
infarction
  anterior communicating artery distribution
  bicerebral
  bone
  brain stem
  capsular
  capsulocaudate
  capsuloputaminal
  capsuloputaminocaudate
  cerebellar
  cerebral
  cerebral artery
  cortical
  dominant-hemisphere
  embolic
  Freiberg so-called
  frontal lobe
  gyral

infarction *(cont.)*
  hemispheric
  hemorrhagic
  hippocampal
  ischemic
  ischemic brain stem
  lacunar
  lacunar brain
  medullary
  mesencephalic
  migrainous
  multifocal
  multiple cortical
  nonembolic
  nonseptic embolic brain
  occipital
  occipital lobe
  old
  pale
  paramedian
  pontine
  posterior cerebral territory
  retinal
  small, deep, recent (SDRI)
  spinal cord
  temporal lobe
  thalamic
  ventral pontine
  watershed
  white matter
infection
  bone
  brucellosis
  central nervous system
  chronic spinal epidural
  chronic spinal intradural
  closed disk-space
  coccidioidomycosis
  cryptococcosis
  disk-space
  felon
  helminthic (of the nervous system)
  Meleney gangrene
  mycotic (of bones and joints)

infection *(cont.)*
  paraspinal
  pin tract
  rickettsial (of central nervous system)
  slow-virus (of the nervous system)
  soft tissue
  syphilis
  tendon sheat space
  tuberculous cold abscess
infectious hepatitis encephalitis
infectious mononucleosis encephalitis
infectious polyneuritis syndrome
inferior cerebellar peduncle
inferior dorsal radioulnar ligament
inferior frontal gyrus
inferior parietal lobule
inferior quadriceps retinaculum
inferior temporal gyrus
inferior temporal lobule
INFH (ischemic necrosis of femoral head)
infiltrate, meningeal
infiltrating tenosynovitis, hypertrophic
infiltration of meninges, leukemic
inflame, inflamed
inflammation
  bursal
  meningeal
  polyarticular symmetric tophaceous joint
inflammatory arthropathy
inflammatory process of the superior orbital fissure
inflate, inflated
inflation
influenza encephalitis
influenza viral encephalitis
information
  fund of
  recall of
infracalcaneal bursitis
infracalcarine gyrus
infraction, Freiberg
infragluteal crease
infraisthmal
infranuclear lesion
infranuclear paralysis
infranuclear weakness
infrapatellar contracture syndrome (IPCS)
infrapatellar fat pad
infrapatellar tendinitis
infrapopliteal artery occlusion
infrared (IR) electronic thermography
infraspinatus tendon
infratemporal fossa
infratentorial approach
infratentorial brain tumor
infratentorial compartment
infratentorial-Lindau tumor
infundibular stalk
infundibulum hypothalami
infundibulum of hypophysis
infundibulum, tumor of the
Infusaid continuous flow drug pump
Infuse-a-port drug delivery system
infusion, Katzman (of radionuclide cisternography)
Inge cervical lamina spreader
Inge laminectomy retractor
Inge laminectomy spreader
Inglis-Cooper technique
Inglis-Pellicci elbow arthroplasty rating system
Inglis-Ranawat-Straub technique
Ingraham-Fowler tantalum clip
Ingraham skull punch forceps
Ingram-Bachynski classification of hip fracture
Ingram osteotomy
Ingram procedure
Ingram-Withers-Speltz motor test
ingrowing toenail
ingrown toenail
ingrowth, bone
inguinal ligament syndrome

inhibition
periodic interneuron
reflex
synchronous interneuron
inhibitory postsynaptic potential (IPSP)
inhomogeneity
iniencephaly
inion
inion bump
initial double support (of gait)
initiation, gait
initiation of movement
injection
Black peroneal tendon sheath
chymopapain
corticosteroid
cortisone
extradural
intraneural phenol
procaine-phenol motor point
steroid
tenosynovial
thecal
trigger point
injection technique
injured excitable cells (epileptic foci)
injury, injuries
acute stretch
ballistic
barked
brachial plexus
burst
cervical spine
closed head (CHI)
cocking
compression flexion
compression-plus-torque theory of cervical
compressive hyperextension
contrecoûp
crush
degloving
digit span test of recall after head
discoligamentous
injury *(cont.)*
distraction hyperflexion
Erb-Duchenne-Klumpke (to brachial plexus)
Erb (to brachial plexus)
extensive head
flexion-distraction
forced flexion
frostbite
growth plate
head (HI)
high-caliber, low-velocity handgun
hyperextension
hyperflexion
hyperflexion/hyperextension cervical
hypertension
inversion
Klumpke (to brachial plexus)
Lisfranc
low back
matrix
mild head
motor vehicle (MVI)
nerve
Ontario Cohort Study of Running-Related
penetrating
perinatal
peripheral nerve
physeal
plexus
postnatal
prenatal
pronation-external rotation (P-ER)
repetitive strain (RSI)
repetitive stress (RSI)
running-related
salient antecedents to
seat belt
severe head
skier's
soft tissue
soft tissue ankle
softball sliding

injury *(cont.)*
  spinal cord (SCI)
  straddle
  strain-sprain
  supination-outward rotation
  three-column (spinal column)
  throwing-arm
  transcutaneous crush
  traumatic
  traumatic brain (TBI)
  traumatic head
  two-column
  ultrasonic assessment of
  weight-bearing rotational
  whiplash
  windup
injury to nerve roots
Inland Super Multi-Hite orthopedic bed
inlay graft
inner stripe of Baillinger (in brain)
inner table
innervate
innervated
innervation
  motor
  parasympathetic
  sympathetic
innervatory dyspraxia
Innomed bone curet
innominate angiography
innominate bone
innominate osteotomy
INO (internuclear ophthalmoplegia) syndrome
inoperable brain tumor
input
  distorted synaptic (in epilepsy)
  limbic
  sensory
  tonic desynchronizing
Inronail finger prosthesis
Insall-Burstein-Freeman knee arthroplasty
Insall-Burstein semiconstrained tricompartmental knee prosthesis
Insall-Burstein total knee prosthesis
Insall-Hood reconstruction technique
Insall ligament reconstruction
Insall patella alta method (or ratio)
Insall-Salvati ratio
insaniens, chorea
insensate foot
insensitivity to painful stimuli, congenital
insert
  Alimed
  cushioned shoe
  NYU (New York University)
  orthosis
  Poly-Dial
  polypropylene
  silicone gel socket
  sole
  Spenco shoe
inserter
  Buck cement restrictor
  C-wire
  CDH cup
  cement restrictor
  cement spacer
  cerclage wire
  Kirschner wire
  Massie
  spacer
  staple
  T-shaped
inserter-extractor, compression
inserter-extractor screw-in instrument
insertion
  anomalous
  Bosworth bone peg
  ligamentous
  percutaneous pin
  tendinous
insertion tendinopathy
inset
insetting

inside-out Bankart shoulder operation
insidious
insidious onset of symptoms
insight and judgment
insight, preservation of
insipidus, diabetes
insole
  Aliplast
  Comforthotic
  Darco moldable
  Hapad metatarsal
insomnia
insonation, Doppler
Inspiron
instability
  anterolateral rotary knee
  articular
  atlantoaxial
  chronic functional
  dorsal intercalary segment (DISI)
  first ray
  hindfoot
  inversion
  joint
  lateral rotatory ankle
  ligamentous
  osseous
  postlaminectomy
  postural
  rotary
  rotary ankle
  rotational
  rotatory
  shoulder joint
  spinal
  subtalar
  sympathetic vascular
  truncal
  varus-valgus
  vasomotor
  volarflexed intercalated segment (VISI)
instability gait
instability while walking
Institute, National
  of Neurological and Communicative Disorders and Stroke (NINCDS)
  on Aging (NIA)
  on Mental Health (NIMH)
instructions, head injury
instrument, instrumentation (see also *device*)
  Accu-Line knee
  Acufex arthroscopic
  Beckman, 20 channel, for EEG
  CD (Cotrel-Dubousset)
  Collis TDR
  Craig vertebral body biopsy
  craniofacial remodeling
  Dwyer spinal
  Dyonics arthroscopic
  Evershears surgical
  Gamma knife (radiosurgical)
  graft-measuring
  Harrington
  hollow mill
  Howmedica knee
  interspinous segmental spinal (ISSI)
  Kinetix
  Kloehn craniofacial
  Luque
  McElroy
  Midas Rex pneumatic
  Millet neurological test
  Nucleotome Endoflex
  Nucleotome Flex II cannula
  Putti-Platt
  Rancho external fixation
  remodeling
  Richmond subarachnoid screw
  segmental spinal (SSI)
  signature
  Surgi-Tron
  Wiet graft-measuring
  Zielke
instrumental ADLs (activities of daily living, IADLs) (cooking, housework, shopping, and work)

insufficiency
  basilar
  cerebrovascular
  vertebrobasilar
insufflate, insufflated
insula, roof of
insular epilepsy
insular gyrus
insular lobe
insular-opercular syndrome
insular region of brain
insulin-like growth factor I
insult
  bihemispheral
  mechanical (to spine)
  occlusive cerebrovascular
intact
  neurologically
  neurovascularly
intact neurologic exam
integrative language processing, higher
integrity and alignment
integrity
  nervous system
  neurologic
  spinal
Integrity acetabular cup prosthesis
integrity of nerve impulse, electrophysiologic
intellectual deterioration
intellectual functioning, discrepant
intensifier, image (x-ray)
intention myoclonus
intention tremor
Inter-Royal frame orthopedic bed
interaction, surface-shoe
interarticular disk
interbody fusion
interburst interval measurement
intercalary defect
intercarpal articulation
intercarpal coalition
intercarpal joints
intercaudate distance
intercollicular groove
intercondylar fossa
intercondylar groove
intercondylar notch
intercostal neuralgia
intercostal space (ICS)
intercostal spasm
intercostobrachial nerve
interdigital clavus
interdigital ligament
interdigital neoplasm
interdigital neuritis
interdigital neuroma
interdigitation of vastus lateral with fascia
interelectrode distance
interelectrode impedance
interface
  acetabular-prosthetic
  bone-cement
  bone-implant
  bony
  cement
  cement-bone
  cement-prosthesis
  electrode-skin
  implant-cement
  joint
  pin-skin
  scalp-electrode
  skin-electrode
interference on EEG
interference pattern, EMG incomplete
interferential therapy
interfragmental compression
interfragmentary plate
interfragmentary screw
intergluteal cleft
interhemispheric cyst
interhemispheric fissure, displacement of
interhemispheric synchrony
interictal behavior
interictal epileptic personality
interictal epileptiform activity

interictal epileptiform pattern
interictal focal epileptiform discharge
interictal paroxysmal sharp waves on EEG
interictal paroxysmal spike waves on EEG
interictal phenomenon
interictal spike discharge
interlaminar clamp system, Halifax
intermediate bursa
intermediate cuneiform fracture-dislocation
intermediate nerve of Wrisberg
Intermediate Care Facilities (ICF)
Intermedics Natural Knee prosthesis
intermediolateral gray column
intermediolateral horn cells
intermedullary guide
intermetacarpal articulation
intermetatarsal angle (IMA)
intermetatarsal angle-reducing procedure
intermetatarsal joint (IM)
intermetatarsal ligament
intermetatarsal space
intermetatarsophalangeal bursa
intermetatarsophalangeal bursitis
intermittent catheterization (IC)
intermittent compression pump (mechanical)
intermittent passive muscle stretch
intermittent pneumatic compression (IPC)
intermittent traction
intermixing of wave upon wave in EEG
intermuscular septum
internal capsule and basal ganglia tumor
internal derangement of the knee (IDK)
internal disk herniation
internal femoral rotation
internal intermuscular septum
internal rotary component of force (in gait)
internal rotation in extension (IRE)
internal rotation in flexion (IRF)
internal speech
internal tibial torsion
internal tibiofibular torsion
International 10-20 System for EEG electrode placement
interneuron, thalamic inhibitory
internuclear ophthalmoplegia
interorbital distance
interosseous, dorsal
interosseous ligament
interosseous membrane
interosseous muscle groups of hand
interosseous nerve
interosseous talocalcaneal ligament
interpedicular distance
interpediculate
interpeduncular notch
interpeduncular space
interphalangeal (IP) joint
interphalangeal articulation
interphalangeal dislocation
interphalangeal fusion
interphalangectomy
Interpore bone replacement material
interposition, soft tissue
interpretation of proverbs test
interpulse time
interscapular aching
intersegmental aberration
interseptal region
intersesamoid ligament
interspace
  ballooning of vertebral
  disk
  wedging of vertebral
interspinal ligament
interspinous distance
interspinous ligament
interspinous process
interspinous pseudarthrosis

interspinous widening
interspinous wiring
interstices, bone
interstitial fluid hydrostatic pressure
interstitial meniscal tear
interstitial myofasciitis
interstitial nucleus of Cajal
interthalamic bridge
intertrabecular hemorrhage
intertrabecular soft tissue
intertransverse process arthrodesis
intertriginous dermatophytosis
intertrigo
intertrochanteric plate
interval
  acromiohumeral (AHI)
  atlantoaxial
  atlantodens (ADI)
  headache-free
  interburst
  lucid (in head trauma)
  supracricoid
interval scale (in rehabilitation testing)
intervention
  nonsurgical
  rehabilitation
interventricular foramen
intervertebral disk
intervertebral disk narrowing
intervertebral disk rongeur
  Cushing
  Wilde
intervertebral disk space
intervertebral foramen
intervertebral joint
intervertebral ligament
interzone
intima
intoeing gait
intorting of eye
intorsion
intoxication
  alcoholic
  anticonvulsant

intoxication *(cont.)*
  carbon dioxide
  carbon monoxide
  glutethimide
  manganese
  water
intra-acetabular
intra-arterial digital subtraction angiography (IADSA)
intra-articular adhesion
intra-articular calcaneal fracture
intra-articular fracture
intra-articular loose body
intra-articular pigmented villonodular synovitis (IPVS)
intra-articular shaver (IAS)
intracapsular osteotomy
intracarotid amobarbital speech test
Intracath needle
intracerebral electrode
intracerebral hematoma
intracerebral hemorrhage
intracerebral lesion
intracerebral lymphoma
intracompartmental ischemia and edema
Intracone intramedullary reamer
intracortical osteogenic sarcoma
intracranial aneurysm
  arteriosclerotic
  congenital
  dissecting
  mycotic
  traumatic
intracranial calcification
intracranial cyst
intracranial glioma
intracranial hemorrhage
intracranial hypertension
intracranial lesion
intracranial malformation
intracranial mass, parasagittal
intracranial monitor
intracranial neoplasm

intracranial pressure
intracranial sinus thrombosis
intracranial tumor
intractable pain
intractable plantar keratoses (IPK)
intractable seizures
intracuticular stitch
intradermal angioma
intradermal pedal nevi
intradermal suture
intradiskal pressure
intradural abscess
intradural anastomosis
intradural arteriovenous fistula
intradural extramedullary tumor of spinal cord
intradural nerve root
intradural retromedullary arteriovenous fistula
Intraflex intramedullary pin
intraforaminal approach
intrafusal fibers
intralaminar thalamus
intramedullary (IM) rodding
intramedullary epidermoid cyst
intramedullary fixation device
intramedullary rasp
intramedullary rod
intramedullary rodding
intramedullary spinal cord tumor
intramedullary spinal lesion
intramedullary tumor
intramuscular injection
intraneural ganglion cyst
intraneural phenol injection
intraneuronal neurofibrillary tangles
intranuclear diskogram
intraoperative autologous transfusion (IAT)
intraoperative complications
intraoperative radiation therapy (IORT)
intraosseous venography
intrapedicular fixation
intraperiosteal fracture
intraprosthetic
intrasellar Rathke cleft cyst (RCC)
intrasellar tumor
intraspinal adenoma
intraspinal lesion
intraspinal tumor
intraspongy nuclear herniation
intratendinous fluid collection
intrathecal administration of drug
intrathecal roots
intrathecal route of drug administration
intrathecal space
intrauterine cytomegalic inclusion disease
intrauterine fracture
intravenous line
intraventricular cannula
intraventricular hemorrhage
Intrel II spinal cord stimulator
intrinsic foot muscles
intrinsic muscle spasm in hand
intrinsic-negative runners
intrinsic plus deformity
intrinsic-positive runners
intrinsics, finger
introducer
  Charnley
  ventricular catheter
inturning
intussusception of vein
invagination, basilar
invasion
  Aspergillus (of the nervous system)
  neoplastic (of meninges)
  neoplastic (of roots)
  Nocardia (of the nervous system)
invasive malignant sheath tumor
Inventory, Wakefield Self-Assessment Depression
inverse Argyll-Robertson pupil
inverse Marcus Gunn syndrome
inversion-eversion
inversion injury of the ankle

inversion recovery
inversion sprain
inversion time (TI)
invertors
involucrum
involuntary flexor spasm
involuntary movement
involvement, cranial nerve
Inyo nail
Ioban 2 skin prep
iodine-125 therapy
iodoform gauze
iodophor solution
Iohexol contrast media
IOM (interosseous membrane)
iontophoresis, acetic acid
iontophoretic drug delivery system
IORT (intraoperative radiation therapy)
Iowa internal prosthesis
Iowa University periosteal elevator
IP (interphalangeal) joint
IPC (intermittent pneumatic compression)
IPCS (infrapatellar contracture syndrome)
IPK (intractable plantar keratoses)
IPL (interpeak latency)
I-Plus humeral brace
IPSF (immediate postsurgical fitting)
ipsilateral approach
ipsilateral cerebellar signs
ipsilateral corticospinal tract signs
ipsilateral facial paralysis
ipsilateral facial paresis
ipsilateral hemianopsia
ipsilateral increase in waveform amplitude
ipsilateral loss
ipsilateral monocular blindness
ipsilateral tonic deviation
IPSP (inhibitory postsynaptic potential)
IPVS (intra-articular pigmented villonodular synovitis)
IR (infrared electronic thermography)
IRDA (intermittent rhythmic delta activity)
IRE (internal rotation in extension)
IRF (internal rotation in flexion)
iridium-192 seed
iridium-192 therapy
iridocyclitis
iridoplegia, reflex
IRM spiral arthrosis
iron, Jewett bending
irradiation
  external beam
  gamma
  heavy-particle
  whole brain
irreducible dorsal dislocation of the metatarsophalanageal joint
irreducible fracture
irregular nystagmus
irrigation
  antibiotic
  ice water
irrigation of wound
  pulse lavage
  syringe (with deionized sterile water)
irrigation with antibiotic solution
irrigator
  Arthro-Flo
  jet
  ophthalmic
  pulse lavage
  Simpulse suction
irritability
  muscle
  nerve root
irritation
  meningeal
  nerve root
  nociceptor
  root
Irvine ankle arthroplasty
Irwin osteotomy
Isaacs syndrome

ISAH stereotactic immobilization
 frame
ISAH stereotactic immobilizing mask
Isch-Dish Plus cushion
ischemia
 anoxic
 brain stem
 cerebral
 cortical
 cortical transient
 foot
 global cerebral
 intracompartmental
 ischemic
 muscle
 myoneural
 rostral brain stem
 transient brain stem
 vertebrobasilar
 Volkmann
ischemia of the optic nerve head
ischemic (stagnant) hypoxia
ischemic attack, transient (TIA)
ischemic brain damage
ischemic foot
ischemic foot ulcer
ischemic forearm exercise test
ischemic gangrene
ischemic hypoxia
ischemic-hypoxic encephalopathy
ischemic infarction
ischemic neuritis
ischemic optic neuropathy
ischial tuberosity
ischiogluteal bursa
ischium, ischial
ISEDP (intraspinal epidural pressure)
Ishihara color plate test for multiple
 sclerosis
Ishizuki unconstrained elbow prosthesis
island, bone (or bony)
island of impaired vision
island of Reil
island pedicle flap
isodense appearance
isodense mass
isoelectric (flat) EEG record
isointense soft tissue on MRI
isokinetic exercise
isokinetic passive mode exercise
Isola fixation system
Isola hook
Isola rod
Isola vertebral screw
Isola wire
isolation syndrome
Isoloss AC material
isometric exercise
isometric muscle strength
isometric position
isometry
isopotential line on EEG
isoprene plastic splint
Isotec patellar tendon graft
isotonic exercise
isotope bone scan
isovalericacidemia
Israel rake retractor
Israel rasp
ISS (inferior sagittal sinus)
Isseis-Aussies scoliosis operation
ISSI (interspinous segmental spinal
 instrumentation)
isthmus of femur
isthmus, temporal
IT (iliotibial) band
ITC radiopaque balloon catheter
ITT (internal tibial torsion)
Ivalon particles
IVC (intracerebral-ventricular)
 administration
IVH (intraventricular hemorrhage)
IVRA (intravenous regional anesthesia)
IWB (Index of Well-Being)

J, j

Jaboulay amputation
Jaccoud arthropathy
Jaccoud (arthritis) syndrome
    (cf. *Jacod*)
JACE shoulder exerciser
JACE-STIM electrotherapy stimulation
    unit
JACE W550 CPM device for wrist
jacket
    Boston soft body
    cervicothoracic
    flexion body
    Frejka
    halo body
    immobilization
    Kydex body
    Lexan
    Minerva cervical
    Ortho-Mold lumbar body
    orthoplast
    Prenyl
    Royalite body
    von Lackum transection shift
    Wilmington
jackknife attack
jackknife position
jackknife seizure
Jackson bone clamp
Jackson bone-extension clamp
Jackson compression test
Jackson disk rongeur
Jackson epilepsy
jacksonian attack
    motor
    sensory
jacksonian epilepsy
jacksonian march
jacksonian (motor) march
jacksonian seizure
Jackson intervertebral disk rongeur
Jackson-Pratt drain
Jackson rongeur
Jackson syndrome
Jackson tendon-seizing forceps
Jacob shift test
Jacobs adapter for neurosurgical
    perforators
Jacobs chuck adapter
Jacobs chuck drive
Jacobs distraction rod
Jacobson bulldog clamp
Jacobson dressing forceps
Jacobson endarterectomy spatula
Jacobson microneurosurgical scissors
Jacobson microprobe
Jacobson microvascular knife
Jacobson mosquito forceps
Jacobson needle holder
Jacobson-Potts vascular clamp
Jacobson probe
Jacobson scissors
Jacobson suture pusher
Jacobson vessel knife
Jacoby bunion splint

Jacod (neuralgia) syndrome
(cf. *Jaccoud*)
jacktatio capitis nocturna
jactitation
Jacuzzi
Jaffe-Capello-Averill hip prosthesis
Jaffe disease
Jaffe procedure
Jahss classification of ankle dislocation
Jahss classification of metatarsophalangeal joint dislocation
jake paralysis (Jamaica ginger)
Jako stimulator
Jakob-Creutzfeldt disease
Jakob-Creutzfeldt viral encephalitis
Jamaica ginger paralysis
jamais entendu (never heard)
jamais vu (never seen)
Jamar grip test
Jamar hand dynamometer
Jameson muscle hook
jamming forces/trauma
Jamshidi needle
Janecki-Nelson shoulder procedure
Janes fracture frame
Jannetta alligator forceps
Jannetta aneurysm neck dissector
Jannetta bayonet forceps
Jannetta dissector
Jannetta duckbill elevator
Jannetta forceps
Jannetta fork
Jannetta hook
Jannetta knife
Jannetta-Kurze dissecting scissors
Jannetta posterior fossa retractor
Jannetta probe
Jansen bone curet
Jansen mastoid retractor
Jansen-Middleton septal forceps
Jansen monopolar forceps
Jansen rasp
Jansen rongeur
Jansen scalp retractor
Jansen test
Jansen-Wagner retractor
Jansky-Bielschowsky disease
Jansky-Bielschowsky syndrome
Janz juvenile myoclonic seizure
Janz response
Japanese B encephalitis
Japanese B viral encephalitis
Japanese fingertrap
Jarcho-Levin syndrome
Jarell forceps
jargon, aphasia
Jarisch-Herxheimer reaction
Jarit brain forceps
Jarit-Kerrison laminectomy rongeur
Jarit-Liston bone rongeur
Jarit rotator
Jarit-Ruskin bone rongeur
Jarit tendon-pulling forceps
Javid carotid clamp
Javid shunt
jaw clenching, repetitive
jaw jerk
jaw jerk reflex
Jebsen hand function test
Jebsen-Taylor hand function test
Jefferson cerival fracture
Jeffery classification of radial fracture
Jelanko splint
jelly
  conductive EEG
  EEG electrolyte
jelly nystagmus
Jendrassik maneuver
Jenet sign
Jergesen I-beam
Jergesen plate
Jergesen tube
jerk, jerking
  Achilles
  ankle
  biceps
  crossed
  elbow
  flurry of myoclonic
  hypnic

jerk *(cont.)*
- jaw
- knee (KJ)
- macro square wave
- myoclonic
- nystagmoid
- paretic
- patellar
- photomyoclonic
- quadriceps
- rhythmical
- sleep
- square wave
- supinator
- tendon
- triceps (TJ)
- triceps surae

jerky incoordinate movement
jersey finger
jet, Ortholav
Jette Functional Status Index
jet wire tightener
Jewett bending iron
Jewett bending tool
Jewett-Benjamin cervical orthosis
Jewett brace
Jewett contraflexion brace
Jewett contraflexion orthosis
Jewett driver
Jewett extractor
Jewett gouge
Jewett hyperextension brace
Jewett hyperextension orthosis
Jewett nail
Jewett plate
Jewett postfusion brace
Jewett postfusion orthosis
jig
- chamfer cut
- Charnley tibial onlay
- drilling
- extramedullary tibial alignment
- femoral alignment

jig *(cont.)*
- intramedullary
- Miller-Galante
- spacer-tensor
- tibial alignment

jitteriness
jittery response
Jobst antithrombotic pump
Jobst brassiere
Jobst stocking
Joerns orthopedic bed
Johannesberg staple
Johannson hip nail
Johannson lag screw
John Barnes myofascial release
John C. Wilson arthrodesis
Johns Hopkins bulldog clamp
Johnson-Boseker scale
Johnson brain tumor forceps
Johnson hemiphalangectomy
Johnson-Jahss classification of posterior tibial tendon tear
Johnson pelvic fracture technique
Johnson resection arthroplasty
Johnson retractor
Johnson-Spiegl hallux varus correction
Johnson tumor forceps
Johnson-Zuck-Wingate motor test
joint
- AC (acromioclavicular)
- acromioclavicular
- atlantoaxial
- bail-lock knee
- ball-and-socket
- basal
- calcaneocuboid
- capitate hamate
- capitolunate
- carpometacarpal
- carpophalangeal
- center of
- Charcot
- Chopart

joint *(cont.)*
- chronic recurrent dislocation of the ankle
- CMC (carpometacarpal)
- costovertebral
- cubonavicular
- cuneiform
- diarthrodial
- DIP (distal interphalangeal)
- distraction of
- double-stem silicone lesser MP
- ellipsoid
- facet
- finger
- flail
- free knee
- Gaffney
- Gillette
- glenohumeral
- gliding
- hallux interphalangeal (IP)
- hinge
- hip capsule
- hyperextensibility of
- immovable
- intercarpal
- intermetatarsal (IM)
- intervertebral
- IP (interphalangeal)
- knee
- lesser metatarsophalangeal
- Lisfranc
- LT (lunotriquetral)
- Luschka
- MCP, MP (metacarpophalangeal)
- metatarsocuneiform (MC)
- metatarsophalangeal (MPJ)
- midcarpal
- midtarsal
- naviculocuneiform
- neuropathic
- neuropathic tarsal-metatarsal
- occipital-axis

joint *(cont.)*
- Oklahoma ankle
- PIP (proximal interphalangeal)
- pisotriquetral
- pivot
- radiocapitellar
- radiocarpal
- radioulnar
- Regnauld degeneration of MTP
- sacroiliac (SI)
- saddle
- scaphocapitate
- scapholunate
- scaphotrapezoid-trapezial (STT)
- Select
- sesamoidometatarsal
- SI (sacroiliac)
- Silastic finger
- SL (scapholunate)
- sternoclavicular
- STT (scaphotrapezoid-trapezial)
- subtalar
- surgeon's tarsal joint
- Swanson finger
- synovial
- talocalcaneal
- talocrural
- talofibular
- talonavicular
- tarsometatarsal
- tibiofibular
- tibiotalar
- transverse tarsal
- trapeziometacarpal
- trapezioscaphoid
- trapeziotrapezoid
- triquetrohamate
- uncovertebral
- unstable
- weightbearing

joint congruency

joint congruity

joint debris

joint depression fracture
joint dislocation
joint fluid aspiration
joint fulcrum
joint immobilization
joint interface
Joint-Jack finger splint
joint laxity
joint line pain, medial
joint line tenderness
joint manipulation, chiropractic
joint mice
joint morphology
joint play, excessive
joint position sense (JPS)
joint segment
joint space
    cartilage
    metatarsal-phalangeal
    subtalar
    tarsal-metatarsal
joint stiffness
joint swelling
joint tenderness
joint warmth
joker periosteal elevator
Jonell splint
Jones abduction frame
Jones-Brackett technique
Jones classification of congenital tibial deficiency
Jones classification of diaphyseal fractures
Jones cock-up toe operation
Jones compression plate
Jones dressing
Jones-Ellison ACL reconstruction
Jones fracture
Jones traction splint
Joplin bunionectomy
Joplin toe prosthesis
Joseph disease
Joseph elevator
Joseph hook
Joseph periosteal elevator
Joseph periosteotome
Joseph splint
JPS (joint position sense)
JRA (juvenile rheumatoid arthritis)
Jude pelvic x-ray
Judet graft
Judet hip prosthesis
Judet hip status system
judgment and insight
Juers-Lempert rongeur forceps
jugal suture
jugular foramen syndrome
jugular venous oxygen saturation
jump graft
jump sign
jumper's knee position
junction
    cervicomedullary
    cervicothoracic
    craniocervical
    gastrocnemius-soleus
    gray-white matter
    meniscosynovial
    metaphyseal-diaphyseal
    musculotendinous
    myoneural
    myotendinous
    neuromuscular
    occipitocervical
    pontomedullary
    pontomesencephalic
    sylvian/rolandic
    temporal-occipital
    TFA
junction separation, costochondral
juncture, myofascial periosteal
Jurgan pin ball
jury-rig
Juvara foot procedure
juvenile bunion
juvenile flatfoot pathomechanics

juvenile myoclonic epilepsy
juvenile rheumatoid arthritis (JRA)
juvenile Tillaux fracture
juxta-articular osteoid osteoma
juxta-articulation
juxtacortical chondroma
juxtacortical sarcoma
juxtapapillary uveitis
juxtarestiform body

K, k

Kaessmann nail
Kaessmann screw
KAFO (knee-ankle-foot orthosis)
Kager triangle
Kahre-Williger periosteal elevator
Kalamchi-Dawe classification of
  congenital tibial deficiency
Kalessy brace
Kalish Duredge wire cutter
Kalish Duredge wire extractor
Kalish osteotomy
kallikrein-kinin (KK) system
Kaltostat dressing
Kampe corset
KAM Super Sucker
Kam Vac suction tube
Kanavel cock-up splint
Kanavel four cardinal symptoms
Kanavel sign
Kaneda distraction device
Kaneda rod
Kannon headframe
Kapel elbow dislocation technique
Kaplan sign
Kaplan technique
Kaposi sarcoma
  classic
  epidemic
kappa rhythm on EEG
Karakousis-Vezeridis resection
Karfoil splint
Karnofsky performance score (KPS)
Kartchner carotid artery clamp
Kasdan retractor
Kashiwagi technique
Kastec mitral valve prosthesis
KAT (Kinesthetic Ability Trainer)
Kates forefoot arthroplasty
Kates-Kessel-Kay technique
Katz ADL Index (KAI) (activities of
  daily living)
Katzman infusion of radionuclide
  cisternography
Kaufer tendon technique
Kayser-Fleischer (K-F) ring
Kazanjian splint
K blade
K-Cap to cover end of Kirschner wire
K complex on EEG
Keane Mobility bed
Kearns-Sayre disease
Kearns-Sayre syndrome (KSS)
Kech and Kelly osteotomy
keel, McNaught
keel of glenoid component
Keen sign
Keene compression hook
Keene obturator
Kehr sign
Keitel index
Keith needle
Kelikian classification of nail deformity
Kelikian-Clayton-Loseff technique
Kelikian-McFarland procedure
Kelikian modified Z bunionectomy
Kelikian-Riashi-Gleason patellar tendon
  repair
Keller arthroplasty

Keller-Blake half-ring splint
Keller-Brandes procedure
Keller bunionectomy
Keller hallux valgus operation
Keller foot procedure
Keller-Mann resection arthroplasty
Keller resection arthroplasty
Kellgren sign
Kellogg-Speed lumbar spinal fusion
Kelly artery forceps
Kelly clamp
Kelly forceps
Kelly-Goerss Compass stereotactic system
Kelly hemostat
keloid
Ken driver-extractor
Ken nail
Kendall A-V Impulse System
Kendrick-Sharma-Hassler-Herndon technique
Kennedy ligament technique
Kennerdell-Maroon dissector
Kennerdell-Maroon elevator
Kennerdell-Maroon hook
Kennerdell-Maroon orbital retractor
Kenny Howard shoulder sling
Kenny Self-Care Questionnaire
keratoderma plantare
keratolytic agents
keratome Beaver blade
keratosis, intractable plantar (IPK)
keratotic lesions
Kerlix bandage
Kerlix cast padding
Kerlix dressing
Kerlix wrap
Kern bone-holding clamp
Kern-Lane bone forceps
kernicterus
Kernig sign
Kernohan classification of astrocytomas and glioblastomas
Kernohan classification of brain tumor
Kernohan grading
Kernohan notch phenomenon
Kernohan notch syndrome
Kerpel bone curet
Kerr-Lagen abdominal support
Kerr sign
Kerr splint
Kerrison curet
Kerrison laminectomy rongeur
Kerrison punch
Kessel-Bonney extension osteotomy
Kessler metacarpal distractor
Kessler posterior tibial tendon transfer operation
Kessler prosthesis
Kessler suture
Kessler traction frame
Ketac cement
ketotic hygerglycemia
key, chuck
Key-Conwell classification of pelvic fracture
keyhole neurosurgery
keyhole tenodesis technique
Key intra-articular knee arthrodesis
Key-loc wrench
Key periosteal elevator
Key rasp
Keys-Kirschner traction
keystone of the calcar arch
key the cement
keyway
K-F (Kayser-Fleischer) ring
Khodadad clip
Kickaldy-Willis arthrodesis
Kidde tourniquet
Kidner flatfoot
Kidner procedure for accessory navicular
kidney rest
Kienböck disease
Kiene bone tamp
Kilfoyle classification of condylar fracture

Killian gouge
Killian septum speculum
Kilner hook
Kiloh-Nevin dystrophy
Kiloh-Nevin ocular form of progressive muscular dystrophy
Kiloh-Nevin ocular myopathy
Kiloh-Nevin syndrome
kilohertz (kHz)
Kimura blink reflex measurement for diagnosis of multiple sclerosis
Kimura disease
KinAir bed
kinase C antiglioma monoclonal antibody
kinase C protein
Kin-Con device
Kin-Con isokinetic exercise system
kindling phenomenon
Kindt carotid clamp
kinematic indices of McMurtry
Kinematic rotating hinge knee prosthesis
kinematics, hindfoot
Kinemax Plus knee prosthesis
kinesigenic attack
kinesiologic testing devices
kinesiology
kinesthesia
Kinesthetic Ability Trainer (KAT)
KineTec clubfoot CPM exerciser
KineTec hip CPM machine
kinetic cervical spine
kinetic chain activities
  closed
  open
kinetic foot pain
kinetic splint
kinetic strabismus
kinetic tremor
Kinetix instrument for carpal tunnel release
Kinetron muscle strengthening apparatus
King brace
King classification of thoracic scoliosis
King intra-articular hip fusion
King-Moe scoliosis
King operation
King-Richards dislocation technique
King-Steelquist technique
King traction
kinins
Kinnier-Wilson disease
Kinsbourne syndrome
Kirby muscle hook
Kirk distal thigh amputation
Kirk mallet
Kirmission periosteal elevator
Kirmission periosteal rasp
Kirner deformity
Kirschner apparatus
Kirschner hand drill
Kirschner Medical Dimension hip replacement
Kirschner stem
Kirschner tightener
Kirschner traction bow nut
Kirschner wire (K wire)
Kirschner wire cutter
Kirschner wire drill
Kirschner wire traction bow
Kistler classification of subarachnoid hemorrhage
kit, Zervas hypophysectomy
kitchen utensils, one-handed
Kite slipper
Kite clubfoot casting
KJ (knee jerk)
Kjellberg 1% risk line
Kjolbe technique
Klagsbrun harvesting technique
Klebsiella pneumoniae meningitis
kleidoscope photopsias
Kleiger test
Klein approach or technique
Kleine-Levin syndrome
Kleinert-Kutz bone cutter
Kleinert-Kutz bone rongeur
Kleinert-Kutz rasp

Kleinert-Kutz rongeur forceps
Kleinert-Kutz synovectomy rongeur
Kleinert-Kutz tendon forceps
Kleinert-Kutz tendon retriever
Kleinert-Ragdell retractor
Kleinert repair
Kleinert splint
Klemme laminectomy retractor
Klengall brace
Klenzak spring brace
Klinefelter syndrome
Kling elastic bandage
Klippel-Feil syndrome
Klippel-Trenaunay-Weber syndrome
Klisic-Jankovic technique
Kloehn craniofacial remodeling
  instrument
Klumpke injury to brachial plexus
Klumpke palsy
Klüver-Bucy ablation syndrome
KMC femoral stem
KMP femoral stem
KMW/PC femoral stem
knee-ankle-foot orthosis (KAFO)
knee
  anterior cruciate deficit
  biocompartmental replacement of
  breaststroker's
  corner of
  dislocated
  floating
  friction rub in (Renee creak sign)
  game
  gimpy
  hamstrung
  housemaid's
  internal derangement of the (IDK)
  jumper's
  locked
  Miller-Galante
  motorcyclist's
  Press-Fit Condylar Total
  runner's
  trick
  wrenched
knee brace (see *brace*)
kneecap
knee drop test
knee extension
knee flexion stress test
knee holder
knee immobilizer
knee jerk, hung-up (sustained)
knee jerk (KJ)
knee knob of Osgood-Schlatter disease
kneeling bench test
knee orthosis (see *orthosis*)
knee prosthesis (see *prosthesis*)
knee support
knife (blade)
  acetabular
  Adson dural
  Adson right-angle
  amputation
  angular
  arachnoid
  arthroscopic
  backward-cutting
  Ballenger swivel
  banana
  Bard-Parker
  bayonet
  Beaver-DeBakey
  Bircher meniscus
  Blount
  Bovie
  Bucy chordotomy (or cordotomy)
  cartilage
  Catlin amputating
  chondroplasty
  chordotomy (cordotomy)
  cobalt-60 gamma
  Collin amputating
  cordotomy (chordotomy)
  Crile gasserian ganglion
  Cushing dural hook
  deep blade
  DeMarneffe meniscotomy
  Down epiphyseal
  Downing cartilage

knife (cont.)
- dural
- epiphyseal
- Esmarch plaster
- flap
- forward-cutting
- Frazier cordotomy
- Frazier pituitary
- Freer-Swanson ganglion
- Freiberg cartilage
- Freiberg meniscectomy
- full-radius resector
- Gamma (radiosurgical instrument)
- ganglion
- Grover meniscus
- Halle dura
- hemilaminectomy
- hook
- Hopkins plaster
- hot
- interosseous
- Jacobson microvascular
- Jacobson vessel
- Jannetta
- Koos microvascular
- Krull acetabular
- Langenbeck flap
- Langenbeck resection
- left-cutting
- Leksell cobalt-60 gamma
- Leksell Gamma
- Lindvall-Stille
- Liston amputating
- Liston phalangeal
- Lowe-Breck cartilage
- Lowe-Breck meniscectomy
- Maltz cartilage
- McKeever cartilage
- meniscotomy
- meniscus
- microvascular
- Midas Rex
- myelotomy
- Neff meniscus

knife (cont.)
- Olivecrona trigeminal
- Oretorp arthroscopy
- pituitary
- plaster
- Rayport dural dissector and
- Reiner plaster
- resection
- retrograde
- Ridlon plaster
- right-angle
- right-cutting
- roentgen
- Salenius meniscus
- semilunar cartilage
- sharp
- skin blade
- Smillie-Beaver
- Smillie cartilage
- Smillie meniscus
- Smith cartilage
- Stecher arachnoid
- Stryker cartilage
- swivel
- tenotomy
- Tiemann Meals tenolysis
- Toennis dura
- 201-source cobalt-60 gamma
- vessel
- Weary cordotomy
- Weck
- Yamanda myelotomy
- Yasargil arachnoid
- Yasargil microvascular

Knight back brace
Knight bone-cutting forceps
Knight-Taylor thoracic brace
Knighton hemilaminectomy retractor
Knighton laminectomy retractor
Knobby-Clark procedure
knock, bladder, in distance runners
knock-knee (genu valgum) deformity
knock-out, knocked-out (KO)
Knodt compression rod

Knodt hook
knot of Henry
knot tier and ligature carrier, Retter
knots, surfer's
knowledge, fund of
Knowles nail
Knowles pin
knuckle bender splint
knuckle-shaped
KO (knock-out, knocked-out)
Koch-Mason dressing
Kocher clamp
Kocher collar incision
Kocher-Cushing sign
Kocher-Debré-Sémélaigne syndrome
Kocher dissector
Kocher elevator
Kocher forceps
Kocher fracture
Kocher lateral J approach
Kocher-Lorenz classification of capitellum fracture
Kocher maneuver
Kocher-McFarland hip arthroplasty
Kocher retractor
Kodel knee sling
Koenig metatarsophalangeal joint arthroplasty
Koenig MPJ implant and arthroplasty
Koenig nail-splitting scissors
Koenig rasp
Koenig-Schaefer approach
Koerber-Salus-Elschnig syndrome
Köhler lines (Koehler)
Kohs block test
Kohs blocks
Komai stereotactic head frame
König disease (Koenig)
Konstram angle
Kool Kit cold therapy pack
Koos microvascular knife
Korn Cage knee brace
Korsakoff amnesia
Korsakoff psychosis
Korsakoff syndrome
Kortzeborn hand procedure
Koshevnikoff epilepsy
Kostuik-Errico classification of spinal stability
Kostuik-Harrington spinal instrumentation
Kostuik rod
Kostuik screw
Koutsogiannis-Fowler-Anderson osteotomy
K pack
K pad
KPS (Karnofsky performance score)
Krabbe diffuse sclerosis
Krabbe disease
Krabbe leukodystrophy
Krackow point
Kramer-Craig-Noel osteotomy technique
Kramer modification of Hohmann osteotomy
Krankendonk pin
Kraske position in surgery
Krause sensory receptor
Krause, suture of
Krause-Wolfe skin graft
Krayenbuehl nerve hook (Krayenbühl)
Krempen-Craig-Sotelo tibia nonunion technique
Kretschmer syndrome
Kreuscher bunionectomy
Kreuscher scissors
Kristiansen eyelet lag screw
Kronecker aneurysm needle
Kronner external fixation
Krukenberg hand procedure
Krull acetabular knife
KSS (Kearns-Sayre syndrome)
KT-1000 joint arthrometer
KT-1000 knee arthrometer
KTP (potassium titanyl phosphate) laser
KTP/532 laser

Kudo unconstrained elbow prosthesis
Kufs disease
Kugelberg-Welander disease
Kugelberg-Welander juvenile spinal muscle atrophy
Kugelberg-Welander syndrome
Kuhlman cervical traction
Kumar-Cowell-Ramsey technique
Kumar spica cast technique
Küntscher (Kuentscher)
Küntscher awl
Küntscher drill
Küntscher finisher
Küntscher hammer
Küntscher impactor
Küntscher nail
Küntscher nail driver
Küntscher traction apparatus
Küntscher reamer
Küntscher rod
Küntscher nail-extracting hook
Kurosaka fixation screw
Kurtzke disability score
kuru viral encephalitis
Kurze dissection scissors
Kurze suction-irrigator
Kussmaul aphasia
Kussmaul coma
Kutler digital flap
Kutler V-Y flap graft
Kveim test
K wire (Kirschner wire)
K wire driver
K wire fixation
K wire skeletal traction
Kwoh-Young stereotactic robot
Kydex body jacket
Kydex brace
Kyle fracture classification system
kyphectomy, Sharrard-type
kyphoscoliosis
kyphosis
  Cobb method of measuring
  lumbar
  lumbosacral
  postlaminectomy
  Scheuermann juvenile
kyphosis brace
kyphotic angulation

L, l

Labbe, vein of
la belle indifférence
labial dysarthria
lability, emotional
labioglossolaryngeal paralysis
labioglossopharyngeal paralysis
labium
labored breathing
labrum
  acetabular
  articular
  glenoid
labyrinthine disorder
labyrinthine hydrops
labyrinthine vertigo
LAC (long arm cast)
lace-on brace
laced blucher of shoe
laceration
  brain
  bursting-type
  chevron
  dural
  stellate
laceration of the spinal cord
lacertus fibrosus
Lacey knee prosthesis
Lachman maneuver
Lachman sign
Lachman test
laciniate ligament of ankle
lack of clear-cut cerebral dominance
LaCrosse virus encephalitis
lactic dehydrogenase of cerebrospinal fluid
lacunae
lacunaire, état (multiple small strokes)
lacunar infarct (infarction)
lacunar state
lacunar stroke
lacunar syndrome
Lafora body disease
Lafora inclusion body epilepsy
lag
  adductive
  extension
  head
  lid
  phase
lag screw
lagophthalmos ("hare's eye")
Lahey clamp
Lahey Clinic dural hook
Lahey Clinic nerve hook
Laing concentric hip cup
Laitinen CT guidance system
Laitinen stereotactic head frame
lalling (babbling)
Lalonde hook forceps
Lalonde tendon approximator
Lamb muscle transfer
lambda wave on EEG
lambdoid suture
Lambert-Eaton myasthenic syndrome (LEMS)
Lambert-Lowman bone clamp
Lambert-Lowman chisel
Lambeth Disability Screening Questionnaire
Lambotte bone-holding forceps

Lambotte bone hook
Lambotte elevator
Lambotte osteotome
Lambotte rasp
Lambrinudi drop foot operation
Lambrinudi splint
Lambrinudi triple arthrodesis
lamb's wool pad
lamella
lamellae, concentric
lamellar reaction, on x-ray
lamina chisel, D'Errico
lamina cribrosa
lamina, medullary
lamina spreader
lamina terminalis
laminaplasty, Tsuji
laminar air flow system
lamination of gyrus
laminectomy
  cervical
  decompressive
  emergency
  multilevel
  osteoplastic
  single-level decompressive
laminectomy frame
laminectomy retractor
  Cloward-Hoen
  Cone
  Meyerding
  Poppen-Gelpi
  Seletz-Gelpi
  Cone
laminectomy rongeur
  Bucy
  Cloward-English
  Codman-Harper
  Codman-Kerrison
  Codman-Leksell
  Codman-Schlesinger cervical
  Echlin
  Ferris Smith-Kerrison
  Fulton
laminectomy rongeur (cont.)
  Hajek-Koffler
  Raney
  Smith-Petersen
  Whitcomb-Kerrison
laminoplasty, open door
laminotomy, suspension
Lamis patellar clamp
lamp
  stroboscopic
  Wood
Lance-Adams syndrome
lancinating pain
land, no man's (in hand)
Landau-Kleffner syndrome
Landau reflex
landmark
  anatomic
  bony
  bony skull
Landolt pituitary speculum
Landolt spreading forceps
Landouzy-Dejerine disease
Landouzy-Dejerine dystrophy
Landry ascending paralysis
Landry-Guillain-Barré-Strohl syndrome
Landsmeer ligament
Lane bending tool
Lane bone-holding clamp
Lane bone-holding forceps
Lane bone lever
Lane bone screw
Lane periosteal elevator
Lane plate
Lane screw-holding forceps
Lanex screen
Lange Achilles tendon reconstruction
Lange bone retractor
Lange hip reduction
Lange-Hohmann bone retractor
Lange tendon lengthening and repair
Langenbeck bone-holding forceps
Langenbeck flap knife
Langenbeck forceps

Langenbeck metacarpal saw
Langenbeck periosteal elevator
Langenbeck rasp
Langenbeck resection knife
Langenbeck retractor
Langenbeck saw
Langenskiöld bony bridge resection
Langer line
Langoria sign
language deficit
language dysfunction
language
  emotive
  executive
  expressive
  global loss of
  receptive
Lansing strain (type II poliomyelitis virus)
lap (laparotomy) sponge
laparoscopy
laparotomy sheet
Lapidus alternating air-pressure mattress
Lapidus bed
Lapidus bunionectomy
Laplacian montage
LaPorte total toe prosthesis
lapse of awareness
lapse of consciousness
large-vessel disease of the diabetic foot
large-vessel thrombosis
Larmon forefoot procedure
Larmor equation
Larmor frequency
Larsen tendon-holding forceps
Larson ligament reconstruction
larval spike-and-slow wave
laryngeal dysarthria
laryngography, double-contrast
Lasègue sign
laser
  argon
  ArthroProbe arthroscopic

laser (cont.)
  CO_2 (carbon dioxide)
  KTP (potassium titanyl phosphate)
  KTP/532
  Nd:YAG (neodymium: yttrium-aluminum-garnet)
  red light neon (for acupressure points) (chiropractic)
  Surgilase CO_2
  VersaPulse
  VersaPulse holmium
laser Doppler velocimetry
Laserflo Doppler probe
laser image custom arthroplasty (LICA)
laser nucleotomy
lashing of first and second metatarsals
lashing suture
lassitude
LAT (left anterior temporal) EEG lead
latah of Malaysia syndrome
LATC (lateral talocalcaneal angle)
late maturers
latency
  decline in
  distal motor
  interpeak (IPL)
  mean sleep
  motor
  short sleep
latent nausea, in migraine
lateral spring ligament of foot
lateral bending views of the spine
lateral column calcaneal fracture
lateral corticospinal tract
lateral entrapment
lateral gaze
lateral gaze center, pontine
lateral gaze mystagmus
lateral gaze palsy
lateral geniculate nucleus, body
lateral head of gastrocnemius
laterality
lateralization

lateralized activity on EEG
lateralized distribution on EEG
lateralized slowing on EEG
lateralizing deficit
lateralizing finding
lateralizing sign
lateral lemniscus, in brain
lateral ligamentous sprain
laterally displaced fracture
lateral mamillary nucleus of Rose
lateral medullary syndrome
lateral motion racket sports
lateral occipital sulcus
lateral occipitotemporal gyrus
lateral pinch testing
lateral spinocerebellar tracts
lateral spinothalamic tract
lateral sulcus
lateral translation force
lateral wedge for sole or heel of foot
lateropulsion
late traumatic epilepsy
latissimus dorsi musculocutaneous free flap
lattice, fibrovascular
latticework
latus, metatarsus
Lauge-Hansen classification of ankle fracture
Lauge-Hansen stage II supination-eversion fracture
laughing and crying, pathologic
laughing seizures (gelastic epilepsy)
laughter, uncontrollable mirthless
Laugier sign
Laugier test
Laurence-Moon-Biedl syndrome
Laurin angle
Lausanne stereotactic robot
lavage
  angled showerhead
  bone
  Exeter bone
  Hi Speed Pulse
lavage (cont.)
  jet
  joint
  pulsatile jet
  pulsatile pressure
  Pulsavac
  Simpulse pulsing
  Simpulse S/I
law
  Bell-Magendie
  Heuter-Volkmann
  Rayleigh scattering
  Semon
  von Schwann
  Wolff
Lawson-Thornton plate
laxity
  joint
  ligament
  ligamentous
laxity of ligament
laxity to varus stress
layer
  Bekhterev
  parietal tendon sheath
  periosteal cambium
  tangential (of hand)
  visceral tendon sheath
Lazarus sign
"lazy eye" (amblyopia ex anopsia)
LB (longitudinal bipolar) montage
L bars
LBP (low back pain)
LC-DCP (low-contact dynamic compression plate)
LCL (lateral collateral ligament)
LCP (Legg-Calvé-Perthes disease)
LCS New Jersey knee prosthesis
LCT (liquid crystal contact thermography)
LDD (laser-assisted disk decompression)
LDF (laser-Doppler flowmetry) probe
L-dopa-induced dyskinesia

Le Dentu suture
Le Fort fibular fracture
Le Fort mandible fracture
LE prep (lupus erythematosus
  preparation)
Leach-Igou step-cut medial osteotomy
lead
  black EEG
  dual electrode
  EEG
  grid
  left-sided EEG
  multi-electrode
  right-sided EEG
  sphenoidal fossae EEG
  white EEG
Leadbetter maneuver
lead encephalopathy (plumbism)
leadpipe fracture
leadpipe rigidity
lead poisoning as cause of some
  neonatal seizures
lead wire
leaf
  inferior
  superior
leak, cerebrospinal fluid (CSF)
leakage of cerebrospinal fluid
leakage headache (of CSF)
lean mass
Leander chiropractic table
Leander motorized flexion table
Leander 790 Series distraction table
LEAP (Lewis expandable adjustable
  prosthesis)
leather lacer gauntlet
Leatherman hook
Leber disease
Leber optic atrophy
Lebsche rongeur
Lebsche saw guide
Lebsche wire saw
lectins
  RCA (*Ricinus communis* agglutinin)
  UE (*Ulex europaeus*)
lectins antibody
Lectron II electrode gel
Lee bone graft
leech
Leeds spinal procedure
Lefferts rib shears
LeFort II fracture
left anterior temporal (LAT) EEG lead
left-bearing nystagmus
left frontal (LF) EEG lead
left-hand dominant
left-handed patient
left hemiplegia
left motor (LM) EEG lead
left occipital (LO) EEG lead
left parietal (LP) EEG lead
left posterior temporal (LPT) EEG
  lead
left respiratory nerve (phrenic)
left-sided weakness
leg, legs
  badger
  baker
  bandy
  bayonet
  bow
  champagne-bottle legs (in Charcot-
    Marie-Tooth disease)
  flaccid
  game
  gimpy
  lusty legs (of tabes dorsalis)
  nonpreferred
  paretic
  preferred
  restless
  rider's
  scissor
  scissoring of
  stork's legs (in Charcot-Marie-
    Tooth disease)
  tennis (plantaris rupture)
  unilateral spastic
leg drift
leg-foot-toe syndrome

leg holder
leg length discrepancy
leg-lengthening device
Legg-Calvé-Perthes disease (LCP)
Legg-Perthes sling
Legg-Perthes shoe extension
Lehman technique
Leibinger Micro Plus plate
Leibinger Micro Plus screw
Leibinger Micro System cranial fixation plate
Leibinger Micro System drill bit
Leibinger Micro System plate cutters
Leibinger Micro System plate-holding forceps
Leibinger Micro System pliers
Leibinger microplate
Leibinger mini-Wurzbach
Leichtenstern encephalitis
Leichtenstern sign
Leigh disease
Leigh necrotizing encephalopathy
Leigh subacute necrotizing encephalomyelitis
Leigh syndrome
Leinbach device
Leinbach femoral prosthesis
Leinbach osteotome
Leinbach screw
leiomyosarcoma
Leksell adapter to Mayfield device
Leksell cobalt-60 Gamma knife
Leksell D-shaped stereotactic frame
Leksell-Elekta stereotactic frame
Leksell Gamma knife
Leksell gamma stereotactic frame
Leksell laminectomy rongeur
Leksell microstereotactic system
Leksell Model G stereotactic frame
Leksell posteroventral pallidotomy
Leksell rongeur forceps
Leksell stereotactic coordinate frame
Leksell stereotaxic system
Leksell-Stille thoracic rongeur
Lelièvre operation to block end-range pronation
Lemmon rib contractor
Lemmon sternal approximator
Lemmon sternal spreader
lemniscus
  lateral (in brain)
  medial
  spinal
Lempert bone curet
Lempert bone rongeur
Lempert periosteal elevator
Lempert rongeur forceps
LEMS (Lambert-Eaton myasthenic syndrome)
Lenart-Kullman technique
length
  limb
  stride
lengthening
  Achilles tendon
  Armistead ulnar
  gastrocnemius
  hamstring
  Ilizarov leg
  Lange tendon (and repair)
  Silfverskiöld Achilles tendoning
  Tachdjian hamstring
  tendon
  tendon Achilles (TAL)
  Vulpius
  Vulpius-Compere Z
  Z-slide lengthening in hallux limitus
lengthening reflex
Lennox-Gastaut syndrome
Lennox syndrome
Lenox Hill derotational knee brace
lenticulostriate artery
lentiform nucleus
Leon strain (type III poliomyelitis virus)
leontiasis ossea
L-Episcopo-Zachary procedure

leptomeningeal carcinomatosis
leptomeningeal disease
leptomeningeal hemangioma
leptomeninges
leptomeningitis
Léri sign
Léri pleonosteosis
Lerman multiligamentous knee control orthosis
LeRoy-Raney scalp clips
LeRoy scalp clip-applying forceps
LEs (lower extremities)
Lesch-Nyhan syndrome
lesion
  acute cerebellar hemispheric
  afferent nerve
  anterior parietal
  anterochiasmatic
  atrophic
  Bankart shoulder
  Bennett
  biparietal
  brain stem
  Brown-Séquard
  callosal
  cartilaginous
  cavernous sinus
  central
  cerebral
  cervical cord
  chiasmal
  chiasmatic
  cleavage
  complete nerve
  conus medullaris
  cortical
  corticospinal pathway
  cyclops
  cystic
  desmoid
  destructive
  disk
  dominant hemisphere
  dorsal root entry zone

lesion *(cont.)*
  DREZ (dorsal root entry zone)
  Duret
  epicortical
  epileptogenic
  excitatory
  extra-axial
  focal
  focal hemispheric
  focal irritative
  focal ischemic
  frank
  frontal lobe
  hamartomatous
  hemorrhagic
  high cervical spinal cord
  high pontine
  high-signal
  Hill-Sachs
  Hill-Sachs shoulder
  homogeneous
  hyperintense
  hyperkeratotic
  hyperkeratotic plantar
  hyperostotic
  hypothalamic
  infranuclear
  intra-axial brain
  intracerebral
  intracranial
  intramedullary
  intramedullary spinal
  intrasellar
  intraspinal
  irregular-shaped
  irregularly shaped
  ischemic
  isointense
  keratotic
  Kidner
  lateral temporal epileptogenic
  low-density
  lower motor neuron
  lytic

lesion *(cont.)*
- lytic bone
- mass
- medial longitudinal fasciculus (MLF)
- median nerve
- mesial temporal epileptogenic
- metabolic
- midbrain
- midline
- Monteggia
- multiple focal
- muscular
- nail bed
- neurogenic
- nondominant hemisphere
- nucleus basalis
- obstructive (of the CSF pathways)
- occipital
- osteocartilaginous
- osteochondral (of the talus)
- parasagittal
- parasellar
- parietal cortex
- parietal lobe
- parieto-occipital
- pedal hyperpigmented
- peripheral
- peripheral nerve
- periventricular
- Perthes-Bankart
- pontine
- posterior column
- posterior compartment
- posterior fossa
- posterior language area
- pretectal
- radiofrequency
- retrochiasmal
- retrochiasmatic
- ring-enhancing (on CT)
- root
- root entry-zone
- signal characteristics of

lesion *(cont.)*
- skin
- SLAP (superior labrum anterior posterior)
- space-occupying
- spinal cord
- Stener
- striatal
- structural
- subchondral
- subcortical
- subtentorial
- supranuclear
- suprasellar
- supratentorial
- synchronous
- tectal
- temporal
- thalamic
- transfer
- transverse cord
- ulnar nerve
- uncommitted metaphyseal
- upper motor neuron
- well-defined
- white matter
- Wolin meniscoid

lesion localization
lesser atrophy of disuse
lesser metatarsophalangeal joint
lesser multangular (trapezoid) bone
Lester muscle forceps
"let-down" migraine
lethargic
lethargica, encephalitis
lethargy
lethica
Letournel guidelines
Letournel plate
letter reversals
Letterer-Siwe disease
leukemia, meningeal
leukemic infiltration of meninges
leukoaraiosis

leukodystrophy
  Canavan
  globoid
  globoid cell
  hereditary cerebral
  Krabbe
  metachromatic (MLD)
  Pelizaeus-Merzbacher
  spongiform
  spongy degeneration
  sudanophilic
leukodystrophy with diffuse Rosenthal fiber formation
leukoencephalitis
  acute hemorrhagic
  acute necrotizing hemorrhagic
  necrotizing hemorrhagic
  postinfectious
  postvaccinial
  van Bogaert sclerosing
  viral
leukoencephalopathy
  multifocal
  necrotizing
  postinfectious
  progressive multifocal (PML)
  subacute sclerosing
leukoencephaly, metachromatic
leukomalacia, periventricular
leukopenia, cerebral
leukotome
leukotomy
leukotriene
Leung thumb loss classification
level
  automatic phrase
  engagement
  occipitocervical
  peak and trough
  pontine-medullary
  sensory
  trough and peak
level of activity
level of alertness
level of consciousness
level of demarcation in sensory testing
level of denervation
level of functioning, premorbid
level of sensory loss
lever, Lane bone
levering
Levin thermocouple cordotomy electrode
Levis splint
levodopa, decarboxylation of
levoscoliosis
Levy & Rappel foot orthosis
Lewin baseball-finger splint
Lewin bone clamp
Lewin bone-holding forceps
Lewin bunion dissector
Lewin finger splint
Lewin-Gaenslen test
Lewin punch test
Lewin reverse Lasègue test
Lewin snuff test
Lewin spinal perforating forceps
Lewin standing test
Lewin-Stern thumb splint
Lewin supine test
Lewis-Chekofsky resection
Lewis expandable adjustable prosthesis (LEAP)
Lewis nail
Lewis periosteal elevator
Lewis rasp
Lewy body
Lexan jacket
Lexer chisel
Lexer gouge
Lexer osteotome
Lex-Ton spinal frame
Leyla bar
Leyla brain retractor
LF (left frontal) EEG lead
LFF (low filter frequency) on EEG
L-5 hydroxytryptophan (L-5HTP)
LGA (low-grade astrocytoma)

LHB (long head of biceps)
Lhermitte-Duclos disease
Lhermitte sign
LIAD (low-impact aerobic dance)
LICA (laser image custom arthroplasty)
Lichtheim aphasia
Lichtheim disease
Lichtman technique
lid flutter on EEG
lid lag
Lidge cement gun
Lido Active Multijoint System
Lido Passive Multijoint System
Lido WorkSET (simulation, evaluation, and training)
Lidoback isokinetic dynamometry system
Liebolt radioulnar technique
Liepmann apraxia
Life-Port drug delivery system
Life Satisfaction Index (LSI)
lifestyle, sedentary
Li-Fraumeni syndrome (LFS)
lift
  chiropractic laser nonsurgical face
  DiPalma shoe
  heel
  Hoyer
lift-off of heel in walk
lifter, Yasargil tissue
Ligaclip clip applier
Ligaclip hemostatic clip
ligament
  accessory collateral
  acromioclavicular
  acromiocoracoid
  alar
  annular
  anterior collateral (ACL)
  anterior cruciate
  anterior fibular
  anterior longitudinal (ALL)
  anterior medial

ligament *(cont.)*
  anterior talofibular (ATF)
  apical
  arcuate
  atlantal
  attenuated
  avulsed
  beak
  calcaneocuboid
  calcaneofibular (CF)
  calcaneonavicular
  capsular
  cervical mover (of ankle)
  check
  check rein
  Cleland
  collateral
  congenital laxity of
  conoid
  coracoacromial
  coracoclavicular
  coracohumeral
  cross
  cruciate
  deep collateral
  deep transverse metacarpal
  deep transverse palmar
  deltoid
  deltoid (of shoulder, of ankle)
  dentate
  dorsal metacarpal
  dorsal wrist
  fibular collateral
  fibulotalar
  fibulotalocalcaneal
  flaval
  floating
  Gerdy
  glenohumeral
  Grayson
  Haines-McDougall medial
  Henle
  inferior dorsal radioulnar
  inferior ilioischial

ligament *(cont.)*
- infrapatellar
- intercarpal
- interdigital
- intermetatarsal
- interosseous talocalcaneal
- intersesamoid
- interspinal
- interspinous
- intervertebral
- laciniate
- Landsmeer
- lateral "spring"
- lateral collateral (LCL)
- limited proteoglycan matrix of
- long fibers of the posterior talofibular
- longitudinal
- LTC (lateral talocalcaneal)
- lunotriquetral
- macroscopic hemorrhage
- medial collateral (MCL)
- meniscotibial
- metacarpoglenoidal
- metacarpophalangeal
- microscopic hemorrhage of
- natatory
- naviculocuneiform
- nuchal
- oblique retinacular
- occipital-atlas-axis
- palmar
- palmar metacarpal
- petroclinoid
- phalangeal glenoidal
- posterior cruciate (PCL)
- posterior longitudinal (PLL)
- posterior medial
- posterior oblique (POL)
- posterior talofibular (PTF)
- posterior tibiofibular
- posterior tibiotalar
- Poupart inguinal
- radial collateral

ligament *(cont.)*
- radial metacarpal
- radiocarpal
- radiolunotriquetral
- radioscaphocapitate
- radioscaphoid
- radioscapholunate
- retinacular
- Rouviere
- sacrotuberous
- scapholunate
- sesamoid
- sesamophalangeal
- spring
- stretched out
- Struthers
- supraspinous
- syndesmotic
- talocalcaneal
- talofibular
- talonavicular
- tectoral
- tibial sesamoid
- tibiocalcaneal
- tibiofibular
- tibionavicular
- torn meniscotibial
- transverse carpal
- transverse intertarsal
- transverse metatarsal
- trapezoid
- triangular
- triquetrohamate
- ulnar collateral (UCL)
- ulnocarpal
- ulnolunate
- ulnotriquetral
- vaginal hand
- volar carpal
- Weitbrecht
- Wrisberg

ligamenta flava
ligament avulsion
ligament laxity

ligament reconstruction
ligamentoplasty
ligamentotaxis
ligamentous bouncing
ligamentous box
ligamentous complex
ligamentous disruption
ligamentous impingement, ankle
ligamentous insertion
ligamentous instability
ligamentous laxity
ligamentous luxation
ligamentous-muscular hypertrophy
ligamentous release
ligamentous sprain
ligamentous strain
ligamentous support
ligamentous thickening
ligamentum cervicis
ligamentum denticulatum
ligamentum flavum, pleating of
ligamentum nuchae
ligamentum teres
Ligamentus Ankle ankle orthotic
ligation, clip
ligature carrier
ligature guide
ligature, stick tie
light conductor
light
  flashes of
  flashing
  intermittent flashes of
  patterned
  photic stimulation during EEG with
    a stroboscopic
  repetitive flashes of
  stroboscopic flashes of
light source, fiberoptic
Light-Veley headrest
lightheaded
lightheadedness
lightning-like flexion spasm of the
  head
LIH (Lars Ingvar Hansson) hook pin
Lilienthal rib spreader
Liliequist membrane
lilliputian disorder of visual perception
  in migraine
limb
  amputated
  congenitally short
  ischemic
  nonischemic
  posture of
limb absence
  congenital intercalary
  congenital terminal
  ischemic
  nonischemic
limb apraxia, pure
limb ataxia
limb bud
limb-girdle dystrophy
limb-girdle-trunk paresis
limb hemodynamics
limb kinetic apraxia
limb length discrepancy (LLD)
limb lengthening operation
limb paresthesia
limb salvage surgery
limbic cortex
limbic encephalitis
limbic encephalopathy
limbic input
limbic structures of the frontal lobe
limbic structures of the temporal lobe
limbic system
limbus annularis
limitation of joint motion
limited proteoglycan matrix of
  ligaments
limitus
  hallux (HL)
  Z-slide lengthening in hallux
limp
  antalgic
  new-onset

LINAC (linear accelerator)
- Boston
- Siemens
- University of Florida
- Varian

LINAC radiosurgery
Lindau syndrome
Lindeman bur
Lindeman procedure
Linder sign
Lindgren oblique osteotomy
Lindholm open surgical tendon repair
Lindholm technique
Lindvall-Stille knife
line
- AC-PC (anterior commissure-posterior commissure)
- Beau
- bisector
- Blumensaat
- central sacral (CSL)
- Chamberlain
- dentate
- divisionary (in a bipartite sesamoid)
- epiphyseal
- equipotential
- Feiss
- Fränkel's white
- fracture
- gluteal
- growth arrest
- Harris hip
- Hawkins
- heel bisector
- Heuter
- Hilgenreiner horizontal Y
- Hilgenreiner-Pauwels
- Hilgenreiner-Perkins (H-P)
- H-P (Hilgenreiner-Perkins)
- Hueter
- isodose
- isopotential
- joint
- Köhler

line *(cont.)*
- Kjellberg 1% risk
- Langer
- large-bore intravenous
- lateral joint
- lead
- lucent (on x-ray)
- McGregor
- medial joint
- metopic suture
- Meyer
- nipple
- Nélaton
- Ogston
- orbitomeatal
- parallel pitch
- Perkins
- Shenton
- soleal
- spinographic
- suture
- Ullman
- vertebral body
- Wagner
- Wineberger
- Zahn
- zero

linea aspera
linear accelerator (see *LINAC*)
linear accelerator radiosurgery
linear analog pain scale
linear and depressed skull fracture
linear skull fracture
linear translation force
linebacker's arm
line imaging
line of Gennari
line scanning
liner
- acetabular
- acetabular prosthetic
- cast
- DePuy acetabular
- Duraloc acetabular

liner *(cont.)*
  Enduron acetabular
  Gore-Tex cast
  grommet bone
  Hylamer acetabular
  polyethylene
  Polysorb
  Spenco
Ling hip prosthesis
lingual airway dysfunction
lingual dysarthria
lingual gyrus
lingula
lining cells, synovial
link, musculotendinous-osseous
Link Stack Split Splint
Linvatec driver
lip of acetabulum
lip of glenoid
lip of navicular
lip of taenia
lip of tibia
lip, osteophytic bone
lip-smacking (with seizures)
lip-smacking automatism
lip-smacking, repetitive
lipid crystals, birefringent (in tendinitis)
lipid droplets, within muscle fibers
lipid storage disease
lipidosis (pl. lipidoses)
  cerebral
  cerebroside
  galactosylceramide
  neuronal
  sphingomyelin
  sulfatide
lipoblastoma
lipoblastomatosis
lipochondrodystrophy
lipodermatosis
lipofibroma
lipofuscinosis, neuronal ceroid
lipoma
lipomyelomeningocele
liposarcoma
  myxoid-type
  pleomorphic
  round cell type
lipoxygenase pathway
lipping, osteophytic
Lippman hip prosthesis
Lippman test
lips of lateral sulcus
Lipscomb modified McKeever arthrodesis
liquid crystal contact thermography (LCT)
Lisfranc amputation
Lisfranc articulation
Lisfranc below-knee prosthesis
Lisfranc dislocation
Lisfranc fracture
Lisfranc fracture-dislocation
Lisfranc injury
Lisfranc joint
Lissauer paralysis
Lissauer tracts of spinal cord
lissencephaly
Lister scissors
Lister tubercle
Listeria monocytogenes meningitis
listhesis
listing gait
Liston amputating knife
Liston bone-cutting forceps
Liston-Key bone-cutting forceps
Liston-Key-Horsley rib shears
Liston knife
Liston-Littauer bone-cutting forceps
Liston-Littauer rongeur
Liston phalangeal knife
Liston splint
Liston-Stille bone-cutting forceps
lists to the right (or left)
LiteNest portable seating system
literal (or phonemic) paraphasia
Littauer-Liston bone-cutting forceps
Littauer-West rongeur

litter, Neal-Robertson
Little disease
Little Leaguer's elbow
Little Leaguer's shoulder
Littler-Cooley transfer of abductor
  digiti quinti
Littler opponensplasty
Littler pollicization
"live flesh" (hemifacial spasm)
Liverpool elbow prosthesis
Liverpool knee prostheses
living
  activities of daily (ADLs)
  normal activities of daily
Livingston intramedullary bar
LLC (long leg cast)
LLD (leg length discrepancy)
LLD (limb length discrepancy)
LLE (left lower extremity)
Llorente dissecting forceps
Lloyd adapter for Smith-Petersen nail
Lloyd chiropractic table
Lloyd nail driver
Lloyd-Roberts fracture technique
LLWBC (long leg weightbearing cast)
LLWC (long leg walking cast)
LM (left motor) EEG lead
LMR (localized magnetic resonance)
LNV (last normal vertebra)
LO (left occipital) EEG lead
Lo Bak spinal support
load, loading
  axial
  carbohydrate
  Dilantin
  rotatory (on spine)
  spinal axial
  torque
LOAF muscles of hand
  lumbricals
  opponens pollicis
  abductor pollicis brevis
  flexor pollicis brevis
Loban adhesive drape
lobar atrophy of Pick
lobe
  anterior tip of temporal
  flocculonodular (of cerebellum)
  frontal
  insular
  medial temporal
  mesial aspect of temporal
  mesial part of frontal
  mesiobasal temporal
  mesiotemporal
  occipital
  orbital aspect of frontal
  orbital part of frontal
  parietal
  temporal
  uncus of temporal
lobectomy
  anterior lobe
  anterior temporal (ATL)
  temporal
lobe signs, parietal
lobotomy, prefrontal
lobster-claw deformity
lobule
  inferior parietal
  inferior temporal
  paracentral
  parietal
local standby (anesthesia) technique
Localio procedure
localization
  electrophysiological l. of nerve
  lesions
  intraoperative lesion
  lesion
  point
localized delta activity (on EEG)
localized muscular atrophy
localizer
  Mayfield fiducial
  Risser
localizing neurologic signs
localizing neurologic symptoms

locator, Berman
lock-stitch
Locke clamp
Locke elevator
locked-in state
locked-in syndrome
locked knee
locking of joint
locking-position test
locomotion (gait)
locomotor ataxia
locomotor mechanisms
locomotor pattern
locus ceruleus of the pons
locus niger
Locus of Control, Recovery
Lofstrand crutch
logrolling of patient in bed
Logan traction
logical memory (paragraph recall) test
after head injury
London unconstrained elbow prosthesis
L1-APo cephalometric measurement
L1-L6 intervertebral disks
L1-NB cephalometric measurement
Long Beach stereotactic robot
long bone osteomyelitis
long fibers of the posterior talofibular
ligament
long leg weightbearing cast (LLWBC)
long-term memory
long thoracic nerve palsy
long tract signs
longette, plaster
longitudinal arch of foot
longitudinal blood supply to ulnar
nerve
longitudinal fasciculus, medial (MLF)
longitudinal magnetization
longitudinal relaxation
longitudinalis medialis fasciculus
long-lived
long-standing
long-suffering
longum, vinculum
longus
extensor hallucis
flexor hallucis (FHL)
loop (not *loupe*)
figure-of-8 wire
Meyer (in brain)
peduncular
vessel
loop-lock cock-up splint
loop of Vieussens
loose associations
loose bodies (of knee)
loose body, osteochondritic
Loose procedure
Lo-Por vascular graft prosthesis
lordosis
cervical
compensatory lumbar
lumbar
occipitocervical
reversal of cervical
thoracic
lordotica, dysbasia
Lord total hip prosthesis
Lore suction tube and tip-holding
forceps
Lorentzian line
Lorenz cast
Lorenz cranial plate
Lorenz cranial screw
Lorenz hip reduction
Lorenz osteosynthesis system
Lorenz sign
Lorenzo screw
lorry driver's fracture
LOS (Lincoln-Ogeretzky Scale) test
Losee modification of MacIntosh
technique
loss
axonal
central sensory
complete visual
contralateral

loss *(cont.)*
  cortical sensory
  dense sensory
  dissociated sensory
  estimated blood (EBL)
  functional
  hemi-field
  hemisensory
  hysterical visual
  ipsilateral
  level of sensory
  mechanical functional
  monocular visual
  motor
  neuronal
  partial visual
  peripheral sensory
  saddle-area sensory
  sensory
  stocking-glove sensory
  visual
loss of consciousness
loss of motion
loss of sphincter control
loss of spontaneity
loss of vision
Lottes pin
Lottes triflanged medullary nail
Lou Gehrig disease
loud bruit
Louis-Bar syndrome
Louisiana State University (LSU) reciprocation-gait orthosis
loupe (not *loop*)
  binocular
  magnification
  magnifying
Loute wire tightener
Love-Adson periosteal elevator
Love-Gruenwald alligator forceps
Love-Gruenwald intervertebral disk forceps
Love-Gruenwald intervertebral disk rongeur
Love-Gruenwald pituitary forceps
Love-Gruenwald pituitary rongeur
Love-Kerrison laminectomy rongeur
Love-Kerrison rongeur forceps
Love nerve root hook
Love nerve root retractor
Lovell clubfoot cast
lovers' paralysis
Lovett clinical scale of strength
Loving Care/Springwall chiropractic mattress
low back pain (LBP)
Low Back Pain Symptom Checklist
low back spinal support (see *Lo Bak*)
low CSF production
LowDye taping technique
Lowe-Breck cartilage knife
Lowe-Breck meniscectomy knife
Lowe-Miller unconstrained elbow prosthesis
Lowe syndrome
Lowenberg sign
lower extremity arterial tree
lower lumbar root compression
lower motor neuron disease
lower motor neuron lesion, remote
lower motor neuron paralysis
lower radial palsy
low-grade astrocytoma tumor
low-grade malignant histiocytoma
low-impact aerobic dance (LIAD)
low-reading thermometer
Lowman bone-holding clamp
Lowman bone-holding forceps
Lowman chisel
Lowman-Gerster bone clamp
Lowman hand retractor
Lowman-Hoglund bone-holding clamp
Lowman-Hoglund chisel
Lowman retractor
Lowman shelf procedure
Low Profile leg holder
low-voltage fast activity
LP (left parietal) EEG lead

LP (lumbar puncture)
LP (lumboperitoneal) shunt
LPCh (lateral posterior choroidal) artery
L plate
LPPS (low-pressure plasma spray)
LPPS hydroxyapatite adhesive
LPT (left posterior temporal) EEG lead
L rod, Luque
LS (lumbosacral) spine
L-shaped incision
LSI (Life Satisfaction Index)
L spine (lumbar spine)
LSU (Louisiana State University) reciprocation-gait orthosis
LSUMC (Louisiana State University Medical College)
LSUMC classification of motor and sensory function
LSUMC classification of nerve injury
LT (lunotriquetral) joint
LTC (lateral talocalcaneal) ligament
Lubinus knee prosthesis
Lucae bone mallet
Lucae nerve hook
Lucas chisel
Lucas-Cottrell osteotomy
Lucas gouge
Lucas-Murray knee arthrodesis
lucency, putaminal
lucent band (on x-ray)
lucent defect
lucent line (on x-ray)
lucid interval, in head trauma
Luck-Bishop bone saw
Luck procedure (of hand)
Ludington test
Ludloff incision
Ludloff sign
Ludloff technique
LUE (left upper extremity)
Luer bone rongeur
Luer-Friedman bone rongeur
Luer-Hartmann rongeur
Luer rongeur forceps
Luer-Whiting rongeur forceps
lues (syphilis)
luetic (syphilitic)
Luhr Microfixation cranial plate
Luhr Microfixation System drill bit
Luhr Microfixation System plate cutters
Luhr Microfixation System plate-holding forceps
Luhr Microfixation System pliers
Luhr microplate
Luhr miniplate
Luhr pan plate
Luhr plate
Luhr screw
lumbago
lumbar arachnoid peritoneal shunt
lumbar component of scoliosis
lumbar lordosis
lumbar plexus
lumbar puncture (LP)
lumbar puncture traumatic tap
lumbar puncture test
lumbar root compression
lumbar spine (L1 to L5 or L6)
lumbar theco-peritoneal shunt syndrome
lumbarization
lumbarized spine
lumbopelvic dysfunction
lumbosacral corset
lumbosacral fusion elevator
lumbosacral kyphosis
lumbosacral plexus
lumbosacral radiculopathy
lumbosacral series (x-rays)
lumbosacral spine strain
lumbosacral traction
lumbrical bar
lumbrical muscles of hand
lumen
Lumina telescope

lunate bone
lunate dislocation
lunate fracture
lunate wrist prosthesis (of acrylic
cement)
lunate-triquetral coalition
lunatomalacia
Lunceford-Pilliar-Engh hip prosthesis
Lunceford total hip replacement
Lundborg epilepsy
Lundholm plate
Lundholm screw
lunocapitate bone
lunotriquetral (LT) joint
lunotriquetral ligament
Luongo hand retractor
lupus erythematosus preparation
(LE prep)
Luque cerclage wire
Luque fixation device
Luque-Galveston rod
Luque II fixation system
Luque II plate
Luque II screw
Luque instrumentation
Luque L-rod
Luque loop fixation
Luque rectangle
Luque rod fixation for kyphosis
Luque segmental fixation
Luque wire
Luque wiring
lurch
abductor
gluteal
Luschka (also von Luschka)
bursa
foramen of
joint of
nerve of
lusty legs of tabes dorsalis
luxated bone
luxatio coxae congenita
luxatio erecta shoulder dislocation
luxatio perinealis
luxation
ligamentous
palmar
luxury collateral perfusion on cerebral
arteriography
luxury perfusion
Luys body
Luys, subthalamic nucleus of
Luysii, corpus
Lyden-Lehman technique
Lyman-Smith brace
Lyman-Smith traction
Lyme disease complex
lymphadenopathy
lymphangiography
lymphedema, familial
lymphocytic choriomeningitis viral
encephalitis
lymphocytic meningitis
lymphocytic pleocytosis (in CSF)
lymphoepithelioma
lymphogranuloma venereum viral
encephalitis
lymphoma
cerebral
intracerebral
intracerebral Hodgkin
intracranial Hodgkin
malignant
primary brain
primary CNS
Lynco foot orthosis
Lynn technique
Lyofoam wound dressing
lyophilization (freeze-drying)
Lysholm-Gillquist score
Lysholm knee function scale
Lysholm score for knee joint instability
Lysholm test

lysosomal absorption of cartilage (in rheumatoid arthritis)
lysosomal enzymes
lysozymes
lytic bone lesion
lytic lesion of the skull
Lytle splint

M, m

MAC cervical collar (Miami Acute Care)
MacAusland lumbar brace
MacAusland procedure
MacCarthy procedure
MacDonald dissector
MacDougall diet for multiple sclerosis
maceration
Macewen-Shands osteotomy
Macewen sign
MacGregor osteotome
machine (see also *apparatus*; *device*)
  Accu-Tron microcurrent
  CPM (continuous passive motion)
  Cybex Trunk Extension Flexion
  KineTec hip CPM
  Nautilus
  Orthion traction
  Orthotron
  Stryker knee joint laxity
  Stryker Surgilav
  Surgilav
MacIntosh extra-articular tenodesis
MacIntosh knee prosthesis
MacIntosh over-the-top ACL reconstruction
MacKenty periosteal elevator
MacKenzie exercises
MacNab-English shoulder prosthesis
MacNichol-Voutsinas classification
macroadenoma
macrocephaly
macrodactyly
Macrofit hip prosthesis
macrographia (in cerebellar disease)
macrogyria
macropsia
macroscopic hemorrhage of ligaments
macroscopic magnetization moment
macroscopic magnetization vector
macular fan
macular sparing
macular star
maculoneural bundle
Maddacrawler Crawler crawling frame
Maddox rod test
Madelung deformity
madness, myxedema
madreporic hip prosthesis
Maffucci syndrome
MAG (transcranial magnetic stimulation)
Magendie, foramen of
magenta tongue ("beefy")
Magerl hook-plate fixation
Magerl screw placement technique
Magerl transarticular screw fixation
Magilligan technique for measuring anteversion
Magnatherm diathermy unit
magnet, Dyonics Golden Retriever
magnetic dipole
magnetic field
magnetic gradient
magnetic induction
magnetic moment
magnetic reaction (grasp reflex)
magnetic resonance

magnetic resonance imaging (MRI)
  (see *MRI terms*)
magnetic resonance signal
magnetic stimulation
magnetic susceptibility
magnetization
magnetoencephalogram (M-EEG)
magnification, loupe
magnifying loupe
magnum, foramen (herniation of)
Magnum 800 bed
Magnuson-Stack shoulder arthrotomy
Ma-Griffith end-to-end anastomosis
Ma-Griffith repair of ruptured Achilles
  tendon
Ma-Griffith tendon anastomosis
main d'accoucheur (obstetrician's
  hand)
main en griffe (clawhand)
Maison retractor
Maisonneuve fibular fracture
Maisonneuve sign
Majestro-Ruda-Frost tendon technique
major causalgia
major cystic malformation
major motor fit
major sprain
mal, impulsive petit
mal perforant diabetic ulcer
Malacarne antrum
malacoplakia
malaise
malalignment syndrome
malangulation
malar fracture
malaria
  cerebellar
  cerebral
Malawer excision technique
Malaysia, latah of
malformation
  angiographically occult vascular
    (AOVM)
  angiographically visualized vascular
    (AVVM)

malformation *(cont.)*
  Arnold-Chiari
  arteriovenous (AVM)
  cavernous
  cerebral arteriovenous
  Chiari
  cryptic arteriovenous
  cryptic vascular (CVM)
  deep-seated arteriovenous
  dural arteriovenous
  dural venous
  familial arteriovenous
  glomus arteriovenous
  glomus-type arteriovenous
  infratentorial arteriovenous
  intracranial
  juvenile arteriovenous
  major cystic
  medullary venous (MVM)
  retromedullary arteriovenous
  Spetzler-Martin classification of
    arteriovenous
  supratentorial arteriovenous
  venous
  Wyburn-Mason arteriovenous
Malgaigne pelvic fracture
malignant glioma tumor
malignant melanoma, plantar
malingering
Malis angled-up bipolar forceps
Malis bipolar cautery forceps
Malis bipolar cautery scissors
Malis brain retractor
Malis CMC-II bipolar coagulator
Malis curet
Malis dissector
Malis elevator
Malis irrigation forceps
Malis-Jensen micro bipolar forceps
Malis Jeweler bipolar forceps
Malis ligature passer
Malis needle holders
Malis nerve hook
Malis neurological scissors
Malis vessel supporter

malleable metal finger splints
malleable template
malleolar torsion
Malleoloc ankle orthosis
malleolus (pl. malleoli)
  collicular fracture of the medial
  lateral
  medial
mallet (see also *hammer*)
  Acufex
  Bergman
  bone
  boxwood
  cervical
  copper
  Cottle
  Crane
  Doyen bone
  Gerzog bone
  Hajek
  Heath
  Henning
  Hibbs
  Kirk
  lead-filled
  Lucae bone
  Mead
  Meyerding
  Ombredanne
  Ralks
  Richards
  Rush
  Steinbach
  Surgical No Bounce
  Swanson
  Williger bone
  Wolfe-Boehler
mallet deformity
mallet finger
mallet fracture
mallet toes
Mallory-Head femoral stem
Mallory-Head rasp
Mallory-Head revision operation
Mallory-Head total hip prosthesis
Malmö hip splint
malrotation
Maltz cartilage knife
Maltz rasp
malum coxae senile
malunion
malunited
mamillary body
mamillary suture
mandibular angle
mandibular fracture
maneuver (see also *reflex*; *sign*; *test*)
  Adson
  Adson modified
  alerting
  Allen
  Bárány-Nylen
  Barlow
  circumduction
  closed manipulative
  costoclavicular
  Dandy
  Dix-Hallpike
  doll's head
  eye opening and closing
  flexion-extension
  flexion-rotation-compression
  Foster-Kennedy
  Fowler
  Gowers
  Hippocratic
  hyperabduction
  Jendrassik
  Kocher
  Lachman
  Leadbetter
  McMurray circumduction
  Meyn and Quigley
  Ortolani
  osteoclasis
  Parvin
  Phalen
  postural fixation back

maneuver *(cont.)*
  provocative
  rotation-compression
  Schreiber
  Slocum
  Spurling
  Stimson
  tripoding
  Valsalva
  vestibulo-ocular
  Walton
manganese intoxication
Mangled Extremity Severity Score (MESS)
mania
  dancing (choreomania)
  epileptic
manifestation, clinical seizure
manipulate
manipulation
  back
  chiropractic joint
  fine
  gross
  Hippocrates
  medical (versus chiropractic)
  opening wedge
manipulation of the articulations and adjacent tissues
manipulation with distraction, bifocal
manipulative procedures (adjustments)
Mankin technique
Manktelow transfer procedure
Mann-Coughlin arthrodesis
Mann-Coughlin-DuVries cheilectomy
Mann-DuVries arthroplasty
Mann modified McKeever arthrodesis
Mann resection arthroplasty
Mann-Thompson-Coughlin arthrodesis
mannerism, speech
manometer, measuring CSF pressure with a
manometric test
Manske technique
mantle
  brain
  cerebral
  shunted
Mantoux test
manual dexterity
manual manipulation of the spine, chiropractic
manual percussion test
manual reduction
manual traction test for cervical radiculitis
manubrium
map
  brain
  topographic
MAPF femoral stem
maple syrup urine disease (MSUD)
mapping (of EEG)
  behavioral
  brain electrical activity (BEAM)
  cerebral
  cortical
  evoked potential (EP)
  frequency domain
  functional
  motor cortex
  statistical
  time domain
  topographic
mapping of apraxia, cerebral
mapping of cortical function
mapping of language areas of brain
mapping the defect
Maquet procedure
marathoner's toe
marble bones
marbré, état
march
  epileptic
  focal motor sign with/without
  jacksonian (motor)
march foot
march fracture

march of cranial nerve palsy
march of scotoma
march of sensory deficit
Marchand-Waterhouse syndrome
marche à petits pas
Marchiafava-Bignami disease
Marchiafava-Bignami syndrome
Marcus-Balourdas-Heiple ankle fusion technique
Marcus grading scale for avascular necrosis
Marcus Gunn pupils
Marfan syndrome
margin
  blurring of disk
  cortical
  disk
  orbital
marginal exostosis
margin of scapula
margo
Marie ataxia
Marie-Bamberger disease
Marie-Charcot-Tooth disease
Marie-Foix sign
Marie hereditary spastic ataxia
Marie sign
Marie-Strümpell disease
Marin-Amat phenomenon
Marin reamer
Marinesco-Sjögren syndrome
Marino transsphenoidal curet
Marino transsphenoidal dissector
Marino transsphenoidal enucleator
Marino transsphenoidal hook
Marion screw
Mark II Chandler retractor
Mark II distal femur retractor
Mark II lateral collateral ligament
Mark II PCL retractor
Mark II S knee retractor
Mark II Sorrells hip arthroplasty retraction system
Mark II Stulberg hip positioner
Mark II Wixson hip positioner
Mark II Z knee retractor
Markell Mobility Healing Clogs
Markell Mobility Shoes
Markell open-toe shoes
Markell tarso medius straight shoe
Markell tarso pronator outflare shoe
marker
  interspace width
  Schoemaker-Burkart
  skin
  tumor
Markham-Meyerding hemilaminectomy retractor
Marks-Bayne technique for thumb duplication
Markwalder bone rongeur
Markwalder rib forceps
Marmor modular knee prosthesis
Marmor replacement
marmoratus, status
Maroon-Jannetta dissector
Maroteaux-Lamy syndrome
Marquardt bone rongeur
marrow
  bone
  red
  yellow
marrow cavity
marrow space, hyperintense
Marshall ligament repair technique
marshmallows
marsupialization
Martin cartilage chisel
Martin cartilage clamp
Martin cartilage forceps
Martin cartilage scissors
Martin diamond wire cutter
Martin-Gruber anastomosis
Martin-Gruber connection
Martin muscle clamp
Martin nerve root retractor
Martin patellar wiring technique
Martin retractor

Martin scissors
Martin Vigorimeter
Martini bone curet
Marval test
Maryland Foot Score Profile
MAS (Motor Assessment scale)
mask facies
mask, ISAH stereotactic immobilizing
masked facies of parkinsonism
Mason-Allen universal splint
Mason fracture classification system
Mason suction tube
mass (see also *lesion*)
  cerebellar
  enhancing
  enhancing (on MRI)
  epidural
  expanding intracranial
  fat-free (body) (FFM)
  fibrin
  hemispheral
  high-density
  intermediate
  isodense
  lean
  low-density
  osteocartilaginous
  parasagittal intracranial
  parasellar
  paraspinal soft tissue
  posterior fossa brain
  presacral
  signal lentiform
  soft-tissue
  suprasellar
  supratentorial
  well-demarcated
  well-encapsulated
massage
  deep
  effleurage
  ice
mass effect of tumor
mass effect (on scan)
masseter-temporalis stretch (jaw jerk) reflex
Massie sliding nail
mass lesion
mass limb reflex
mass motor reflex response
Masson fasciatome
Masson-Fontana stain
Masson vegetant intravascular hemangioendothelioma
MAST (medical antishock trousers)
MAST pressure trousers
master knot of Henry
masticatory attack
Mastin muscle clamp
mastoid, retractor
mat
  Harris and Beath footprint
  silicone
Matchett-Brown internal prosthesis
matchsticked
mater
  dura
  pia
material
  bioceramic joint replacement
  bone replacement
  extraneous
  flexible splinting
  nidus of embolic
  Plasti-Pore prosthetic
  Polysplint A flexible splinting
  Porocoat prosthetic
  porous prosthetic material
  Proplast prosthetic
  splinting
  Synergy flexible splinting
  tophaceous, in gout
Maternal Kradle support for pregnant women
Mathews drill points
Mathieu rasp
Mathys prosthesis
matricectomy, phenol

matrix
  collagen
  germinal
  nail
  tumor
matrix injury
Matroc femoral head
Matson-Alexander rib elevator
matter
  central gray
  cortical gray
  dorsal gray
  gray (of central nervous system)
  long spinal white
  midbrain
  periventricular white
  PVG (periventricular gray)
  subcortical white
  white (of central nervous system)
Matthew cross-leg clamp
Matti-Russe technique
mattress
  air
  Akros extended care
  Akros pressure
  alternating pressure
  chiropractic
  Clinisert
  egg-crate
  egg-crate foam
  foam
  KinAir flotation
  Lapidus alternating air-pressure
  Loving Care/Springwall chiropractic
  pressure
maturation, electrographic (on EEG)
maturation index
maturers, late
maturity, skeletal
Mauck procedure
MaxCast casting tape
Maxidriver
maxillary fracture
Maxima II TENS unit
maximal assist
maximal cervical compression test
Maxon suture
May-White syndrome
Mayeda shelf
Mayer reflex
Mayer splint
Mayfield adaptor
Mayfield aneurysm clips
Mayfield brain spatula
Mayfield cranial aneurysm set
Mayfield curet
Mayfield fixation frame
Mayfield forceps
Mayfield head holder
Mayfield horseshoe headrest
Mayfield incision
Mayfield-Kees headrest
Mayfield-Larsen table
Mayfield miniature clip applier
Mayfield neurosurgical headrest
Mayfield neurosurgical skull clamp
Mayfield pinion
Mayfield rongeur
Mayfield skull clamp pin
Mayfield skull-pin head holder
Mayfield spinal curet
Mayfield temporary aneurysm clip applier
Mayfield tic headrest
Mayfield tongs
Mayo ankle arthroplasty
Mayo ankle prosthesis
Mayo block anesthesia
Mayo bunionectomy
Mayo Clinic stereotactic robot
Mayo-Collins retractor
Mayo hallux valgus operation, modified
Mayo-Hegar needle holder
Mayo metatarsal head resection
Mayo resection arthroplasty
Mayo scissors

Mayo semiconstrained elbow prosthesis
Mayo Thomas collar
Mazas totally constrained elbow prosthesis
Mazet technique
Mazur ankle evaluation system
Mazur ankle fusion grading system
Mazur ankle rating system
MB&J knee positioner
MCA (middle cerebral artery)
MCA (motorcycle accident)
McArdle disease
McArdle syndrome
McAtee-Tharias-Blazina arthroplasty
McBride bunionectomy
McBride femoral prosthesis
McBride hallux valgus reduction
McCabe-Farrior rasp
McCain TMJ arthroscopic system
McCarroll-Baker procedure
McCash hand surgery
McCauley foot procedure
McClintoch brace
McCollough internal tibial torsion brace
McConnell capsular artery
McCullough internal tibial torsion brace
McCune-Albright syndrome
McCutchen implant
McCutchen SLT hip prosthesis
McDavid ankle guard
McDavid hinged knee guard
McDowell Impairment Index (MII)
McElfresh-Dobyns-O'Brien technique
McElroy curet
McElroy instrumentation
McElvenny foot procedure
McFadden temporary aneurysm clips
McFarland-Osborne technique
McGee-Priest wire forceps
McGee splint
McGee wire-crimping forceps
McGill neurological percussor
McGill pain checklist
McGill Pain Questionnaire
McGlamry elevator
McGregor line
McIndoe bone rongeur
McIndoe rongeur forceps
McIndoe scissors
McIntire splint
McIntosh test
McKay-Simons clubfoot operation
McKay-Simons CSR (complete subtalar release) operation
McKee-Farrar acetabular cup
McKee-Farrar cartilage knife
McKee-Farrar total hip arthroplasty
McKee totally constrained elbow prosthesis
McKeever arthrodesis for hallux limitus
McKeever-Buck elbow technique
McKeever cartilage knife
McKeever metatarsophalangeal fusion
McKeever Vitallium knee prosthesis
McKenzie brain clip forceps
McKenzie clip-applying forceps
McKenzie clip-bending forceps
McKenzie clip-introducing forceps
McKenzie enlarging bur
McKenzie exercises
McKenzie forceps
McKenzie hemostasis clip
McKenzie perforating twist drill
McKenzie reservoir
McKenzie silver clip
McKittrick transmetatarsal amputation
MCL (medial collateral ligament)
McLain-Weinstein classification of spinal tumors
McLaughlin-Hay technique
McLaughlin intertrochanteric plate
McLaughlin modification of Bunnell pull-out suture
McLaughlin nail
McLaughlin osteosynthesis apparatus
McLaughlin plate
McLaughlin screw

McLeod splint
McMaster bone graft
McMaster Health Index Questionnaire
McMurray maneuver for torn knee cartilage
McMurray osteotomy
McMurray sign
McMurray test
McMurtry, kinematic indices of
McNaught keel
MCP (metacarpophalangeal) joint
MCR (midcarpal radial) portal
McReynolds driver-extractor
McReynolds open reduction technique
MCTC (metrizamide CT cisternogram)
MCTD (mixed connective tissue disease)
MCU (midcarpal ulnar) portal
McWhorter shoulder approach
MD (muscular dystrophy)
MDP ^{99m}Tc-methylene diphosphonate for bone scanning
Mead bone rongeur
Mead mallet
Mead periosteal elevator
Mead rongeur
mean maximal compression
Mears sacroiliac plate
Meary metatarsotalar angle
measles encephalitis
measles viral encephalitis
measure, measures
  APACHE II measure of disease severity
  modified self-report measure of social adjustment
  Functional Independence (FIM)
measurement
  ANB cephalometric
  FMA cephalometric
  foot pressure
  F wave
  global (of disability)

measurement *(cont.)*
  IMPA cephalometric
  impairment-based
  instrumental ADL
  interburst interval
  L1-APo cephalometric
  L1-NB cephalometric
  motor (to test sensory disturbance)
  NPo-FH cephalometric
  Schober
  SISI (short increments sensitivity index)
  skin fluorescence
  SN-MPA cephalometric
  SN tissue pressure
  SNA cephalometric
  SNB cephalometric
  true ratio
  U1-L1 cephalometric
  U1-NA cephalometric
  Wits cephalometric
  xenon washout technique
measurer
  Bunnell digital exertion
  digital exertion
measures of disability
mechanical functional loss
mechanical insult to spine
mechanics, body
mechanism
  Adjustable Leg and Ankle Repositioning
  central extensor (CEM)
  extensor
  extensor hood
  flexor
  locomotor
  Midas Rex (MB)
  plantar fascia as windlass
  quadriceps
  screw-home
  swallowing
  tendo Achillis
  terminal extensor (TEM)

mechanism *(cont.)*
  triggering
  video fluoroscopy of swallowing
  windlass
mechanoreceptor
  Pacinian
  Ruffini
Meckel cave
Meckel cavity
Mecring acetabular prosthesis
Medasonics transcranial Doppler
media, ocular
medial column calcaneal fracture
medial compartment
medial eminence
medial facial spasm of Meige
medial femoral condyle
medial heel wedge shoe modification
medial joint line pain
medial meniscus
medial longitudinal fasciculus (MLF) lesion
medial longitudinal fasciculus syndrome
medial malleolar fracture
medial malleolus
medial metatarsal drift
medial nucleus, dorsal (of the thalamus)
medial occipitotemporal gyrus
medial physis
medial retinaculum of the knee, reefing of the
medial shelf
medial sole wedge shoe modification
medial V-Y capsulotomy
medialis, fasciculus longitudinalis
medialization
median duo
median fissure, anterior
median nerve compression
median nerve disorder
median nerve lesion
median nucleus of Perlia
Medic Alert ID bracelets for memory-impaired persons
medical manipulation (versus chiropractic)
medical [or military] antishock trousers (MAST)
Medical Research Council (MRC) classification of muscle function
Medicare
medications (see also *drugs*)
  ABLC (amphotericin B lipid complex)
  Abrodil (methiodal sodium)
  absolute alcohol
  acecarbromal
  acetaminophen
  acetazolamide
  acetazolamide sodium
  acetylcarbromal (acecarbromal)
  acetylcholine chloride
  acetylcysteine
  acetylcysteine sodium
  acetyl-L-carnitine
  acetylsalicylic acid (ASA; aspirin)
  ACTH (adrenocorticotropic hormone; corticotropin)
  Adalat (nifedipine)
  Adapin (doxepin HCl)
  adrenocorticotropic hormone (ACTH; corticotropin)
  Advil (ibuprofen)
  A-hydroCort (hydrocortisone sodium succinate)
  Akineton (biperiden lactate)
  Alcar (acetyl-L-carnitine)
  alfacalcidol
  alfa interferon
  allopurinol
  Alpha Chymar (chymotrypsin)
  alpha-chymotrypsin (chymotrypsin)
  alpha-galactosidase A
  alprazolam
  aluminum chloride solution
  Alurate (aprobarbital)

medications *(cont.)*
- Alzene
- amantadine HCl
- ambenonium chloride
- Ambien (zolpidem tartrate)
- A-methaPred (methylprednisolone sodium succinate)
- Amicar (aminocaproic acid)
- Amigesic (salsalate)
- aminobenzoate sodium
- aminocaproic acid
- 4-aminopyridine (4-AP)
- amitriptyline HCl
- amobarbital
- amobarbital sodium
- amoxapine
- amphetamine
- amphetamine aspartate
- amphetamine complex
- amphetamine sulfate
- amphotericin B lipid complex (ABLC)
- ampicillin
- Amytal (amobarbital)
- Amytal Sodium (amobarbital sodium)
- Anacin (aspirin, caffeine)
- Anacin-3 (acetaminophen)
- Anaprox (naproxen sodium)
- Anaprox DS (naproxen sodium)
- Ancef (cefazolin sodium)
- ancrod
- Anexsia (hydrocodone bitartrate, acetaminophen)
- Anodynos (aspirin, salicylamide, caffeine)
- Anodynos DHC (hydrocodone bitartrate, acetaminophen)
- Ansaid (flurbiprofen)
- antiepilepsirine
- Antilirium (physostigmine salicylate)
- antipyrine
- Antivert (meclizine)

medications *(cont.)*
- Anturane (sulfinpyrazone)
- aprobarbital
- arecholine hydrobromide
- Aristocort (triamcinolone acetonide)
- Aristospan (triamcinolone hexacetonide)
- Armacodone
- Artane (trihexyphenidyl HCl)
- Artha-G (salsalate)
- Arthropan (choline salicylate)
- Arvin (ancrod)
- ASA (acetylsalicylic acid; aspirin)
- A.S.A. Enseals (aspirin)
- ascorbic acid (vitamin C)
- Ascriptin (buffered aspirin)
- Ascriptin A/D (buffered aspirin)
- ASD (azaspirodecanediones)
- aspirin
- Asproject (sodium thiosalicylate)
- atenolol
- Ativan (lorazepam)
- atracurium besylate
- atropine
- atropine sulfate
- auranofin
- Aurorix (moclobemide)
- aurothioglucose
- Avan (idebenone)
- Aventyl (nortriptyline HCl)
- Aviva (linopridine)
- Axotal (aspirin, butalbital)
- azathioprine
- Azdone (hydrocodone bitartrate, aspirin)
- Azolid (phenylbutazone)
- baclofen
- Bancap (acetaminophen caffeine, butalbital)
- Bayer Aspirin
- belladonna extract
- Bellergal-S (belladonna extract, phenobarbital, ergotamine tartrate)

medications *(cont.)*
- Benemid (probenecid)
- benztropine mesylate
- Betadine (povidone-iodine)
- beta interferon
- betamethasone
- Betaseron (beta interferon)
- biperiden
- biperiden lactate
- Biphetamine (dextroamphetamine, amphetamine)
- Blocadren (timolol maleate)
- botulinum toxin
- botulinum toxin type A
- bromocriptine
- bromocriptine mesylate
- Brompton cocktail
- buffered aspirin
- Bufferin (buffered aspirin)
- bupivacaine HCl
- Buprenex (buprenorphine HCl)
- buprenorphine HCl
- bupropion HCl
- butabarbital
- butabarbital sodium
- Butalan (butabarbital sodium)
- butalbital
- Butazolidin (phenylbutazone)
- Buticaps (butabarbital sodium)
- Butisol Sodium (butabarbital sodium)
- butorphanol tartrate
- Cafergot (ergotamine tartrate, caffeine, belladonna extract, pentobarbital)
- caffeine
- Calan (verapamil HCl)
- Calcimar (calcitonin)
- calcitonin
- calcitriol
- calcium gluconate
- calcium pyrophosphate
- Cama (buffered aspirin)
- cantharidin
- Cantharone (cantharidin)

medications *(cont.)*
- carbamazepine
- carbidopa
- Cardizem (diltiazem HCl)
- carisoprodol
- carprofen
- cefazolin
- cefazolin sodium
- Celestone (betamethisone)
- Celontin Kapseals (methsuximide)
- Centrax (prazepam)
- cephalexin
- Cervene
- chloral hydrate
- chloramphenicol
- chlordiazepoxide
- chlordiazepoxide HCl
- chlorphenesin carbamate
- chlorpromazine
- chlorzoxazone
- choline magnesium trisalicylate (choline salicylate, magnesium salicylate)
- choline salicylate
- Chymodiactin (chymopapain)
- chymopapain
- chymotrypsin
- Cibacalcin (calcitonin)
- clindamycin
- Clinoril (sulindac)
- clobazam
- clomipramine HCl
- clonazepam
- clopidogrel
- clorazepate dipotassium
- clorazepate monopotassium
- clotrimazole
- Co-Gesic (hydrocodone bitartrate, acetaminophen)
- Codalan No. 1 (codeine phosphate, acetaminophen, aspirin, caffeine)
- Codalan No. 2 (codeine phosphate, acetaminophen, aspirin, caffeine)

medications *(cont.)*
Codalan No. 3 (codeine phosphate, acetaminophen, aspirin, caffeine)
codeine
codeine phosphate
Cogentin (benztropine mesylate)
Cognex (tacrine HCl)
ColBenemid (probenecid, colchicine)
colchicine
commercial dry ice for plantar wart treatment
Compoz (diphenhydramine HCl)
COP 1 (copolymer 1)
Cope (aspirin, caffeine, magnesium hydroxide, aluminum hydroxide)
copolymer 1 (COP 1)
Corgard (nadolol)
Cortef (hydrocortisone)
corticosteroid
corticotropin
cortisone acetate
Cortone Acetate (cortisone acetate)
Cuprimine (penicillamine)
curare (tubocurarine chloride)
cyclobenzaprine HCl
cycloserine
cyclophosphamide
Cylert (pemoline)
cyproheptadine HCl
Cytotec (misoprostol)
D-penicillamine
D.H.E. 45 (dihydroergotamine mesylate)
Dalgan (dezocine)
Dalmane (flurazepam HCl)
danaproid
Dantrium (dantrolene sodium)
dantrolene
dantrolene sodium
Darvon Compound-65 Puvules (propoxyphene HCl, aspirin, caffeine)

medications *(cont.)*
Darvon Puvules (propoxyphene HCl)
Darvon with A.S.A. Puvules (propoxyphene HCl, aspirin)
Darvon-N (propoxyphene napsylate)
Dasin (aspirin, caffeine, atropine sulfate, ipecac)
Datril (acetaminophen)
Daypro (oxaprozin)
DDAVP (deamino-D-arginine-vasopressin; desmopressin acetate)
Decadron (dexamethasone)
Delta-Cortef (prednisolone)
Deltasone (prednisone)
Demerol HCl (meperidine HCl)
Depakene (valproic acid)
Depakote Sprinkles (divalproex sodium)
Depo-Medrol (methylprednisolone acetate)
deprenyl (selegiline HCl)
desipramine HCl
desmopressin acetate (DDAVP)
Desoxyn (methamphetamine HCl)
desoxyribonuclease
dexamethasone
Dexedrine (dextroamphetamine sulfate)
dextroamphetamine
dextroamphetamine saccharate
dextroamphetamine sulfate
dezocine
DHE (dihydroergotamine)
Diamox (acetazolamide sodium)
diazepam
diaziquone
dichloralphenazone (chloral hydrate, phenazone)
diclofenac sodium
Didronel (etidronate disodium)
diflunisal

medications *(cont.)*
- dihydrocodeine bitartrate
- dihydroergotamine (DHE) mesylate
- dihydroxycholecalciferol (calcitonin)
- Dilantin (phenytoin sodium)
- Dilantin Infatabs (phenytoin)
- Dilaudid (hydromorphone HCl)
- diltiazem HCl
- diphenhydramine HCl
- Disalcid (salsalate)
- divalproex sodium
- Doan's Pills (magnesium salicylate)
- Dolacet (hydrocodone bitartrate, acetaminophen)
- Dolene (propoxyphene HCl, acetaminophen)
- Dolene AP (propoxyphene HCl, acetaminophen)
- Dolobid (diflunisal)
- dopamine agonist
- Dopar (levodopa)
- Dopram (doxapram)
- Doral (quazepam)
- Doriden (glutethimide)
- doxapram
- doxepin HCl
- doxylamine succinate
- Duocet (hydrocodone bitartrate, acetaminophen)
- Duradyne (acetaminophen, aspirin, caffeine)
- Duradyne DHC (hydrocodone bitartrate, acetaminophen)
- Duragesic (fentanyl citrate)
- Duramorph (morphine sulfate)
- dynamine
- EACA (epsilon aminocaproic acid)
- Easprin (aspirin)
- Ecotrin (aspirin)
- edrophonium chloride
- EHDP (etidronate disodium)
- Elase (fibrinolysin, desoxyribonuclease)

medications *(cont.)*
- Elase-Chloromycetin (fibrinolysin, desoxyribonuclease, chloramphenicol)
- Elavil (amitriptyline HCl)
- Eldepryl (selegiline HCl)
- Empirin with Codeine No. 2 (aspirin, codeine phosphate)
- Empirin with Codeine No. 3
- Empirin with Codeine No. 4
- Endep (amitriptyline HCl)
- Enlon (edrophonium chloride)
- Enlon-Plus (edrophonium chloride, atropine sulfate)
- enoxaparin (Lovenox)
- ephedrine
- epinephrine
- epsilon aminocaproic acid (EACA)
- Equagesic (meprobamate, aspirin)
- Equizine M
- ergoloid mesylates
- Ergomar (ergotamine tartrate)
- Ergostat (ergotamine tartrate)
- ergotamine tartrate
- Esgic (acetaminophen, aspirin, butalbital)
- estazolam
- ethchlorvynol
- ethinamate
- ethopropazine HCl
- ethosuximide
- ethotoin
- ethyl chloride
- etidronate disodium
- etodolac
- Eucalyptamint (menthol)
- Excedrin (acetaminophen, aspirin, caffeine)
- Excedrin P.M. (acetaminophen, diphenhydramine HCl)
- FABRase (alpha-galactosidase A)
- felbamate
- Felbatol (felbamate)
- Feldene (piroxicam)

medications *(cont.)*
fenoprofen
fenoprofen calcium
fentanyl citrate
fibrinolysin (plasmin)
Fioricet (acetaminophen, caffeine, butalbital)
Fiorinal (aspirin, caffeine, butalbital)
Fiorinal with Codeine No. 3 (aspirin, caffeine, butalbital, codeine phosphate)
Flex-all 454 (menthol, methyl salicylate, trolamine)
Flexeril (cyclobenzaprine HCl)
Flexon (orphenadrine citrate)
flunarizine HCl
fluoxetine
fluoxetine HCl
flupirtine maleate
flurazepam HCl
flurbiprofen
fluvoxamine
fosphenytion
4-aminopyridine (4-AP)
fractionalized fish oil
Freedox (tirilazad mesylate)
gabapentin
gadodiamide
gadopentetate dimeglumine
gadoteridol
gamma-hydroxybutyrate sodium
ganglioside GM1
Gedocarnil
Gemnisyn (acetaminophen, aspirin)
Gemonil (metharbital)
Genagesic (propoxyphene HCl, acetaminophen)
gepirone HCl
Gerimal (ergoloid mesylates)
Gliadel implant
glutethimide
gold salts
gold sodium thiomalate

medications *(cont.)*
Gramalil
guanethidine monosulfate
Haemophilus influenzae type B vaccine
halazepam
Halcion (triazolam)
Halfprin (aspirin)
haloperidol (Haldol)
Haltran (ibuprofen)
HCl (hydrochloride)
hexachlorophene
Hexadrol (dexamethasone)
Hy-Phen (hydrocodone bitartrate, acetaminophen)
Hydergine (ergoloid mesylates)
Hydrocet (hydrocodone bitartrate, acetaminophen)
hydrochloride (HCl)
hydrocodone bitartrate
hydrocodone sodium succinate
hydrocortisone
hydrocortisone sodium succinate
Hydrocortone (hydrocortisone)
Hydrogesic (hydrocodone bitartrate, acetaminophen)
hydromorphone HCl
hydroxychloroquine sulfate
L-5-hydroxytryptophan (L-5HTP)
ibuprofen
idebenone
Ifex (ifosfamide)
ifosfamide
imipramine HCl
Imitrex (sumatriptan succinate)
Inderal (propranolol HCl)
Indocin (indomethacin)
Indocin SR (indomethacin)
indomethacin
Infumorph (morphine sulfate)
inosine pranobex
insulin-like growth factor
interferon
interferon alfa

medications *(cont.)*
- interferon beta
- Ismelin Sulfate (guanethidine monosulfate)
- isocarboxazid
- isometheptene mucate
- Isoprinosine (inosine pranobex)
- isopropyl alcohol
- Isoptin (verapamil HCl)
- isoxicam
- Janimine (imipramine HCl)
- kanamycin sulfate
- Kantrex (kanamycin sulfate)
- Kefzol (cefazolin sodium)
- Kemadrin (procyclidine HCl)
- Kenacort (triamcinolone)
- Kenalog (triamcinolone acetonide)
- ketoprofen
- ketorolac tromethamine
- Klonopin (clonazepam)
- Lamictal (lamotrigine)
- lamotrigine
- lanolin
- Largon (propiomazine HCl)
- Larodopa (levodopa)
- L-baclofen
- L-dopa (levodopa)
- lecithin
- levemopamil
- Levo-Dromoran (levorphanol tartrate)
- levodopa
- Levoprome (methotrimeprazine)
- levorphanol tartrate
- L-5HTP (L-5-hydroxytryptophan)
- Librium (chlordiazepoxide HCl)
- lidocaine
- lidocaine HCl
- lidopridine
- Life-Port drug delivery
- lignocaine (lidocaine)
- Lioresal (baclofen)
- liquid nitrogen
- Liquiprin (acetaminophen)

medications *(cont.)*
- lithium carbonate
- Lodine (etodolac)
- Lodosyn (carbidopa)
- Lopressor (metoprolol tartrate)
- Lopurin (allopurinol)
- lorazepam
- Lorcet (hydrocodone bitartrate, acetaminophen)
- Lortab (hydrocodone bitartrate, acetaminophen)
- Lotusate (talbutal)
- Lovenox (enoxaparin)
- L-threonine
- L-tryptophan
- Luminal Sodium (phenobarbital sodium)
- LY233053 neuroprotector
- Magan (magnesium salicylate)
- magnesium salicylate
- magnesium sulfate
- Magnevist (gadopentetate dimeglumine)
- Magsal (magnesium salicylate, phenyltoloxamine citrate)
- MAOI (monoamine oxidase inhibitor)
- Maolate (chlorphenesin carbamate)
- maprotiline
- maprotiline HCl
- Marazine
- Marcaine (bupivacaine HCl)
- Marplan (isocarboxazid)
- Maxicam (isoxicam)
- mazindol
- Mebaral (mephobarbital)
- meclizine
- meclofenamate sodium
- Meclomen (meclofenamate sodium)
- Medigesic (acetaminophen, caffeine, butalbital)
- Medihaler Ergotamine (ergotamine tartrate)
- Medipren (ibuprofen)

medications *(cont.)*
- Medrol Dosepak (methyl-prednisolone)
- Mentane (velnacrine)
- menthol
- Mepergan (meperidine HCl, promethazine HCl)
- meperidine HCl
- mephenytoin
- mephobarbital
- meprobamate
- merbromin
- Mercurochrome (merbromin)
- Mesantoin (mephenytoin)
- Mestinon (pyridostigmine bromide)
- metaxalone
- methamphetamine HCl
- metharbital
- methiodal sodium
- methocarbamol
- methohexital
- methotrexate (MTX)
- methotrexate sodium
- methotrimeprazine
- methsuximide
- methylglyoxal-bis-guanylhydrazone (MGBG)
- methylphenidate HCl
- methylprednisolone
- methylprednisolone acetate
- methylprednisolone sodium succinate
- methyl salicylate
- methylsergide maleate
- methyprylon
- methysergide maleate
- metoprolol tartrate
- MGBG (methylglyoxal-bis-guanylhydrazone)
- midazolam HCl
- midazolam maleate
- midodrine HCl
- Midrin (isometheptene mucate, dichloralphenazone, acetaminophen)

medications *(cont.)*
- Migratine (isometheptene mucate, dichloralphenazone, acetaminophen)
- Milontin Kapseals (phensuximide)
- misoprostol
- Mivacron (mivacurium chloride)
- mivacurium chloride
- Mobidin (magnesium salicylate)
- Mobigesic (magnesium salicylate, phenyltoloxamine citrate)
- moclobemide
- molecusol-carbamazepine
- Momentum (aspirin, phenyltoloxamine citrate)
- monoamine oxidase inhibitors (MAOIs)
- Mono-Gesic (salsalate)
- Morphine Rhotard
- morphine sulfate
- Motrin (ibuprofen)
- Motrin IB (ibuprofen)
- MS Contin (morphine sulfate)
- MTX (methotrexate)
- Mucomyst (acetylcysteine sodium)
- Myochrysine (gold sodium thiomalate)
- Myotrophin (insulin-like growth factor)
- Mysoline (primidone)
- Mytelase (ambenonium chloride)
- nabumetone
- nadolol
- nalbuphine HCl
- Nalfon (fenoprofen calcium)
- naloxone HCl
- Naprosyn (naproxen)
- naproxen
- naproxen sodium
- Nardil (phenelzine sulfate)
- Nembutal (pentobarbital)
- neostigmine bromide
- neostigmine methylsulfate
- Nervine (diphenhydramine HCl)
- Neurontin (gabapentin)

medications *(cont.)*
nifedipine
nimodipine
Nimotop (nimodipine)
nitrofurazone
Noctec (chloral hydrate)
Nodoz (caffeine)
Noludar (methyprylon)
nomifensine maleate
Nootropil (piracetam)
Noradex (orphenadrine citrate)
Norcet (hydrocodone bitartrate, acetaminophen)
Norflex (orphenadrine citrate)
Norgesic (orphenadrine citrate, aspirin, caffeine)
Norpramin (desipramine HCl)
nortriptyline HCl
Novocain (procaine HCl)
Nubain (nalbuphine HCl)
Numorphan (oxymorphone HCl)
Nuprin (ibuprofen)
Nytol (diphenhydramine HCl)
Obetrol (dextroamphetamine sulfate, dextroamphetamine saccharate, amphetamine aspartate, amphetamine sulfate)
Oculinum (botulinum toxin type A)
omega-3 fatty acids
Omniscan (gadodiamide)
One-Alpha (alfacalcidol)
1,25-dihydroxycholecalciferol (calcitonin)
opium
Orgaran (danaproid)
orphenadrine citrate
Ortholinum (botulinum toxin)
Orudis (ketoprofen)
osmic acid
oxcarbazepine
oxaprozin
oxazepam
oxycodone
oxycodone HCl

medications *(cont.)*
oxycodone terephthalate
oxymorphone HCl
oxyphenbutazone
Pabalate (sodium salicylate,
P-A-C (aspirin, caffeine)
aminobenzoate sodium)
Panadol (acetaminophen)
Pantopon (opium)
Paradione (paramethadione)
Paraflex (chlorzoxazone)
Parafon Forte DSC (chlorzoxazone)
Paral (paraldehyde)
paraldehyde
paramethadione
Parlodel (bromocriptine mesylate)
paroxetine
paroxetine HCl
Parsidol (ethopropazine HCl)
Paxarel (acetylcarbromal)
Paxil (paroxetine HCl)
Paxipam (halazepam)
Peganone (ethotoin)
PEG-SOD (polyethylene glycol-superoxide dismutase)
pemoline
penicillamine
pentazocine
pentazocine HCl
pentazocine lactate
pentobarbital
pentoxifylline
pentylenetetrazol
Percocet (oxycodone HCl, acetaminophen)
Percodan (oxycodone HCl, oxycodone terephthalate, aspirin)
Percodan-Demi (oxycodone HCl, oxycodone terephthalate, aspirin)
Percogesic (acetaminophen, phenyltoloxamine citrate)
pergolide mesylate

medications *(cont.)*
Periactin (cyproheptadine HCl)
Permax (pergolide mesylate)
Pertofrane (desipramine HCl)
phenacemide
phenazone (antipyrine)
phenelzine sulfate
phenobarbital
phenobarbital sodium
phenol
phensuximide
Phenurone (phenacemide)
phenylbutazone
phenytoin
phenytoin sodium
physostigmine
physostigmine salicylate
piracetam
piroxicam
Placidyl (ethchlorvynol)
Plaquenil Sulfate (hydroxychloroquine sulfate)
plasmin (fibrinolysin)
polyethylene glycol-superoxide dismutase (PEG-SOD)
povidone-iodine
pramipexole
prazepam
Predate S
Prednicen-M (prednisone)
prednisolone
prednisone
Presalin (acetaminophen, aspirin, salicylamide, aluminum hydroxide)
primidone
probenecid
procaine HCl
Procardia (nifedipine)
procyclidine HCl
ProHance (gadoteridol)
promethazine HCl
Propacet (propoxyphene napsylate, acetaminophen)

medications *(cont.)*
propiomazine
propiomazine HCl
propoxyphene HCl
propoxyphene napsylate
propranolol HCl
ProSom (estazolam)
Prostigmin (neostigmine methylsulfate)
protirelin
protriptyline HCl
pyridostigmine bromide
pyrilamine maleate
pyritinol
quazepam
Quiet World (pyrilamine maleate, acetaminophen, aspirin)
Relafen (nabumetone)
Repan (butalbital, acetaminophen, caffeine)
Restoril (temazepam)
Rexolate (sodium thiosalicylate)
Rheumatrex Dose Pack (methotrexate sodium)
Ridaura (auranofin)
Rimadyl (carprofen)
Ritalin-SR (methylphenidate HCl)
Robaxin (methocarbamol)
Robaxisal (methocarbamol, aspirin)
Rocaltrol (calcitriol)
Ropinirole
Roxanol (morphine sulfate)
Roxicet (oxycodone HCl, acetaminophen)
Roxicodone Intensol (oxycodone HCl)
Roxiprin (oxycodone HCl, oxy codone terephthalate, aspirin)
Rufen (ibuprofen)
sabeluzole
Sabril
Saleto (acetaminophen, aspirin, salicylamide, caffeine)
Salflex (salsalate)

medications *(cont.)*
salicylamide
salicylic acid liquid
salicylic acid plaster
salicylic acid tape
saline
salsalate
Salsitab (salsalate)
Sanorex (mazindol)
Sansert (methylsergide maleate)
secobarbital
secobarbital sodium
Seconal Sodium (secobarbital sodium)
selegiline HCl
Serax (oxazepam)
Serratia marcescens extract
sertraline HCl
Sibelium (flunarizine HCl)
silver nitrate
Sinemet (carbidopa, levodopa)
Sinequan (doxepin HCl)
Skelaxin (metaxalone)
Sleep-Eze 3 (diphenhydramine HCl)
sodium oxybate
sodium salicylate
sodium tetradecyl sulfate
sodium thiosalicylate
Solganal (aurothioglucose)
Solu-Cortef (hydrocortisone sodium succinate)
Solu-Medrol (methylprednisolone sodium succinate)
Soma (carisoprodol)
Soma Compound (carisoprodol, aspirin)
Sominex (diphenhydramine HCl)
Stadol NS (butorphanol tartrate)
sulfinpyrazone
sulindac
sumatriptan succinate
Supac (acetaminophen, aspirin, caffeine, calcium gluconate)

medications *(cont.)*
suprofen
Suprol (suprofen)
Symmetrel (amantadine HCl)
sympathomimetic stumulants
Synalgos (aspirin, caffeine)
Synalgos-DC (dihydrocodeine bitartrate, aspirin, caffeine)
Synapton (physostigmine)
Synchromed programmable drug pump
T-Gesic (hydrocodone bitartrate, acetaminophen)
tacrine HCl
Talacen (pentazocine HCl, acetaminophen)
talbutal
Talwin (pentazocine lactate)
Talwin Compound (pentazocine HCl, aspirin)
Talwin NX (pentazocine HCl, naloxone HCl)
Tandearil (oxyphenbutazone)
Tegretol (carbamazepine)
temazepam
Tempra (acetaminophen)
Tenormin (atenolol)
Tensilon (edrophonium chloride)
tetanus antitoxin
tetanus immune globulin
tetanus toxoid
tetrahydroaminoacridine (THA; tacrine HCl)
TGF-B (transforming growth factor-beta)
THA (tetrahydroaminoacridine; tacrine HCl)
Thorazine (chlorpromazine)
threonine
Threostat (threonine)
Thymone (protirelin)
tiagabine
Ticlid (ticlopidine HCl)
ticlopidine HCl

medications *(cont.)*
timolol maleate
Tirend (caffeine)
tirilazad mesylate
TLC ABLC (amphotericin B lipid complex)
tocopherol (vitamin E)
Tofranil (imipramine HCl)
Tolectin DS (tolmetin sodium)
tolmetin sodium
Toradol (ketorolac tromethamine)
Tracium (atracurium besylate)
transforming growth factor-beta (TGF-B)
Tranxene (clorazepate dipotassium)
tranylcypromine sulfate
trazodone HCl
triamcinolone
triamcinolone acetonide
triamcinolone hexacetonide
Triapin (acetominophen, caffeine, butalbital)
triazolam
trichloroacetic acid
Tridione (trimethadoine)
Trigesic (acetaminophen, aspirin, caffeine)
trihexyphenidyl HCl
Trilisate (choline salicylate, magnesium salicylate)
trimethadione
trimipramine
trimipramine maleate
trolamine
trypsin, crystallized
tubocurarine chloride
Tuinal (amobarbital sodium, secobarbital sodium)
Tusal (sodium thiosalicylate)
24,25-dihydroxycholecalciferol
Twilite (diphenhydramine HCl)
Tylenol (acetaminophen)
Tylenol with Codeine No. 1 (acetaminophen, codeine phosphate)

medications *(cont.)*
Tylenol with Codeine No. 2 (acetaminophen, codeine phosphate)
Tylenol with Codeine No. 3 (acetaminophen, codeine phosphate)
Tylenol with Codeine No. 4 (acetaminophen, codeine phosphate)
Tylox (oxycodone HCl, acetaminophen)
Ultradol (etodolac)
Unisom (doxylamine succinate)
Valesin (acetaminophen, aspirin, salicylamide)
Valium (diazepam)
Valmid Pulvules (ethinamate)
valproic acid
Valrelease (diazepam)
Vanquish (acetaminophen, aspirin, caffeine, magnesium hydroxide, aluminum hydroxide)
vasopressin (VP)
velnacrine maleate
verapamil
verapamil HCl
Versed (midazolam HCl)
Vicodin (hydrocodone bitartrate, acetaminophen)
vigabatrin
viloxazine HCl
vitamin C (ascorbic acid)
vitamin E (tocopherol)
Vivactil (protriptyline HCl)
Vivalan (viloxazine HCl)
Vivarin (caffeine)
Voltaren (diclofenac sodium)
VP (vasopressin)
Wellbutrin (bupropion HCl)
Wigraine (ergotamine tartrate, tartaric acid)
Wigrettes (ergotamine tartrate)
Wygesic (propoxyphene HCl, acetaminophen)
Xanax (alprazolam)
Xylocaine (lidocaine HCl)

medications *(cont.)*
- Zarontin (ethosuximide)
- zinc oxide
- Zoloft (sertraline HCl)
- zolpidem tartrate
- Zydone (hydrocodone bitartrate)
- Zyloprim (allopurinol)

medicine, sports
Medicus bed
Mediloy implant metal
mediolateral stress
mediopatellaris, plica synovalis
Medipedic Multicentric knee brace
Medi plaster scissors
Medi-Quet tourniquet
medium-voltage beta activity on EEG
Medmetric KT-1000 knee laxity arthrometer
Medtronic neuromuscular stimulator
Medtronic programmable drug pump
Medtronic spinal cord stimulator
medulla
- postrema of
- rostral

medulla oblongata syndrome
medullaris thalami
medullary grafting
medullary infarction
medullary syndrome, lateral
medullary tumors
medulloblast
medulloblastoma
- desmoplastic
- familial
- vermian

Meek clavicle strap
Meek pelvic traction belt
Mega-Air bed
megacephaly
Mega Tilt and Turn bed
megalencephaly, benign familial
megalocephaly
meglumine diatrizoate contrast media
megrim (migraine)
Meige, medial facial spasm of
Meige syndrome
Meissner corpuscle sensory receptor
melanocytoma, meningeal
melanoma
- leptomeningeal
- plantar malignant
- subungual amelanotic

melanosome
melanotic whitlow
MELAS (mitochondrial encephalomyopathy with lactic acidosis and strokelike) episodes
melena
Meleney infection
Meleney synergistic gangrene
Melkersson-Rosenthal syndrome
melorheostosis
membrane
- atlantoaxial (posterior)
- atlanto-occipital
- basement
- blood behind tympanic
- depolarization of neuronal
- interosseous (IOM)
- Liliequist
- neuronal
- posterior (atlantoaxial)
- synovial
- thickened synovial

membrane permeability
membrane potential
memory
- figural
- gaps in
- immediate
- impaired
- long-term
- loss of
- recent
- recognition
- remote
- semantic
- sequence

memory *(cont.)*
  short-term
  verbal
  visual
  visual-spatial
Memory for Designs Test
memory for digits test
memory-impaired person
memory impairment
Mendel-Bekhterev reflex
Mendel-Bekhterev sign
Ménière syndrome
meningeal carcinomatosis
meningeal enhancement
meningeal fibrosis
meningeal infiltrate
meningeal inflammation
meningeal irritation
meningeal leukemia
meningeal sign
meningeal spread of tumor
meningeal streak
meningeal tumor
meninges (pl. of *meninx*)
meningioma
  angioplastic
  cavernous sinus
  clival
  clivus
  cutaneous
  dermal
  endotheliomatous
  epidural
  falx
  fibroblastic
  intracranial
  intradural-extradural
  intraspinal
  metastasizing
  olfactory groove
  parasagittal
  posterior fossa
  psammomatous
  sphenoid ridge
meningioma *(cont.)*
  subdural
  subfrontal
  suprasellar
  tentorial
  tuberculum sellae
meningioma en plaque
meningioma of the cribriform plate
meningioma of the olfactory groove
meningioma tumor
meningiosarcoma
meningism
meningismus
meningitic neurosyphilis
meningitic stria
meningitis (pl. meningitides)
  actinomycosis lymphocytic
  acute
  acute purulent
  Aerobacter aerogenes purulent
  aseptic
  aseptic uremic
  bacterial
  Bacterium anitratum
  beta-hemolytic streptococcus
  beta strep
  Brucella abortus purulent
  Brucella melitensis purulent
  Brucella suis purulent
  Candida
  candidal
  carcinomatous
  cerebrospinal (CSM)
  chemical
  chronic
  chronic basal, with cranial nerve
    paralysis
  CMV (cytomegalovirus)
  Corynebacterium diphtheriae
    purulent
  coxsackievirus
  cryptococcal
  diffuse syphilitic
  echinomycosis lymphocytic

meningitis *(cont.)*
echovirus
enterovirus
Escherichia coli purulent (E. coli)
fungal
group B streptococcal
herpes simplex virus type 2
Haemophilus influenzae (H. influenzae)
Histoplasma
Histoplasma capsulatum
HIV (human immunodeficiency virus)
Klebsiella pneumoniae purulent
leptospirosis lymphocytic
Listeria monocytogenes purulent
lymphocytic
lymphomatous
meningococcal purulent
Meningococcus
Mollaret
mumps
mycotic
Naegleria
Neisseria
Neisseria catarrhalis purulent
Neisseria gonorrhoeae purulent
neonatal
neoplastic
Nocardia
ornithosis lymphocytic
otogenic
paragonimiasis lymphocytic
pneumococcal purulent
Pneumococcus
posterior basic
Proteus vulgaris purulent
Pseudomonas aeruginosa purulent
purulent
pyogenic
rabies lymphocytic
Rich theory of tuberculous
Salmonella
Salmonella choleraesuis purulent

meningitis *(cont.)*
sinogenic
staphylococcal purulent
Staphylococcus aureus
streptococcal purulent
Streptococcus pneumoniae
subacute
subacute granulomatous
syphilitic
Toxoplasma
toxoplasmosis lymphocytic
Treponema pallidum
trichinosis
Trypanosoma gambiense
tuberculous
uremic aseptic
Vibrio fetus
viral
meningocele, sacral
meningococcal meningitis
meningoencephalitis (pl. meningoencephalitides)
arbo- (arthropod-borne)
murine typhus
Rocky Mountain spotted fever
Trichinella spiralis
meningoencephalocele
basal
ethmoidal
sphenoethmoidal
spheno-orbital
sphenopharyngeal
stalk of
transsphenoidal
meningoencephalocystocele
meningoencephalomyelitis
meningohypophyseal artery
meningomyelitis
meningomyelocele
meningomyelocystocele
meningothelioma
meningovascular neurosyphilis
meningovascular syphilis
meninx (pl. meninges)

- meniscal injury
- meniscal tear (see *tear*)
- meniscal trimmer blade
- meniscectomy
  - arthroscopic
  - medial
  - partial
  - Patel medial
  - subtotal
  - subtotal lateral
  - total
- meniscectomy blade
- meniscitis
- meniscorrhexis
- meniscosynovial junction
- meniscotibial ligament
- meniscotome
  - Bircher
  - Bowen-Grover
  - Grover
  - Storz
- meniscus
  - bridge of
  - clefting of
  - degenerative
  - discoid
  - frayed
  - fraying of
  - lateral
  - medial
  - menisci
  - torn
- Menkes disease
- Menkes syndrome
- Mennell sign
- Mensor-Scheck technique
- *mentagrophytes, Tricophyton*
- mental changes
- mental deficiency
- mental faculty
- mental retardation
- mental status changes
- mental status examination
- mental status questionnaire
- mentation
  - change in
  - normal
- Mentor tissue expander
- Menzel olivopontocerebellar atrophy
- Menzel olivopontocerebellar degeneration
- MEP (motor evoked potential)
- MEPP (miniature endplate potential)
- MERA (minor emergency room area)
- MERAC (Musculoskeletal Evaluation Rehabilitation and Conditioning) system
- meralgia paresthetica
- Merchant angle
- Merchant views (x-rays)
- mercury poisoning
- meridian, vertical visual
- Merkel disc sensory receptor
- Merland classification of perimedullary arteriovenous fistulas
- Merle D'Aubigné pain and mobility rating scale
- Merocel packing
- MERRF (myoclonic epilepsy with ragged red fibers)
- Mersilene suture
- Mersilene tape
- mesencephalic infarct
- mesencephalic reticular formation
- mesencephalon aqueduct
- mesenchymal chondrosarcoma
- mesenchymoma, pluripotential
- mesh
  - Dumbach cranial titanium
  - metal
  - titanium
- mesial frontal lobe damage
- mesial hemisphere
- mesial part of brain
- mesial temporal sclerosis
- mesialward
- mesiotemporal lobe
- mesocephalic head shape

mesotenon (or mesotendon)
MESS (Mangled Extremity Severity
  Score)
metabolic bone disease
metabolic encephalopathy
metabolic lesion
metabolic tremor
metabolism
  myelin
  neuronal
metabolites, washing out of accumulated
metacarpal, base of
metacarpal ligament, dorsal
metacarpoglenoidal ligament
metacarpophalangeal (MCP or MP)
  dislocation
metacarpophalangeal (MCP) joint
metacarpus
metachromatic leukodystrophy
metadductus
metal (see *implant metal*)
metal locator, Berman-Moorhead
metamorphopsia of Amsler grid
metaphyseal-diaphyseal junction
metaphyseal-epiphyseal angle
metaphysis
metaplasia
  cartilaginous
  osteocartilaginous
metastasis (pl. metastases)
  bony
  brain
  cerebral
  distant
  extradural spinal
  intramedullary
  Picker Magnascanner for bone
  spinal cord
metastatic bone survey
metastatic brain tumor
metastatic tumor to the brain
metastatic tumor to the cord
metatarsal bar shoe modification
metatarsal bars
metatarsal head
metatarsal head osteotomy
metatarsal lashing of first and second
metatarsal neck osteotomy
metatarsal overload syndromes
metatarsal pads (shoe modification)
metatarsal parabola
metatarsal-phalangeal joint space
metatarsalgia
  Morton
  secondary
metatarsocuneiform (MC) arthrodesis
metatarsocuneiform joint
metatarsophalangeal (MTP) joint
  arthrodesis
metatarsotalar angle
metatarsus adductovarus
metatarsus adductus (MTA)
metatarsus atavicus
metatarsus elevatus
metatarsus equinus
metatarsus internus
metatarsus latus
metatarsus primus adductus
metatarsus primus angle
metatarsus primus elevatus
metatarsus primus varus (MPV)
metatarsus supinatus
metatarsus valgus
metatarsus varus (MTV)
meter
  impedance
  pinch
methacrylate, methyl
method
  Abbott
  Bleck
  Borggreve
  Budin-Chandler
  bundle-nailing
  Cobb
  Ferguson scoliosis measuring
  hydrogen washout
  Insall patella alta

method *(cont.)*
  Kocher
  Mose
  Mosley
  Stullberg (in Perthes disease)
methyl alcohol poisoning
methyl bromide, neurologic
  complications of
methyl methacrylate
  beads of
  centrifuged
methyl methacrylate cement
methylene blue dye
methylmalonic aciduria
metopic craniectomy
metopic suture
metopodynia
metopon
metrizamide contrast media
metrizamide CT cisternogram
  (MCTC)
metrizamide myelogram
metronomic eye movements
Metzenbaum chisel
Metzenbaum gouge
Metzenbaum scissors
Meurig Williams spinal fusion plate
Meyer cervical orthosis
Meyer line
Meyer loop in brain
Meyer sublaminar wiring technique
Meyerding bone skid
Meyerding chisel
Meyerding curved gouge
Meyerding finger retractor
Meyerding laminectomy blade
Meyerding laminectomy retractor
Meyerding mallet
Meyerding osteotome
Meyerding-Scoville blade
Meyerding-Van Demark technique
Meyers-McKeever classification of
  tibial fracture
Meyhoefer bone curet
Meynert, nucleus basalis of
Meynet node
Meyn-Quigley maneuver
MFD (monorhythmic frontal delta)
  activity
MFD waves
MG (myasthenia gravis) antibody
MG II knee prosthesis
MGH osteotome
MHAQ (Modified Health Assessment
  Questionnaire)
MHT (meningohypophyseal trunk
  artery)
Miami Acute Care (MAC) cervical
  collar
Miami J cervical collar
Miami TLSO scoliosis brace
mice, joint
Michael Reese articulated prosthesis
Michel clip
Michele vertebral biopsy
Michele vertebral body trephine
microabscess
microadenoma, pituitary
Micro-Aire blade
Micro-Aire debridement of bone
  surfaces
Micro-Aire drill
Micro-Aire oscillating saw
Micro-Aire osteotome
Micro-Aire pulse lavage system
Micro-Aire reamer
microaneurysm, Charcot-Bouchard
microangiopathy
microatheroma
microballoon
  embolization
  Rand
microbipolar forceps
microcatheter
Microcell-puff material
microcephalic
microcephaly
microcirculation

microclip
microcuret
microcurrent therapy
microdialysis, intracerebral
microdiscectomy (or microdiskectomy)
microdiskectomy, arthroscopic (AMD)
microdrill
microelectrode recording
microembolus (pl. microemboli)
microendarterectomy, carotid
microfibrillar collagen hemostat
microfibrils of connective tissue
Microfoam dressing
microforceps
microfracture
microfreer
microglioblastoma tumor
microgliomata
microgyria in parkinsonism
microgyrus
microhemorrhage
microinfarction
microirrigation
micro-Kerrison rongeur
Microknit vascular graft prosthesis
Microloc knee prosthesis
micromanipulator
micromovement (wiggling and
  fidgeting)
microneurography
micronucleator
Micro-One dissecting forceps
Micro-One hook
Micro-One needle holder
Micro-One scissors
micro-pin, Pischel
microplate
  C-shaped
  H-shaped
  half-circle
  L-shaped
  Leibinger
  Luhr
  Storz Microsystem

microplate *(cont.)*
  Synthes Microsystem
  T-shaped
  X-shaped
  Y-shaped
micropolygyria
microport
micropsia
microreamer
microrongeur
microsaw
  oscillating
  Zimmer
microscissors
  Decker
  Yasargil
microscope
  double binocular operating
  Grenoble-Paris-Rennes (GPR) robot
  operating
  robot neurosurgical
  stereotactic operating (or
    stereotaxic)
  Zeiss OPMI surgical
microscopic hemorrhage of ligaments
microscopy, nail fold
microsomia
  craniofacial
  hemifacial
microscrew, Barouk
Micro Series wire driver
microsphere
microstaple, Barouk
microsurgery
  computer-assisted
  guided
  stereotactic laser
microsurgical decompression
microsurgical dissection
microsurgical DREZ-otomy
microsurgical free flap
microsuture
MicroTeq portable belt
Micro-Three microsurgery instruments

micro tear
Micro-Two forceps
Micro-Two needle holder
Micro-Two scissors
microtraumas, repeated
microvascular decompression
microvascular hemodynamics
microvasculature
microvolts (μV)
micturition syncope
mid-dorsal back pain
mid-tarsal movement test
MID (multi-infarct dementia)
Midas Rex craniotomy bur
Midas Rex craniotomy saw
Midas Rex knife
Midas Rex mechanism (MB)
Midas Rex pneumatic instruments
Midas Rex saw
midaxillary line incision
midbody of vertebra
midbrain
  paramedian
  tegmentum of
midbrain aqueduct
midbrain compression, destruction
midbrain displacement syndrome
midbrain dysfunction
midbrain lesions
midbrain reticular formation (MRF)
midbrain stroke
midbrain subthalamic region
midbrain syndrome
midbrain tumors
midcalf
midcarpal joints
Middeldorpf splint
Middeldorpf triangle
middle cerebral artery syndrome
middle cerebral artery territory stroke
middle frontal gyrus
middle medial palsy
middle-path regimen for spinal TB
middle radial palsy
middle temporal gyrus
midfacial fracture
midfemur
midfoot
midfoot cavus
midfoot, swivel dislocation of
midline cerebellum
midline shift on skull x-ray
midline tumors of the anterior lobe
midpalmar abscess
midpalmar space
midpatellar tendon
midpons
midshaft fracture
midshaft of femur
midshaft of humerus
midstance, of gait
midswing phase of gait
midtarsal joint
midthigh
migraine accompaniments
migraine aura
migraine diathesis
migraine equivalent
migraine headache
  abdominal
  acephalalgic
  acute confusional (ACM)
  aphasic
  basilar
  basilar artery
  Bickerstaff
  bilateral
  catamenial
  ciliary
  circumstantial
  classic
  classical
  classical abdominal
  cluster
  common
  complicated
  conditions that precipitate a
  confusional

migraine headache *(cont.)*
 deficits of ideation and speech in
 dislocations of time and space
  perception in
 facioplegic
 familial
 familial hemiplegic
 hemiparesthetic
 hemiplegic
 late-life
 let-down
 ocular
 ophthalmic
 ophthalmoplegic
 paroxysmal
 pectoralgic
 predisposition to
 recurrent
 recurring
 red
 retinal
 seasonal
 syncopal
 unilateral
 vestibular
 white
migraine headache prodrome
migrainelike headache
migraine precipitated by birth control
 pills
migraine precipitated by coitus
migraine precipitated by emotional
 tension
migraine precipitated by exercise
migraine precipitated by food
migraine precipitated by menstruation
migraine precipitated by nasal
 congestion
migraine precipitated by pregnancy
migraine precipitated by temperature
 changes
migraine precipitated premenstrually
migraine predisposition
migraine spectra
migraineur
migrainoid neuralgia
migrainous constitution
migrainous disorder
migrainous infarction
migrainous neuralgia
migrainous reaction
migrainous stroke
migrainous symptom
migrainous syncope
migrainous syndrome
migralepsy
migration
 hallux
 sesamoid
 staple
migration of acetabular cup
migration of prosthesis
migratory arthralgia
MII (McDowell Impairment Index)
Mik pad (slang for Mikulicz pad)
Mikhail bone block
Mikulicz angle
Mikulicz pad
Mikulicz sponge
Milch cuff resection of ulna technique
Milch fracture classification syndrome
mild ataxia
Miles bone chisel
milestone
 delayed motor
 developmental of infants
Milgram test
miliary aneurysm
military [or medical] antishock
 trousers (MAST)
milk-alkali disease
milk-alkali syndrome
milk leg disease
milking of vessel
Milkman syndrome
Millard-Gubler syndrome
Millender-Nalebuff wrist arthrodesis
Miller-Fisher syndrome

Miller-Fisher test
Miller-Fisher variant of Guillain-Barré syndrome
Miller-Galante hip prosthesis
Miller-Galante knee arthroplasty
Miller-Gubler syndrome
Miller foot procedure
Miller rasp
Miller-Senn retractor
Millesi modified technique
Millet neurological test instrument
Milligan dissector
Milliknit vascular graft prosthesis
millimeters of mercury (mmHg)
milling-cutter
millisecond pulses per second
millivolts (mV)
Mills dressing
Mills test
Milroy disease
Miltex rib spreader
Milwaukee cervicothoracolumbosacral orthosis
Milwaukee scoliosis brace
mimocausalgia
Minaar classification of coalition
MindSet toe splint
Miner osteotome
mineralization
miners' nystagmus
Minerva cast
Minerva fixation
Minerva jacket
Minerva orthosis
Minerva vest
miniangiogram
miniblink on EEG
minicatheter
minidriver
mini-Hoffmann external fixator
mini-Hohmann retractor
minimal assist
minimal brain dysfunction
minimal incision technique
miniplate
  C-shaped
  H-shaped
  half-circle
  L-shaped
  Storz Microsystem
  T-shaped
  X-shaped
  Y-shaped
Miniport drug delivery system
miniscrewdriver
minisponge
mini-squat
Minneapolis prosthesis
Minnesota rate of manipulation test
Minnesota Test for Differential Diagnosis of Aphasia (MTDDA)
Minnesota Test of Aphasia
minor causalgia
minor chorea
minor motor seizures
minor reflex dystrophy
minor reflex sympathetic dystrophies
minor sprain
minor syndrome, pectoralis
Minor sign
Mira cautery
Mira Mark III cranial drill
Mira Mark V craniotome set
Mira reamer
mirror
  Apfelbaum
  dental
mirroring
MIS (minimum incision surgery)
Mishler flush valve
Miskimon cerebellar retractor
misplaced objects test
misshapen
missiles, fully-jacketed (handgun)
Mital elbow release technique
Mitchell osteotomy bunionectomy
Mitchell step-down osteotomy
Mitek bone anchor

Mitek staples
mitotic figures
Mittlemeir broach
Mittlemeir ceramic hip prosthesis
Mittlemeir non-cemented femoral
  prosthesis
Mitutoyo digital calipers
mixed tumors
MixEvac bone-cement mixer
Mixter forceps
Mixter hemostat
Mixter ventricular needles
Miyakawa knee procedure
Mizuno technique
MKG knee support
MLD (metachromatic leukodystrophy)
MLF (medial longitudinal fasciculus)
MLF lesion
MLF syndrome
MLSI (multiple line-scan imaging)
mmHg (millimeters of mercury)
MMT (manual muscle test)
MNCV (motor nerve conduction
  velocity)
MND (motor neuron disease)
Moberg arthrodesis
Moberg-Gedda open reduction fracture
Moberg osteotome
mobile, mobility
Mobilimb CPM (continuous passive
  motion) device
mobility
  fundamental aspects of
  independent in bed
  joint
  normal
mobility disability
mobility handicap
Mobility Healing Clogs
Mobility Shoes
mobilization, soft tissue
Möbius syndrome (Moebius)
modality
  sensory
  therapeutic
moderate ataxia
moderate dysarthria
modification
  Green-Laird m. of the Reverdin
  osteotomy
  medial heel wedge shoe
  metatarsal bar shoe
  shoe
modified Ashworth Scale, for grading
  spasticity
modified dorsalis pedis myofascial flap
modified Mau bunionectomy
modified McBride bunionectomy
modified Oppenheimer splint
modified self-report measure of social
  adjustment (rehab)
Modified Health Assessment
  Questionnaire (MHAQ)
Modny pin
modulus of elasticity
Moe bone curet
Moe distraction rod
Moe gouge
Moe impactor
Moe-Kettleson distribution of curves
  in scoliosis
Moe modified Cotrel cast
Moe osteotome
Moe spinal hook
Moe square-ended hook
Moe modified Harrington rod
Moebius (Möbius) syndrome
Moeltgen flexometer
mogi postop shoe cover
Mohr splint
moist heat
mold, Aufranc concentric hip
molding (or moulding) of skull
moleskin dressing
moleskin patch
moleskin strips
Molesworth-Campbell elbow approach
Mollaret meningitis
Mollaret triangle
Molt periosteal elevator

monarthric process
monarticular
Mönckeberg sclerosis
mongolian idiocy
monitor
  Camino ICP
  eye movement (EM)
  ICP (intracranial pressure)
  intracranial
  nerve integrity (Xomed NIM-2)
  Phoenix ICP
  Polar Vantage XL heart rate
  pressure
  subdural pressure
  submental EMG activity
  Tekscan in-shoe
  thoracic strain gauge (in EEG)
Monitor-2, Nicolet Nerve Integrity (NIM-2)
monitoring
  fluorescein perfusion
  skinfold thickness
Monk hip prosthesis
monoarticular
monoclonal gammopathy
monocular acuity change
monocular blindness
monocular visual loss
monofilament nylon drain
Monofixateur external fixator
monomorphic wave on EEG
monomyoplegia
monomyositis multiplex
mononeural
mononeuritis multiplex
mononeuropathy
  cranial
  diabetic
  diabetic third nerve
  entrapment
  ischemic
  ocular
  sensory
mononeuropathy multiplex
monoparesis
monophasic sharp wave on EEG
monoplegia, crural
monorhythmic frontal delta (MFD) activity
monorhythmic frontal delta (MFD) waves
monorhythmic frontal slowing on EEG
monorhythmic pattern on EEG
monorhythmic waves on EEG
monosodium urate crystal deposition, in gout
monostotic fibrous dysplasia
monosyllabic speech
monosynaptic reflex arc
Monro
  aqueduct of
  foramen of
Monro-Kellie doctrine
montage (on EEG)
  bipolar
  circumferential bipolar
  common average reference
  common reference
  coronal bipolar
  Cz reference
  double-banana
  ear reference
  8-channel
  18-channel
  ipsilateral reference
  Laplacian
  LB (longitudinal bipolar)
  linked ear reference
  longitudinal bipolar (LB)
  noncephalic reference
  referential alternating
  referential block
  reformatting
  scalp-scalp
  16-channel
  source derivation
  TB (transverse bipolar)
  transverse bipolar (TB)
  unipolar
Monteggia fracture-dislocation of ulna

Monteggia lesion
Montenovesi rongeur
Montercaux fracture
Monticelli-Spinelli distractor
Monticelli-Spinelli fixator
Monticelli-Spinelli frame
Montreal hip positioner
mood swing
Moon Boot brace
Mooney brace
Mooney cast
Moore bone elevator
Moore bone reamer
Moore fracture
Moore hand drill
Moore nail set
Moore osteotomy-osteoclasis
Moore pin
Moore plate
Moore stem
mooring
morcel (or morsel)
morcellation, Robinson-Chung-Farahvar clavicular
morcelize (or morselize)
Moreira bolt
Moreira plate
Morel syndrome
Morgan-Casscells meniscus suturing technique
Morgan disk pad
moria
moribund appearance
moribund state
morning shakes
Moro reflex
morphology
  fused alpha wave
  joint
morphology of EEG complex
morphology of wave
Morquio sign
Morquio syndrome
Morrey arthritis grading system
Morrey-Bryan total elbow arthroplasty
Morris biphase screw
Morris retractor
Morrison technique
Morrissy percutaneous fixation of slipped epiphysis
Morscher cervical plate
morsel (or morcel)
morselize (or morcelize)
morsellation (or morcellation)
Morse sternal spreader
Morse tape
Morse tapered prosthetic post
mortise
  ankle
  axis of ankle
  cuneiform
  diaphyseal cortical
  mortised
  widening of the ankle, on x-ray
mortise cut
mortise view
mortising chisel
Morton foot
Morton-Horwitz nerve cross-over sign
Morton metatarsalgia
Morton neuralgia
Morton neuroma
Morton sign
Morton syndrome
Morton test
Morvan chorea
Morvan disease
Morvan syndrome
mosaic disorder of visual perception in migraine
mosaic plantar verruca
mosaic plantar wart
Mose concentric rings
Mose method
Moseley bone age graph
Moseley fasciatome
Moseley straight line graph
Mosley method

Moss fixation system
Moss hook
Moss rod
Moss screw
mother-daughter type plantar warts
Mother Jones dressing
motility
  extraocular
  ocular
motion
  active ankle joint complex range of (AAROM)
  active-assistive range of
  active integral range of (AIROM)
  ankle dorsiflexion range of (ADROM)
  ankle inversion-eversion range of
  arc of
  continuous passive (CPM)
  end-range limitation of
  full range of (FROM)
  limitation of
  passive range of (PROM)
  plantarflexory
  protective limitation of range of
  range of
  scapulothoracic
  shear
  toe range of
  uninhibited ankle
motor (EEG lead)
  left (LM)
  right (RM)
motor activity
motor aphasia
motor apraxia
motor cortex mapping
motor delay
motor disorder
motor dysphasia
motor evoked potential
motor fibers
motor hemiplegia, pure
motor impairment
  anterior horn cell level
  peripheral nerve level
  root level
  spinal nerve level
motor impersistence
motor jacksonian attack
motor loss
motor march, jacksonian
motor measures, to test sensory disturbance
motor negativism
motor nerve conduction study
motor neurofibrils
motor neuron disease (MND)
motor nuclei in the lower brain stem
motor output
motor paralytic bladder
motor paresis
motor phenomena
motor potentials on EMG
motor power
motor problem, high level
motor sign
motor skills
motor speech area of the brain, Broca
motor strip
motor symptoms
motor tic
motor transcortical aphasias
motor vehicle accident (MVA)
motor vehicle injury (MVI)
Motor Assessment scale (MAS)
Motor Club assessment of motor impairment
motorcyclist's knee
motorized bur
motorized shaver
Motoricity Index
Mount laminectomy rongeur
Mouradian rod
Mouradian screw
mouse, joint

mouth, tapir's (bouche de tapir) (in muscular dystrophy)
mouthing phenomenon (pathological reflex)
movement
  adventitious
  anomalous
  arcuate
  automatic hand
  bread-crumbling
  choreic limb
  choreiform
  choreoathetoid
  choreoathetotic
  clonic
  conjugate eye
  decomposition of
  dysconjugate eye
  dysjunctive eye
  dysmetric overshoot of eye
  dyspractic
  dysrhythmic
  dystonic
  fine finger
  fly-catching of the tongue
  following
  freezing of
  functional
  horizontal metronomic eye
  hyperkinetic
  Independent Living
  initiation of
  involuntary limb
  irregular
  jerking
  jerky incoordinate
  mouthing
  nystagmoid
  objective limited
  organization of ocular, in infants
  poverty of
  prehensile hand
  pseudoathetoid
  purposeless

movement *(cont.)*
  pursuit
  quasipurposive
  random
  rapid
  rapid-alternating (RAM)
  rapid eye (REM)
  reflex eye
  reflexive
  rhythmic slow eye
  roving eye
  roving ocular
  saccadic eye
  slow lateral eye (SEMs)
  smooth pursuit eye
  subjective limited
  supranuclear disorders of ocular
  symmetry of limb, in infants
  synkinetic motor
  tonic-clonic
  tremulous
  uncontrollable
  vermicular
  visual pursuit
  visual tracking
  volitional
  voluntary
  withdrawal
movement artifact, on EEG
movement disorder
movers
  capital
  cervical
  prime
moyamoya disease
Moynihan forceps
Moynihan towel clamp
MP (metatarsophalangeal or metacarpophalangeal) (MTP or MCP) joint
MP articulation
MP35N implant metal prosthesis
MPAP (multipurpose access port), Cordis

MPCh (medial posterior choroidal) artery
MPJ (metatarsophalangeal joint)
MPS (myofascial pain syndrome)
MPV (metatarsus primus varus)
MRC (Medical Research Council) classification of muscle function
MRF (midbrain reticular formation)
MRI terms (magnetic resonance image)
  acquisition time
  adiabatic fast passage
  analog to digital converter
  angular frequency
  angular momentum
  antenna
  array processor
  artifact
  Bloch equation
  Boltzmann distribution
  Carr-Purcell sequence
  Carr-Purcell-Meiboom-Gill sequence
  chemical shift
  coherence
  coil
  continuous wave
  crossed coil
  cryomagnet
  cryostat
  demodulator
  detector
  diamagnetic
  diffusion
  digital to analog converter
  echo planar imaging
  echo time (TE)
  echo, echoes
  eddy currents; eddies
  excitation
  Faraday shield
  fast-Fourier transform
  ferromagnetic
  FID (free induction decay)

MRI terms *(cont.)*
  field gradient
  field lock
  filling factor
  filtered-back projection
  flip angle
  Fourier transform
  free induction decay (FID)
  free induction signal
  frequency
  gadolinium enhancement
  gauss
  Golay coil
  gradient coil
  gradient magnetic field
  gyromagnetic ratio
  Helmholtz coil
  hertz (Hz)
  homogeneity
  image acquisition time
  inductance
  inhomogeneity
  interface
  interpulse time
  inversion
  inversion recovery
  inversion time (TI)
  kilohertz (kHz)
  Larmor equation
  Larmor frequency
  lattice
  line imaging
  line scanning
  line width
  LMR (localized magnetic resonance)
  longitudinal magnetization
  longitudinal relaxation
  Lorentzian line
  macroscopic magnetization moment
  macroscopic magnetization vector
  magnetic dipole
  magnetic field
  magnetic gradient
  magnetic induction

MRI terms (*cont.*)
- magnetic moment
- magnetic resonance
- magnetic resonance signal
- magnetic susceptibility
- magnetization
- multiple line-scan imaging (MLSI)
- multiple plane imaging
- multiple sensitive point
- nuclear magnetic resonance
- nuclear signal
- nuclear spin
- nuclear spin quantum number
- nucleon
- nutation
- orientation: coronal; sagittal; transverse
- paramagnetic
- partial saturation
- permanent magnet
- permeability
- phantom
- phase
- phase sensitive detector
- pixel (picture element)
- planar spin imaging
- point imaging
- point scanning
- precession
- precessional frequency
- proton
- pulse length
- pulse sequences
- pulse width
- pulse, radiofrequency
- pulsed gradients
- quadrature detector
- quality factor
- quenching
- radian
- radiofrequency (RF)
- radiofrequency coil
- radiofrequency pulse
- readout delay

MRI terms (*cont.*)
- receiver
- receiver coil
- reconstruction
- relaxation rate
- relaxation time
- repeated FID (free induction decay)
- repetition time (TR)
- rephasing gradient
- resistive magnet
- resolution, spatial
- resonance
- resonant frequency
- RF (radiofrequency)
- RF coil
- RF pulse
- rotating frame of reference
- S/N ratio (signal-to-noise)
- saddle coil
- saturation recovery
- saturation transfer
- selective excitation
- selective irradiation
- sensitive plane
- sensitive point
- sensitive volume
- sequence time
- sequential plane imaging
- sequential point imaging
- shim coil
- shimming
- signal-to-noise ratio (SNR or S/N ratio)
- simultaneous volume imaging
- skin depth
- SNR (signal-to-noise ratio)
- solenoid coil
- spectrometer
- spectrum
- spin
- spin density
- spin echo
- spin-echo imaging
- spin-lattice relaxation time

MRI terms (*cont.)*
  spin-spin relaxation time
  spin-warp imaging
  steady state free precession (SSFP)
  stereotactic
  superconducting magnet
  surface coil MR
  T1 (spin-lattice or longitudinal relaxation time)
  T2 (spin-spin or transverse relaxation time)
  TE (echo time)
  tesla (T)
  three-dimensional Fourier transform imaging
  TI (inversion time)
  TR (repetition time)
  transverse magnetization
  tuning
  tunnel
  two-dimensional Fourier transform imaging
  vector
  volume imaging
  voxel (volume element)
  zeugmatography, Fourier transformation
MRI with gadolinium enhancement
MS (multiple sclerosis)
MSC cold pack
MSD (midsagittal diameter)
MSLT (multiple sleep latency test)
MST (multifocal sharp transient)
MST-6A1-4V implant metal prosthesis
MSUD (maple syrup urine disease)
MT (or MTP) joint (metatarso-phalangeal)
MTA (metatarsus adductus)
MTDDA (Minnesota Test for Differential Diagnoss of Aphasia)
MTM 2 bur
MTP (metatarsophalangeal) capsule
MTV (metatarsus varus)
MUAP (motor unit action potential)
Mubarak-Hargens decompression technique
mucolipidosis III (pseudo-Hurler deformity)
mucopolysaccharides
mucopolysaccharidosis
mucormycosis
mucopurulent drainage
mud pack bath
Mueli wrist prosthesis
Mueller Duo-Lock hip prosthesis
Muhlberger orbital implant prosthesis
Mulder sign
Mulholland and Gunn criteria
Müller (Mueller)
Müller arthrodesis
Müller classification of humerus fractures
Müller muscle
Müller knee procedure
Müller saw
multangular, greater (or lesser)
multi-infarct dementia (MID)
multi-item indices in rehabilitation testing
Multi-Lock knee brace
multifocal leukoencephalopathy, progressive (PML)
multifocal myoclonus
multifocal seizures
multiforme, glioblastoma
Multileaf Collimator
Multipaks, Ortho-Ice
multiplanar compression
multiplanar ligamentotaxis
multiple cortical infarcts
multiple focal lesions of the spinal cord
multiple line-scan imaging (MLSI)
multiple plane imaging
multiple sclerosis (MS)
  benign form
  chronic-progressive form
  chronic-relapsing form

multiple sclerosis (*cont.)*
 exacerbating-remitting form
 graying of vision in
 Ishihara color plate test for
 MacDougall diet for
multiple sclerosis plateau
multiple sensitive point
multiple small strokes (état lacunaire)
multiple, symphalangism
multiplex
 mononeuritis
 paramyoclonus
Multipoise headrest
multisystem disease
mumbling automatism
Mumford-Gurd arthroplasty
Mumford-Gurd procedure
mumps encephalitis
mumps viral encephalitis
Mundinger-Reichert stereotactic frame
murine typhus meningoencephalitis
"murmuring a perpetual litany"
murmurs (thrills)
Murphy gouge
Murphy heel cord advancement
Murphy-Lane bone skid
Murphy osteotome
Murphy punch test
Murray-Jones splint
Murray-Thomas splint
Murray Valley (Australian X) viral encephalitis
muscle
 abdominis rectus
 abductor
 abductor hallucis
 accelerator urinae
 adductor
 adductor pollicis
 ADQ (abductor digiti quinti)
 anconeus
 antagonistic
 anterior papillary
 antigravity

muscle (*cont.)*
 antistriated
 APB (abductor pollicis brevis)
 APL (abductor pollicis longus)
 appendicular
 articular
 aryepiglotticus
 ascending oblique
 atrophied
 BBC (biceps, brachialis, coracobrachialis)
 belly of
 biceps brachii
 biceps femoris
 biopsy
 bipennate
 bipenniform
 brachial
 brachialis
 brachioradialis
 broad
 bronchoesophageal
 calf
 cardiac
 cervical interspinal
 cervical rotator
 cheek
 ciliary
 circumpennate
 coccygeal
 compressor
 coracobrachial
 corrugator
 cowl
 cremaster
 cricothyroid
 cruciate
 cucullaris
 cutaneomucous
 cutaneous
 degeneration of muscle
 deltoid
 denervated
 denervation of

muscle (*cont.*)
- depressor
- digastric
- dilator
- dorsal interosseous
- DRAM (de-epithelialized rectus abdominis)
- ECRB (extensor carpi radialis brevis)
- ECRL (extensor carpi radialis longus)
- ECU (extensor carpi ulnaris)
- EDB (extensor digitorum brevis)
- EDC (extensor digitorum communis)
- EDL (extensor digitorum longus)
- EDQ (extensor digitorum quinti)
- EHL (extensor hallucis longus)
- EIP (extensor indicis proprius)
- enlarged calf
- EPB (extensor pollicis brevis)
- epicranial
- EPL (extensor pollicis longus)
- EQP (extensor quinti proprius)
- erector
- external oblique
- extraocular
- extrinsic
- facial
- fan-shaped
- fasciculations of
- FCR (flexor carpi radialis)
- FCU (flexor carpi ulnaris)
- FDC (flexor digitorum communis)
- FDI (first digital interosseous)
- FDL (flexor digitorum longus)
- FDP (flexor digitorum profundus)
- FDQ (flexor digiti quinti)
- FDS (flexor digitorum sublimis)
- FDS (flexor digitorum superficialis)
- femoral
- FHB (flexor hallucis brevis)
- FHL (flexor hallucis longus)
- fibrosed
- finger flexor

muscle (*cont.*)
- flat
- flat abdominal
- flexor
- FPB (flexor pollicis brevis)
- FPL (flexor pollicis longus)
- fusiform
- gastrocnemius
- ghost muscle
- gluteus
- gluteus maximus
- gluteus medius
- gluteus minimus
- gracilis
- hamstring
- humeroperoneal
- hypothenar
- iliopsoas
- infraspinatus
- internal oblique
- interosseous
- intraspinous
- intrinsic foot
- involuntary
- ischiocavernosus
- isometric
- latissimus dorsi
- LOAF (**l**umbricals, **o**pponens pollicis, **a**bductor pollicis brevis, **f**lexor pollicis brevis)
- lumbrical
- motor point of
- Muller
- multipennate
- nonstriated
- oblique
- obturator internus
- occipitofrontal
- occipitofrontalis
- ODQ (opponens digiti quinti)
- opponens pollicis
- overpull of
- overwhelming of extensor
- palmar interosseous

muscle (*cont.*)
papillary
paraspinal
paravertebral
pectoral
pectoralis major
pennate
peroneal
piriformis
plantaris
platysma
popliteal
postvertebral
profundus
progressive neuropathic
pronator
psoas
pubococcygeal
quadratus femoris
quadriceps
rectus abdominis
rectus femoris
regeneration of
release of abductor hallucis
retronuchal
sartorius
scalene
scalenus anterior
scalenus anticus
semitendinosus
septal papillary
serratus anterior
serratus posterior
sheath of
skeletal
skeletal striated
smooth
spasticity of
sternocleidomastoid
sternohyoid
sternothyroid
strap
straplike
stretching of

muscle (*cont.*)
striated
striated cardiac
subcostal
subscapularis
supinator
supraspinatus
synergistic
tensing of
teres major
thenar
thigh
tibial
tibialis anterior
tibialis posterior
toe extensor
toe flexor
TRAM (transverse rectus abdominis myocutaneous)
transversus abdominis
trapezius
triangular
triceps
trunk
twigs to the piriformis
vastus lateralis
vastus medialis
vastus medialis obliquus
viscoelastic property of
muscle action in arthritis
muscle action potential
muscle anatomy
muscle artifact on EEG
muscle atrophy
muscle attachment
muscle belly
muscle biopsy
muscle bulk
muscle clamp
muscle contractility
muscle contraction
muscle contracture
muscle coordination
muscle cramp

muscle denervation
muscle disorder
muscle dissection
muscle dystrophy
muscle fascicle
muscle fiber action potential
muscle fiber conduction velocity
muscle fiber wasting
muscle flap
muscle forceps
muscle function
muscle glycogen supersaturation
muscle group
muscle guarding
muscle hook
muscle imbalance
muscle insufficiency
muscle interference pattern
muscle irritability
muscle ischemia
muscle origin
muscle palsy, extraocular
muscle-paretic nystagmus
muscle-pedicle bone graft
muscleplasty
muscle potential
muscle power
muscle pump (anatomical)
muscle relaxant
muscle-setting exercises
muscle sheath
muscle soreness
muscle spasm
muscle-splitting incision
muscle sprain
muscle stimulator
muscle strain
muscle strength
muscle stretch
muscle-tendon injury
muscle tissue
muscle tone
muscle training
  concentric
  eccentric
muscle transfer
muscle wasting
muscle-wasting fasciculations
muscular atrophy
  scapuloperoneal
  Vulpian-Bernhardt spinal
  Welander distal
  Werdnig-Hoffmann spinal
muscular dystrophy
muscular dystrophy (MD)
  Becker
  benign X-linked recessive
  Duchenne
  Erb
  Gowers
  Kiloh-Nevin ocular form of
    progressive
  oculopharyngeal
muscular lesion
muscular tonus
musculature
  axial
  cervical
  paraspinal
  paraspinous
  paretic
  scalene
musculocutaneous free flaps
musculocutaneous nerve
musculorum deformans, dystonia
musculoskeletal trauma
musculotendinous cuff
musculotendinous junction
musculotendinous-osseous link
Musgrave footprint pedobarograph
musicogenic epilepsy
muslin sling
Mustard iliopsoas transfer
mute, akinetically
mute toe signs
mutism
  akinetic
  elective
  hyperpathic akinetic

mutism (*cont.*)
  hysterical
  postictal
muzzle velocity, in handgun injury
mV (millivolt)
MVA (motor vehicle accident)
MVD (microvascular decompression)
MVI (motor vehicle injury)
MVM (medullary venous malformation)
MVR blade
MWD (microwave diathermy)
myalgia
myasthenia
  congenital
  ocular
myasthenia gravis (MG)
  familial infantile
  transient neonatal
myasthenic crisis
myasthenic ptosis
myasthenic symptom
myasthenic syndrome
Mycoplasma pneumoniae encephalitis
mycotic aneurysm
mycotic infections of bones and joints
mycotic intracranial aneurysm
mycotic meningitis
myectomy
myelalgia
myelanalosis
myelapoplexy
myelasthenia
myelatelia
myelatrophy
myelauxe
myelencephalon
myeleterosis
myelin
  subcortical
  subependymal
myelin basic protein
myelin bleb
myelin damage
myelin metabolism
myelin sheath
myelinated nerve fiber
myelinoclasis, acute perivascular
myelinolysis
  central pontine
  pontine
myelitis
  acute transverse
  ascending
  herpes simplex
  herpes zoster
  postinfectious
  subacute necrotizing
  transverse
myeloblastoma
myelocele
myelocystocele
myelocystomeningocele
myelocytoma
myelodiastasis
myelodysplasia
myelofibrosis
myelogram
  cervical
  corduroy cloth pattern on
  metrizamide
myelographic block
myelography
  air
  contrast
  Hypaque
  metrizamide
  Pantopaque
myelography dye
myelolipoma
myeloma
  multiple
  plasma cell
myelomalacia
myelomeningitis
myelomeningocele
myelomere
myeloneuritis
myelo-opticoneuropathy, subacute (SMON)

myeloparalysis
myelopathy
  AIDS
  cervical
  cervical spondylotic (CSM)
  CMV (cytomegalovirus)
  compression
  necrotizing
  noncompressive
  progressive subacute
  radiation
  radiation-induced
  spinal stenotic
  spondylitic
  spondylotic
  subacute necrotizing
  transverse
  vacuolar
myelopathy of the spinal cord
myelophthisis
myeloplegia
myeloradiculitis
myeloradiculopathy
myelorrhagia
myelorrhaphy, commissural
myeloschisis, dorsal
myelosclerosis
myelosyphilis
myelosyringosis
myelotomy, midline
Myers-Briggs Type Indicator (MBTI) test
Myers knee retractor
Myerson sign
myoasthenia
myoblast
myoblastoma, granular cell
Myobock artificial hand
myobradia
myocele
myocelialgia
myocelitis
myocellulitis
myocerosis
myocervical rigid collar
myoclasis
myoclonia
  eyelid
  facial
  Ramsey Hunt dyssynergia cerebellaris
myoclonic epilepsy
myoclonic jerk
myoclonic seizure
myoclonic spells
myoclonic triangle
myoclonus
  action
  Baltic
  benign
  branchial
  cherry red spot
  epileptic
  essential
  familial essential
  focal
  generalized
  hereditary essential
  infantile
  intention
  multifocal
  nocturnal (NM)
  nonepileptic
  nonprogressive
  ocular
  palatal
  palate
  palatopharyngolaryngo-oculodiaphragmatic
  partial
  postanoxic intention
  postaxonic
  posthypoxic
  precipitated by sensory stimulation
  progressive
  rhythmical
  segmental
  spinal

myoclonus (*cont.*)
  spiral
  spontaneous generalized
  startle
  static
  stimulus-induced
  stimulus-sensitive
  subcortical segmental
  symptomatic
  transient
myoclonus epilepsy
myocutaneous flap
myocytoma
myodegeneration
myodemia
myodesis, suture
myodiastasis
myodynia
myodystonia
myoedema
myoelectric control for upper arm
  prosthesis
myofascial flap
myofascial muscular tissues
myofascial pain syndrome (MPS)
myofascial periosteal juncture
myofascial stretching exercises
myofasciitis, interstitial
myofibril
  disorganized
  striated
myofibroma
myofibrosis
myofibrositis
MyoForce test
myofusio-periostitis
myogelosis
myoglobinuria, march
myohypertrophia
myointimal proliferation
myoischemia
myokerosis
myokymia
  exercise-induced
  facial

myokymia (*cont.*)
  limb
  superior oblique
myokymic discharge
myolipoma
myolysis
myoma
myomalacia
myomatosis
myomectomy (myomatectomy)
myomelanosis
myoneural ischemia
myoneural junction
myoneural necrosis
myoneuralgia
myoneurasthenia
myoneurectomy
myoneuroma
myoneurosis
myopachynsis
myopalmus
myoparalysis
myoparesis
myopathic dystrophy
myopathic weakness
myopathy (pl. myopathies)
  acquired
  alcoholic
  centronuclear
  congenital
  dystrophic
  endocrine
  entrapment
  fingerprint body
  hereditary
  idiopathic polymyositis
  Kiloh-Nevin ocular
  metabolic
  mitochondrial
  myotubular
  nemaline rod
  ocular
  polymyositis
  postinfectious

myopathy (*cont.*)
  primary
  reducing body
  sarcoid
  sarcotubular
  steroid
  storage
  subclinical
  thyroid
  thyrotoxic
  zebra body
  zidovudine-induced
myophagism
myoplasty
myopsychopathy
Myo rigid cervical collar
myorrhaphy
myorrhexis
myosalgia
myosarcoma
myosclerosis
myoseism
myositis
  clostridial
  focal nodular
  granulomatous
  inclusion body (IBM)
  inflammatory
  ischemic
  myositides
  ossificans
  proliferative
  streptococcal
  tension
  viral
myositis fibrosa
myositis ossificans circumscripta
myositis ossificans progressiva
myositis ossificans traumatica
myospasm
myospasmia
myostasis
myostatic contracture
myosteoma
myosynizesis
myotendinous junction
myotenontoplasty
myotenositis
myotenotomy
myotomal diagram of pain
myotomal distribution
myotomal muscular pain
myotomal pattern
myotome
myotomy
myotonia
  chondrodystrophic
  congenital
myotonia atrophica
myotonia congenita
myotonia intermittens
myotonia paradoxica
myotonic discharge
myotonic dystrophy
myotonic facies
myotonic pupil
myotonic syndrome
myotube
myotubular myopathy
mytenositis
myxedema coma
myxedema madness
myxofibroma
myxoma, soft tissue
myxosarcoma

N, n

NA (neuropathic arthropathy)
Naden-Rieth hip prosthesis
Naegleria meningitis
Naffziger sign
Naffziger syndrome
nail, nailing
  adjustable
  Ainsworth modification of Massie
  AO slotted medullary
  AP
  Augustine boat
  Bailey-Dubow
  Barr
  Bickel intramedullary
  blind medullary
  boat
  Brooker femoral
  Brooker-Wills
  cannulated
  Chick
  Christensen interlocking
  closed
  closed Küntscher
  closed unlocked
  cloverleaf intramedullary
  cloverleaf Küntscher
  condylocephalic
  crutch and belt femoral closed
  Curry hip
  Derby
  Deyerle pin
  diamond-shaped medullary
  Dooley
  double-ended

nail *(cont.)*
  dynamic locking
  elastic stable intramedullary (ESIN)
  Ender
  Ender flexible medullary
  Engel-May
  extension
  femoral neck
  fluted titanium
  four-flanged
  gamma locking
  Grosse-Kempf
  Grosse-Kempf interlocking
    medullary
  Hagie pin
  Hahn bone
  half and half
  hallux
  Hansen-Street
  Harris condylocephalic
  Harris hip
  Harris medullary
  Holt
  hooked intramedullary
  hooked medullary
  Huckstep
  ingrown (onychocryptosis)
  interlocking
  interlocking intramedullary
  intramedullary
  Inyo
  Jewett
  Johannson hip
  Kaessmann

nail *(cont.)*
 Ken sliding
 Knowles
 Küntscher medullary
 left-sided
 Lewis
 locking
 Lottes triflanged medullary
 Massie II
 Massie sliding
 McKee tri-fin
 McLaughlin
 medullary
 Moore
 nested
 Neufeld
 noncannulated
 Nylok self-locking
 open
 OrthoSorb pin
 Palmer bone
 PGP
 Pidcock
 prebent
 Pugh sliding
 reconstruction
 Richards reconstruction
 right-sided
 Rush flexible medullary
 Rush pin
 Russell-Taylor interlocking medullary
 Rydell
 Sage triangular
 Sampson medullary
 Sarmiento
 Schneider medullary
 Seidel humeral locking
 self-broaching
 self-locking
 Slocum
 Smillie
 Smith-Petersen femoral neck
 Smith-Petersen transarticular

nail *(cont.)*
 spring-loaded
 static locking
 Steinmann extension
 Street
 Sven-Johansson femoral neck
 telescoping
 Temple University
 Terry nails
 Thatcher
 Thornton
 Tiemann
 triangular medullary
 triflange
 triflanged Lottes
 V-medullary
 Venable-Stuck
 Vesely-Street split
 Vitallium Küntscher
 Watson-Jones
 Webb
 Z fixation
 Zickel intramedullary
 Zickel subtrochanteric
 Zickel supracondylar medullary
nail assembly, Massie
nail base
nail bed
nail bed lesion
nail fold microscopy
nail matrix
nail starter, Ritchie
nail sulcus
Nalebuff arthrodesis
Nalebuff-Millender technique
Namaqualand hip dysplasia
NAP (nerve-action potential)
narcolepsy cataplexy syndrome
narcoleptic
narcotics, blood screen for
narrowing
 disk space
 joint space
 neural foramina

narrowing *(cont.)*
  segmental
  thecal sac
nasal fracture
nasal septum hematoma
nasal thermistor for EEG
Nashold biopsy needle
Nashold TC electrode
nasion
nasociliary neuralgia
nasoethmoidal encephalocele
nasofrontal encephalocele
nasolabial fold, flat
nasopharyngeal EEG leads
nasopharyngeal electrode
natatory ligament
National Association for Mental Health
National Association for the Deaf
National Association for the Visually Handicapped
National Collegiate Athletic Association (NCAA)
National Institute of Mental Health (NIMH)
National Institute of Neurological and Communicative Disorders and Stroke (NINCDS)
National Institute on Aging (NIA)
National Institute on Mental Health (NIMH)
National Multiple Sclerosis Society (NMSS)
National Operating Committee on Standards for Athletic Equipment (NOCSAE)
National Society for the Prevention of Blindness
National Special Olympics
National Technical Institute for the Deaf (NTID)
Natural-Knee prosthesis
Naughton-Dunn triple arthrodesis
Nauth traction apparatus
Nautilus machine
navicular (scaphoid) bone
  accessory
  cartilaginous
  lip of
navicular body fracture
  dorsal cortical avulsion
  medial tuberosity
navicular cookie in shoe
navicularis, os
naviculectomy
naviculocapitate fracture syndrome
naviculocuneiform joint
naviculocuneiform ligament
NCAA (National Collegiate Athletic Association)
NCCU (neurological critical care unit)
NCS (nerve conduction study)
NCV (nerve conduction velocity)
Nd:YAG laser (neodymium: yttrium-aluminum-garnet)
Neal-Robertson litter
near reflex
NEB (New England Baptist) hip prosthesis
neck
  basal
  crick in the
  femoral
  metatarsal
  stiff
  supple
  surgical
  swan
  talar
  webbed
neck ache
neck compression test
neck fracture
Neck-Huggar cervical support pillow
neck of aneurysm
neck of femur
neck of metatarsal
neck reflex, tonic

neck school
neck stiffness
NECKSYS home neck care system
Nec Loc cervical collar
necrosis
  aseptic
  avascular (AVN)
  cerebral radiation (CRN)
  epiphyseal ischemic
  femoral head
  gangrenous
  hemorrhagic
  ischemic needle of femoral head (INFH)
  Marcus grading scale for avascular
  muscle
  myoneural
  neuronal
  pressure (from bed rest)
  septic
  skin
  soft-tissue
necrotic bone
necrotizing encephalitis
necrotizing fasciitis
NED (no evidence of disease)
needle
  Adson aneurysm
  Adson scalp
  aneurysm
  Backlund biopsy
  band circling
  Beath
  Bier lumbar puncture
  biopsy
  bone biopsy
  bore
  Bouge
  Bunnell tendon
  cone biopsy
  cone ventricular
  Cournand arteriogram
  Cournand-Grino arteriogram
  Cushing ventricular

needle *(cont.)*
  D'Errico ventricular
  Dandy ventricular
  dural
  EMG (electromyogram)
  Estridge biopsy
  eye
  Feild-Lee brain biopsy
  Framer tendon-passing
  Frazier ventricular
  Gallie
  Hawkeye suture (for arthroscopy)
  Hemo-Drain
  Hoen ventricular
  hubbed
  Huber
  Intracath
  Jamshidi
  Keith
  Kronecker aneurysm
  lumbar puncture
  micro
  Mixter ventricular
  Nashold biopsy
  Pace ventricular
  Parhad-Poppen arteriogram
  Parham band circling
  P-4
  PMT biopsy
  Poppen ventricular
  Protect Point
  Quincke lumbar puncture
  Reichert-Mundinger biopsy
  Retter aneurysm
  Rhoton
  scalp
  Scoville ventricular
  Shaw aneurysm
  Sheldon-Spatz vertebral arteriogram
  side-aspirating biopsy
  Smiley-Williams arteriogram
  spinal
  stereotactic biopsy
  tendon-passing

needle *(cont.)*
  TruCut
  Tuohy lumbar puncture
  ventricular
  ventriculostomy
  Verbrugge
  wire circling
needle electrode
needle electromyography
needle holder (also see *holder*)
  Adson dural
  Ayers
  Donaghy angled suture
  Micro-One
  titanium microsurgical
  Wangensteen
  Webster
needlescope
Neer acromioplasty for rotator cuff tear
Neer classification of shoulder fractures (I, II, III)
Neer hemiarthroplasty
Neer-Horowitz fracture classification
Neer impingement sign
Neer lateral view
Neer shoulder replacement prosthesis
Neer trans-scapular view
Neer-Vitallium humeral prosthesis
Neff meniscus knife
negative scotoma
negativism, motor (gegenhalten)
neglect
  auditory
  left/right side of body
  organic unilateral
  polymodal
  spatial
  tactile
  unilateral
  unilateral organic
  unilateral visual
  visual
neglect syndrome
Negri bodies (seen in rabies)
Negro sign
Neisseria meningitidis meningitis
Neivert osteotome
Nélaton dislocation of the ankle
Nélaton line
Nélaton rubber tube drain
N_z electrode
Nelson finger exerciser
Nelson rib retractor
Nelson rib spreader
Nelson scissors
Nelson sign
Nelson syndrome
nemaline body
nemaline myopathy
neocortex
neodymium: yttrium-aluminum-garnet laser (Nd:YAG laser)
neoformans, Cryptococcus
neologisms (nonsensical words)
neologistic paraphasia
neonatal EEG recording
neonatal flatfoot
neonatal Horner syndrome
neonatal meningitis
neonatal neurological syndrome
neonatal reflex
neonatal seizures
neonatal tyrosinemia
neonatal withdrawal seizures
neopallium
neoplasm
  CNS
  frontal
  interdigital
  intracranial
  temporal horn
  spinal cord
neoplasm of the spinal cord
neoplastic cord damage
neoplastic destruction of spinal elements
neoplastic disorder
  benign
  malignant

neoplastic invasion of meninges
neoplastic invasion of roots
neoplastic process of the superior
orbital fissure
neoprene patellar brace
neoprene support brace
neotendon
Neri bowing sign
nerve
abducens (sixth cranial nerve)
acoustic
afferent digital
atrophy of optic
auditory division of the eighth
cranial
calcaneal
circumflex
cluneal
common peroneal
compression of
corticopontocerebellar
course of
cranial, I-XII
deep peroneal
demyelinated
digital
efferent digital
eighth cranial (auditory and
vestibular divisions)
eleventh cranial (spinal accessory
nerve)
entrapped
ethmoidal
facial (seventh cranial nerve)
femoral cutaneous
fifth cranial (trigeminal nerve)
first cranial (olfactory nerve)
fourth cranial (trochlear nerve)
glossopharyngeal (ninth cranial
nerve)
head of optic
hypoglossal (twelfth cranial nerve)
iliohypogastric
ilioinguinal

nerve *(cont.)*
intact cranial
intermediate n. of Wrisberg
lateral antebrachial cutaneous
lateral femoral cutaneous
left respiratory (phrenic)
Luschka (also von Luschka)
medial cutaneous
medial plantar
median
musculocutaneous
myelinated
nasociliary
neurofibroma of interdigital
ninth cranial (glossopharyngeal
nerve)
obturator
oculomotor (third cranial nerve)
olfactory (first cranial nerve)
olivocerebellar
optic (second cranial nerve)
palmar digital
parolfactory (callosal area)
percutaneous interosseous (PIN)
peripheral
peripheral third
periradicular
phrenic (right and left respiratory
nerves)
pinched
posterior tibial
preservation of
proper digital
recurrent meningeal (Luschka
nerve)
right respiratory (phrenic nerve)
root of
rootlets of
rostral cervical
saphenous
sciatic
second cranial (optic nerve)
sensory branch of the radial
(SBRN)

nerve *(cont.)*
  seventh cranial (facial nerve)
  sinuvertebral (of Luschka)
  sixth cranial (abducens nerve)
  spinal accessory (eleventh cranial nerve)
  spinocerebellar
  superficial peroneal
  supraspinatus
  sural
  tectocerebellar
  tenth cranial (vagus nerve)
  tethering of
  third cranial (oculomotor nerve)
  tract of
  transection of
  trigeminal (fifth cranial nerve)
  trigeminocerebellar
  trochlear (fourth cranial nerve)
  twelfth cranial (hypoglossal nerve)
  ulnar
  ulnar digital
  unroofing of
  vagus (tenth cranial nerve)
  vestibular division of the eighth cranial
  vestibulocerebellar
nerve-action potential (NAP)
nerve biopsy
nerve conduction study (NCS)
nerve conduction velocity (NCV)
nerve disorder, vestibular
nerve entrapment
nerve entrapment syndrome
nerve fascicle
nerve fiber membrane depolarization
nerve growth factor (NGF)
nerve head, ischemia of the
nerve hook
  Dandy
  Lahey Clinic
  Malis
  Scoville
  Smithwick
nerve injury
nerve of Wrisberg
nerve pain from cervical or brachial plexus injury ("stinger")
NervePace nerve conduction monitor
nerve palsy, tardive ulnar
nerve paralysis
nerve plexus
nerve root
  extrathecal
  intradural
nerve root compression
nerve root cutoff
nerve root dissector
nerve root edema
nerve root embarrassment
nerve root fila
nerve root gutter
nerve root, injury to
nerve root retractor
nerve root sheath
nerve root sheath effacement
nerve root sleeve
nerve root syndrome
nerve separator-spatula
nerve sheath tumor
nerve terminal
nerve transfer
nerve trunk
nerve twig
nervous system
  parasympathetic
  sympathetic
nervous system integrity
nervousness
nervus intermedius neuralgia
nest, bees' (in angiomatous malformations of the retina)
nests of tumor cells
Neubeiser splint
Neufeld cast
Neufeld nail
Neufeld traction
Neurairtome

neural arch resection technique
neural deficit
  peripheral
  radicular
  spinal
  thalamic
neural foramina
  narrowing of
  widely patent
neuralgia
  abdominal
  ciliary
  cranial
  geniculate
  glossopharyngeal
  Hunt
  hypoglossal
  intercostal
  migrainous
  migrainous cranial
  Morton
  nasociliary
  nerve entrapment
  nervus intermedius
  occipital
  paratrigeminal
  petrosal
  postherpetic
  pterygopalatine
  Sluder
  sphenopalatine
  Trélat-Charlin
  trigeminal (tic douloureux)
  trigger point
  vidian
neuralgic amyotrophy
neuralgic pain
neural regeneration
neural-tube defect
neurapraxia
neurasthenia
neuraxis, spinal
neurectomy
  chemical
  obturator
neurilemmoma, hourglass-type of
neurilemmoma tumor
neurinoma, acoustic
neuritic plaque
neuritic senile plaques
neuritis (see also *polyneuritis*)
  axial
  brachial
  brachial neuritis
  brachial plexus
  heavy-metal
  idiopathic plexus
  interdigital
  ischemic
  ischemic optic
  lumbosacral plexus
  multiple
  optic
  relapsing hypertrophic
  retrobulbar
  traction
neuroacanthocytosis
neuroanatomic correlate
neuroanatomy
neuroanesthesia
neuroarthropathy
  atrophic
  diabetic (of the foot and ankle)
neuroastrocytoma
neuroaxis radiotherapy
neuroaxonal dystrophy
neurobehavioral syndrome
Neurobehavioral Cognitive Status
  Examination
Neurobehavioral Rating Scale
neuroblastoma
  dumbbell-type
  Hutchinson type of
  intra-abdominal
  occipital
  Pepper
neurochemical
neurocirculatory check
neurocirculatory status
neurocranium

neurocutaneous syndrome
neurocysticercosis
neurocytoma
  central
  intraventricular
neurodegenerative disease
neurodevelopment
neurodiagnostic imaging
neurodissector, Penfield
NeuroDrape surgical drape
neuroectodermal tumor, primitive
neuroendoscope
neurofibrillary degeneration
neurofibrillary tangle
neurofibrils, motor
neurofibroma
  dumbbell
  nonplexiform cutaneous
  plexiform
  solitary
neurofibroma of interdigital nerve
neurofibroma tumor
neurofibromatosa, elephantiasis
neurofibromatosis
neurogenic bladder
  refluxing spastic
  spastic
neurogenic bowel
neurogenic disorder
neurogenic hyperventilation, central
neurogenic lesion
neuroglia
neurohormone
neurohypophyseal germinoma
neurohypophysectomy
neurohypophysial
neurohypophysis
neuroimaging procedure
neuroleptic malignant syndrome
neuroleptic medication
neuroleptics
Neurolite (technetium-99m bicisate)
neurologic or neurological
neurologic complications of antibiotics
neurologic complications of anti-psychotic and phenothiazine drugs
neurologic complications of griseofulvin
neurologic complications of methyl bromide
neurologic deficit
neurologic deterioration
neurologic disease, emotional lability following infectious
neurologic dysfunction
neurologic exam, physiologic
neurologic integrity
neurologic symptom
neurological critical care unit (NCCU)
neurological deficit
neurological deterioration
neurological examination
neurological improvement
neurological rehabilitation
neurological scissors, Strully
neurologically intact
neurologist
neurology, behavioral
neurolysis
  interfascicular
  intramuscular
neuroma
  acoustic
  amputation
  gasserian ganglion
  incisional
  interdigital
  Morton
  neuromata
  peripheral nerve
  plexiform
  posttraumatic
neuromechanical spinal chiropractic management
Neuromed stimulator
neuromotor dysfunction
neuromuscular disease
neuromuscular electrical stimulation (NMES)

neuromuscular facilitation, proprioceptive (PNF)
neuromuscular junction
neuromuscular re-education
neuromuscular transmission
neuromyasthenia, epidemic
neuromyelitis optica
neuromyopathy
  carcinomatous
  uremic
neuromyotonia
neuron, neurons
  abnormal epileptic
  afferent
  alpha motor
  collateral sprouting
  cortical
  corticobulbar motor
  corticospinal motor
  epileptic
  firing of
  foci of abnormal epileptic
  gamma motor
  giant
  lower motor
  motor
  pedunculopontine
  pyramidal
  striatal
  thalamocortical relay (TCR)
  upper motor
neuronal aggregate
neuronal dropout
neuronal dysfunction
  cortical
  subcortical
neuronal loss
neuronal membrane
neuronal membrane depolarization
neuronal metabolism
neuronal necrosis
neuronavigator attachment to Mayfield head holder
neuronitis, vestibular
neuronopathy, subacute motor
neuronophagy
neuron-specific enolase (NSE) antibody
neuro-ophthalmic
neuro-ophthalmologic function
neuro-ophthalmological test
neuro-ophthalmology
neuro-otologist
neuro-otology
neuropathic ankle
neuropathic arthropathy (NA)
neuropathic joint
neuropathic tarsal-metatarsal joint
neuropathic ulcerations
neuropathology
neuropathophysiology
neuropathy (see also *peripheral neuropathy*)
  acquired demyelinative
  acute autonomic
  AIDS
  alcoholic
  amyloid
  anterograde fast component
  autonomic
  autosympathectomy secondary to diabetic
  axonal
  B vitamin deficiency
  carcinomatous
  chronic alcoholism
  compression
  compressive
  congenital hypomyelination
  cranial
  demyelinating
  Denny-Brown
  diabetic
  diabetic autonomic
  diabetic ischemic
  diabetic peripheral
  diabetic sensory
  diabetic thoracoabdominal

neuropathy *(cont.)*
  distal
  dying-back
  entrapment
  familial
  familial amyloid
  familial sensory radicular
  familial visceral
  femoral
  focal
  giant axonal
  handcuff
  heavy metal
  hereditary motor and sensory (HMSN)
  hereditary peripheral
  hereditary sensorimotor (HSMN)
  hereditary sensory (HSN)
  hereditary sensory radicular
  heredofamilial
  hypertrophic interstitial
  inflammatory demyelinating
  ischemic
  ischemic optic
  isoniazid-induced
  lead
  metachromatic leukodystrophy
  multifocal
  nonprogressive
  nutritional
  occupational
  onion bulb formation of
  optic
  paraproteinemic
  peripheral
  progressive
  progressive hypertrophic
  progressive hypertrophic interstitial
  pure sensory
  radicular
  relapsing
  retrograde fast component
  rheumatoid
  sensorimotor

neuropathy *(cont.)*
  sensorimotor peripheral
  sensory
  sensory-motor-autonomic
  Shy-Drager
  slow component
  steroid-sensitive
  subclinical
  symmetrical diffuse
  traumatic
  Wegener granulomatosis-associated peripheral
neuropeptide K
neuropharmacology
neurophysiologic
neurophysiology
neuroplasticity
neuroplasty
neuropsychiatric syndrome
neuropsychologic battery of tests
neuropsychological evaluation
neuropsychological impairment
neuropsychological testing
neuropsychology, clinical
neuropsychometric test
neuropsychopharmacology
neuroradiologist
neurorrhaphy
  epineurial
  perineurial
NeuroSectOR
neurosheet
neurosis, traumatic
neurosonographer
neurosonography
neurosonology
neurosurgeon
  endoscopic
  key-hole
  pediatric
  stereotaxic
neurosurgical evaluation
neurosurgical skull clamp, Gardner

neurosyphilis
  Argyll Robertson pupils of tabetic
  meningitic
  meningovascular
  parenchymatous
  paretic
  tabetic
neurotensin
neurotmesis
neurotologic surgery
neurotomy, Spiller-Frazier
neurotoxic drugs
neurotoxicity
Neuro-Trace
neurotransmission, adrenergic
neurotransmitter
neurotraumatic evolution of Charcot joint disease
neurotripsy
neurovascular bundle
neurovascular corn
neurovascular impairment
neurovascular island pedicle flaps
neurovascular status
neurovascular structures
neutral calcaneal stance position
neutral hip position
nevi
  intradermal pedal
  pedal intradermal
Neviaser acromioclavicular technique
Neviaser classification of frozen shoulder
Neviaser-Wilson-Gardner transfer
Neville tracheal and tracheobronchial prosthesis
Nevin-Jones subacute spongiform encephalopathy
new bone formation (incorporation)
New England Baptist (NEB) acetabular cup
New England Baptist arthroplasty
New Jersey LCS knee prosthesis
New Mind Set toe splint
new-onset limp
New Orleans endarterectomy stripper
New York diagnostic criteria for rheumatoid arthritis
New York Glass suction tubes
New York Orthopedic front-opening orthosis
New York University insert for orthosis
Newington brace
Newman classification of radial fracture
Newton ankle prosthesis
newtons of force (SI units)
Newvicon vacuum chamber pickup
Nextep knee brace
Nexus hip prosthesis
Nexus implant
N fiducial localization stereotactic system
NGF (nerve growth factor)
NHP (Nottingham Health Profile)
NHPT (Nine Hole Peg Test)
NIA (National Institute on Aging)
Nicholas five-in-one reconstruction technique
Nicholas ligament technique
Nicola forceps
Nicola pituitary rongeur
Nicola shoulder procedure
Nicola rasp
Nicola scissors
Nicolet Nerve Integrity Monitor-2 (NIM-2)
Nicoll bone replacement material
Nicoll cancellous bone graft
Nicoll plate
NICU (neurological intensive care unit)
nidus
  diameter of
  volume of
nidus obliteration
nidus of embolic material
nidus of osteoid osteoma
Niebauer-King technique

Niebauer metacarpophalangeal joint Silastic prosthesis
Niebauer prosthesis
Niemann-Pick disease
Niemann-Pick syndrome
Nievergelt syndrome
niger, Aspergillus
night nurse's paralysis
night terror (pavor nocturnus)
nightstick fracture
nigra, substantia
nigrostriatal pathway
nigrostriatal system
NIH (National Institutes of Health) Stroke Scale
NIM-2 (Nicolet Nerve Integrity Monitor-2)
NIMH (National Institute of Mental Health)
NINCDS (National Institute of Neurological and Communicative Disorders and Stroke)
Nine Hole Peg Test (NHPT)
ninety-ninety (90/90) intraosseous wiring
Ninhydrin print test
ninth cranial nerve (glossopharyngeal nerve)
nipper
  House-Dieter malleus
  nail
nipplelike osteophyte formation
Niro bone-cutting forceps
Niro wire-twister forceps
Niro wire-twisting forceps
Nirschl technique
Nissl degeneration
Nitinol flexible guide wire
nitrite, headaches from
nitrogen, compressed
N-K 330 BRQ exercise tables
NM (nocturnal myoclonus)
NMES (neuromuscular electrical stimulation)
NMR (nuclear magnetic resonance)
NMS unit
NMSS (National Multiple Sclerosis Society)
no man's land area of hand
Nocardia invasion of the nervous system
nocardiosis, cerebral
nociception
nociceptive afferent system
nociceptive tissues
nociceptor agents
nociceptor irritation
nociceptor sites
nociperception
NOCSAE (National Operating Committee on Standard for Athletic Equipment)
nocturnal epilepsy
nocturnal leg muscle spasticity
nocturnal paresthesia
nocturnus, pavor (night terror)
nodding, head
node, nodes
  Bouchard
  gouty
  Haygarth
  Heberden
  Meynet
  Osler
  Parrot
  Ranvier
  Schmorl
nodular fasciitis
nodule
  glial
  Lisch
  rheumatoid
  Schmorl
  synovial
  tendon
nodulus
Noiles fully constrained tricompartmental knee prosthesis
noise, startling

NoLok screw
Nomad electromyogram
nominal aphasia
nonambulant individual
nonambulatory patient
nonbeveled
non-coma, in head injury
noncommunicating hydrocephalus
nonconvulsive status epilepticus
nondominant hemisphere lesion
nondominant putaminal hemorrhage
nonelaborative speech
nonembolic cerebral infarction
nonepileptic myoclonic contraction
nonepileptiform activity (on EEG)
nonepileptiform sharp transient
nonfenestrated stem
nonfluent aphasic speech
nonfocal neurologic exam
nonfunctioning
nongerminomatous germ-cell tumor
nonglial tumor
nonhinged linked prosthesis
nonhomonymous field defect
nonicteric sclerae
noninvasive brain tests
noninvasive soft tissue evaluation
nonketotic hyperglycemia
nonneoplastic tumors
nonoperative orthopedic management: traction, weights, bedrest
nonossified tarsal navicular cartilage
nonossifying fibroma
nonosteoconductive bone-void filler
nonosteogenic fibroma
nonparalytic poliomyelitis
nonphasic forms of nystagmus
nonresponsive
nonresponsiveness
nonresponsive state
nonsensical words (neologisms)
nonspecific activating thalamic nuclei
nonsteroidal anti-inflammatory drug (NSAID)
nonsuppurative osteomyelitis
nontender
nonunion
  diaphyseal
  elephant foot
  fibrous
  horse-hoof
  oligotrophic
  torsion wedge
nonunion of fracture site
nonweightbearing (NWB) brace
nonweightbearing x-ray
NordiCare Back Therapy System (BTS)
NordiCare Enabler exerciser
NordiCare Strider exerciser
normal affect
normal, cosmetically and functionally
normalization of EEG
Normalize hip prosthesis
normal last shoes
normal mechanical tension (in hand)
normal mobility
normal motor potentials on EMG
normal-pressure hydrocephalus (NPH)
normal, upper limits of
North-South retractor
Northwick Park Index of Independence in ADLs
Norton ball reamer
Norwood tenodesis
nosebleed (epistaxis)
notch
  clavicular
  coracoid
  costal
  cotyloid
  intercondylar
  interpeduncular
  intervertebral
  Kernohan
  scapular
  sciatic
  sigmoid

notch *(cont.)*
  spinoglenoid
  tentorial
  trochlear
notchplasty blade
Nothnagel syndrome
notochord
notochordal remnants
Nottingham Extended ADL Index (domestic, kitchen, leisure, mobility)
Nottingham Health Profile (NHP) for quality of life
Nottingham Ten-Point ADL Scale
noxious stimulus
Noyes flexion rotation drawer test
Noyes knee rating scale
NPH (normal pressure hydrocephalus)
NPo-FH cephalometric measurement
NREM (nonrapid eye movement) sleep
NSAID (nonsteroidal anti-inflammatory drug)
NSE (neuron-specific enolase) antibody
NTID (National Technical Institute for the Deaf)
nubbin
nuchal ligament
nuchal rigidity
nuchal stiffness
nuchocephalic reflex
nuclear arrangement, string of pearls
nuclear bone imaging scan
nuclear magnetic resonance (NMR)
nuclear paralysis
nuclear signal
nuclear spin quantum number
nuclear weakness
nucleoli, eosinophilic
nucleon
Nucleotome aspiration probe
Nucleotome Endoflex instrument
Nucleotome Flex II flexible cutting probe
Nucleotome system for lumbar diskectomy
nucleotomy, laser
nucleus (pl. nuclei)
  abducens (or abducent)
  accessory oculomotor
  ambiguous
  amygdaloid
  arcuate
  autonomic oculomotor
  Cajal interstitial
  caudate
  centromedian
  cochlear, dorsal
  contralateral dentate
  Darkshevitch (Darkschewitsch)
  Deiter (in brain)
  dentate
  dorsal cochlear
  dorsal medial (of the thalamus)
  Edinger-Westphal
  facial
  fastigial
  geniculate
  habenular
  head of caudate
  inferior olivary
  interstitial (of Cajal)
  intralaminar thalamic
  lateral geniculate
  lateral mamillary (of Rose)
  lenticular
  lentiform
  median (of Perlia)
  motor
  motor (in the lower brain stem)
  nonspecific activating (of the thalamus)
  nonspecific thalamic
  oculomotor-trochlear
  olivary
  ossific
  Perlia medial
  PF (parafascicular)
  pigmentary
  pontine
  pontis

nucleus *(cont.)*
- prerubral field
- pretectal
- prominent
- raphe
- red
- Schwalbe (of cerebellum)
- septal
- specific thalamic
- subthalamic (in brain)
- subthalamic (of Luys)
- suprachiasmatic
- tractus solitarius
- ventral
- ventral cochlear
- ventral intermedius (VIM)
- vestibular
- vestibulocochlear
- Westphal-Edinger

nucleus basalis of Meynert
nucleus centromedianus
nucleus cuneatus
nucleus dentatus
nucleus gracilis
nucleus lateralis of Le Gros Clark
nucleus locus ceruleus
nucleus of Cajal
nucleus of cerebellum, Deiter
nucleus of Darkschewitsch
nucleus of Gudden
nucleus of tractus solitarius
nucleus of trigeminal nerve
nucleus of vagus, dorsal
nucleus pulposus, herniated (HNP)
nucleus subthalamic
nucleus ventralis intermedius
nucleus ventralis oralis
nudge control for prosthesis
Nu Gauze dressing
Nu Gauze sterile gauze bandage
NuKO knee orthosis
null cell adenoma
null position nystagmus
numb
numbness
- circumoral
- transient

Nurick classification of spondylosis
Nurolon suture
nurse, circulating
nut
- conical tapered
- hex
- jam
- Kirschner traction bow
- lock
- ring
- traction bow
- umbrella
- VDS (ventral derotating spinal) hex

nutans, spasmus
nutation
Nu-Tip disposable scissor tip with reusable handle and shaft
nutrient flap
NWB (nonweightbearing)
Nylatex nylon-latex wrap
Nylen-Bárány test
Nylok self-locking nail
nylon threads as drains
nystagmogram
nystagmoid beating
nystagmoid jerk
nystagmoid movement
nystagmoid quaver
nystagmologist
nystagmus
- abduction
- acquired
- alternating
- apogeotropic
- asymmetric
- Bruns
- caloric
- central
- central vestibular
- centrally caused
- cerebellar

nystagmus *(cont.)*
- circular
- coarse
- congenital
- congenital idiopathic
- congenital latent
- conjugate
- contralateral monocular
- convergence-evoked
- convergence-retraction
- diagonal
- dissociated (ataxic)
- downbeat
- downbeating
- drug-induced
- dysjunctive
- elliptical
- end-gaze jerk
- end point (physiologic)
- fast component of
- fine rapid
- fixation
- gaze-evoked
- gaze-paretic
- irregular
- jelly
- jerk (rhythmic)
- lateral gaze
- left-bearing
- lid
- manifest latent
- miners'
- muscle-paretic
- nonphasic forms of
- null position
- oblique
- ocular
- optokinetic (OKN)

nystagmus *(cont.)*
- palatal
- party
- pendular (nonphasic) forms of
- periodic
- periodic alternating
- phasic
- physiologic (end point)
- physiologic (railway)
- positional
- positional (of central origin)
- positional (of peripheral origin)
- postrotational
- railway (physiological)
- rapid
- rebound
- retraction-convergence
- retractory
- reversed optokinetic
- rhythmic (jerk)
- right-bearing
- rotary
- rotatory
- see-saw
- sensory-deprivation
- torsional
- toxic
- transient
- true
- unidirectional
- upbeat
- upbeating
- vertical
- vestibular
- vestibular end-organ
- voluntary

NYU (New York University) orthosis

O, o

OA (osteoarthritis)
O&M (orientation and mobility)
oasthouse urine disease
oath hand
OAV (oculoauriculovertebral) dysplasia
OAWO (opening abductory wedge osteotomy)
OBD (organic brain disease)
Ober-Barr procedure for brachioradialis transfer
Ober tendon technique
Ober test
Oberhill laminectomy retractor
object agnosia
objective limited movement
objective symptoms of impairment
objective vertigo
oblique displacement osteotomy
oblique metaphyseal osteotomy
oblique radiograms
oblique retinacular ligament
oblique slide osteotomy
oblique wiring technique
obliquity, pelvic
obliteration
  nidus
  sulcal
  surgical
O'Brien classification of radial fracture
O'Brien rib hook
obscuration of vision
obstetrician's hand
obstruction of flow of cerebrospinal fluid
obstructive lesion of the CSF pathways
OBT stereotactic frame
obtundation
obtunded
obturator
  conical
  core biopsy
  Keene
obturator internus muscle
obturator neurectomy
obturator sign
Obwegeser sagittal mandibular osteotomy technique
occipital (EEG lead)
  left (LO)
  right (RO)
occipital-atlas-axis ligaments
occipital-axis joint
occipital condyle
occipital gyrus
occipital lesion
occipital lobe contusion
occipital lobe tumor
occipital negative sharp transient on EEG
occipital neuralgia
occipital neuroblastoma
occipital-temporal sulcus
occipital tip
occipitoatlantoaxial fusion
occipitocervical articulation
occipitocervical level
occipitofrontalis muscle
occipitomastoid suture
occipitoparietal suture
occipitosphenoid suture

occipitotemporal gyrus
occipitotemporal, medial
occipitotemporal sulcus
occipitotemporopontine tract
occiput
occlusal segment
occlusion
  aqueductal
  arterial
  balloon
  basilar
  bilateral carotid artery
  carotid artery
  carotid cavernous fistula
  deep venous
  infrapopliteal artery
  intracranial vascular
  subclavian artery
  unilateral carotid artery
  vascular
  vertebral artery
  vertebrobasilar
occlusion of artery
occlusive cerebrovascular insult
occult fracture
occult hydrocephalus
occult seizure
occult spinal dysraphism
occult subluxation
occulta, spina bifida (SBO)
occultum, cranium bifidum
occupational therapist, registered (OTR)
occupational therapy (OT)
ochronosis
O'Connor finger dexterity test
OctreoScan (indium-111 pentetreotide)
ocular bobbing
ocular flutter
ocular mononeuropathy
ocular motility
ocular motor nucleus
ocular movements, roving
ocular muscle paresis
ocular myasthenia
ocular myoclonus
ocular myopathy
ocular nystagmus
ocular vertigo
oculoauriculovertebral (OAV)
oculocephalic reflex
oculocephalic response
oculocerebrorenal syndrome
oculogyric crisis
oculomotor apparatus
oculomotor apraxia
oculomotor disturbance
oculomotor dysfunction
oculomotor nerve (third cranial nerve)
oculomotor nucleus
oculomotor paresis
oculomotor sign
oculomotor-trochlear nucleus
oculopharyngeal dystrophy
oculopharyngeal muscular dystrophy
oculoplethysmography (OPG)
oculosubcutaneous syndrome of Yuge
oculovestibular reflex
OD (osteochondritis dissecans)
Oden classification of peroneal tendon subluxation
Odland ankle prostheses
ODN (ophthalmodynamometry)
odontoid (dens) process
  fractured
  pannus deformity of
O'Donoghue facetectomy
O'Donoghue splint
O'Donoghue's Unhappy Triad (OUT)
O'Rahilly classification of limb deficiency
ODQ (opponens digiti quinti) muscle
OEC knee immobilizer
OEC popliteal pad
OEC wrist/forearm support
OEIS (omphalocele, cloacal exstrophy, imperforate anus, spinal deformity) complex

O electrode (occipital)
  (O_1, O_2, O_z)
Office of Vocational Rehabilitation
  (OVR)
offset, head-stem
Ogden classification of epiphyseal
  fracture
Ogden plate
Ogston line
Oh hip prosthesis
ohmmeter
ohms impedance
ointment
  Pickles
  Whitfield
OIRDA (occipital dominant intermittent rhythmic delta activity)
Oklahoma ankle joint orthosis
OKN (optokinetic nystagmus) testing
Oldberg brain retractor
Oldberg dissector
Oldberg intervertebral disk rongeur
Oldberg pituitary forceps
Oldberg pituitary rongeur
Olds pin
olecranon bursitis
olecranon fossa
olecranon tip fracture
Olerud internal fixator
Olerud PSF fixation system
Olerud PSF rod
Olerud PSF screw
olfaction, a function of the first cranial
  nerve
olfactory aura
olfactory bulb
olfactory groove, meningioma of the
olfactory hallucination
olfactory nerve (first cranial nerve)
olfactory psychomotor seizures
olfactory seizure
olfactory symptoms
oligoclonal IgG bands in CSF
oligodendroglial cell
oligodendroglioma, anaplastic
oligodendroglioma-astrocytoma
oligodendroglioma tumor
oligodendroma
olisthesis
olisthetic vertebra, wedging of
olisthy
olivary hypertrophy
olivary nucleus
olive
  inferior
  posterior (in brain)
  superior (in brain)
olive ring
olive wire
Olivecrona aneurysm clips
Olivecrona brain spatula
Olivecrona clip-applying and removing
  forceps
Olivecrona dural dissector
Olivecrona dural scissors
Olivecrona-Gigli saw
Olivecrona rasp
Olivecrona rongeur
Olivecrona saw
Olivecrona scissors
Olivecrona-Toennis clip-applying forceps
Olivecrona trigeminal knife
Olivecrona trigeminal scissors
Olivecrona wire saw
Olivier-Bertrand-Talairach stereotactic
  head frame
olivopontocerebellar atrophy
olivopontocerebellar degeneration
Ollier approach to hips, modified
Ollier disease
Ollier rake retractor
Ollier-Thiersch skin graft
Olympics, National Special
omagra
omalgia
omarthritis
Ombredanne mallet

OMC (short orientation-memory-concentration) test
Omega compression hip screw system
Omer-Capen technique
omitis
Ommaya ventriculoperitoneal shunt
Ommaya ventriculostomy reservoir
Omni-Flexor physical therapy device
Omni-Flexor wrist exerciser
Omni Prep electrolyte gel for EEG
Omnifit HA hip stem prosthesis
Omnifit knee prosthesis
omoclavicular
omodynia
omohyoid
omoplata
omosternum
on-off effect of L-dopa in parkinsonism
on-off phenomenon
oncocytoma
Ondine curse
one and a half syndrome
one-handed kitchen utensils
ONI (old nerve injury)
onion bulb appearance of myelin sheaths
onion bulb changes on biopsy
onion bulb formation of neuropathy
onion peel appearance on x-ray
onion skin distribution of sensation
onlay cancellous iliac graft
onset
  latency of
  new (of pain)
  short latency to sleep
  sleep
onset of sleep
Ontario Cohort Study of Running-Related Injuries
onychectomy
onycho-osteodysplasia
onychocryptosis (ingrown nail)
onychomycosis
onychotomy
Op-Site dressing
open fracture
open-mouth view on x-ray exam
open reduction and internal fixation (ORIF)
open tendon repair
opening osteotomy
opening pressure on lumbar puncture (spinal tap)
opening wedge manipulation and reapplication of plaster
opera glass hand
operations (also *approach*; *procedure*; *repair*; *technique*)
  Abbott knee approach
  Abbott-Fischer-Lucas hip arthrodesis
  Abbott-Gill osteotomy
  Abbott-Lucas shoulder
  Abbott-Lucas shoulder approach
  abduction osteotomy
  ablation
  ablative arthroplasty
  ablative surgery
  abrasion arthroplasty
  ACF (anterior cervical fusion)
  Achilles tendon lengthening
  ACL (anterior cruciate ligament) repair
  acromioclavicular arthroplasty
  Adams arthrodesis
  Adams hip
  adduction osteotomy
  adductor tenotomy
  Adkins spinal fusion
  adrenal medulla transplantation
  Akin phalangeal osteotomy
  Albee spinal fusion
  Albee-Delbert
  Albert procedure
  Allen open reduction of calcaneal fracture
  Allman modification of Evans ankle reconstruction
  AMBI fixation

operations *(cont.)*
Amspacher-Messenbaugh technique
Amstutz resurfacing
Amstutz total hip replacement
Amstutz-Wilson osteotomy
AMTR (anteromedial temporal lobe resection)
amygdalohippocampectomy
Anderson-Fowler procedure
Anderson-Hutchins technique
Andrews iliotibial band reconstruction
aneurysmal clipping
ankle-level arteriotomy
anterior capsular shift
anterior capsulolabral reconstruction (ACLR)
anterior corpectomy
anterior lobectomy
anterior retropharyngeal approach
anterior transcallosal approach
AO/ASIF compression technique
AO group shoulder arthrodesis
APR cement fixation
Arafiles elbow arthrodesis
Arana-Iniquez intracranial cyst removal
Armistead ulnar lengthening
arthrodesis
arthroplasty
arthroscopic acromioplasty
arthroscopic debridement
arthroscopic resection
arthroscopic screw fixation
arthroscopy
arthrotomy
articular reconstruction
Ashworth hand arthroplasty
ASIF screw fixation technique
Aston cartilage reduction
Atasoy V-Y technique
atlanto-occipital fusion
Aufranc cup arthroplasty
Austin Moore arthroplasty

operations *(cont.)*
Austin Moore hemiarthroplasty
Auto-Implant procedure
autoadrenal transplantation for Parkinson disease
autogenous bone graft
autograft of adrenal medulla tissue
automated percutaneous lumbar diskectomy (APLD)
Averill total hip replacement
Avila technique
avulsion technique
Axer-Clark procedure
Axer varus derotational osteotomy
B.H. Moore procedure
Baciu-Filibiu dowel ankle arthrodesis
Badgley iliac wing resection
Bailey-Badgley anterior cervical approach
Bailey-Badgley cervical spine fusion
Bailey-Dubow osteotomy
Baker patellar advancement
Baker translocation
Baker-Hill osteotomy
Balacescu-Golden technique
balloon embolization
balloon occlusion
Bandi technique
Bankart shoulder repair
Bankart-Putti-Platt
Banks-Laufman technique
Barnhart repair
Barr open reduction and internal fixation
Barr tendon transfer
Barr tibial fracture fixation
Barr-Record arthrodesis
Barrasso-Wile-Gage arthrodesis
Barsky technique
Bartlett nail fold
basal osteotomy
base wedge osteotomy

operations *(cont.)*
- basilar crescentic osteotomy
- Batch-Spittler-McFaddin technique
- Batchelor-Brown arthrodesis
- Bateman hemiarthroplasty
- Bateman modification of Mayer transfer
- Bateman shoulder
- Bauer-Tondra-Trusler
- Baumgard-Schwartz tennis elbow technique
- Beall-Webel-Bailey technique
- Bechtol arthroplasty
- Beckenbaugh technique
- Becker tendon repair
- Becton technique
- Bell-Tawse open reduction technique
- Bellemore-Barrett-Middleton-Scougall-Whiteway technique
- Bennett posterior shoulder approach
- Bennett quadriceps plastic
- Berman-Gartland metatarsal osteotomy
- Bickel-Moe procedure
- bimalleolar approach to ankle arthrodesis
- biocompartmental replacement of knee
- bioelectrical repair of delayed union or nonunion
- Bircher-Weber technique
- Black-Bröstrom staple technique
- Blair ankle fusion
- Blair tibiotalar arthrodesis
- Blair-Morris-Dunn-Hand ankle arthrodesis
- Bleck recession technique
- Bloom-Raney modification
- Blount displacement osteotomy
- Blount tracing technique
- Blundell-Jones technique
- Bohlman cervical fusion technique
- bone graft repair

operations *(cont.)*
- bone-blocking
- Bonfiglio modification
- Bora technique
- Borggreve limb rotation
- Bose nail fold excision
- Bosworth bone peg insertion
- Bosworth shelf
- Bosworth spinal fusion
- Bowers radial arthroplasty
- Boyd amputation
- Boyd approach
- Boyd-Anderson biceps tendon repair
- Boyd-Anderson technique
- Boyd-Bosworth procedure
- Boyd-McLeod tennis elbow technique
- Boyd-Sisk posterior capsulorrhaphy
- Boyes brachioradialis transfer technique
- Brackett-Osgood knee approach
- Brackett-Osgood-Putti-Abbott
- Brady-Jewett technique
- Bragg-peak radiosurgery
- Brahms foot
- brain biopsy
- Brain arthroplasty
- Brand tendon transfer technique
- Brannon-Wickstrom technique
- Brantigan-Voshell procedure
- Braun procedure
- Brett-Campbell tibial osteotomy
- bridle posterior tibial tendon transfer
- Bristow shoulder reconstruction
- Bristow-Helfet procedure
- Bristow-May procedure
- Brittain arthrodesis
- Brockman foot
- Brooker-Jones tendon transfer
- Brooks cervical fusion
- Brooks-Gallie cervical
- Brooks-Jenkins atlantoaxial fusion
- Brooks-Jenkins cervical

operations *(cont.)*
- Brooks-Seddon transfer technique
- Broomhead approach
- Brostrom procedure
- Brostrom-Gould lateral ankle instability
- Brown knee approach
- Brown knee joint reconstruction
- Bruser knee approach
- Bryan arthroplasty
- Bryan-Morrey elbow approach
- Bryan-Morrey technique
- Buck-Gramcko technique
- Bugg-Boyd technique
- Buncke technique
- bunionectomy, tricorrectional
- bunionette excision
- Bunnell posterior tibial tendon transfer
- Bunnell tendon repair
- Burgess technique
- Burkhalter transfer technique
- Burow skin flap technique
- Butler fifth toe
- Calandriello hip reduction
- Calandruccio fixation
- calcaneal resection
- calcanectomy
- calcaneocuboid arthrodesis
- calcaneonavicular bar resection
- calcaneotibial fusion
- Caldwell-Coleman flatfoot
- Caldwell-Durham tendon
- Callahan approach
- Callahan fusion
- Camitz
- Campbell-Akbarnia arthrodesis
- Campbell ankle procedure
- Campbell elbow approach
- Campbell-Goldthwait procedure
- Campbell posterior bone block
- Campbell posterior shoulder approach
- Canale osteotomy
- Capello total hip replacement

operations *(cont.)*
- capitellocondylar arthroplasty
- capsular release
- capsular-shift reconstruction
- capsulotomy
- Carceau-Brahms ankle arthrodesis
- Carnesale hip approach
- carotid artery ligation
- carotid bifurcation endarterectomy
- carotid ligation
- Carrell fibular substitution
- Caspari repair
- Castle procedure
- Cave hip approach
- Cave knee approach
- Cave-Rowe shoulder dislocation
- central commissurotomy
- centralization of radius
- centralization procedure
- cervical sympathectomy
- cervico-occipital fusion
- Chandler arthrodesis
- Chandler hip fusion
- Chapchal knee arthrodesis
- Charcot hip arthrodesis
- charged-particle radiosurgery
- Charnley ankle arthrodesis
- Charnley compression-type knee fusion
- Charnley hip replacement
- Charnley-Houston arthrodesis
- Chaves-Rapp muscle transfer
- cheilectomy
- cheilotomy
- chemical rhizotomy
- chemonucleolysis
- chevron osteotomy
- Chiari innominate osteotomy
- Childress ankle fixation technique
- Cho cruciate ligament reconstruction
- Chrisman-Snook reconstruction of ankle ligaments
- Chuinard autogenous bone graft
- Chuinard-Petersen ankle arthrodesis

operations *(cont.)*
- cingulotomy
- Clancy-Andrews reconstruction
- Clancy ligament technique
- Clark transfer technique
- Clayton-Fowler technique
- Clayton resection arthroplasty
- Cleveland-Bosworth-Thompson
- clip ligation of aneurysm
- clipping of aneurysm
- closed base wedge osteotomy (CBWO)
- closed manipulative
- closing wedge osteotomy
- Cloward back fusion
- Cloward cervical arthrodesis
- Cloward cervical disk approach
- clubfoot release
- coating of aneurysm
- Cobb scoliosis measuring technique
- coccygeal
- Cocklin toe
- Codivilla tendon lengthening
- Codman saber-cut shoulder approach
- Coleman flatfoot technique
- Cole tendon fixation
- Collis broken femoral stem technique
- Colonna-Ralston ankle approach
- Colonna shelf
- Colonna trochanteric arthroplasty
- Coltart fracture technique
- Compere-Thompson arthrodesis
- compression screw arthrodesis
- computer-assisted microsurgery
- condylectomy
- cone arthrodesis
- Contour DF-80 total hip
- contoured loop fixation
- Coonrad total elbow arthroplasty
- Coonse-Adam knee approach
- Copeland-Howard shoulder
- cordotomy

operations *(cont.)*
- corrective lengthening osteotomy
- corrective osteotomy
- corticotomy
- costotransversectomy technique
- Cotrel-Dubousset derotation
- Couch-Derosa-Throop transfer
- countersinking osteotomy
- Coventry vagus osteotomy
- Cozen-Brockway technique
- Cracchiolo forefoot arthroplasty
- Cracchiolo-Sculco implant
- craniofacial reconstruction
- cranioplasty
- craniotomy
- Crawford-Adams cup arthroplasty
- Crego hip reduction
- Crego tendon transfer technique
- crescentic osteotomy
- cruciate ligament reconstruction
- cryohypophysectomy
- CSR (complete subtalar release)
- CT-assisted stereotactic craniotomy
- CT-guided stereotactic procedure
- Cubbins arthroplasty
- Cubbins shoulder approach
- cup on cup arthroplasty of the hip
- Curtin plantar fibromatosis excision
- Curtis-Fisher knee technique
- Curtis PIP joint capsulotomy
- D'Aubigné femoral reconstruction
- Darrach
- Darrach-McLaughlin technique
- Das Gupta procedure
- Davey-Rorabeck-Fowler decompression technique
- Davis drainage technique
- De Andrade-MacNab occipito-cervical arthrodesis
- Debeyre-Patte-Elmelik rotator cuff
- decompression fasciotomy
- decompression technique
- decompressive craniectomy
- decompressive laminectomy

operations *(cont.)*
- degloving procedure
- deltoid-splitting shoulder approach
- Dennyson-Fulford subtalar arthrodesis
- Dewar-Barrington arthroplasty
- Dewar cervical procedure
- Dewar-Harris shoulder technique
- Deyerle femoral fracture technique
- Diamond-Gould syndactyly
- diaphyseal osteotomy
- diaphysectomy
- Dias-Giegerich fracture technique
- Dickinson-Coutts-Woodward-Handler osteotomy
- Dickson-Diveley foot
- Dickson transplant technique
- Dimon-Hughston fracture fixation
- diskectomy (or discectomy)
- distal metatarsal osteotomy
- distraction-compression bone graft arthrodesis
- distraction lengthening
- division of corpus callosum
- Doll trochanteric reattachment
- Domen laminoplasty
- dome osteotomy
- Dorrance procedure
- dorsal pedal bypass
- dowel arthrodesis
- dowel graft technique
- doweling spondylolisthesis
- Dowling intracranial cyst removal
- DREZ (dorsal root entry zone) modification of Eriksson technique
- Drummond wire technique
- Dunn-Brittain foot stabilization
- Dunn-Hess trochanteric osteotomy
- Dunn hip
- Durham flatfoot
- duToit-Roux arthroplasty
- duToit-Roux staple capsulorrhaphy
- DuVries arthroplasty

operations *(cont.)*
- DuVries hammer toe repair
- DuVries modified McBride hallux valgus
- DuVries phalangeal condylectomy
- DuVries reconstruction technique
- DuVries technique for overlapping toe
- Dwyer clawfoot
- Eaton arthroplasty
- Eaton-Littler technique
- Eaton-Malerich fracture-dislocation
- Eberle contracture release
- Ecker-Lotke-Glazer tendon reconstruction
- ECT (European compression technique) fixation
- Eden-Hybbinette arthroplasty
- Eden-Lange procedure
- Edward procedure
- Eftekhar broken femoral stem technique
- Eggers tendon transfer technique
- Elizabethtown osteotomy
- Ellis Jones peroneal tendon
- Ellison lateral knee reconstruction
- Elmslie peroneal tendon procedure
- Elmslie-Cholmeley foot
- Elmslie-Trillat patellar
- Elmslie-Trillat transplant
- Emmon osteotomy
- en bloc resection
- endarterectomy
- Ender rod fixation of fracture
- endoscopic neurosurgery
- Engh total hip replacement
- Enneking knee arthrodesis
- epineural repair
- epiphysiodesis
- Eppright dial osteotomy
- Erickson-Leider-Brown technique
- Eriksson cruciate ligament reconstruction
- Essex-Lopresti axial fixation

operations *(cont.)*
- Essex-Lopresti fixation of calcaneal fracture
- Essex-Lopresti open reduction
- evacuation of blood clot
- Evans ankle joint instability
- Evans ankle reconstruction technique
- Evans calcaneal lengthening
- Evans lateral ankle reconstruction
- Evans osteotomy
- Evans tenodesis
- eversion endarterectomy
- Ewald total elbow replacement
- Ewald-Walker knee arthroplasty
- excision arthroplasty
- extended tibial in situ bypass
- extensor brevis arthroplasty
- extensor tenotomy
- Eyler flexorplasty
- facet fusion
- facetectomy
- Fahey approach
- Fahey-O'Brien
- failed joint replacement
- Fairbanks technique with Sever modification
- Farmer
- fascial release
- fascicular repair
- fasciectomy
- femorodistal bypass
- Ferciot-Thomson excision
- Ferguson hip reduction
- Ferguson-Thompson-King two-stage osteotomy
- Ferkel torticollis
- Fernandez osteotomy
- fetal substantia nigra transplantation
- fibular osteotomy
- Ficat procedure
- first rib resection
- first-toe Jones repair
- Fish cuneiform osteotomy

operations *(cont.)*
- five-in-one knee ligament repair
- five-in-one knee reconstruction
- flexor tendon transfer
- flexor tenotomy
- Flynn procedure
- forage
- foraminotomy
- Forbes modification of Phemister graft
- forefoot arthroplasty
- four-bar external fixation
- Fowler tendon transfer
- Fowles dislocation
- Fox-Blazina knee procedure
- fracture repair
- free body fusion technique
- French supracondylar fracture
- Fried-Green foot
- Fried-Hendel tendon
- Froimson-Oh arm procedure
- frontal craniotomy
- frontotemporal craniotomy
- Frost foot procedure
- Frost posterior tibialis tendon lengthening
- Furnas-Haq-Somers technique
- fusion
- Gaenslen technique
- Galeazzi patellar
- Gallie ankle arthrodesis
- Gallie cervical fusion
- Gallie subtalar fusion
- Gallis foot
- Galveston sacral fixation
- gangliolysis
- Ganley modification of Keller arthroplasty
- Gant osteotomy
- Garceau-Brahms arthrodesis
- Gardner procedure
- Gartland procedure
- Gatellier-Chastang ankle approach
- Gelman foot procedure

operations *(cont.)*
Gerard resurfacing procedure
Getty decompression technique
Ghormley arthrodesis
Ghormley shelf procedure
Giannestras metatarsal oblique osteotomy
Giannestras step-down modified osteotomy
Gibson approach
Gibson-Piggott osteotomy
Gigli saw osteotomy
Gilbert-Tamai-Weiland technique
Gillies-Millard cocked-hat technique
Gill-Manning-White spondylolisthesis
Gill modification of Campbell ankle procedure
Gill shelf procedure
Gill-Stein arthrodesis
Girdlestone pseudarthrosis
Girdlestone-Taylor procedure
Girdlestone tendon transfer
Glynn-Neibauer technique
Goldner-Clippinger technique
Goldstein spinal fusion
Goldthwait-Hauser procedure
Gordon-Brostrom technique
Gordon-Taylor technique
Gouffon fixation
Graber-Devernay hip
Green-Banks technique
Greenfield osteotomy
Greulich-Pyle technique
Grice-Green extra-articular subtalar arthrodesis
Gristina-Webb shoulder arthroplasty
Gritti-Stokes distal thigh procedure
Grosse-Kempf tibial technique
grouped fascicular repair
Groves-Goldner technique
Gruca lower leg procedure
Guleke-Stookey approach
Guller resection

operations *(cont.)*
Gustilo-Kyle cementless total hip arthroplasty
guttering
Guttmann subtalar arthrodesis
Guyon tunnel release
Haddad-Riordan arthrodesis
Hall facet fusion
hallux interphalanageal joint arthrodesis
hammer toe correction with interphalangeal fusion
Hammon foot procedure
hamstring lengthening
hamstring release
hanging toe procedure
Hardinge femoral approach
Hardinge vastus lateralis procedure
Hark foot procedure
Harmon cervical approach
Harmon shoulder approach
Harmon transfer technique
Harrington rod fixation
Harrington total hip arthroplasty
Harris-Beath arthrodesis
Harris-Smith cervical fusion
Hass procedure
Hassmann-Brunn-Neer elbow technique
Hastings bipolar hemiarthroplasty
Hauser bunionectomy
Hauser heel cord procedure
Hauser patellar technique
Hay-Groves shelf procedure
heel cord advancement
hemiarthroplasty
hemicraniectomy
hemicraniotomy
hemilaminectomy
hemiphalangectomy
Henderson approach
Henderson arthrodesis
Henry radial approach
Henry-Geist spinal fusion

operations *(cont.)*
Herbert screw fixation
Hermodsson internal rotation
Herndon-Heyman foot
Hey-Groves-Kirk technique
Heyman-Herndon clubfoot
Heyman-Herndon-Strong technique
Hibbs-Jones spinal fusion
Hill-Nahai-Vasconez-Mathes technique
hindfoot arthrodesis
hip pinning
Hirschhorn compression approach
His-Haas procedure
Hitchcock arm procedure
Hitchcock tendon technique
Hoffer ankle procedure
Hoffmann-Clayton procedure
Hoffmann metatarsal procedure
Hohmann osteotomy
Hoke Achilles tendon lengthening
Hoke arthrodesis
Hoke tibial palsy procedure
holistic approach
hook pin fixation
Hoppenfeld-Deboer technique
Horwitz-Adams ankle fusion
Houghton-Akroyd technique
Hovnanian transfer technique
Howard technique
Howorth approach
Howse total hip replacement
Hughston-Degenhardt reconstruction
Hughston-Hauser procedure
Hughston-Jacobson technique
Hungerford-Krackow-Kenna knee arthroplasty
hunterian ligation of aneurysm
Huntington tibial technique
I-beam hemiarthroplasty
I-beam hip
ICLH double cup arthroplasty
Ilizarov ankle arthrodesis
Ilizarov corticotomy

operations *(cont.)*
Ilizarov leg lengthening
Ilizarov limb lengthening
implant arthroplasty
Inclan modification of Campbell ankle procedure
Inclan-Ober procedure
infratemporal approach
infratentorial approach
Inglis-Cooper technique
Inglis-Ranawat-Straub technique
Ingram bony bridge resection
Insall-Burstein-Freeman knee arthroplasty
inside-out Bankart shoulder instability
in situ vein bypass to ankle
interbody arthrodesis
interbody fusion
interhemispheric approach
intermetatarsal angle-reducing
internal fixation compression arthrodesis of the ankle
interphalangeal fusion
interpositional arthroplasty of foot
interpositional elbow arthroplasty
interstitial radiosurgery
intertransverse process arthrodesis
intra-articular knee fusion
intracranial arterial bypass
intraforaminal approach
ipsilateral approach
Irvine ankle arthroplasty
Isseis-Aussies scoliosis
Jaffe procedure
Janecki-Nelson shoulder
Jansey technique
Japas osteotomy
Jeffery technique
John Barnes myofascial release
John C. Wilson arthrodesis
Johnson hemiphalangectomy
Johnson pelvic fracture technique
Johnson-Spiegl hallux varus correction

operations *(cont.)*
- joint fluid aspiration
- Jones cock-up toe
- Jones-Brackett technique
- Jones-Ellison ACL reconstruction
- J.R. Moore procedure
- Juvara foot
- Kapel elbow dislocation technique
- Kaplan technique
- Karakousis-Vezeridis procedure
- Kashiwagi technique
- Kates forefoot arthroplasty
- Kates-Kessel-Kay technique
- Kaufer tendon technique
- Kelikian-Clayton-Loseff technique
- Kelikian-McFarland procedure
- Kelikian-Riashi-Gleason technique
- Keller arthroplasty
- Keller bunionectomy
- Keller foot
- Keller hallux valgus
- Keller resection arthroplasty
- Keller-Brandes procedure
- Kellogg-Speed fusion technique
- Kendrick-Sharma-Hassler-Herndon
- Kennedy ligament technique
- Kessel-Bonney extension osteotomy
- Kessler posterior tibial tendon transfer
- Key intra-articular knee arthrodesis
- keyhole tenodesis
- Kickaldy-Willis arthrodesis
- Kidner foot procedure
- King-Richards dislocation technique
- King-Steelquist technique
- Kirk distal thigh
- Kirschner wire fixation (K wire)
- Klein approach
- Kleinert repair
- Klisic-Jankovic technique
- Knobby-Clark procedure
- Kocher lateral J approach
- Kocher-McFarland hip arthroplasty
- Koenig arthroplasty

operations *(cont.)*
- Koenig-Schaefer approach
- Kortzeborn hand
- Koutsogiannis-Fowler-Anderson osteotomy
- Kramer-Craig-Noel osteotomy
- Krempen-Silver-Sotelo nonunion
- Kronner external fixation
- Krukenberg hand
- Kumar-Cowell-Ramsey technique
- Kumar spica cast technique
- Lamb muscle transfer
- Lambrinudi drop foot
- laminectomy
- laminoplasty
- laminotomy
- Lange Achilles tendon reconstruction
- Lange hip reduction
- Lange tendon lengthening and repair
- Lapidus hammertoe technique
- Larmon forefoot procedure
- Larson ligament reconstruction
- laser microsurgery
- lateral approach
- lateral cerebellopontine angle approach
- lateral extracavitary approach
- Leach-Igou step-cut medial osteotomy
- Leeds spine
- leg compartment release
- Lehman procedure
- Lelièvre (to block end-range pronation)
- Lenart-Kullman technique
- L'Episcopo-Zachary technique
- Lewis-Chekofsky resection
- Lichtman technique
- Liebolt radioulnar technique
- ligament reconstruction
- ligamentous release
- limb lengthening
- limb salvage

operations *(cont.)*
- limb sparing
- LINAC (linear accelerator) radiosurgery
- Lindeman procedure
- Lindgren oblique osteotomy
- Lindholm open surgical tendon repair
- Lipscomb modified McKeever arthrodesis
- Littler-Cooley technique
- Lloyd-Roberts fracture technique
- Localio procedure
- Loose procedure
- Lorenz hip reduction
- Losee modification of MacIntosh
- Lowman shelf procedure
- L-shaped capsulotomy
- Lucas-Murray knee arthrodesis
- Luck hand procedure
- Ludloff approach
- Lunceford total hip replacement
- Luque rod fixation
- MacAusland procedure
- MacCarthy procedure
- MacEwen-Shands osteotomy
- MacIntosh over-the-top repair
- MacIntosh tenodesis
- MacNab shoulder repair
- Magilligan measuring technique
- Magnuson-Stack shoulder arthrotomy
- Ma-Griffith ruptured Achilles tendon repair
- Ma-Griffith tendon anastomosis
- Majestro-Ruda-Frost tendon
- Malawer excision technique
- Mallory-Head total hip revision
- Mankin technique
- Manktelow transfer procedure
- Mann-Coughlin arthrodesis
- Mann-DuVries arthroplasty
- Mann modified McKeever arthrodesis
- Mann resection arthroplasty
- Mann-Thompson-Coughlin arthrodesis

operations *(cont.)*
- Manske technique
- Maquet technique
- Marcus-Balourdas-Heiple ankle fusion
- Marks-Bayne thumb duplication
- Marmor replacement
- Marshall ligament repair
- Martin osteotomy
- Matchett-Brown hip arthroplasty
- Matti-Russe technique
- Mauck (reverse) knee procedure
- Mayo bunionectomy
- Mayo hallux valgus modified
- Mayo metatarsal head resection
- Mayo total elbow arthroplasty
- Mazet technique
- McBride bunionectomy
- McBride hallux abductovalgus reduction
- McCarroll-Baker procedure
- McCarty hip procedure
- McCash hand procedure
- McCauley foot procedure
- McConnell technique
- McElfresh-Dobyns-O'Brien
- McElvenny foot procedure
- McFarland-Osborne technique
- McKay-Simons clubfoot
- McKay-Simons CSR (complete subtalar release)
- McKeever arthrodesis for hallux limitus
- McKeever-Buck elbow technique
- McKeever medullary clavicle fixation
- McKeever metatarsophalangeal fusion
- McKittrick transmetatarsal amputation
- McLaughlin-Hay procedure
- McReynolds open reduction
- McWhorter posterior shoulder approach
- medial parapatellar arthrotomy
- medial V-Y capsulotomy
- Mensor-Scheck procedure

operations *(cont.)*
- metatarasocuneiform fusion
- metatarsal neck osteotomy
- metatarsocuneiform joint fusion
- metatarsophalangeal joint fusion
- Meyerding-Van Demark procedure
- microdiskectomy
- microlumbar diskectomy
- microsurgery
- microsurgical diskectomy
- middle fossa transtentorial trans-labyrinthine approach
- Milch cuff resection
- Milch elbow technique
- Millender-Nalebuff wrist arthrodesis
- Miller flatfoot procedure
- Miller-Galante arthroplasty
- Millesi modified
- mini-fragment plate fixation
- minimal incision technique
- Mital elbow release
- Mitchell bunionectomy
- Mitchell hallux valgus procedure
- Mitchell osteotomy
- Miyakawa knee
- Mizuno technique
- Moberg-Gedda open reduction
- modified Bristow
- modified Brostrom lateral ankle instability
- modified Hoke-Miller flatfoot procedure
- modified Kessler procedure
- modified McBride bunionectomy
- modified mold and surface replacement arthroplasty
- modified Watson-Jones ankle tenodesis
- modified Wilson osteotomy
- Moe scoliosis
- Molesworth-Campbell elbow approach
- monofilament wire fixation
- monospherical shoulder arthroplasty
- Monticelli-Spinelli distraction

operations *(cont.)*
- Moore approach
- Morgan-Casscells meniscus suturing
- Morrey-Bryan elbow arthroplasty
- Morrison technique
- Morrissy percutaneous slipped epiphysis fixation
- Mubarak-Hargens decompression
- Mueller (Müller) hip arthroplasty
- Mueller knee procedure
- multiarc LINAC radiosurgery
- multilevel laminectomy
- Mumford-Gurd acromioclavicular
- Mumford-Gurd arthroplasty
- Murphy heel cord advancement
- muscle shortening
- Nalebuff-Millender technique
- Naughton-Dunn triple arthrodesis
- Neer unconstrained shoulder arthroplasty
- neural arch resection
- neurectomy
- neurolysis
- Neviaser-Wilson-Gardner procedure
- New England Baptist hip arthroplasty
- Nicholas five-in-one reconstruction
- Nicola shoulder procedure
- Nicoll fracture repair
- Niebauer-King technique
- Nirschl procedure
- Ober-Barr transfer technique
- oblique osteotomy
- O'Brien pelvic halo procedure
- obturator neurectomy
- Obwegeser sagittal mandibular osteotomy
- occipital interhemispheric approach
- occipitoatlantoaxial fusion
- occipitocervical arthrodesis
- occipitocervical fusion
- O'Donoghue ACL reconstruction
- Ollier arthrodesis approach
- Omer-Capen technique
- open door laminoplasty

operations *(cont.)*
- open tendon repair
- opercular cortex
- ORIF (open reduction, internal fixation)
- Osborne-Cotterill elbow dislocation
- Osgood rotational osteotomy
- Osmone-Clarke foot procedure
- osteoclasis
- osteoplastic craniotomy
- osteoplastic laminectomy
- Ostrup technique
- over-the-top knee procedure
- Pack technique
- Paddu knee
- Palmer-Widen shoulder technique
- Paltrinieri-Trentani resurfacing
- panmetatarsal head resection
- pantalar arthrodesis
- pantalar fusion
- pants-over-vest technique
- Papineau technique
- parapatellar arthrotomy
- parietal cortectomy
- Patel medial meniscectomy
- patellar tendon substitution
- patellar tendon transfer (PTT)
- Paterson technique
- Paulos ligament technique
- Pauwels proximal osteotomy
- Pauwels Y osteotomy
- Peacock transposing technique
- pedicle screw fixation
- Pemberton pericapsular osteotomy
- percutaneous corticotomy
- percutaneous heel cord lengthening
- percutaneous high-frequency rhizotomy
- percutaneous lengthening of Achilles tendon
- percutaneous osteotomy
- percutaneous pin insertion
- percutaneous pinning
- percutaneous radiofrequency coagulation

operations *(cont.)*
- percutaneous repair
- percutaneous tenotomy
- Perry-Nickel technique
- Perry-O'Brien-Hodgson technique
- Perry-Robinson cervical technique
- phalangeal condylectomy
- Pheasant elbow technique
- Phemister onlay bone graft
- Pilliar total hip replacement
- plantar fasciotomy
- plantar flexor proximal metatarsal
- Platou osteotomy
- PMR (posteromedial release) for clubfoot
- polyethylene femoral buck plug
- porous coated total hip replacement
- portmanteau procedure
- Post shoulder arthroplasty
- posterior fossa exploration
- posterior lumbar interbody fusion (PLIF)
- posterior tibialis tendon lengthening
- posterolateral approach
- Potts eversion osteotomy
- primary repair
- proximal metatarsal approach
- proximal phalanx osteotomy
- pseudarthrosis
- pterional approach
- PTT (posterior tibialis tendon transfer)
- pulp plasty
- Putti knee arthrodesis
- Putti-Platt arthroplasty
- radialization of club hand
- radical nail bed ablation of ingrowing toenail
- radiosurgery
- Radley-Liebig-Brown resection
- ray resection
- reefing
- reefing of the medial retinaculum of the knee

operations *(cont.)*
Regnauld free phalangeal base autograft for hallux limitus
Regnauld modification of Keller arthroplasty
Reichenheim-King procedure
release of abductor hallucis muscle
resection arthroplasty
resection of epileptogenic focus
resection of iliopsoas tendon
resurfacing
retrogeniculate hamstring release
retromastoid craniotomy
retrosigmoid transmeatal approach
Reverdin-Green foot procedure
Reverdin-Green osteotomy
reverse Mauck knee procedure
revision arthroplasty
revision total hip
rhachotomy
rhizotomy
Ridlon hip reduction
Ring UPM total hip replacement
Ring UPM total knee replacement
Robinson anterior cervical diskectomy
Robinson anterior cervical fusion
Robinson-Chung-Farahvar morcellation
Robinson-Riley cervical arthrodesis
Robinson-Southwick fusion
Rockwood-Green technique
Rogers cervical fusion technique
Roos approach
Root-Siegal osteotomy
Rose foot procedure
rotational osteotomy
rotational scarf bunionectomy
rotator cuff repair
Roux-duToit staple capsulorrhaphy
Roux-Goldthwait procedure
Rowe posterior shoulder approach
Rowe-Zarins shoulder immobilization

operations *(cont.)*
Ruiz-Mora procedure
Russe approach
Ryerson triple arthrodesis
saber-cut approach
SAF hip (self-articulating femoral) replacement
Sage-Clark technique
Saha transfer technique
Salter pelvic osteotomy
salvage
Salzer resurfacing
Samilson osteotomy
Sargent knee
Sarmiento trochanteric fracture technique
Scaglietti closed reduction technique
Scarborough total hip replacement
scarf bunionectomy, rotational
Schaberg-Harper-Allen technique
Schanz angulation osteotomy
Schauwecker patellar wiring
Schlein elbow arthroplasty
Schneider hip arthrodesis
Schnute wedge resection technique
Schrock procedure
Scott glenoplasty
screw fixation
Scuderi technique
SDR (selective dorsal rhizotomy)
Seddon modification
segmental epidural nerve block with local anesthesia
segmental spinal fixation
self-bearing ceramic total hip replacement
Selig hip
Sell-Frank-Johnson extensor shift
Senegas hip approach
sesamoidectomy
Sever-L'Episcopo shoulder repair
Sharrard transfer technique
shelf procedure

operations *(cont.)*
- Sherk-Probst technique
- shish kebab technique
- shortening collectomy
- shortening osteotomy
- Shriver-Johnson arthrodesis
- Siffert-Forster-Nachamie arthrodesis
- Siffert-Storen intraepiphyseal osteotomy
- Silfverskiöld Achilles tendon reconstruction
- silicone implant arthroplasty
- Silver bunionectomy
- Simmonds-Menelaus metatarsal osteotomy
- Simmons cervical spine fusion
- sinus tarsi peg
- Skoog technique
- Slocum fusion technique
- Slocum knee procedure
- Smith-Petersen cup arthroplasty
- Smith-Petersen sacroiliac joint fusion
- Smith-Robinson cervical fusion
- Smith-Robinson diskectomy
- Sofield femoral deficiency
- soft tissue reconstruction
- somatectomy
- Somerville technique
- Souter hip procedure
- Southwick slide procedure
- Southwick-Robinson cervical approach
- Speed arthroplasty
- Speed-Boyd radial-ulnar technique
- Spencer tendon lengthening
- Spier elbow arthrodesis
- Spiller-Frazier neurotomy
- Spira procedure
- Spittler procedure
- SPLATT (split anterior tibial tendon transfer)
- split patellar approach
- split posterior tibial tendon transfer
- split-thickness skin excision (STSE)

operations *(cont.)*
- spondylectomy
- Sponsel oblique osteotomy
- Stack shoulder procedure
- Staheli shelf procedure
- Stamm procedure
- Stanmore knee replacement
- Stanmore shoulder arthroplasty
- Stanmore total hip replacement
- staple arthroereisis
- staple fixation
- Staples-Black-Brostrom ligament repair
- Staples elbow arthrodesis
- Stark-Moore-Ashworth-Boyes technique
- Steel shelf
- Steel triple innominate osteotomy
- Steindler flexorplasty
- Steindler stripping
- Stener-Gunterberg hip
- step-cut osteotomy
- stereotactic biopsy
- stereotactic laser microsurgery
- stereotactic placement of depth electrodes
- stereotactic radiosurgery
- stereotactic thalamotomy
- sternal-splitting approach
- Stewart arm
- Stewart-Harley ankle arthrodesis
- Stiles-Bunnell transfer technique
- Stone bunionectomy
- Strayer tendon technique
- Strickland tendon repair
- subcutaneous palmar fasciotomy
- subfrontal transbasal approach
- suboccipital craniectomy
- suboccipital craniotomy
- suboccipital muscle release
- suboccipital posterior fossa approach
- subtalar arthrodesis
- subtalar arthrotomy
- subtalar capsulotomy

operations *(cont.)*
subtalar release
subtalar stabilization
subtemporal approach
subtotal vertebrectomy
subtraction osteotomy
Sugioka transtrochanteric osteotomy
Sundaresan approach
Suppan foot
supracerebellar approach
supracondylar femoral derotational osteotomy
supramalleolar osteotomy
suprasyndesmotic screw fixation
supratentorial approach
surface replacement
surgical decompression
suspension laminotomy
Sutherland-Greenfield osteotomy
Sutherland hip procedure
Swanson Convex condylar arthroplasty
Swanson interpositional wrist arthroplasty
Swanson metatarsophalangeal joint arthroplasty
Swanson silicone wrist arthroplasty
Swedish approach
Syme amputation
symmetric vertebral fusion
sympathectomy
syndactylization
synovectomy
synovial biopsy
T-plasty modification of Bankart shoulder
Tachdjian hamstring lengthening
TAL (tendo Achillis lengthening)
talonavicular arthrodesis
talonavicular capsulotomy
talonavicular cuneiform arthrodesis
tarsal tunnel release (TTR)
Taylor-Daniel-Weiland technique
TCR (tethered cord release)

operations *(cont.)*
temporo-occipital approach
tendon interposition arthroplasty
tendon lengthening
tendon transfer
tendon transplant
tendonplasty
tenectomy
tenodesis of the heel cord
tenoplastic reconstruction
tenotomy
tension band fixation
terminal Syme procedure
Teuffer technique
THA (total hip arthroplasty)
Thackery
thalamectomy
thalamotomy
Tharies hip replacement
Thomas-Thompson-Straub transfer
Thompson-Henry technique
Thompson posterior radial approach
Thompson telescoping V osteotomy
tibiocalcaneal fusion
tibiotalar arthrodesis
tibiotalar fusion
tibiotalocalcaneal fusion
Tikhoff-Linberg radical arm procedure
Tikhoff-Linberg shoulder resection
TKA (total knee arthroplasty)
Tohen tendon technique
tongue and trough technique
Torgerson-Leach modified technique
Torg knee reconstruction
Torkildsen shunt
total articular resurfacing arthroplasty (TARA)
total hip arthroplasty
total hip replacement (THR)
total knee arthroplasty
total synovectomy

operations *(cont.)*
TPL-6 total hip replacement
TR-28 total hip replacement
transarticular screw fixation
transcallosal approach
transcerebellar approach
transchoroidal approach
transclival approach
transcranial approach
transfibular approach for arthrodesis
transfibular fusion
transfrontal approach
transfrontonaso-orbital approach
translabyrinthine approach
translational osteotomy
transmalleolar ankle arthrodesis
transmaxillosphenoidal approach
transmetatarsal amputation
transnaso-orbital approach
transoral approach
transpedicular approach
transpetrosal approach
transplantation of autologous adrenal medullary tissue
transsphenoidal approach
transsternal approach
transsylvian transventricular approach
transsyndesmotic screw fixation
transtemporal approach
transtentorial approach
transthoracic approach
transtrochanteric approach
transverse chevron osteotomy
transzygomatic approach
trephination
trephine craniotomy
Trethowan-Stamm-Simmonds, Menelaus-Haddad triangulation
triad knee repair
triangular external ankle fixation
triaxial total elbow arthroplasty
trigger thumb release
Trillat osteotomy

operations *(cont.)*
triple arthrodesis
triple tarsal fusion
Trumble arthrodesis
Tsuge tendon repair
Turco clubfoot release
Turco posteromedial release
Turco repair of talipes equinovarus
twist drill craniostomy
two-sleeve technique
two-stage hip fusion
two-strut tibial graft technique
Uematsu shoulder arthrodesis
ulnocarpal arthrodesis
ultrasound-guided echo biopsy
ultrasound-guided stereotactic biopsy
U osteotomy
V osteotomy
Valenti arthroplasty
valgus-extension osteotomy
Vandenbos and Bowers procedure
Vastamaki technique
vastus medialis advancement
Veleanu-Rosianu-Ionescu technique
Verdan technique
vertebrectomy
vest-over-pants technique
veterinary approach
Vidal-Adrey fracture technique
Vitallium cup arthroplasty
volar plate repair
volumetric stereotactic surgical resection
Volz total wrist arthroplasty
Volz-Turner reattachment
VSP (variable screw placement) fixation
Vulpius Achilles tendon reconstruction
Vulpius-Compere tendon technique
Vulpius equinus deformity
V-Y plasty correction of varus toes
Wadsworth elbow approach
Wagner open reduction technique
Wagoner cervical technique

operations *(cont.)*
- Warner-Farber ankle fixation
- Warren White Achilles tendon lengthening
- Watkins fusion technique
- Watson-Cheyne technique
- Watson-Jones ankle tenodesis
- Watson-Jones arthrodesis
- Weaver-Dunn acromioclavicular
- Weber-Brunner-Freuler-Boitzy
- Weber-Vasey traction-absorption
- wedge excision of ingrowing toe nail
- West and Soto-Hall patella technique
- White arthrodesis
- Whitecloud-LaRocca arthrodesis
- Whitesides-Kelly cervical technique
- Whitman osteotomy
- Williams-Haddad technique
- Wilson double oblique osteotomy
- Wilson-Jacobs tibial fixation
- Wilson-Johansson-Barrington arthrodesis
- Wilson-McKeever arthroplasty
- Wiltberger anterior cervical approach
- Wiltse ankle osteotomy
- Winograd ingrown nail technique
- Winston-Lutz LINAC-based radiosurgery
- Winter spondylolisthesis
- wire fixation
- Wirth-Jager tendon technique
- Wisconsin wire fixation
- Woodward technique
- wrapping of aneurysm
- Wu bunionectomy
- Yee posterior shoulder approach
- Yoke transposition procedure
- Yount procedure
- Zadik foot
- Zadik total nail bed ablation
- Zancolli rerouting technique

operations *(cont.)*
- Zaricznyj ligament technique
- Zarins-Rowe ligament technique
- Zazepen-Gamidov technique
- Zeier transfer technique
- Zickel nail fixation
- Zickel subtrochanteric fracture
- Z-lengthening of tendon
- Z-plasty
- Z-plasty release
- Z-slide lengthening

opercular epilepsy

operculum
- frontal
- frontoparietal
- insula
- medial
- occipital
- sylvian
- temporal

OPG (ophthalmoplethysmography)

ophthalmic migraine

ophthalmodynamometry (ODN)

ophthalmoplegia
- internuclear (INO)
- progressive external
- pseudo-internuclear
- supranuclear

ophthalmoplegic migraine

ophthalmoplethysmography (OPG)

ophthalmoscopic examination

opisthotonic position

opisthotonic posture (posturing)

opisthotonos

OPLL (opacification of posterior longitudinal ligament)

Opmi microscope drape

Oppenheim brace

Oppenheim disease

Oppenheim gait

Oppenheim reflex

Oppenheim sign

Oppenheimer knuckle-bender splint

Oppenheimer splint, modified

Oppenheimer spring wire splint
opponens bar
opponensplasty
  Goldmar
  Groves
  Littler
  Phalen-Miller
  Riordan finger
opposite foot strike phase of gait
opposite toe-off phase of gait
opposition, finger
opposition of hand or thumb muscles
  hard
  soft
Opraflex incise drape
opsoclonia (opsoclonus, or dancing eyes)
opsoclonus-myoclonus syndrome
optic atrophy, Leber
optic chiasm tumors
optic disk, pallor of the
optic glioma tumor
optic nerve (second cranial nerve)
optic nerve atrophy
optic nerve defect
optic nerve head, ischemia of the
optic neuritis
optic pathway tumor
optic radiation of Gratiolet
optic tract
optic-type spongiform encephalopathy
optica, neuromyelitis
optico-chiasmatic cistern, arachnoiditis of the
Opti-Curve therapeutic pillow
Opti-Fix II acetabular cup
optokinetic nystagmus (OKN)
optokinetic response
optokinetic testing
oral apraxia
oral-buccal-lingual dyskinesia
oral petit mal
oral thermistor (used during EEG)
orbit, angular process of
orbital mass compression
orbital pseudo-tumor
orbital rim stepoff
orbitofrontal region
orbitotomy, open sky
Oregon ankle prosthesis
Oregon Poly II ankle prosthesis
Oretorp arthroscopy knife
Orfit splints
organ, organs
  Corti
  proprioceptive end
organic brain disease (OBD)
organic brain syndrome with psychosis
organic brain with psychosis syndrome
organic denial
organic headache
organic inattention
organic mental syndrome
organic signs (of brain damage)
organic unilateral neglect
organization of ocular movements in infants
organomegaly
organophosphorus insecticide poisoning
orientation
  coronal
  disturbed
  sagittal
  spatial
  temporal
  transverse
orientation and mobility (O&M)
orientation-memory-contraction (OMC) test
orientation to person, place, and time
oriented and alert x 3 (times 3) (to person, place, and time)
oriented and alert x 4 (times 4) (to person, place, time, and future plans)
oriented, fully
oriented in all spheres
oriented x 3 (to person, place, time)

oriented; awake, alert and (AAO)
ORIF (open reduction and internal fixation)
origin, muscle
Oris pin
ORLAU (Orthotic Research and Locomotor Assessment Unit)
ORLAU swivel walker orthosis
Orozco cervical plate
Orr-Buck traction
Orthacor material
Orthair oscillating saw
Orthairtome wire driver
Orthawear antiembolism stockings
Orth-evac autotransfusion system
Orthion traction machine
Ortho-Cel padding
Orthochrome implant metal
orthodromic sensory study
orthodromic velocity
Orthofix external fixator
Orthofix M-100 distractor
Orthofix miniature fixator
Orthofix prosthesis
Orthofix screw
Ortho-Foam elbow/heel pad
Ortho-Foam protector
OrthoGen implantable stimulator for nonunion of fracture
OrthoGen/OsteoGen
Ortho-Ice Multipaks
Ortholav jet lavage
Ortholoc implant metal
Orthomet
Ortho-Mold lumbar body jacket
orthopaedic or orthopedic
orthopaedic oxford
OrthoPak II bone growth stimulator
orthopedic bed
orthopedic evaluation
orthopedic hardware
Orthopedic Trauma Association, fracture classification of
orthoplast jacket
orthopedist (also orthopaedist)
orthopod
orthoptic evaluation
orthoroentgenogram
orthosis (see also *prosthesis*; *splint*)
  abduction hip
  accommodative
  A-frame
  airplane splint
  Alden CDI
  ankle-foot (AFO)
  ankle-foot plastic
  articulated AFO
  Atlanta brace
  bail-lock knee joint
  balance padding
  bar and shoe
  Biothotic foot
  Boston brace thoracolumbosacral
  C-bar
  cable twister
  calcaneal spur cookie
  CASH thoracolumbosacral
  cervical
  cervicothoracic
  cervicothoracolumbosacral (CTLSO)
  chairback
  cock-up splint
  copolymer ankle-foot
  custom
  custom-fabricated
  Denis Browne bar foot
  dermoplast/plastizote
  Diabetic D-Sole foot
  dial lock
  elastic knee cage
  elastic twister
  elbow-wrist-hand (EWHO)
  Engen palmar finger
  figure-of-8 thoracic
  Fillauer bar foot
  FirmFlex custom
  flexion-extension control cervical
  floor-reaction ankle-foot

orthosis *(cont.)*
- foot (FO)
- Foot Levelers
- four-poster cervical
- Frejka pillow
- gator plastic
- Gilette modification of ankle-foot
- Gillette joint
- GunSlinger shoulder
- G/W Heel Lift, Inc.
- halo cervical
- halo extension
- halo traction
- halo-vest
- heat-molded petroplastic ankle-foot
- heel lift
- hip-knee-ankle-foot (HKAFO)
- Ilfield splint
- J-24 cervical
- J-35 hyperextension
- J-45 contraflexion
- J-55 postfusion
- Jewett-Benjamin cervical
- Jewett contraflexion
- Jewett hyperextension
- Jewett postfusion
- Jewett thoracolumbosacral
- Klenzak
- knee extension
- knee-ankle-foot (KAFO)
- Knight-Taylor thoracolumbosacral
- lateral heel wedge
- Legg-Perthes disease
- Lenox Hill knee
- Lerman multiligamentous knee control
- Levy & Rappel foot
- Ligamentus Ankle
- long leg
- long opponens
- LSU reciprocation-gait (Louisiana State University)
- Lynco foot
- Malleoloc ankle

orthosis *(cont.)*
- medial heel wedge
- medial sole wedge
- metatarsal bar
- metatarsal pads
- Meyer cervical
- Milwaukee cervicothoraco-lumbosacral
- Minerva
- molded AFO
- molded ankle-foot
- New York Orthopedic front-opening
- New York University insert for
- Newington
- NuKO knee
- Oklahoma ankle joint
- ORLAU swivel walker
- orthotic coiled spring twisters
- outrigger upper limb
- parapodium
- Phelps
- plantar arch support
- plastic floor reaction ankle-foot
- Plastizote arch support
- Plastizote collar cervical
- polypropylene
- polypropylene ankle-foot
- posterior leaf spring
- posterior leaf spring ankle-foot
- PSA thermoplastic
- PTB (patellar tendon bearing) ankle-foot
- PTB plastic
- PTS (patellar tendon stabilization)
- reciprocating gait (RGO)
- rib belt
- Rochester hip-knee-ankle-foot
- Rochester HKAFO (hip-knee-ankle-foot)
- rubber ischial lift
- safety pin
- Scottish Rite hip
- Seattle

orthosis *(cont.)*
 Select joint
 semirigid
 semirigid polypropylene ankle-foot
 Shaeffer rigid
 short opponens
 shoulder-elbow-wrist-hand (SEWHO)
 SMO (supramalleolar)
 soft collar cervical
 SOMI (sternal occipital mandibular immobilization)
 spring wire ankle-foot
 spring-loaded lock
 standard shell ankle-foot (AFO)
 standing frame
 steel sole plate
 supramalleolar (SMO)
 Swedish knee cage
 Tachdhian
 Taylor thoracolumbosacral
 Thera-Band Resistive Therapy System
 thermoplastic ankle-foot
 Thomas collar cervical
 Thomas heel
 thoracolumbosacral (TLSO)
 thumb
 TIRR foot-ankle
 TLSO (thoracolumbosacral)
 tone-reducing ankle-foot (TRAFO)
 Toronto
 Toronto parapodium
 total contact (TCO)
 TPE ankle-foot
 TPE biomechanical foot orthosis
 trilateral knee-ankle-foot
 trimlines for ankle-foot
 twister cable brace
 two-poster cervical
 UCB foot
 underarm
 Viscoheel K
 Viscoheel N

orthosis *(cont.)*
 Viscoheel SofSpot
 Viscolas
 Von Rosen splint hip
 Whitman arch support
 Williams
 wrist-driven flexor hinge
 Zinco ankle
OrthoSorb absorbable fixation pin
orthostatic syncope
orthotic plate
Orthotic Research and Locomotor Assessment Unit (ORLAU)
orthotic twisters to treat internal or external rotation
orthotics
orthotist
orthotome resector
Ortho-Trac adhesive bandage
Orthotron exerciser machine
Ortho-Vent nonadhesive bandage
Ortho-Vent traction
OrthoVision orthopedic table
Ortolani click
Ortolani maneuver
Ortolani sign
os calcis
Osborne-Cotterill elbow technique
oscillating saw
oscillating tremor
oscillation, macro saccadic
oscillograph
oscillopsia, torsional monocular
OS-5/Plus 2 knee brace
Osgood modified technique
Osgood-Schlatter disease
OSI Arthroscopic Leg Holder
OSI Extremity Elevator
os intermetatarseum
OSI Well Leg Support
Osler nodes
Osmone-Clarke foot procedure
os naviculare
ossea, leontiasis

osseous bridge
osseous destructive process
osseous dysplasia
osseous outgrowth
osseous union
ossicle
ossiferous
ossific nucleus of navicular
ossification
  enchondral
  endochondral
  heterotopic
  peripheral (on x-ray)
ossification center
ossification of soft tissue, on x-ray
ossified body
ossifying fibroma of long bone
ossimeter
Ossotome bur
osteal
ostealgia
ostectomy, fibular
osteitis
  condensing (of clavicle)
  sclerosing nonsuppurative
osteitis deformans
osteitis fibrosa cystica
osteitis fragilitans
osteitis ossificans
osteitis pubis
ostemia
ostempyesis
osteoaneurysm
osteoarthritic change
osteoarthritic spur
osteoarthritis (OA)
  degenerative
  erosive
  generalized
  posttraumatic
  traumatic
osteoarthropathy
osteoarthrosis
osteoarthrotomy
osteoarticular
osteoarticular graft
osteoblastic bone regeneration
osteoblastic tumor
osteoblastoma
osteocachexia
osteocalcin
OsteoCap hip prosthesis
osteocartilaginous graft
osteocartilaginous lesion
osteocartilaginous mass
osteocartilaginous metaplasia
osteochondral fractures of the dome of the talus
osteochondral graft
osteochondral lesion of the talus
osteochondritic loose body
osteochondritis
  crushing
  epiphyseal
  juvenile
  puncture wound
osteochondritis deformans juvenilis
osteochondritis dissecans (OD)
osteochondritis ischiopubica
osteochondritis juvenilis
osteochondritis necroticans
osteochondrofibroma
osteochondrolysis
osteochondroma
  epiphyseal
  soft tissue
osteochondromatosis, synovial
osteochondromatous dysplasia, epiarticular
osteochondropathy
osteochondrophyte
osteochondrosarcoma
osteochondrosis deformans tibiae
osteochondrosis dissecans
osteoclasis
osteoclast
osteoclastic erosion
osteoclastic giant cell

osteoclastoma
osteocope
osteocystoma
osteocyte
osteodiastasis
osteodynia
osteodystrophy
  azotemic
  renal
  uremic
osteoenchondroma
osteofibrochondrosarcoma
osteofibromatosis
osteogenesis, distraction
osteogenesis imperfecta
osteogenic sarcoma
OsteoGen implantable bone growth stimulator
osteohalisteresis
osteoid osteoma, juxta-articular
osteolipochondroma
osteolipoma
Osteolock femoral prosthesis
Osteolock hip prosthesis
Osteolock, Precision
osteology
osteolysis
osteolysis, scalloping
osteoma
  juxta-articular osteoid
  parosteal
osteomalacia
osteomatosis
osteomesopyknosis
osteomized
osteomyelitic sinus
osteomyelitis
  Ackerman criteria for
  acute hematogenous (AHO)
  blastomycotic
  Brucella
  chronic pyogenic
  Garré sclerosing
  hematogenous

osteomyelitis *(cont.)*
  hyperbaric oxygen for
  iatrogenic
  long bone
  nonsuppurative
  nonunion
  pedal
  pin-track
  postfracture
  posttraumatic chronic
  Pseudomonas aeruginosa
  Salmonella
  secondary or acute hematogenous
  Staphylococcus aureus spinal
osteomyelodysplasia
osteon
osteonal bone
osteonecrosis
  dysbaric
  Ficat classification of femoral head
osteoneuralgia
Osteonics hip prosthesis
osteopathia striata
osteopathy, doctor of (D.O.)
osteopenia, generalized
osteopenic bone stock
osteoperiosteal graft
osteoperiostitis
osteopetrosis
osteophyte
  bony
  bridging
  cervical
  fringe of
  horseshoe
  marginal
osteophyte formation
  beaklike
  hooklike
  nipplelike
osteophytic bone lip
osteophytic lipping
osteophytic proliferation
osteophytosis

osteoplastica
osteoplasty
osteopoikilosis
osteoporosis
  corticosteroid-induced
  disuse
  senile
osteoporotic bone
osteopsathyrosis idiopathica
osteoradionecrosis
osteosarcoma
  parosteal
  periosteal
  telangiectatic
osteosclerosis fragilis
osteosis
osteospongioma
Osteo Stim implantable bone growth stimulator
osteosynovitis
osteosynthesis, biological
osteotabes
osteotelangiectasia
osteothrombophlebitis
osteothrombosis
osteotome (also periosteotome)
  Acufex
  Albee
  Alexander costal
  Alexander-Farabeuf periosteotome
  Anderson-Neivert
  Andrews
  Army
  Aufranc
  Ballender periosteotome
  bayonet
  Blount
  Bowen
  box
  Brown periosteotome
  Campbell
  Carroll-Legg
  Carroll-Smith-Petersen
  Cavin

osteotome *(cont.)*
  Cherry
  Cinelli
  Clayton
  Cloward spinal fusion
  Cobb
  Compere
  costal periosteotome
  Cottle
  Crane
  curved
  Dautery
  Dawson-Yuhl
  Dingman
  fine
  Fomon periosteotome
  Furnas bayonet
  grooving
  guarded
  guided
  Hardt-Delima
  Hendel guided
  Hibbs curved
  Hibbs straight
  Hoke
  Joseph
  Joseph periosteotome
  Lambotte
  Leinbach
  Lexer
  MacGregor
  Meyerding curved
  Meyerding straight
  MGH
  Micro-Aire
  Miner
  mini-Lambotte
  mini-Lexer
  Mitchell
  Moberg
  Moe
  Murphy
  Neivert
  Padgett

osteotome *(cont.)*
- Parkes
- Peck
- Rhoton
- Rish
- rotary
- Sheehan
- Silver
- Simmons
- Smith-Petersen curved
- Smith-Petersen straight
- Stille
- straight
- Swanson
- thin
- U.S. Army
- unguarded
- Weck
- West

osteotomized

osteotomy (see also *operations)*
- abduction (hip)
- adduction (hip)
- Akin
- angulation
- arcuate
- Austin
- ball-and-socket
- basal
- base wedge
- basilar crescentic
- basilar metatarsal
- basilar wedge
- bicorrectional Austin
- bifurcation
- biplane trochanteric
- biplaning of
- block
- Blount displacement
- Blundell-Jones hip
- Bonney-Kessel dorsiflexionary tilt-up
- Borden-Spencer-Herman
- Brackett

osteotomy *(cont.)*
- calcaneal
- calcaneus dome
- Campbell tibial
- chevron metatarsal
- closing abductory wedge (CAWO)
- closing base wedge (CBWO)
- Cole
- corrective lengthening
- countersinking
- crescent-shaped
- crescentic base wedge
- cuneiform
- cup-and-ball
- curved
- cutting jig for chevron
- decompressive
- delayed femoral
- derotational
- dial pelvic
- diaphyseal
- Dickson
- Dimon
- displacement
- distal Akin phalangeal
- distal first metatarsal osteotomy
- distal L
- distal metatarsal
- dome
- dome-shaped
- dorsal closing wedge metatarsal
- double
- Dwyer
- extension
- femoral derotation
- fibular
- flexion
- free-floating
- geometric extension
- Giannestras step-down modified
- Gigli saw
- Green-Laird modification of Reverdin procedure
- Haas

osteotomy *(cont.)*
- Helal
- Hohmann
- Ingram
- innominate
- intertrochanteric
- intracapsular
- Irwin
- Kalish
- Keck and Kelly
- Kelikian modified Z
- Kramer modification of Hohmann
- lateral closing wedge
- Lindgren oblique
- Lucas-Cottrell
- malleolar
- McMurray
- medial displacement
- medial opening wedge
- metatarsal
- metatarsal head
- metatarsal neck
- Mitchell distal
- Mitchell posterior dispacement
- Mitchell step-down
- modified Mau
- modified Wilson
- oblique displacement
- oblique metaphyseal
- oblique slide
- oblique, with derotation
- Obwegeser's sagittal mandibular
- open base wedge
- open wedge
- opening
- opening abductory wedge (OAWO)
- opening wedge
- peg-in-hole
- pelvic
- percutaneous
- plantarflexory proximal metatarsal
- posterior displacement (of the calcaneus)
- Potts tibial

osteotomy *(cont.)*
- proximal first metatarsal
- proximal phalangeal
- proximal phalanx
- reduction
- Reverdin-Green
- rotational
- rotational scarf
- Salter innominate
- Samilson
- scarf
- Schede hip
- shortening
- Sofield
- Southwick
- spike
- step
- step-cut
- subtalar posterior displacement (of the calcaneus)
- subtraction
- Sugioka
- supracondylar femoral derotational
- supracondylar varus
- supramalleolar
- supratubercular wedge
- Swanson
- talar
- talar neck
- talocalcaneal
- tarsal wedge
- through-and-through V-shaped horizontal
- tibial
- translational
- transverse
- transverse chevron
- trapezoidal
- Trillat
- triplane
- U
- V
- valgus
- valgus-extension

osteotomy *(cont.)*
  varus derotational
  Waterman
  wedge-shaped
  Wilson double oblique
osteotomy-osteoclasis
osteotomy sigmoid cavity of radius
osteotribe (rasp)
osteotripsy
os tibiale externum
os trapezium
os trapezoideum
os trigonum
os trigonum syndrome
Ostrup technique
Oswestry Low Back Pain Disability Questionnaire
OT (occupational therapy)
otic ganglion
otocerebritis
otocranial
otocranium
otoencephalitis
otogenic meningitis
otoneurologic
otoneurology
otorrhea, cerebrospinal fluid (CSF)
OTR (occupational therapist, registered)
OTR (ocular tilt reaction)
Otto Bock modular PTB prosthesis
Otto pelvis dislocation
OUT (O'Donoghue's Unhappy Triad)
outburst, aggressive
Outerbridge ridge
Outerbridge scale for joint or articular surface damage in chondromalacia
Outerbridge staging of degenerative arthritis
outflow of ventricle
outgrowth, osseous patellar
outlet, ventricular
outlet view
out-of-cast ankle brace
out-of-phase signal on EEG
outpatient communication/cognition treatment
outpatient physical therapy
output, motor
outrigger, Harrington distraction
outrigger upper limb orthosis
outrigger with splint
out-toeing
Ovadia-Beals classification of tibial plafond fracture
ovale, foramen
over-dependent attitude
over-the-top procedure of knee
overactivity, sympathetic
overbreathing, voluntary hysterical
overcorrection of hallux valgus
overdrilled
Overdyke hip prosthesis
overextension
overgrowth, bony
overhanging edges, or margins, on x-ray in gout
overhead suspension
Overholt clip-applying forceps
overlap of toes
overlap
  talocalcaneal
  tibiofibular
overlapped uprights in orthosis
overlapping of toes
overlay, functional
overpronator
overpull of muscle
overreading of EEG
overriding of fracture fragments
overriding toes
oversampling on EEG
oversewn
Overton dowel graft
overtraining
overuse injuries
overuse syndrome of the foot and lower leg in athletes
overuse syndrome of the wrist
overwhelming of extensor muscles

OVR (oculovestibular reflex)
OVR (Office of Vocational Rehabilitation)
Owen gauze dressing
Owen silk
Owen suture
Owestry staple
"ox-eye" (buphthalmos)
oxford shoe, orthopaedic
Oxford fixator
Oxford scale measuring muscle strength
Oxford unicompartmental devices
oxycephaly
oxygen cisternography
oxygen, hyperbaric (for osteomyelitis)

P, p

pacchionian bodies
pacchionian granulations
Pace ventricular needle
Paced Auditory Serial Addition Test (PASAT)
pacemaker
  subcortical
  thalamic
pacemaker theory, facultative
pachygyria
pachymeninges
pachymeningitis cervicalis hypertrophica
pachyonychia
pacinian corpuscle
pacinian nerve endings of hand
pacinian mechanoreceptor
pack, packing
  Adaptic
  Avitene
  cold
  Gelfoam
  hot
  Hydrocollator
  Kool Kit cold therapy
  Merocel
  MSC cold
  steam
  vaginal
packer, Woodson dura
Pack technique
PACs (picture archive and communication system) for x-rays
PACU (postanesthesia care unit)
pad, padding
  ABD (abdominal) lap
  Aquatech cast
  Arthropor
  balance
  buttock
  calcaneal fat
  cast
  Charnley foam suture
  contoured felt
  cotton cast
  digital
  fat
  fatty heel
  felt
  finger
  fingertip
  Hapad heel
  Hapad medial arch
  heel ("cookies")
  horseshoe heel
  horseshoe-shaped felt
  Hydrocollator
  J
  Kerlix cast
  knee-control orthosis
  knuckle
  lamb's wool
  metatarsal (shoe modification)
  Mik
  Mikulicz
  Morgan disk
  navicular shoe

pad *(cont.)*
- OEC popliteal
- Ortho-Cel
- Ortho-Foam elbow/heel
- painful heel
- patellar orthosis
- Pedifix hammertoe
- plantar fat
- proximal
- pubic
- Redigrip knee
- reticulated polyurethane
- scalene fat
- scaphoid shoe
- Scholl
- shock-absorbent heel
- shoe heel
- Silopad friction
- Sof-Rol cast
- spur
- thickness of heel
- Vac-Pac
- velvet foam
- Zimfoam

padded bolsters
Paddu knee procedure
Padgett osteotome
pad/protector, Decubinex
Paget associated osteogenic sarcoma
Paget disease, "fluffy rarefaction" of (on x-ray)
Paget osteitis deformans
pagetoid bone
pain
- aching
- acute
- atypical
- band-like
- boring
- bright
- burning
- calcaneal
- causalgic
- central

pain *(cont.)*
- chronic
- chronic low back (CLBP)
- chronic subtalar joint
- continuous
- contralateral
- cramping
- deafferentation
- dermatomal distribution of
- diffuse
- diskogenic
- dull
- dull aching
- electric shock-like
- endogenous
- exacerbation of
- fibromyalgia joint
- fibromyalgic
- gouty
- intense
- intermittent
- intractable
- jabbing
- joint line
- kinetic foot
- lancinating
- low back (LBP)
- machine gun-like
- medial joint line
- mid-dorsal back
- myofascial
- myotomal muscular
- nerve root
- neuralgic
- perimalleolar
- periscapulitis shoulder
- persistent
- phantom
- phantom limb
- plantar
- postherpetic
- postherpetic facial
- posttraumatic neck
- pounding

pain *(cont.)*
  pricking
  prickling
  pulsating
  radiation of
  radicular
  recalcitrant
  referred
  referred neuritic
  residual
  responded purposefully to
  Roland index of low back
  sclerotomal
  searing
  shooting
  splint-like
  stabbing
  static foot (when standing)
  steady
  stinging
  tearing
  throbbing
  ticlike
  vise-like
  volleys of
pain and temperature pathways
pain at rest
pain behaviors
painful-arc syndrome
painful heel pad
painter's encephalopathy
pain syndrome
pain threshold
pain with weightbearing
Pais fracture
Palacos bone cement
palatal myoclonus
palatal nystagmus
palatopharyngo-oculodiaphragmatic myoclonus
palatopharyngolaryngo-oculo-diaphragmatic myoclonus
pale disk
pale infarct
paleencephalon
paleocerebellar
paleocortex
paleokinetic
Paley classification of complications
paliacusis
palilalia
palindromic rheumatism
palinopsia
palipraxia
palisade formation
Palister-Hall syndrome
pallesthesia (vibratory sense)
pallidal syndrome
pallidotomy
  Leksell posteroventral
  stereotaxic
pallidum, Treponema
pallidus, globus
pallium
pallor of the optic disk
palmar aponeurosis
palmar crease
palmar fascia
palmar fasciotomy
palmar fibrous fasciculi
palmar ganglion
palmar ligaments
palmar luxation
palmar metacarpal ligament
"palmar migraine"
palmar plates
palmaris longus tendon
Palmer bone nail
Palmer-Widen shoulder technique
palmomental reflex
palpation
palsy
  abducens
  ataxic cerebral
  backpack
  Bell
  bilateral gaze
  bridegroom's

palsy *(cont.)*
- bulbar
- cerebral (CP)
- common peroneal nerve
- complete ulnar nerve
- cranial nerve
- crossed-leg
- Dejerine-Klumpke
- diabetic third-nerve
- Duchenne-Erb
- dyskinetic cerebral
- Erb
- Erb-Duchenne
- extraocular muscle
- facial nerve
- fourth nerve
- gaze
- handlebar
- Hoke procedure for tibial
- honeymoon
- horizontal gaze
- hypotonic cerebral
- idiopathic facial nerve
- ipsilateral
- ipsilateral facial
- ipsilateral gaze
- juvenile progressive bulbar
- Klumpke
- labioglossolaryngeal
- lateral gaze
- long thoracic nerve
- lower radial
- march of cranial nerve
- median nerve
- middle medial
- middle radial
- peripheral seventh nerve
- peroneal
- persistent facial
- postganglionic oculosympathetic
- progressive
- progressive bulbar
- progressive supranuclear (PSP)
- pseudobulbar

palsy *(cont.)*
- pure athetoid
- pure spastic
- pursuit
- radial nerve
- saccadic
- "Saturday night" radial
- sciatic
- shaking
- sixth nerve
- spastic cerebral
- supranuclear
- supranuclear gaze
- tardive median nerve
- tardive ulnar nerve
- third nerve
- Todd
- turnip planter's
- ulnar nerve
- upper median
- vertical-gaze

Paltrinieri-Trentani resurfacing procedure
Palumbo knee brace
Palumbo stabilizing brace
Pancoast (thoracic inlet) syndrome
pancytokeratin immunostain
P&O (prosthetics and orthotics)
pandiculation
Pandy test
pandysautonomia
panencephalitis
- rubella
- subacute sclerosing (SSPE)

panfacial fracture
panhypopituitarism
Panje voice button prosthesis
panmetatarsal head resection
Panner disease
pannus deformity of odontoid
pannus of synovium
pantalar arthrodesis
pantalar fusion
Panthers, Gray

Pantopaque myelography
panty girdle, Cadenza
paper
  Shutrack carbon
  tracing
Papez circuit
papilledema
  high-grade
  long-standing
  marked
papilloma, choroid plexus
papilloma of the fourth ventricle
papilloma of the fourth ventricle tumor
Papineau grafting
PAR (postanesthesia recovery) room
para-articular bone remodeling
para-articular calcification
parabola, metatarsal
paracentral lobule
paracentral scotoma (pl. scotomata)
paracervical region
paracusis
paradoxical ipsilateral hemiparesis
paradoxical sleep (REM sleep)
paraepilepsy
parafascicular nucleus
parafascicular thalamotomy (PFT)
parafascicularis of the thalamus
paraffin-oil bath
paraganglioma
paragrammatism
paragraph recall test (after head injury)
paragraphias
parahippocampal gyrus
paralexic errors
parallel bars
parallelism of articular surface
paralysis
  acute ascending motor
  ascending
  backpack
  Benedikt's ipsilateral oculomotor
  bilateral

paralysis *(cont.)*
  Chaves-Rapp
  chronic basal meningitis with cranial nerve
  contralateral facial
  convergence
  deglutition
  Dejerine-Klumpke
  Dewar-Harris
  Dickson
  equinovarus of spastic
  Erb
  Erb-Duchenne
  facial
  familial hypokalemic periodic
  familial periodic
  flaccid
  frank
  gaze
  Haas
  Henry
  hyperkalemic periodic
  hypokalemic periodic
  infranuclear
  ipsilateral
  ipsilateral facial
  jake (Jamaica ginger)
  "night nurse's"
  labioglossolaryngeal
  labioglossopharyngeal
  Landry ascending
  Lissauer
  lovers'
  lower motor neuron
  nerve
  normokalemic familial periodic
  nuclear
  periodic
  peripheral nerve
  peroneal
  postepileptic
  postictal
  rucksack
  sleep (postdormital)

paralysis *(cont.)*
  sleep (predormital)
  spastic
  supranuclear
  thyrotoxic periodic
  tick
  Todd motor (postepileptic)
  ulnar nerve
  unilateral
  upper motor neuron
  Vastamaki
  vesical (as response to spinal trauma)
  Volkmann ischemic
  Wernicke-Mann predilection
  Whitman
paralysis agitans
  Hunt juvenile
  juvenile
paralytic calcaneus
paramagnetic
paramalleolar arteries
Paramax angled driver
paramedian sagittal plane
parameningeal
paramyoclonus multiplex
paramyotonia congenita
paraneoplastic cerebellar degeneration
paranoia
paraparesis
  flaccid
  spastic
parapatellar plica
paraphasia (not paraphrasia)
  formal verbal
  literal
  neologistic
  phonemic (or literal)
  semantic
  verbal
paraphasic error
paraphasic speech, fluent
paraphrasia (not paraphasia)
paraphyseal cysts
paraplegia
  cerebral
  Erb spastic
  familial amyotrophic dystonic
  familial spastic
  hereditary spastic
  Pott
  spastic
  spinal
paraplegic
parapodium orthosis
parapodium, Toronto
parapraxia
pararthrosis
parasagittal head region
parasagittal intracranial mass
parasagittal lesion
parasagittal meningioma
parasagittal region
parasagittal scar
parasagittal tumor
parasellar mass
parasellar tumor
parasomniac conscious state
paraspinal abnormality
paraspinal infection
paraspinal muscles
paraspinal musculature
paraspinal soft tissue mass
paraspinal soft tissue shadowing
paraspinous musculature
parasternal heave
parasthesia, facial
parastriate cortex
parasympathetic innervation
parasympathetic nervous system
parasympathetic pupillary constrictor fibers
parasympathin
paratendinitis, Achilles
paratenon
P:A ratio (peroneal to anterior compartment)

paratonia
paratrigeminal syndrome of Raeder
paratrooper fracture
paravermian region
paravertebral musculature
paravertebral nerve plexus
paravertebral region
paraxial hemimelia (complete and incomplete)
parenchyma
  cerebral
  spinal cord
parenchymal brain cysticercosis
parenchymal hemorrhage
parenchymatous atrophy
parenchymatous cerebellar degeneration
parenchymatous hemorrhage
parenchymatous neurosyphilis
paresis
  abducens nerve
  canal
  central facial
  complete ptosis of third nerve
  crural
  early ulnar nerve
  extraocular muscle
  gaze
  general
  ipsilateral facial
  limb-girdle-trunk
  motor
  ocular muscle
  oculomotor
  partial ptosis of third nerve
  radial nerve
  spastic
  "watershed" area
paresis of gaze
paresis of up gaze
paresthesia
  bandlike
  digital
  facial

paresthesia *(cont.)*
  intermittent
  limb
  nocturnal
  transient
paresthetica
  cheiralgia
  meralgia
paretic jerks
paretic leg
paretic musculature
paretic neurosyphilis
Parhad-Poppen arteriogram needle
Parham band
Parham band circling needle
Parham band tightener
Parham-Martin bone clamp
Parham-Martin fracture apparatus
Parham metal band
parietal association areas
parietal cephalohematoma
parietal cortex lesion
parietal cortex, post-rolandic
parietal EEG lead (P)
  left (LP)
  right (RP)
parietal gyrus
parietal lesion
parietal lobe contusion
parietal lobe disease
parietal lobe lesion
parietal lobe sign
parietal lobe tumors
parietal pleura
parietal signs
parietal suture
parietal tendon sheath layer
parietomastoid suture
parieto-occipital aphasia
parieto-occipital lesion
parieto-occipital sulcus
parieto-occipital suture
parietotemporal area
Parinaud syndrome

park bench position
Parkes osteotome
Parkinson disease
parkinsonian hypokinesia
parkinsonian symptoms
parkinsonian tremor
parkinsonism
  drug-induced
  en bloc turning in
  encephalopathic
  masked facies of
  postencephalitic
parkinsonism-dementia complex of Guam
parolfactory nerve (callosal area)
Parona space (subtendinous)
paronychia
parosmia
parosteal chondrosarcoma
parosteal osteogenic sarcoma
parosteal osteoma tumor
parosteal sarcoma tumor
parotitis
paroxysm of a seizure
paroxysmal changes on EEG
paroxysmal choreoathetosis seizure
paroxysmal convulsions
paroxysmal discharge on EEG
paroxysmal migraine
paroxysmal patterns of epilepsy
Parquetry Block Test
Parrish-Mann hammertoe technique
parrot-beak meniscus tears
Parrot node
Parrot sign
pars interarticularis
pars planitis
Parsonage-Turner disease
Parsonage-Turner syndrome
partial amnesia
partial closure
partial complex seizure
partial elementary seizures with motor symptoms
partial obliteration of a lateral ventricle (on scan)
partial ossicular replacement prosthesis (PORP)
partial ptosis of third nerve paresis
partial saturation technique (on MRI)
partial tonic seizure
particles, Ivalon
particles of bone
particulate debris
Partridge band
Partsch chisel
Partsch gouge
Parvin maneuver
PASA (proximal articular set angle)
PASAT (Paced Auditory Serial Addition Test)
pascals of force (SI units)
passage, adiabatic fast
passer
  Batzdorf cervical wire
  Brand tendon
  Bunnell tendon
  Charnley wire
  curved
  Framer tendon
  Hewson suture
  ligature
  Malis ligature
  suture
  tendon
passing out
passive head rotation
passive range of motion (PROM) exercise
passive traction table
Passow chisel
paste
  conductive EEG
  EEG electrolyte
  electrode
  Unna
past-pointing

patch
  ash leaf
  blood patch for post-LP headache
  epidural blood
  periosteal
  postsynaptic neuronal membrane
  shagreen patch in tuberous sclerosis
  vein
patella
  apex of head of
  bipartite
  dislocated
  high-riding
  minima
  skyline x-ray view of
  subluxing
  undersurface of
patella alta
patella baja
patella infera
patella minima
patellae, chondromalacia
patellae OUT (O'Donoghue's Unhappy Triad)
patellapexy
patellaplasty
patellar advancement
patellar aligner
patellar apprehension test
patellar bursitis
patellar button
patellar contour
patellar dislocation
patellar edge
patellar entrapment
patellar fat pad
patellar groove
patellar inhibition test
patellar instability
patellar jerk
patellar orthosis pad
patellar pole
patellar reflex (quadriceps stretch reflex)
patellar retraction test
patellar shaving
patellar subluxation
patellar tendon bearing cast (PTB)
patellar tracking
patellectomy
patellofemoral arthritis
patellofemoral crepitation
patellofemoral joint space
patellofemoral realignment
patellofemoral region
patelloquadriceps tendon
Patel medial meniscectomy
Paterson procedure
pathognomonic sign
pathologic dislocation
pathologic fracture
pathologic fracture dislocation
pathologic hyperreflexia
pathologic laughing and crying
pathologic reflexes
  Babinski
  frontal lobe
  grasp
  root
  snout
  suck
pathologist, speech
pathomechanical process
pathomechanics
  gait
  juvenile flatfoot
pathway
  amygdalofugal
  cerebellar
  corticifugal
  corticobulbar
  corticospinal motor
  CSF (cerebrospinal fluid)
  CSF outflow
  dentato-olivary
  frontopontocerebellar
  geniculocortical
  lipoxygenase

pathway *(cont.)*
- nigrostriatal
- obstructive lesion of the CSF
- pain and temperature
- perforant
- pyramidal
- reticulocortical
- retinal
- retrochiasmal visual
- stretch reflex
- subcortical
- synaptic
- thalamocortical
- visual

patient
- agitated
- ambulatory
- apallic
- aphasic
- arousable
- brain-dead
- comatose
- combative
- disoriented
- distractible
- docile
- floppy (infant)
- fully conscious
- head-injured
- hydrocephalic
- hypotonic
- incoherent
- labile
- left-handed
- lethargic
- moribund
- nonambulatory
- nonresponsive
- obtunded
- posturing
- rapidly deteriorating
- right-handed
- spinal cord-injured
- stuporous

patient *(cont.)*
- unresponsive
- vegetative

Patil stereotactic head frame
Patil stereotactic head holder
Patrick fabere sign
Patrick test
pattern
- alpha blocking
- alpha coma
- beta coma
- bilateral benign epileptiform
- burst-suppression EEG
- checkerboard (for VEP testing)
- Collimator plugging
- continuous slow wave
- corduroy cloth (on myelogram)
- delta brush
- dermatomal
- desynchronized
- diffuse delta
- diffusely low-voltage
- dimple-dimple hand
- discontinuous
- DISI collapse
- disorganized
- EMG incomplete interference
- epileptiform
- focal periodic
- full recruitment
- gait
- generalized periodic
- gyral
- high-voltage slow
- hypsarrhythmic
- ictal epileptiform
- infantile EEG
- interictal epileptiform
- intermixed focal and multifocal
- intermixed spike
- invariant EEG
- isoelectric
- knuckle-knuckle hand
- locomotor

pattern *(cont.)*
- low-voltage
- monorhythmic
- myotomal
- occipital delta
- paroxysmal
- phantom spike-and-wave
- pneumoencephalographic
- polyspike and wave EEG
  - paroxysmal
- pseudoepileptiform EEG
- rhythmic theta
- seizure
- sigmoid hair (on spine)
- sigmoid scalp hair
- sleep
- slow spike and wave EEG
- spindle coma
- storiform
- subclinical seizure
- suppression-burst
- surface convexity
- temporal sawtooth
- theta coma
- triphasic wave
- vertebral body picture frame

pattern-induced epilepsy
"patterning" (to cue a demented person how to eat)
pattern reversal visual evoked response
pattie or patty
- cement
- cotton
- cottonoid

pattie tray
patting automatism
pauciarticular
paucity
Paufique blade
Paulos ligament technique
Paulson knee retractor
Paulus plate
Paulus trocar
Pauwels angle of femoral neck fracture
Pauwels fracture classification
Pauwels Y osteotomy
Pavlik bandage
Pavlik harness
Pavlik sling
Pavlik splint
pavor nocturnus (night terror)
Payr sign
PB (paraffin bath)
PC (posterior commissure)
PCA (patient-controlled analgesia)
PCA (porous-coated anatomic) prosthesis
PCA (posterior cerebral artery)
PCA (posterior communicating artery)
PCA E-Series femoral prosthesis
PCA knee prosthesis
PCL (posterior cruciate ligament)
PCoA (posterior communicating artery)
PDA (polymorphic delta activity) on EEG
PDLs (physical daily living skills)
PDS (polydioxanone) suture
PE (pulmonary embolism)
Peabody splint
Peacock transposing technique
peak height velocity
peak of wave on EEG
Pean clamp
Pean forceps
peapod intervertebral disk rongeur
"pearls, string of," nuclear arrangement
Pearson attachment to Thomas frame or splint
Pease bone drill
Pease-Thomson traction
Peck osteotome
Pecquet, cistern of
pectoral reflex
pectoralgic migraine
pectoralis minor syndrome
pectus carinatum

pectus excavatum
pedal disability
pedal hyperpigmented lesions
pedal intradermal nevi
pedal osteomyelitis
Pedestal, IMP Surgical Leg
pedicle
  congenital skin tube
  spinal
  vascular
pedicle bone grafts
pedicle cover
pedicle erosion (on x-ray)
pedicle finder
pedicle finger
pedicle of vertebra
pedicle probe
pedicle sclerosis (on x-ray)
pedicle screw
Pedifix hammertoe pad
pedis
  dorsalis
  tinea
pedobarography
  Biokinetics
  dynamic
  foil
  Musgrave footprint
pedobarographic technique
pedorthist
pedorthotist
peduncle
  cerebellar
  cerebral
  inferior cerebellar
peduncular segment of superior
  cerebellar artery
pedunculated
pedunculi, basis
pedunculopontine neuron
pedunculopontine nucleus pars
  compacta
peg
  beef bone intramedullary
  bone

peg *(cont.)*
  fixation
  Harrison-Nicolle polypropylene
peg and socket bone
pegboard, Purdue
peg graft (grafting)
peg test of arm disability
PEG (pneumoencephalogram)
pegged tibial prosthesis
pegging
Peiper-Beyer laminectomy rongeur
P electrode (parietal) (P_1-P_{10} and P_z)
Pelite shoe liner
Pelizaeus-Merzbacher disease
  adult form
  infantile form
Pelizaeus-Merzbacher leukodystrophy
Pellegrini-Stieda disease
Pelourus stereotactic frame
pelvic brim
pelvic fracture frame, Slatis
pelvic girdle
pelvic obliquity
pelvic rock test
pelvic sling
pelvic tilt, bent knee
pelvic traction
pelvic unleveling
pelvis, Otto
Pemberton pericapsular osteotomy
Pemberton spur-crushing clamp
PEMF (pulsating or pulsed electro-
  magnetic field) therapy
pencil
  electrosurgical
  grease
  skin
pencil test (for Morton neuroma)
penciling of ribs on x-ray
pendular nystagmus
penetrating injury
Penfield elevator
Penfield neurodissector
Penfield No. 1 (to 5) dissector
pen galvanometer on EEG

Penn fingernail drill
Penn wire-cutting scissors
Pennig dynamic wrist fixator
Pennsylvania bimanual work sample
Penrose drain
pen, skin-marking
penta-acetic acid
pen writer on EEG
People-Finder
Pepper neuroblastoma
percent of total disability
perception
  constant-touch
  light touch
  threshold
  vibratory
perceptual disturbance, high level
percussion sign
percussor, McGill neurological
percutaneous autogenous dowel bone graft
percutaneous automated diskectomy
percutaneous cordotomy
percutaneous interosseous nerve (PIN)
percutaneous Kirschner (K) wire
percutaneous repair
Percy amputating saw
Percy amputation retractor
perencephaly
Perfecta hip prosthesis
perforating fracture
perforator
  Acra-Cut cranial
  cranial
  Cushing cranial
  D'Errico
  DGR cranial
  Heifetz cranial
  McKenzie
perforator bur, Adson
perforator vessel
Performance knee prosthesis
perfusion
  luxury
  misery
  regional cerebral
perfusion of brain
perfusion pressure
periaqueductal gray matter
periaqueductal region
periaqueductal structures
periarteritis nodosa
periarticular calcification
periarticular fibrositis
periarticular fracture
pericallosal artery
pericyte, Zimmerman
perikaryon
perilesional bone
perilunate dislocation
perimalleolar pain
perimetry test
perimysiitis
perimysium
perineural
perineurial fibroblastoma tumor
perineurial neurorrhaphy
perineurium
period
  apneic
  apneustic
  ictal
  interictal
  non-REM
  postictal
  REM (rapid eye movements)
  sleep onset REM
  sleep onset REM (SOREMP)
period between complexes on EEG
periodic alternating nystagmus
periodic lateralized epileptiform discharges (PLEDs) on EEG
periodic paralysis
periodicity, internal transverse

perioperative antibiotic therapy
perioral tremor
periorbital ecchymosis
periosteal bone formation
periosteal elevator (see *elevator*)
periosteal fibroma
periosteal osteosarcoma
periosteal reaction (on x-ray)
periosteal reflex
periosteal stripping
periosteotome (see *osteotome*)
periosteotomy
periosteum
periostitis
  florid reactive
  suppurative
  traumatic
periostomy
peripheral facial spasm
peripheral fields (of vision)
peripheral gangrene
peripheral lesion
peripheral nerve function deficits
peripheral nerve injury
peripheral nerve lesion
peripheral nerve level motor impairment
peripheral neural deficit
peripheral neuropathy (see also *neuropathy*)
  acrylamide
  alcohol
  amyloidosis
  arsenic
  avitaminosis B_1
  avitaminosis B_6
  avitaminosis B_{12}
  bacterial
  barbiturates
  Bassen-Kornzweig
  botulism
  brucellosis
  carcinoma
  chronic hepatitic failure

peripheral neuropathy *(cont.)*
  chronic ischemia due to atherosclerosis
  Dejerine-Sottas
  diabetes mellitus
  dinitrophenol
  diphtheria
  emetine
  ethyl alcohol
  gastrointestinal shunts
  gold
  griseofulvin
  Guillain-Barré postinfectious
  hypoglycemia
  infectious hepatitis
  insecticides
  isonicotinic acid
  leprosy
  lupus erythematosus (LE)
  macrocryoglobulinemia
  macroglobulinemia
  malabsorption syndrome
  measles
  mercury
  methyl alcohol
  mononucleosis
  multiple myeloma
  mumps
  myxedema
  pantothenic acid deficiency
  polyarteritis nodosa
  porphyria
  Refsum
  sarcoidosis
  serum sickness
  sprue
  sulfonamides
  Tangier
  thallium
  tricresyl phosphate
  tuberculosis
  typhoid
  uremia
  vaccination

peripheral neuropathy *(cont.)*
  vincristine
  Whipple disease
peripheral origin weakness
peripheral ossification (on x-ray)
peripheral pulses symmetrical and intact
peripheral sensory deficit
peripheral sensory loss
peripheral seventh nerve palsy
periradicular nerve
periradicular sheath
perirolandic cortex
periscapulitis shoulder pain
peristriate cortex
peritendinitis
peritenon
peritoneal catheter, Raimondi
peritonitis, CSF-induced (via catheter)
periulcer venous channels in venous stasis ulcers
periungual
perivascular plane
periventricular density
periventricular gray (PVG) matter
periventricular lesion
periventricular white matter
Perkins line
Perkins test
Perkins traction
Perlia medial nucleus
Perma-Hand braided silk suture
Perman cartilage forceps
permanent magnet
permeability, membrane
peroneal muscular atrophy
peroneal nerve palsy, common
peroneal obliterative thrombi
peroneal paralysis
peroneal spastic flatfoot
peroneal tendon dislocation
peronei muscles
peroneus brevis
peroneus longus
peroneus tertius
peroxide flush
perpendicular
per primam healing
Perry-Nickel technique
Perry-O'Brien-Hodgson technique
Perry-Robinson cervical technique
perseveration of speech
perseverative disorder
persistence of rhythm on EEG
persistent facial palsy
persistent vegetative state
person, memory-impaired
personality
  frontal lobe
  interictal epileptic
personality disorder
Perthes-Bankart lesion
Perthes disease
Perthes epiphysis
Perthes reamer
Perthes test
pertrochanteric fracture
perturbers
pes anserinus
pes arcuatus
pes calcaneocavus
pes calcaneovalgus
pes calcaneus
pes cavovalgus
pes cavovarus
pes cavus
pes cavus-type deformity
pes equinovalgus
pes equinus
pes planovalgus
pes plantigrade planus
pes planus deformity
pes planus, rigid
pes pronation
pes valgus
PET scan (positron emission tomography)
petaling edges of cast

petechia (pl. petechiae)
petit mal 3-per-second spike and wave
 EEG complexes
petit mal epilepsy, glassy stare of
petit mal, oral
petit mal seizure
petit mal status
petit mal variant
Petit triangle
Petren gait
Petrie spica cast
petrobasilar suture
petroccipital
petroclinoid ligament
petroclival region
petromastoid
petro-occipital synchondrosis
petrosal ganglion
petrosal neuralgia
petrosal sinus
petrosectomy
petrositis (petrousitis)
petrosomastoid
petrosphenobasilar suture
petrosphenoid
petrospheno-occipital suture
petrosquamosal
petrosquamous suture
petrous bone
petrous portion of temporal bone
petrous pyramid
petrous region
petrous segment of carotid artery
petrousitis (petrositis)
pexis
Peyronie disease
Peyton brain spatula
PF Night splint
PF nucleus (parafascicular)
PFC femoral prosthesis
PFC total hip system
PFD (polyurethane foam dressing)
Pfeiffer syndrome
PFFD (proximal focal femoral
 deficiency)
PFS (primary fibromyalgia syndrome)
PFT (parafascicular thalamotomy)
PFT (postop flexor tendon) traction
 brace
PGK (Panos G. Koutrouvelis, M.D.)
 stereotactic device
PGP nail
phakomatoses
phalangeal branches
phalangeal glenoidal ligament of hand
phalangeal herniation
phalangectomy, partial proximal
phalanx (pl. phalanges)
 base of
 waist of the
Phalen maneuver
Phalen-Miller opponensplasty
Phalen position
Phalen sign
Phalen test
phantom limb pain
phantom pain
phantom sensation
phantom spike-and-wave pattern on
 EEG
pharyngeal dysarthria
phase
 burst
 heel contact phase of gait
 heel-off phase of gait
 in
 midswing phase of gait
 out of
 toe-off phase of gait
phase angle
phase difference
phase lag on EEG
phase relation
phase reversal on EEG
phase reversing slow wave on EEG
phase sensitive detector
phase shift of sleep-wake cycle
phase spike on EEG
phasic nystagmus

plate and screw system
  MRI-compatible
  titanium
Pheasant elbow technique
Phelps brace
Phelps orthosis
Phelps scapulectomy
Phemister-Bonfiglio technique
Phemister elevator
Phemister onlay bone graft technique
Phemister rasp
phenol matricectomy
phenol nerve blocks
phenolization
phenomenon (pl. phenomena)
  A
  baked brain
  Bancaud
  Bell
  combined-flexion
  crus
  doll's eye (oculocephalic reflex)
  extinction
  freezing
  "glued to the floor" (with Parkinson disease)
  Gordon knee
  Gowers
  Kernohan notch
  kindling
  Marin-Amat
  mouthing (pathological reflex)
  on-off
  paroxysmal
  Piltz-Westphal
  psychomotor
  Raynaud
  Robin Hood (steal syndrome)
  Schiff-Sherrington
  setting-sun
  steal syndrome
  Uhthoff
  unilateral Raynaud

phenomenon *(cont.)*
  V
  vertebral steal
  zone (on x-ray)
phenylketonuria (PKU)
phenytoin-induced choreoathetosis
Philadelphia collar cervical support
Philadelphia halo
Philadelphia neck stabilizer
Philadelphia Plastizote cervical brace
Philips linear accelerator (LINAC)
Philips toe force gauge
Phillips screwdriver
phlebogram
phleborheography (PRG)
phlebothrombosis
phocomelia
  complete
  distal
  proximal
Phoenix cranial drill
Phoenix hip prosthesis
Phoenix ICP monitor
Phoenix ventriculostomy catheter
phonatory seizure
phonemic (or literal) paraphasia
phonophobia in migraine
phonophoresis
Phoresor drug delivery system
Phoresor II iontophoretic drug delivery system
phosphenes (in migraine aura)
phospholipids
phosphoproteins
phosphorus-32 therapy
phosphorylase deficiency
photic driving with EEG
photic epilepsy
photic pattern-evoked responses
photic response
photic stimulation during EEG
photocell plethysmography
photoconvulsive response on EEG

photometrazol test
photomotogram
photomyoclonic jerking
photomyoclonic response on EEG
photon densitometry
photoparoxysmal response on EEG
photophobia in migraine
photoplethysmographic digit
photoplethysmography
photopsia
  Christmas-tree
  kleidoscope
photosensitivity on EEG
phrase-completion difficulties
phrase level, automatic
phrenic nerve
physeal arrest of growth
physeal cartilage
physeal closure
physeal damage
physeal distraction
physeal fracture
physeal injury
physes (see *physis*)
physiatrist
physiatry
physical daily living skills (PDLs)
physical dependence
physical medicine and rehabilitation (PM&R)
physical therapist
physical therapy (PT)
physiologic neurologic exam
physiologic nystagmus
  end point
  railway
physiologic tremor
physiology, cyber
physiotherapist
physiotherapy
physis (pl. physes)
  distal tibial
  fibular
  fused
physis *(cont.)*
  medial
  unfused
physocephaly
phytanic acid storage disease
phytosis
pi, locating
pia mater
pial vessels
piano key sign
piano-wire dorsiflexion brace
PICA (Porch Index of Communicative Ability)
PICA (posterior inferior cerebellar artery) syndrome
Pick body
Pick chisel
Pick dementia
Pick disease
Picker Magnascanner for bone metastases
Picket Fence fiducial localization stereotactic system
Picket Fence leg positioner
Pickles ointment
pickup, Newvicon vacuum chamber
pickwickian syndrome
picture archive and communication system (PACs) for x-rays
picture, complex thematic
picture element (pixel)
picture frame pattern of vertebral bodies
Pidcock check pin
piece, chin-occiput
piecemeal, removed
Piedmont fracture
piercer, triangular bone
Pierrot-Murphy tendon technique
piezoelectric potentials
"pigeon toeing" gait
pigmentary degeneration of the globus pallidus
pigmented villonodular synovitis (PVS)

pigmentosa, retinitis
Pillet hand prosthesis
Pilliar total hip replacement
Pilling-Liston rongeur
pillion fracture
Pillo-Pedic cervical traction pillow
pillow (cushion)
  abduction
  Bio-Gel decubitus
  Carter elevation
  Carter foam
  cervical
  cervical support
  elevate on
  foam
  Frejka
  immobilization
  Neck-Huggar cervical support
  Opti-Curve therapeutic
  Pillo-Pedic cervical traction
  PRN
  Sacro-ease (HMR)
  wedge
pillow orthosis for hip
pill-rolling tremor of parkinsonism
piloerection prior to seizure
pilonidal cyst
pilonidal dimple
pilonidal sinus
Piltz-Westphal phenomenon
pin, pinning
  absorbable
  absorbable polyparadioxanone
  Acufex distractor
  alignment
  Austin Moore
  ball guide
  ball-point guide
  ball-tip guide
  beaded hip
  beaded reamer guide
  Beath
  Bilos
  biodegradable

pin *(cont.)*
  Biofix system
  Böhler (Boehler)
  Bohlman
  breakaway
  Breck
  calcaneal
  calibrated
  Canakis
  Charnley
  clavicle
  closed
  collapsible
  Compere threaded
  Compton clavicle
  Conley
  Crego-McCarroll
  Crowe pilot point on Steinmann
  Davis
  Day
  Denham
  DePuy
  Deyerle II
  distractor
  drawing
  drill
  Ender
  Fahey-Compere
  femoral guide
  Fischer transfixing
  Fisher half
  fixation
  Gardner skull clamp
  Gouffon hip
  guide
  Hagie
  Hagie hip
  half
  halo
  Hansen-Street
  Hare
  Hatcher
  Haynes
  Hessel-Nystrom

pin *(cont.)*
- hip
- hook
- hook-end intramedullary
- in situ
- Intraflex intramedullary
- intramedullary
- Jones compression
- Knowles
- Krankendonk
- Küntscher
- LIH (Lars Ingvar Hansson) hook
- locating
- Lottes
- marble bone
- Mayfield skull clamp
- McBride
- metallic
- Modny
- Moore
- Olds
- open
- Oris
- OrthoSorb absorbable fixation
- partially threaded
- percutaneous
- Pidcock check
- polyparadioxanone, absorbable
- precurved ball-tipped guide
- Pritchard Mark II
- rasp
- resorbable
- Rhinelander
- Riordan
- Roger Anderson
- Rush
- Schanz
- Schneider
- Schweitzer
- self-broaching
- Serrato forearm
- Shriner
- skeletal traction
- skull

pin *(cont.)*
- Smith-Petersen
- smooth Steinmann
- socket
- Sofield
- Stader
- Steinmann
- Steinmann (with ball-bearing)
- Street medullary
- strut-type
- tapered
- threaded
- threaded Steinmann
- titanium half
- traction
- transarticular
- transfixing
- transfixion
- Turner
- Varney
- Venable-Stuck
- Vom Saal
- Wagner closed
- wrench
- Zimmer

PIN (percutaneous interosseous nerve)
PIN (posterior interosseous nerve)
- entrapment

pinched nerve
pinch, key
pinch power, thumb
pinch strength
pineal body, calcified, shift of
pineal gland tumors
pineal region
pinealoma, ectopic
pinealoma tumor
pineoblastoma
pineocytoma
pin fixation
ping-pong fracture
pin headrest
pinion, Mayfield
pin length

pinpoint pupils
pinprick sensation
pinprick test of sensation
  absent
  impaired
  normal
pins and needles sensation
pin-site infection
pin-skin interface
Pinto distractor
pin-tract infection
pin traction
pin-tract sepsis
pinwheel testing
pinwheel, Wartenberg neurological
PION (posterior interosseous nerve)
  syndrome
Piotrowski sign
PIP (proximal interphalangeal)
PIP articulation
PIP flexion crease
PIP joint
PIPJ (proximal interphalangeal joint)
pipe stemming of ankle-brachial index
Pipkin classification of femoral fracture
Pirogoff amputation
Pisces spinal cord stimulation system
Pischel micropin
pisiform bone of wrist
pisotriquetral joint
pistol grip (of hand)
piston, cannulated expulsion
pistoning
piston sign (on x-ray)
pitch-fork retractor
pitch of threads on screw
Pittsburgh collimator helmet
Pittsburgh Gamma knife unit
Pittsburgh pelvic frame
pituitary ablation, total
pituitary adenoma
  ACTH-producing
  chromophobe
pituitary apoplexy
pituitary cachexia
pituitary curet
pituitary gland
pituitary microadenoma
pituitary rongeur
pituitary stalk
pituitary tumor
pivot, Accu-Line dual
pivot of calcar
pivot-shift sign
pivot-shift test
pivot transfers
pixel (picture element)
PKU (phenylketonuria)
placebo response
placement, EEG electrode
placode, neural
plafond fracture
plafond, tibial
plagiocephalic
plagiocephaly
plain tomograms
plain x-ray films
planar spin imaging
plane
  anatomic
  areolar
  axial
  capsular
  coronal
  E
  fascial
  flexion-extension
  frontal
  gonion-gnathion
  Hensen
  Hodge
  horizontal
  internervous
  intertubercular
  Ludwig
  median sagittal
  mesiodistal
  midsagittal

plane *(cont.)*
- paramedian sagittal
- pelvic
- perivascular
- sagittal
- sella-nasion
- spinous
- sternoxiphoid
- subcostal
- suprasternal
- thoracic
- transverse
- tumor cleavage
- varus-valgus
- vertical

plane of cleavage of tumor
planer
- Rubin bone
- Rubin cartilage

planigrams
planigraphy
planning, rehabilitation
planovalgus
- pes
- talipes

planovalgus deformity
planovalgus foot
plantar aponeurosis
plantar arterial arch
plantar axial view
plantar callosities
plantare, keratoderma
plantar fascia as windlass mechanism
plantar fasciitis
plantar fasciotomy
plantar flexed
plantar flexion-inversion deformity
plantar flexion, forced
plantar flexor motion
plantar flexor proximal metatarsal osteotomy
plantar keratosis
plantar malignant melanoma
plantar pain
plantar puncture wounds
plantar reflex, equivocal
plantar response
plantar spur
plantar vault
plantaris muscle
plantaris rupture (tennis leg)
plantarward
plantar wart
- mother-daughter type
- mosaic
- satellite
- single

plantigrade foot
planum temporale
planus, talipes
plaque
- MS (multiple sclerosis)
- neuritic
- neuritic senile
- senile

plasma cell myeloma tumor
plasma cells
plasmacytoma, extramedullary
plasmapheresis to treat Guillain-Barré syndrome
plasmatomas, solitary
Plasmodium falciparum
Plastalume finger splint
plaster
- corn removal
- salicylic acid (for plantar warts)
- Velpeau
- Zoroc

plaster-of-Paris (POP) bandage
plaster-of-Paris cast
plaster slab splint
plaster splint
plaster toe cap
plastic, thermolabile
Plastiport TORP prosthesis
Plastizote arch support
Plastizote cervical collar orthosis
Plastizote material

plate
- acetabular reconstruction
- AcroMed VSP
- anchor
- AO blade
- AO condylar blade
- AO contoured T
- AO hook
- AOI blade
- AO reconstruction
- AO semitubular
- AO small fragment
- Armstrong
- ASIF right-angle blade
- Badgley
- Bagby angled compression
- Batchelor
- biodegradable
- blade
- Blount blade
- bone
- bone flap fixation
- Bosworth spine
- Burns
- buttress
- C-shaped
- Calandruccio side
- cap-and-anchor
- cartilaginous growth
- CASP (contoured anterior spinal)
- Caspar cervical
- cervical locking
- cloverleaf
- coaptation
- cobra-head
- Collison
- compression
- condylar
- conical tectal
- connecting
- contoured T-plate
- cortical
- cranial bone fixation
- cribriform

plate *(cont.)*
- DCP (dynamic compression)
- deck
- DePuy
- Deyerle
- dorsal
- double-H
- Driessen hinged
- dual
- Duopress
- Dwyer-Hall
- dynamic compression (DCP)
- E-Z Flap cranial bone
- eccentric dynamic compression (EDCP)
- Eggers bone
- 11-hole
- Elliott femoral condyle blade
- epiphyseal
- femoral
- fibrocartilaginous
- five-hole (5-hole)
- fixed-angle blade
- flexor palmar
- foot
- four-hole (4-hole)
- fusion
- gait
- Gallannaugh bone
- growth
- Hagie sliding nail
- Haid cervical
- half-circle
- Hansen-Street
- Harlow
- Harm posterior cervical
- Harris
- heavy side
- heavy-duty femur
- Hicks lugged
- Hoen skull
- Holt nail
- Howmedica Microfixation cranial
- H-shaped

plate *(cont.)*
- Hubbard
- I plate of Yuan
- interfragmentary
- intertrochanteric
- Jergesen I-beam
- Jergesen tapered
- Jewett nail overlay
- Jones compression
- Kaneda
- Kessel
- L-shaped
- Laing
- Lane
- Lawson-Thornton
- Leibinger 3-D
- Leibinger Micro Plus
- Leibinger Micro System cranial fixation
- Letournel
- Lorenz cranial
- Louis
- low-contact dynamic compression (LC-DCP)
- L-shaped
- Luhr micro
- Luhr Microfixation cranial
- Luhr mini
- Luhr pan
- Lundholm
- Luque-Galveston
- Luque II
- malleable
- Massie
- McBride
- McLaughlin intertrochanteric
- Mears sacroiliac
- meningioma of the cribriform
- Meurig Williams
- microfixation
- Milch
- minifragment
- Moe intertrochanteric
- Moore sliding nail

plate *(cont.)*
- Moreira
- Morscher cervical
- Müller (Mueller) compression blade
- nail
- Neufeld
- neutralization
- Newman
- Nicoll
- occipitocervical
- Ogden
- orbital
- Orozco cervical
- orthotic
- Osborne
- overlay
- palmar
- Paulus
- pedicle
- peg-base
- plain pattern
- planar
- plantar
- pterygoid
- Pugh
- pylon attachment
- quadrangular positioning plate
- quadrigeminal
- reconstruction
- resorbable
- Richards side
- Richards-Hirschhorn
- roof
- Roy-Camille cervical
- Roy-Camille occipitocervical
- Roy-Camille pedicle
- Schweitzer spring
- semitubular compression
- Senn
- serpentine
- seven-hole
- 17-hole
- Sherman bone
- side

plate *(cont.)*
  Simmons
  six-hole (6-hole)
  skull
  slide
  slotted femur
  Smith-Petersen
  Smith-Petersen intertrochanteric
  SMO (supramalleolar orthosis)
  spoon
  stabilization
  stainless steel
  stainless steel preformed skull
  steel sole
  Steffee
  Steffee pedicle
  Steffee screw
  stem base
  Storz Microsystems cranial fixation
  subchondral bone
  supracondylar
  Synthes cervical
  Synthes Microsystem cranial fixation
  Syracuse I
  T
  T buttress
  T-shaped
  T-shaped AO
  tantalum preformed skull
  tarsal
  tectal
  Temple University
  tendon
  Thornton nail
  3-D (three-dimensional)
  three-hole (3-hole)
  titanium
  toe
  Townley tibial plateau
  Townsend-Gilfillan
  trial base
  tubular
  Tupman
  twisted

plate *(cont.)*
  two-hole (2-hole)
  UCP compression
  Uslenghi
  V blade
  V nail
  Venable
  vertebral body
  Vitallium
  volar
  VSP (variable screw placement)
  Wainwright
  Wenger
  Whitman
  Wilson
  wing
  Wright
  Wurzburg
  X-shaped
  Y bone
  Y-shaped
  Zimmer femoral condyle blade
  Zimmer side
  Zimmer Y
  Z-shaped
  Zuelzer hook
plateau
  multiple sclerosis
  tibial
plating technique
Platou osteotomy
platybasia
platyspondylosis
play, excessive joint
PLC (posterolateral corner) of knee
pleating of ligamentum flavum
PLED (periodic lateralized epileptiform discharge) syndrome
pledget, Betadine-soaked
pledget of gauze
Plenk-Matson rasp
pleocytosis
  CSF
  lymphocytic (in CSF)

pleomorphic
pleomorphism, nuclear
pleonosteosis, Léri's
plerocephalic edema (or papilledema)
plethysmography
  air
  digital
  impedance
  photocell
plexiform neurofibromas
Plexiglas splint
plexitis, brachial
plexopathy
  brachial
  idiopathic
  lumbar
  neoplastic
  radiation
  radiation-induced
plexus
  Batson
  brachial
  calcification of choroid
  carotid
  choroid
  lumbar
  lumbosacral
  nerve
  paravertebral nerve
  paravertebral venous
  sciatic
  spinal nerve
  subdermal
  venous
plexus injury
plexus papilloma, choroid
plica (pl. plicae)
  medial
  parapatellar
  suprapatellar
  synovial
plica alaris elongata
plica synovialis mediopatellaris
plicated dural sheaths
plication
  disk
  soft tissue
plicectomy
pliers
  flat nose
  Howmedica Microfixation System
  Leibinger Micro System
  Luhr Microfixation System
  needle-nose
  pair of
  Power-Grip
  Storz Microsystems
  Synthes Microsystem
  taper-nose
  wire-cutting
PLIF (posterior lumbar interbody fusion)
PLL (posterior longitudinal ligament)
plombage, bone
PLSA (posterolateral spinal artery)
plug
  bone
  bone graft
  Buck
  cement
  patellar
plumbism (lead poisoning)
Plummer sign
Plus, Richards Solcotrans
PM&R (physical medicine and rehabilitation)
PMH (pure motor hemiparesis)
PMI-6A1-4V implant metal
PML (progressive multifocal leuko-encephalopathy) viral encephalitis
PMMA (antibiotic-impregnated polymethyl methacrylate) beads
PMMA bone cement
PMR (posteromedial release) for clubfoot
PMS (periodic movements [of the legs] syndrome)
PMS (primary fibromyalgia syndrome)

PMT biopsy needle
PNET (primitive neuroectodermal
 tumor)
pneumatic drill
pneumatic foot pump (mechanical)
pneumatic tourniquet cuff
pneumoarthrogram
pneumocephalus, tension
pneumoencephalitis
pneumoencephalogram (PEG)
pneumoencephalographic pattern
pneumoencephalography
pneumoencephalomyelogram
pneumoencephalomyelography
pneumoencephalos
pneumogram, impedance (used in
 EEG)
PNF (proprioceptive neuromuscular
 facilitation) exercise
pocket, subfascial
podagra
podiatrist
podiatry
PO electrode (parieto-occipital)
 (P_3, P_4, P_7, P_8, P_z)
Pogan buggy
poikilothermia
point
 bleeding
 Crowe pilot
 dorsal
 drill
 electrode insertion
 end
 entry
 Erb
 frontopolar
 glenoid
 Krackow
 Mathews drill
 Pauly
 preauricular
 pressure
 target
point *(cont.)*
 trigger
 twist drill
 Universal drill
pointer
 hip
 shoulder
point imaging
point localization
point scanning
point tenderness
Poirier, space of
poisoning
 barbiturate
 carbon tetrachloride
 Jamaica ginger
 lead
 mercury
 methyl alcohol
 organophosphorus insecticide
Poisson ratio
POL (posterior oblique ligament)
Poland classification of epiphyseal
 fracture
Poland syndrome
Polar-Mate coagulator
Polar-Med postop shoe cover
polar moment of inertia
Polar Vantage XL heart rate monitor
Polar Wrap cold therapy
polarity
 electrical
 negative
 opposite signal
 positive
 reversal of
 simultaneous opposite (on EEG)
polarity of EEG wave
polarization, electrode
pole
 frontal
 patellar
 temporal
pole of scaphoid

poliodystrophy, progressive cerebral
polioencephalitis hemorrhagica superior
polioencephalopathy
poliomyelitis
  nonparalytic
  pseudo-Babinski sign in
poliomyelitis encephalitis
poliomyelitis viral encephalitis
Polk finger goniometer
Polley-Bickel biopsy trephine
pollicization
  Buck-Gramcko
  Gillies
  Littler
  Riordan finger
pollicization of finger
Poly-Dial acetabular cup prosthesis
polyacetal resin
polyarteritis
  alcoholic
  nonalcoholic
polyarteritis nodosa
polyarthritis
polyarthropathy
polyarticular symmetric tophaceous joint inflammation
polycarbonate eyeguards
Polycentric and Wide-Track knee system
polydactyly, thumb
Polydek suture
polyethylene button
polyethylene femoral buck plug procedure
polyethylene liner
polyethylene proximal brims in quadrilateral contour
polyglactin rods
polyglactin sutures
polyglycolide rods, self-reinforced
polygyria
polyimages, visual
polymer
  cold-curing
  self-curing
polymerized
polymethyl methacrylate (PMMA)
polymicrogyria
polymodal neglect
polymorphic activity on EEG
polymorphic waves on EEG
polymyalgia rheumatica
polymyopathy (see also *myopathy*)
  alcoholic
  centronuclear
  rod body
polymyositis, idiopathic
polymyositis myopathy
polyneuritiformis, heredopathia atactica
polyneuritis (see also *neuritis*)
  acute febrile
  acute infectious
  chronic relapsing
  idiopathic
  infectious (Guillain-Barré syndrome)
polyneuritis cranialis
polyneuropathy (see also *neuropathy*)
  acute inflammatory
  chronic inflammatory demyelinating (CIDPN)
  chronic relapsing
  diabetic sensorimotor
  distal
  dying-back
  dysimmune
  gestational
  idiopathic
  peripheral
  recurrent
  sarcoid
  sensorimotor
  sensorimotor axonal
  subacute
  symmetric
  symmetrical

polyneuropathy *(cont.)*
  thallium
  uremic
polyopsia of cerebral origin
polyostotic fibrous dysplasia
polyparadioxanone pin, absorbable
polyphasic sharp wave on EEG
polypropylene insert
polypropylene orthosis
polyradiculoneuropathy
  chronic inflammatory (CIP)
  demyelinating
  inflammatory
  inflammatory demyelinating
polyradiculopathy
  acute inflammatory
  acute inflammatory demyelinating (AIDP)
  chronic inflammatory demyelinating (CIDP)
  diabetic
polyradioculoneuropathy
polyrhythmic activity on EEG
polyrhythmic waves on EEG
Polysar splint
Polysit drug delivery system
polysomnogram, 48-hour
polysomnography
Polysorb liner
polyspike and slow-wave complex on EEG
polyspike and wave paroxysmal pattern on EEG
Polysplint A flexible splinting material
polysynaptic
Polytechnic foot pressure measuring plate
polytetrafluoroethylene graft (PTFE)
polytomography
polytrauma
polyurethane cast
polyurethane foam dressing (PFD)
polyurethane foam embolus
polyvinyl alcohol (PVA) splinting material
Pompe disease
Pond adjustable splint
P_1-P_4 segments of posterior cerebral artery (PCA)
pongid posture
pons (pl. pontes)
  caudal
  infarctions of the
pons and midbrain, tegmentum of
Ponseti splint
pontine
pontine contusion
pontine gaze center
pontine glioma
pontine glioma tumor
pontine hemorrhage
pontine infarct
pontine infarction
pontine lateral gaze center
pontine lesion, high
pontine-medullary levels
pontine parareticular formation (PPRF)
pontis, nucleus
pontocerebellar fibers
pontocerebellar glioma
pontomedullary junction
pontomedullary region
pontomesencephalic junction
pontotegmental syndromes
pool, hydrotherapy
pool therapy
poorly differentiated tumor
pop, popping
POP bandage (plaster-of-Paris)
popeye arm
popliteal fossa
popliteal recess
Poppen-Blalock carotid clamp
Poppen forceps
Poppen-Gelpi laminectomy retractor
Poppen Gigli saw guide
Poppen intervertebral disk rongeur
Poppen ventricular needle
popping of joint

popping sensation
Porch Index of Communicative Ability (PICA)
porcine heterografts
porencephalia
porencephalic cyst
porencephalous
porencephaly, cystic
Porocoat AML noncemented prosthesis
porocoating
porokeratosis palmaris, plantaris et disseminata
porokeratosis plantaris discreta
Porometal noncemented femoral prosthesis
poroplastic splint
porosis, cerebral
porous-coated anatomic (PCA) knee prosthesis
porous coated total hip replacement
porous ingrowth
PORP (partial ossicular replacement) prosthesis
Port-A-Cath
portable C-arm image intensifier fluoroscopy
portable commode
portal
  anterior aspect of ankle
  anterocentral arthroscopic
  anterolateral
  anteromedial arthroscopic
  arthroscopic entry
  arthroscopy
  Caspari arthroscopic
  distal radioulnar joint
  MCR (midcarpal radial)
  MCU (midcarpal ulnar)
  midcarpal radial (MCR)
  midcarpal ulnar (MCU)
  midlateral
  patellar
  posterior aspect of ankle
  posterolateral arthroscopic

portal *(cont.)*
  posteromedial arthroscopic
  radiocarpal
  subacromial arthroscopic
  superolateral
  superomedial
  Swedish
  trans-Achilles arthroscopic
  transmalleolar arthroscopic
Porter-Richardson-Vainio technique
Porteus Maze Test
porthole
portion
  accessory
  cord
portmanteau procedure
Portnoy ventricular cannula
Portnoy ventricular catheter
Porzett splint
Posey belt
Posey restraint
position
  barber chair
  bayonet fracture
  beach chair
  Bonner
  Brickner
  conjugate forward gaze
  decubitus
  dorsal
  dorsal lithotomy
  dorsal recumbent
  figure 4
  Fowler
  frogleg
  full lateral
  Gaynor-Hart
  horizontal
  intrinsic plus
  jackknife
  Jones
  jumper's knee
  kneeling
  Kraske (in surgery)

position *(cont.)*
lateral decubitus
lateral park-bench
lithotomy
lotus
medial genicular
neutral calcaneal stance
neutral hip
normal anatomic
opisthotonic
park bench
Phalen
prayer
prone
proximal bow
rectus
resting calcaneal stance
reverse Trendelenburg
scissor-leg
semi-Fowler
semisitting
side-lying
Sims
spinal fusion
supine
three-quarters prone
Trendelenburg
W-sitting
position of function, splinted in
position sense
positional nystagmus of central origin
positional nystagmus of peripheral origin
positional tremor
positioner (holder)
acetabular cup
Allen
Allen arthroscopic elbow
Allen arthroscopic knee
Allen arthroscopic wrist
arm
Bareskin knee
cup
Hold-and-Hold

positioner *(cont.)*
knee
leg
Mark II Stulberg hip
Mark II Wixson hip
MB&J knee
Montreal hip
Picket Fence leg
Prep-Assist
Profex arthroscopic leg
Stulberg hip
Stulberg Mark II leg
Surg-Assist leg
Wixson hip
positive abilities
positive bottle sign
positron emission tomography scan (PET)
post
Morse tapered prosthetic
perineal
status
thumb
postactivation exhaustion on electromyogram
postactivation increment on electromyogram
postanesthesia recovery (PAR)
postanoxic coma
postanoxic encephalopathy
postauricular ecchymosis
postaxonic myoclonus
postcalcaneal bursitis (posterior calcaneal bursitis)
postcast compression reflex, sympathetic dystrophy
postcasting syndrome
postcentral (sensory) gyrus
postcentral sulcus
postconcussion syndrome
postdialysis seizure
postdiuresis seizure
postdormital sleep paralysis
Postel hip status system

postencephalitic parkinsonism
postepileptic paralysis
posterior (atlantoaxial) membrane
posterior calcaneal bursitis
(postcalcaneal bursitis)
posterior circulation stroke
posterior colliculus
posterior column deficits (of spine)
posterior column disease
posterior column lesions
posterior commissure
posterior communicating artery (PCA)
posterior compartment lesion
posterior displacement osteotomy of
the calcaneus
posterior drawer test
posterior fossa
posterior fossa brain mass
posterior fossa brain tumor
posterior fossa lesion
posterior fossa stare
posterior fossa tumor
posterior fracture-dislocation
posterior gray column of cord
posterior gray horns of the spinal
canal
posterior inferior cerebellar artery
(PICA)
posterior interosseous nerve syndrome
posterior joint syndrome
posterior language area lesion
posterior leaf spring orthosis
posterior lobe tumors
posterior lumbar interbody fusion
(PLIF)
posterior medial ankle ligaments
posterior medial ligament
posterior median septum, of cord
posterior metatarsal arch
posterior olive, in brain
posterior root ganglia
posterior roots
posterior shin splint
posterior spinocerebellar tract
posterior subluxation
posterior talofibular ligament
posterior third frontal gyrus
posterior tibial nerve entrapment
posterior tibiofibular ligament
posterior tibiotalar ligament
posterolateral aspect
posterolateral sclerosis disease
posterolateral sclerosis of the spinal
cord
posterolateral spinal artery (PLSA)
posteromedial release (PMR)
postfracture osteomyelitis
postfracture swelling
postfracture syndrome
postganglionic fibers
postganglionic gray fibers
posthemiparesis syndrome
postherpetic facial pain
posthypoxic myoclonic seizures
posthypoxic myoclonus
postictal alpha slowing on EEG
postictal bisynchronous slow wave
postictal confusion
postictal depression
postictal drowsiness
postictally
postictal mutism
postictal paralysis
postictal period
postictal slowing on EEG
postictal state
postinfectious encephalitis
postinfectious encephalopathy
postinfectious leukoencephalopathy
postinjection reflex sympathetic
dystrophy
postlaminectomy instability
post-LP (lumbar puncture) headache
postmenopausal
postmetrizamide CT scan
postneuritic atrophy
postneurosurgical evaluation
postoperative wound care

postpoliomyelitic muscle contracture
postreduction x-ray
postrema of medulla
post-rolandic parietal cortex
POSTS (positive occipital sharp transients) on EEG
poststress ankle/arm Doppler index
postsynaptic cortical neuronal potential
postsynaptic neuronal membrane patch
postsynaptic potential (PSP)
postsynaptic receptor
post-tetanic potentiation
Post total shoulder arthroplasty
posttraumatic amnesia (PTA)
posttraumatic angulation
posttraumatic apoplexy of Bollinger
posttraumatic arthritis
posttraumatic cavus
posttraumatic cerebral syndrome
posttraumatic chronic disability
posttraumatic chronic osteomyelitis
posttraumatic cortical dysfunction
posttraumatic encephalopathy
posttraumatic epilepsy
posttraumatic fibrosis
posttraumatic headache
posttraumatic neck pain
posttraumatic neuroma
posttraumatic osteoarthritis
posttraumatic vertigo
posttreatment evaluation
posttreatment neuropsychologic evaluation
postural awareness
postural fixation
postural instability
postural seizure
postural tone
postural tremor
posture, posturing
  batrachian
  benediction (of hand)
  benedictory
  decerebrate

posture *(cont.)*
  decorticate and decerebrate
  dystonic
  extensor
  flexor dystonic
  forward-head
  good
  opisthotonic
  poor
  round back
  stooped
  tonic
posture of limbs
Posture Curve lumbar cushion
Posture Training Support (PTS)
Posturite paper holder
postvaccinial leukoencephalitis
potential
  acoustic evoked
  action
  attack-specific
  auditory evoked
  bias
  biphasic
  brain stem auditory evoked (BAEP)
  brain stem evoked
  bursts of muscle
  cerebral
  compound motor action (CMAP)
  compound muscle action (CMAP)
  compound nerve action (CNAP)
  cortical evoked
  cortical somatosensory evoked (CSSEP)
  denervation
  difference between
  EEG
  electrical
  EMG
  evoked
  excitatory postsynaptic (EPSP)
  extracerebral (on EEG)
  far-field
  fasciculation

potential *(cont.)*
  fibrillation
  glossokinetic
  high-frequency
  inhibitory postsynaptic (IPSP)
  localized evoked
  long-duration
  median mixed nerve action
  membrane
  microvolts of sensory
  millivolts of motor response
  miniature endplate (MEPP)
  motor evoked (MEP)
  motor nerve-evoked
  motor unit action (MUAP)
  near-field
  nerve action (NAP)
  normal motor (on EMG)
  P100
  piezoelectric
  polyphasic
  polyphasic motor unit
  posterior tibial nerve-evoked
  postsynaptic (PSP)
  postsynaptic cortical neuronal
  propagated volley
  recruitment of motor unit
  resting
  satellite
  scalp
  sensory evoked (SEP)
  sensory nerve action (SNAP)
  sensory nerve action potential (SNAP)
  serrated
  short-duration motor unit
  skin
  somatosensory
  somatosensory evoked (SEP, SSEP)
  spinal dorsal horn
  spinal evoked (SEP)
  spinal sensory evoked
  visual evoked (VEP)
  voluntary motor unit
potential cumulative trauma disorders
potential P300 latency
potentiation, post-tetanic
Potenza arthrodesis
Pott (18th century British surgeon)
Pott abscess
Pott disease
Pott fracture of fibula
Pott paraplegia
Pott puffy tumor
Potter arthrodesis
Potts (20th century pediatric surgeon)
Potts eversion osteotomy
Potts rib shears
Potts scissors
Potts-Smith dressing forceps
Potts-Smith scissors
Potts splint
Potts tenotomy scissors
Potts tibial osteotomy
Potts-Yasargil scissors
pouce flottant (floating thumb)
pouch
  dural root
  Rathke (in the brain)
  suprapatellar
pound, foot
pounds of traction
Poupart inguinal ligament
Pourfour du Petit syndrome
poverty of movement
powder
  bone
  cranioplastic
  thrombin
  zinc peroxide
power-driven saw
power grip, of hand
power
  motor
  muscle
PowerCut drill blade
Powered Metaphyseal Stapler
powered shaver

Powerflex CPM exerciser
Power-Grip pliers
power-train
PPPMA (progressive post-polio muscle atrophy)
PPRF (paramedian pontine reticular formation)
PPRF (pontine parareticular formation)
PRA (proximal reference axis)
Prader-Willi syndrome
pragmatics
Pratt technique
praxis
  constructional
  ideational
  ideomotor
praxis testing
preauricular point
precentral gyrus
precentral seizures
precentral sulcus
precession
precessional frequency
precipitate a migraine
precision grips, of hand
Precision Osteolock femoral prosthesis
Precision Osteolock hip prosthesis
Precision total hip
precoated layer
precommunicating segment of anterior cerebral artery
precuneate
precuneus
precursor, serotonin
precursor sign to rupture of aneurysm
predisposition to migraine
predominance
  anterior
  posterior
  temporal
predormital sleep paralysis
predormition
predrilling
preexisting
preferential use of right/left hand
prehensile hand movements
prehension
premature suture synostosis
premedullary arteriovenous fistula
premonition of seizure
premonitory sign
premonitory symptoms (of seizures)
premorbid level of functioning
premorbid traits
premotor area
preneurosurgical evaluation
Prenyl jacket
Prep-Assist leg holder
Prep-Assist leg positioner
preparation, Sayk (of CSF cells)
prepared and draped
prepatellar bursa
prepatellar bursitis
prepontine cistern
prep, 3M
prereduction x-ray
prerubral field nucleus
PREs (progressive resistive exercises)
presacral mass
presacral neurectomy
presbyophrenia
Presbyterian Hospital staphylorrhaphy elevator
prescapula
presenile dementia
presenile onset of dementia
preservation of insight
preservation of nerve
pre-slip changes (on x-ray)
Press-Fit component
Press-Fit Condylar Total Knee
Press-Fit design
Press-Fit stem
pressor reflexes
pressoreceptor

pressure
  ankle systolic
  bone marrow (BMP)
  central venous (CVP)
  cerebral perfusion (CPP)
  cerebrospinal fluid
  closing pressure on lumbar puncture
  colloid oncotic
  compartmental
  continuous positive airway (CPAP)
  cranial perfusion (CPP)
  Doppler ankle systolic
  Doppler calf systolic
  Doppler thigh systolic
  elevated intracranial
  increased intracranial
  interstitial fluid hydrostatic
  intracranial (ICP)
  intracranial epidural (ICEDP)
  intradiskal
  intraspinal epidural (ISEDP)
  manual
  opening pressure on lumbar puncture
  perfusion
  photoelectric skin
  regional cerebral perfusion (rCPP)
  spinal tap opening
  TMA
  toe systolic
  tourniquet
pressure fracture
pressure monitor, subdural
pressure necrosis, from bed rest
pressure sella
pressure sore
pressure wave
Preston ligamentum flavum forceps
Preston Traveler CPM exerciser
presynaptic terminal
presyncope
pretectal area
pretectal lesion
pretectal nucleus (region of midbrain)
pretectal region
pretendinous bands (of hand)
pretendinous cord
pretibial edema
pretibial region
pretreatment evaluation
pretreatment neuropsychologic
  evaluation
PRE 2 suture
prevertebral soft tissue
Prévost sign
pre-walking treatment of pronated feet
  in infancy
PRG (phleborheography)
Pribham suction tubes
Price muscle biopsy clamp
prickling
Prieser disease
primary aminoaciduria
primary auditory cortex
primary brain tumor
primary, cancer of unknown (CUP)
primary closure
primary craniosynostosis
primary degenerative dementia
primary fibromyalgia syndrome (PFS)
primary gain
primary intention, healing by
primary metallic fixation
primary myopathies
primary optic atrophy
primary rigid fixation
primary sarcoma
primary suture of ruptured tendons
primary visual cortex
prime movers (agonist muscle groups)
primitive dislocation
primitive neuroectodermal tumor
primitive reflexes
principle
  axial compression
  Enneking
prion (slow virus)
prism, Fresnel
Pritchard Mark II pin

Pritchard-Walker total elbow prosthesis
probe
  Acufex
  angled
  arthroscopic
  bipolar cautery (BICAP)
  Bunnell
  Bunnell dissecting
  Bunnell forwarding
  Dandy
  dissecting
  electromagnetic focusing field (EFF)
  forwarding
  hemispherical contact
  intraosseous
  Jacobson
  Jacobson micro
  Jannetta
  laser Doppler
  Laserflo Doppler
  LDF (laser-Doppler flowmetry)
  McCain TMJ
  micro
  Nucleotome aspiration
  Nucleotome Flex II cutting
  pedicle
  radiofrequency
  skin temperature monitoring
  Steffee
  Surgical Dynamics aspiration
  tulip
  ultrasonic
problem, high level motor
procaine-phenol motor point injection
procedure (see also *operations*)
  ablative
  activating (on EEG)
  chiropractice adjustment
  debulking
  magnetic source imaging (MSI)
  manipulative (chiropractic adjustments)
  porte manteau
  salvage
procedure time
process
  angular orbital
  clinoid
  concrete thought
  cytoplasmic
  diffuse encephalopathic
  inflammatory process of the superior orbital fissure
  interspinous
  monarthric
  neoplastic process of the superior orbital fissure
  odontoid (dens)
  osseous destructive
  pathomechanical
  processes
  radiostyloid
  SinterLock CSTi bonding
  spinous
  Ti-Nidium surface hardening
  transverse vertebral
  uncinate
  vertebral
processing, higher integrative language
ProCol bovine bioprosthesis tendon
procurvature deformity
prodromal symptom
prodrome
  affective (of epilepsy or migraine)
  epileptic
  irritability
  migraine headache
  visual
Pro-8 ankle brace
Profex arthroscopic leg positioner
Profex arthroscopic tourniquet
profile, Profile
  Functional Limitation (FLP)
  Maryland Foot Score
  Nottingham Health (NHP)
  PULSES
  rotational
  Sickness Impact (SIP)
  Staheli rotational

Profile hip prosthesis
profound
prognosticator, classification system as
program
  exercise
  home exercise
  treatment
  weight-training
  Williams exercise
progression to full weightbearing
progressive cerebral poliodystrophy
progressive dementing illness
progressive diaphyseal dysplasia
progressive external ophthalmoplegia
progressive multifocal leuko-encephalopathy (PML) viral encephalitis
progressive myoclonic epilepsy
progressive resistance
progressive resistive exercises (PREs)
progressive rostral-caudal brain stem dysfunction
progressive supranuclear palsy
progressive weights
Progressive Matrices Test
Prohance contrast medium
projection system, diffuse thalamic
prolactin-secreting adenoma
prolactinoma
Prolene suture
proliferation
  angiofibroblastic
  myointimal
  osteophytic
  synovial
  villous
proliferation of Schwann cells
PROM (passive range of motion) exercise
prominence
  bony (spur)
  tibial tubercle
prominence of forehead
pronated foot
pronated straight flatfoot
pronation and supination
pronation
  hallucal
  rearfoot
  subtalar joint
pronation-external rotation (P-ER) injury
pronation sign
pronator
  round (pronator radii teres)
  square (pronator quadratus)
pronator drift
pronator quadratus
pronator reflex test
pronator sign
pronator syndrome
pronator teres syndrome
prone scapular retraction exercises
prong, modified tonsil
ProOsteon synthetic bone implant
propagation, seizure
prophylactic antibiotic therapy
prophylactic anticoagulation
Proplast prosthesis
proportionality, cephalofacial
proprioception, foot
proprioceptive end organs
proprioceptive neuromuscular facilitation (PNF)
proprioceptive sense of muscles and ligaments
proprioceptive vertigo
proprius, nucleus
propulsion of gait
propulsive foot
propulsive forces
prosencephalon
prosody
prosopagnosia
prostaglandin E_1
prosthesis, prostheses
  acetabular
  Aesculap-PM noncemented femoral

prosthesis *(cont.)*
AFI total hip replacement
AGC (anatomically graduated component)
AGC femoral
AGC knee
AGC tibial
AHP (American Hand Prosthesis)
AHP digital
AHSC (Arizona Health Science Center-Volz) elbow
Aliplast insoles
Alivium implant metal
AMC total wrist
AML (anatomic medullary locking) hip
AML Tang femoral
Amstutz cemented hip (TR-28)
Anametric total knee
anatomic surface
Anderson acetabular
Angelchik anti-reflux
ankle
aortic valve
APR (anatomic porous replacement)
APR acetabular
APR femoral
APR II
APRL hand
Arafiles elbow
Arizona Health Science Center-Volz (AHSC) elbow
Arthopor acetabular cup
Arthopor cup (I, II, III)
Atkinson endoprosthesis
Attenborough knee
Aufranc cobra hip
Aufranc-Turner
Aufranc-Turner cemented hip
Austin Moore hip
Autophor ceramic total hip
Autophor femoral
Averett hip
ball-and-socket ankle

prosthesis *(cont.)*
Bankart shoulder
Bateman UPF
Bateman UPF II bipolar hip
Bateman UPF II shoulder
BDH (biologically designed hip)
Bechtol hip
Bechtol shoulder
Beck-Steffee total ankle
Becker hand
Bi-Angular shoulder
Bi-Metric hip
Bias hip
bicentric
bicompartmental knee implant
bicondylar ankle
bicondylar knee
Bio-Chromatic hand
biodegradable implants
biodegradable self-reinforced polyglycolide rods
Biofit press-fit acetabular
Bio-Groove Macrobond HA femoral
Biomet
Biomet AGC
Biomet hip
Biometric
Biophase implant metal
Biotex implant metal
bipolar femoral head
bipolar hip replacement
Blazina
Bock knee
Bombelli-Mathys-Morscher hip
bovine collagen material
Brigham
Bryan total knee implant
Buchholz ankle
Buchholz hip
C-2 OsteoCap hip
CAD (computer-assisted design) femoral
CAD femoral stem

prosthesis *(cont.)*
- Caffinière
- Calandruccio cemented hip
- calcar replacement femoral
- Callender hip
- Calnan-Nicolle metatarsophalangeal
- Calnan-Nicolle synthetic joint
- capitellocondylar unconstrained elbow
- carpal lunate implant
- carpal scaphoid implant
- Cathcart Orthocentric hip
- Centralign hip
- ceramic femoral head
- Ceramion
- Charnley cemented
- Charnley low friction hip
- Charnley-Hastings
- Charnley-Mueller hip
- Chatzidakis hinged Vitallium implant
- Chopart partial foot
- Christiansen hip
- Cintor knee
- CKS (Continuum knee system)
- Cloutier unconstrained knee
- Coballoy implant metal
- CoCr alloy (cobalt-chromium)
- Co-Cr-Mo alloy (cobalt-chromium-tungsten-nickel)
- Co-Cr-W-Ni alloy (cobalt-chromium-tungsten-nickel)
- Cofield shoulder
- cold-mold
- cold-weld
- collar-calcar support femoral
- Compartmental II
- compression-molded
- Conaxial total ankle
- constrained hinged
- Continuum knee system (CKS)
- Contour internal
- Coonrad hinge
- Coonrad semiconstrained elbow

prosthesis *(cont.)*
- CSF (contoured femoral stem) hip
- custom-threaded
- Cutter-Smeloff cardiac valve
- D'Aubigné femoral
- DANA shoulder
- Deane unconstrained knee
- Dee totally constrained elbow
- Deon hip
- De La Caffinière trapezio-metacarpal
- DePalma
- DePuy AML Porocoat stem
- DF80 (Wilson-Burstein) hip
- digital
- Dimension hip
- Dimension/C femoral stem
- doffing (taking it off)
- donning (putting it on)
- Dorrance hand
- Dow Corning implant
- Dow Corning Wright finger joint
- dual-lock hip
- Dupaco knee
- Duracon
- Dynaplex knee
- Eaton
- Eaton finger joint replacement
- Eicher femoral
- elbow
- ELP femoral
- Endo-Model rotating knee joint
- endoprosthesis
- Engelhardt femoral
- Eriksson knee
- Evolution hip
- Ewald unconstrained elbow
- Exeter cemented hip
- femoral
- Fett
- finger
- finger joint implant
- FIRST knee
- fixed femoral head

prosthesis *(cont.)*
- Flatt finger joint
- Flatt finger/thumb
- Flexfoot foot
- forearm lift-assist
- forged cobalt-chromium alloy
- four-bar linkage on knee
- Freeman modular total hip
- Freeman-Samuelson
- Freeman-Swanson knee
- F.R. Thompson femoral
- fully constrained tricompartmental knee
- Gaffney ankle
- Gemini hip system
- Genesis knee
- Geomedic total knee
- Geometric total knee
- Gerard
- Gianturco
- Giliberty femoral
- Giliberty hip
- Gillette joint
- Gore-Tex knee
- great toe implant
- Gripper acetabular cup
- Gritti-Stokes knee
- GSB (Gschwind-Scheier-Bahler) elbow
- Guepar hinged knee
- Gunston knee
- Gunston-Hult knee
- Gustilo hip
- Gustilo knee
- HA 65101 implant metal
- Hamas
- hand
- Harris Design 1 (or 2) femoral
- Harris-CDH hip
- Harris (HD-2) cemented hip
- Harris-Galante hip
- Hastings hip
- Haynes-Stellite (HS) implant metal
- Hedley-Hungerford hip

prosthesis *(cont.)*
- Henschke-Mauch SNS knee
- Herbert knee
- Hexcel knee
- HG Multilock hip
- hinged implant
- hinged knee
- hip replacement
- Hittenberger
- Howmedica Kinematic II knee
- HPS II hip
- HSS knee
- Hunter tendon
- Hydra-Cadence knee
- Hydroxial hip
- ICLH (Imperial College London Hospital)
- ICLH ankle
- ICLH knee
- Impact total hip
- Indiana conservative
- Indong Oh
- Insall-Burstein II knee
- Insall-Burstein semiconstrained tricompartmental knee
- Insall-Burstein total knee
- Integrity acetabular cup
- Intermedics Natural-Knee knee
- Iowa
- Ishizuki unconstrained elbow
- Jaffe-Capello-Averill hip
- Joplin toe
- Judet press-fit hip
- Kastec mitral valve
- Kessler
- Kinematic fully constrained tricompartmental knee
- Kinematic II rotating hinge total knee
- Kinemax Plus knee
- Kirschner Medical Dimension
- KMC femoral stem
- KMP femoral stem
- KMW/PC femoral

prosthesis *(cont.)*
- knee
- Koenig MPJ
- Kudo unconstrained elbow
- Küntscher humeral
- Lacey fully constrained tricompart mental knee
- LaPorte total toe
- LCS New Jersey knee prosthesis
- Leinbach femoral
- Lewis expandable adjustable (LEAP)
- Lewis Trapezio
- Ling cemented hip
- Lippman hip
- Lisfranc below-knee
- Liverpool elbow
- Liverpool knee
- Lo Bak spinal support
- locking
- Lo-Por vascular graft
- London unconstrained elbow
- Lord Press-Fit hip
- Lord total hip
- Lowe-Miller unconstrained elbow
- low-neck femoral
- low-profile femoral
- Lubinus knee
- lunate acrylic cement wrist
- Lunceford-Pilliar-Engh hip
- MacIntosh knee
- MacNab-English shoulder
- Macrofit hip
- madreporic hip
- Mallory-Head total hip
- manual locking knee
- MAPF femoral stem
- Marmor modular knee
- Matchett-Brown cemented hip
- Mathys
- Matrol femoral head
- Mayo ankle
- Mayo semiconstrained elbow
- Mazas totally constrained elbow

prosthesis *(cont.)*
- McBride femoral
- McCutcheon SLT hip
- McGehee elbow
- McKee-Farrar total hip
- McKeever Vitallium cap
- McKeever Vitallium knee
- Mecring acetabular
- Mediloy implant metal
- medium profile femoral
- metal
- metal femoral head
- MG II knee
- Michael Reese articulated
- Microknit vascular graft
- Microloc knee
- migration of
- Miller-Galante hip
- Miller-Galante knee
- Milliknit vascular graft
- Minneapolis
- Mittlemeir ceramic hip
- Mittlemeir noncemented femoral
- modular total hip
- modular unicompartmental knee
- Monk hip
- Moore femoral
- Moore hip
- MP35N implant metal
- MST-6A1-4V
- Mueli wrist
- Mueller (Müller) Duo-Lock hip
- Mueller total hip replacement
- Muhlberger orbital implant
- multiaxis
- myoelectric control for upper arm
- Naden-Rieth hip
- Natural-Knee knee
- NEB (New England Baptist) hip
- Neer I and II shoulder replacement
- Neer umbrella
- Neer Vitallium humeral
- Neville tracheal and tracheo-bronchial

prosthesis *(cont.)*
New Jersey LCS knee
Newton ankle
Nexus hip
Niebauer
Noiles fully constrained
nonhinged knee
nonhinged linked
Normalize press-fit hip
nudge control on
Odland ankle
Oh cemented hip
Oh press-fit hip
Oklahoma ankle
Omnifit HA hip stem
Omnifit knee
Optifix femoral
Oregon Poly II ankle
Orthochrome implant metal
Orthofix
Ortholoc implant metal
orthopedic
OsteoCap hip
Osteolock femoral
Osteonics hip
Otto Bock modular PTB
Overdyke hip
Panje voice button
partial ossicular replacement
patellar
PCA E-Series femoral
PCA knee (porous-coated anatomic)
PCA unconstrained tricompartmental
PCA unicompartmental knee
pegged tibial
Perfecta hip
Performance knee
Phoenix hip
Pillet hand
Plastiport TORP
PMI-6A1-4V implant metal
polycentric knee
Poly-Dial acetabular cup
polyethylene patellar implant

prosthesis *(cont.)*
Porocoated AML noncemented
Porometal noncemented femoral
porous coated anatomic (PCA) knee
porous surfaced
porous-coated hip
PORP (partial ossicular replacement)
Precision Osteolock femoral
Precision Osteolock hip
precoat hip
Press-Fit condylar total knee
Press-Fit implant
Pritchard-Walker semiconstrained elbow
ProCol bovine bioprosthesis
Profile hip
Protasul-10 noncemented femoral
Protasul-64 WF Zweymuller
provisional
PTB (patellar tendon-bearing) strap of
PTB supracondylar (SC)
PTB suprapatellar (SP)
PTS soft wedge
radial head implant
RAM knee
Ranawat-Burstein hip
Richards hip
Richards hydroxyapatite PORP
Richards Spectron metal-backed
Richards Zirconia femoral head
Ring total hip
RM isoelastic hip
Robert Brigham total knee
Rosenfeld hip
rotating femoral head
rotating hinge
Rothman Institute femoral
S-ROM femoral stem
SACH (solid-ankle, cushioned heel) foot
SAF (self-articulating femoral)
Sarmiento (STH-2) hip
Sauerbach

prosthesis *(cont.)*
- Savastano Hemi-Knee
- Sbarbaro hip
- Sbarbaro tibial plateau
- Schlein elbow
- Schlein semiconstrained elbow
- seated
- seating of the
- Seattle foot
- Select ankle
- Select shoulder
- self-bearing ceramic hip
- semiconstrained tricompartmental
- Sharrard-Trentani
- Sheehan knee
- Sheehy incus replacement
- Sherfee
- Shier total knee
- Silastic
- Silastic ball spacer
- Silastic radial head
- Silflex intramedullary
- silicone elastomer rubber ball
- silicone trapezium
- single-axis ankle
- sintered implant
- SinterLock implant metal
- Sivash hip
- SKI knee
- SMA
- Smith ankle
- Smith-Petersen
- Souter unconstrained elbow
- Spectron hip
- Speed
- spherocentric fully constrained
- spherocentric knee
- stainless steel implant metal
- Stanmore elbow
- Stanmore totally constrained
- Starr-Edwards Silastic ball valve
- STD hip
- stemmed
- stemmed tibial

prosthesis *(cont.)*
- Stevens-Street elbow
- St. George-Buchholz ankle
- St. George total elbow
- St. Jude Medical valve
- STH-2 (Sarmiento) hip
- Street-Stevens humeral
- SuperCup acetabular cup
- Surgitek
- Sutter double-stem silicone implant
- Sutter MCP joint
- Sutter-Smeloff heart valve
- Swanson great toe
- Swanson metacarpal
- Swanson metatarsal
- Swanson T-shaped great toe
- Swanson wrist
- Syme amputation
- Syme foot
- Synatomic knee
- synthetic
- talar part of ankle
- Taperloc femoral
- TARA (total articular replacement arthroplasty) hip
- Tavernetti-Tennant
- TCCK unconstrained knee
- Thackray hip
- Tharies hip replacement
- thermomechanical implant metal
- Thompson femoral neck
- Thompson hip
- threaded titanium acetabular (TTAP)
- Thurst plate femoral
- Ti-BAC II hip prosthesis
- Ti-Con
- tibial part of ankle
- tibial plateau
- Tilastin hip
- Tillman
- Titan cemented hip
- titanium hip
- titanium implant
- Tivanium implant metal

prosthesis *(cont.)*
- TORP (total ossicular replacement)
- Total Condylar Knee
- Total Condylar semiconstrained tricompartmental
- total hip replacement
- total joint replacement
- total knee replacement
- Townley TARA
- TPR ankle
- TR-28 hip
- trapezium implant
- Trapezoidal-28 hip
- Triad hip
- trial
- Tri-Axial
- triaxial semiconstrained elbow
- tricompartmental knee
- Tricon-M patellar
- Tri-Lock
- TTAP-ST acetabular
- two-prong stem finger
- UCI ankle
- UHMWPE (ultrahigh molecular weight polyethylene)
- ulnar head implant
- unconstrained tricompartmental knee
- unicompartmental knee
- Universal hip
- UPF (universal proximal femur)
- Valls hip
- Vanghetti
- Varikopf
- Vinertia implant metal
- Vitallium-W implant metal
- Volz wrist
- Wada valve
- Wadsworth unconstrained elbow
- Wagner
- Wall stent biliary endoprosthesis
- Walldius knee
- Waugh ankle
- Waugh knee

prosthesis *(cont.)*
- Waugh total ankle replacement
- Wehrs incus
- well-seated
- Whiteside knee
- Whiteside Ortholoc II condylar femoral
- William Harris hip
- Wilson-Burstein (DF80) hip
- wrist joint implant
- wrought cobalt-chromium alloy
- Xenophor femoral
- YIS knee
- Young hinged knee
- Young-Vitallium hinged
- Zimalite implant metal
- Zimaloy implant metal
- Zimmer shoulder
- Zirconia femoral head
- Zirconia orthopedic
- zirconium oxide ceramic
- Z stent
- Zweymuller cementless hip

prosthesis cup

prosthetic femorodistal graft

prosthetic hook

prosthetic sheath/liner, Silipos Distal Dip

prosthetic support

Prosthetic Problem Inventory Scale

prosthetics and orthotics (P&O)

prosthetist

Protasul implant metal

protection, radiologic
- adequate collimation
- filtration
- gonadal shielding

protective limitation of range of motion

protective spasm

protector
- Adson drill guide and dura
- Adson dural
- Alvarado collateral ligament

protector *(cont.)*
  Ankle Ligament (ALP)
  collateral ligament
  dural
  grooved
  heel
  Heelbo decubitus heel/elbow
  M-F Athletic heel
  Ortho-Foam
  PRN
  self-retaining
  tissue
Protecto splint
Protect Point needle
protein
  antiglial fibrillary acidic
  Bence Jones
  C-reactive (CRP)
  glial fibrillary acidic (GFAP)
protein kinase C
protein S deficiency
proteoglycan gel of nucleus pulposus
proteoglycans, disk matrix
proteolytic enzymes in rheumatoid arthritis
Proteus syndrome
protocol, Bruce
proton
Protoplast cement
Protouch synthetic orthopedic padding
Pro-Trac cruciate reconstruction system
Pro-Trac measurement device
Pro-Trac system for knee surgery
protrusio acetabuli
protrusion
  disk
  hip
protrusion of the navicular
protrusio shill
protuberance, occipital
proud flesh
proverb interpretation testing
  abstract responses
  concrete responses
proverb interpretation testing *(cont.)*
  semi-abstract responses
provocative maneuvers
provocative test for epilepsy
prow effect
proximal articular set angle (PASA)
proximal bow position
proximal carpal row
proximal denervation
proximal first metatarsal osteotomy
proximal focal femoral deficiency (PFFD)
proximal phalangeal osteotomy
proximal phocomelia
proximal weakness
proximally
Pruitt-Inahara shunt
PSA (power spectral analysis)
PSA thermoplastic orthosis
psammoma body
psammomatous meningiomas
PSE (portal-systemic encephalopathy)
pseudarthrosis
  congenital
  Girdlestone
  interspinous
pseudo-Argyll Robertson pupil
pseudoarthrosis (see *pseudarthrosis*)
pseudoathetosis
pseudo-Babinski sign in poliomyelitis
pseudobulbar palsy
pseudobulbar signs
pseudocapsule
pseudocapsulectomy
pseudocholinesterase syndrome
pseudoclaudication
pseudocoma
pseudodementia, hysterical
pseudodura
pseudoepileptogenic pattern on EEG
pseudofacilitation on electromyogram
pseudo-Foster-Kennedy sign
pseudo-Foster-Kennedy syndrome
pseudogout

pseudo-Hurler deformity
  (mucolipidosis III)
pseudohypertrophic dystrophy
pseudohypertrophic musculature in
  myotonia congenita
pseudohypertrophy of calves
pseudohypoparathyroidism
pseudo-internuclear ophthalmoplegia
pseudojoints
pseudomalignant, non-neoplastic
  osseous soft tissue tumors
pseudomeningocele
pseudomigraine
Pseudomonas aeruginosa osteomyelitis
pseudomyasthenic symptom
pseudomyotonia, Debré-Sémélaigne
pseudomyotonic reflex
pseudonephritis, athlete's
pseudoneurasthenic syndrome
pseudoneuroma
pseudopapilledema
pseudosclerosis, spastic
pseudoseizure
pseudosheath
pseudotabes, diabetic
pseudothrombophlebitis
pseudotumor cerebri (PTC)
pseudotumor, orbital
pseudoxanthoma elasticum
psittacosis encephalitis
psittacosis viral encephalitis
psoas abscess
PSP (postsynaptic potential)
PSP (progressive supranuclear palsy)
psyche, tumor
psychiatry, rehabilitation (RP)
psychic disturbance
psychic equivalent
psychic seizure
psychogenic amnesia
psychogenic hyperventilation
psychogenic rheumatism
psychogenic seizure
psychogenic unresponsiveness
psychogenic vertigo
psychometric testing
psychomotor activity
psychomotor attacks
psychomotor epilepsy
psychomotor fit
psychomotor phenomena
psychomotor retardation
psychomotor seizure
psychomotor slowing
psychomotor symptom
psychomotor variant of epilepsy
psycho-optical reflex controls
psychosensory aphasia
psychosensory stimuli
psychosensory symptom
psychosis, Korsakoff
PT (physical therapy)
PT (prothrombin time)
PTA (posttraumatic amnesia)
PTB ankle-foot orthosis
  (patellar tendon-bearing)
PTB brace
PTB-SC-SP prosthesis
PTB supracondylar (SC) prosthesis
PTB suprapatellar (SP) prosthesis
PTC (pseudotumor cerebri)
pterion
pterional approach
pterional craniotomy
pterygopalatine neuralgia
PTFE graft (polytetrafluoroethylene)
PTF ligament (posterior talofibular)
P-3 suture
P300 latency, potential
ptosis
  bilateral
  ipsilateral
  myasthenic
  unilateral
  upside-down
ptosis of eyelid
ptosis of third nerve paresis
  complete
  partial
PTS (patellar tendon stabilization)

PTS (Posture Training Support)
PTS soft wedge prosthesis
PTT (partial thromboplastin time)
PTT (patellar tendon transfer)
PTTT (posterior tibialis tendon transfer)
PTV (posterior terminal vein)
P-type (persistent) alpha rhythm
puberty, precocious
pubic rami
pubic symphysis
puboischial area
Puddu tendon technique
Pudenz flushing chamber
Pudenz flushing valve
Pudenz peritoneal catheter
Pudenz shunt
Pugh plate
Pugh sliding nail
Pugh traction
pugilistica, dementia
Puka chisel
pulley
  A1 (first annular)
  cruciate
pulley exercises
pulleys of fingers
pull-out technique
Pulmonair 40-bed
pulmonary embolism (PE)
pulp
  finger
  thumb
pulp plasty
pulp space
pulposus
  nucleus
  proteoglycan gel of nucleus
pulsation
Pulsavac lavage
pulse, pulses
  carotid
  dorsalis pedis
  EEG calibration
  radiofrequency
pulse lavage irrigation
pulse lavage system
pulse length
pulse sequences
pulse volume waveforms
pulse width
pulsed electromagnetic field (PEMF) therapy
pulsed gradients
pulsed ultrasound
pulseless disease
PULSES disability profile
  P physical condition
  U upper extremity function
  L lower extremity function
  S sensory and communication abilities
  E excretory control
  S social support
pulsing current (electrostimulation) for nonunion of fracture
Pulver-Taft fish-mouth stitch
Pulver-Taft weave
pulvinar region
pumice stone
pump
  ankle
  antithrombotic
  calf muscle (anatomical)
  cement
  Infusaid continuous flow drug
  intermittent compression (mechanical)
  Jobst antithrombotic
  knee
  Medtronic programmable drug
  pneumatic foot (mechanical)
  programmable drug
  Secor drug (I or II)
  Servo
  Synchromed programmable drug
  Therex programmable drug
  Vacu-Mix cement
  venous pump of the foot (anatomical)
pump bump (retrocalcaneal exostosis)

pump standby
punch
  Acufex rotary
  bone
  boxer's (fracture of the fifth
    metacarpal)
  cervical laminectomy
  Charnley femoral prosthesis neck
  Cone skull
  disk
  dural
  DyoVac suction
  Hajek-Koffler
  Hajek laminectomy
  Hardy sellar
  Hirsch hypophyseal
  intervertebral disk
  Kerrison
  laminectomy
  Raney laminectomy
  Rhoton sellar
  rotary basket
  Rowe glenoid
  Sauerbruch-Frey bone
  Schlesinger
  sellar
  skull
  tibial
  tubular
punch-drunk syndrome of boxers
punch forceps
puncta dolorosa of Valleix (trigeminal
  neuralgia)
puncture
  bloody lumbar
  cisternal
  dry lumbar
  dural
  intraventricular
  lumbar (LP) (spinal tap)
  opening pressure on lumbar
    puncture
  stereotactic
  traumatic lumbar
puncture fracture
puncture-wound osteochondritis
puncture wounds (types I-IV)
pupil, pupils
  Adie
  Adie-Holmes
  Adie tonic
  Argyll-Robertson (of tabetic
    neurosyphilis)
  bilaterally dilated
  bilaterally fixed (dilated)
  blown
  briskly reactive
  consensual response
  corn-picker's
  curtsying
  dilated
  dilated and fixed
  fixed
  Holmes-Adie
  Hutchinson
  inequality of
  inverse Argyll Robertson
  isocoric
  light reaction of opposite
  Marcus Gunn
  midposition
  moderately dilated
  myotonic
  nonreactive to light
  nonresponsive to light
  pinpoint
  poorly reactive
  pseudo-Argyll Robertson
  reactive
  reactivity of
  responsive to light
  sluggishly reactive
  tonic
  tonically dilated
  tonohaptic reaction of
  unequal
  unilaterally fixed, dilated
  unreactive to light
  unresponsive to light
pupil check

pupillary areflexia
pupillary change
pupillary constriction
pupillary dilatation
pupillary escape
pupillary light reaction
pupillary light response
pupillary near-reflex
pupillary reaction
pupillary reflex
pupillary response
pupillary sign
pupillary-skin or ciliary reflex
pupillomotor fibers
purchase, bicortical
Purdue pegboard
pure athetoid palsy
pure hemisensory stroke
pure limb apraxia
pure motor hemiplegia
pure sensory stroke
pure spastic palsy
pure word deafness
purine-free diet
purines, diet low in
Purkinje cells of cerebellum
purse-string closure (or pursestring)
pursuit movements
pursuit movements, visual
purulent drainage
purulent material
purulent meningitis
pus, puric
pusher
  Charnley femoral prosthesis
  femoral
  femoral component
  femoral prosthesis
  Jacobson suture
  suture
  trochanter position
  trochanteric
push-off by great toe
push-off during walking
push-off of the foot in gait
push-off phase of gait
push-off strength
push-off velocity
putamen
  medial
  posterior
putaminal hemorrhage, nondominant
Putnam-Dana syndrome
Putti arthrodesis
Putti bone plast
Putti bone rasp
Putti-Platt arthroplasty
Putti-Platt shoulder procedure
putty, BeOK hand exercise
PVA (polyvinyl alcohol) splinting
  material
PVA strip
PVB (pigmented villonodular bursitis)
PVG matter (periventricular gray)
PVS (persistent vegetative state)
PVS (pigmented villonodular synovitis)
PWB (Puno-Winter-Byrd)
PWB awl
PWB fixation system
PWB rod
PWB screw
pyarthrosis
pyencephalus
pygalgia
pyknodysostosis
pyknoepilepsy
pyknolepsy
pyknomorphous
pyknophrasia
pylon attachment plate
pylon, metal
pyocephalus
pyogenic arthritis
pyogenic granuloma
pyogenic meningitis
pyoventricle
pyramid, petrous
pyramidal cells, Betz

pyramidal layer of cerebral cortex
pyramidal neurons
pyramidal sign
pyramidal tract
pyramis
pyranocarboxylic acid class
pyridoxine dependency
pyriform cortex
Pyrost bone graft material

Q, q

Q angle test
QALYs (Quality Adjusted Life Years)
QEEG (quantitative electroencephalogram)
QL Index
quad cane
quad (quadriceps) sets
quadrangle cartilage
quadrant of death (anterosuperior quadrant of hip)
quadrant on EEG
quadrant-position test
quadrantanopia
quadrantanopsia
  contralateral homonymous inferior
  contralateral homonymous superior
  homonymous
quadrantic hemianopia
quadrapod cane
quadrate gyrus
quadrature detector
quadratus femoris muscle
quadratus fascia
quadratus, pronator
quadriceps apron
quadriceps mechanism
quadriceps muscle
quadriceps retinaculum
  inferior
  superior
quadriceps stretch reflex
quadriceps wasting
quadricepsplasty
  Thompson
  V-Y
quadrigeminal plate
quadrilateral brim
quadriparesis, spastic
quadriphasic wave on EEG
quadriplegia
  high-level
  spastic
  traumatic
quality factor
quality of gait
quality of life assessment
Quality Adjusted Life Years (QALYs)
Quality of Well-Being Scale
quantitative EEG (QEEG)
quantitative electroencephalogram (QEEG)
Quantum foot
quarter (part of shoe)
quartets, digital flexor tendon
quasipurposive movement
quaver, nystagmoid
Queckenstedt sign
Queckenstedt test
quenching
Quengel cast
Quengel hinge
Quenu nail plate removal technique
Quervain disease
Quervain fracture
questionnaire, Questionnaire
  Beck
  cognitive failures (CFQ)
  everyday memory
  Functional Status (FSQ)
  General Health (GHQ)

questionnaire *(cont.)*
  Health Assessment (HAQ)
  Kenny Self-Care
  Lambeth Disability Screening
  McGill Pain
  McMaster Health Index
  mental status
  Modified Health Assessment
    (MHAQ)
  Oswestry Low Back Pain Disability
  Speech Questionnaire
  Toronto Functional Capacity (TFCQ)
quiescence
quiescent
Quigley traction
Quincke lumbar puncture needle
quiritarian epilepsy

R, r

RAB (remote afterloading brachy-therapy)
rabies (hydrophobia)
rabies encephalitis
rabies viral encephalitis
Rabiner neurological hammer
Rabot disease
raccoon eyes sign (periorbital ecchymosis)
rachialgia
rachicentesis
rachiocampsis
rachiochysis
rachiodynia
rachiokyphosis
rachiomyelitis
rachioparalysis
rachiopathy
rachioplegia
rachioscoliosis
rachiotomy
rachisagra
rachischisis
rachitic rosary sign
rachitomy
racquetball
radial bursa
radial collateral ligament
radial deviation
radial drift
radial epiphyseal displacement
radial extensors
radial facing of metacarpal heads
radial forearm flap
radial head dislocation
radial head fracture
radial head subluxation
radial metacarpal ligament
radial nerve palsy
radial nerve paresis
radial styloid process fracture
radial ray defect
radial trio
radialis sign
radialized
radian
radiata, corona
radiating "burner" down an extremity (paresthesia)
radiation
  auditory
  myelopathy
  neutron capture
  optic
  whole brain
  visual
radical nail bed ablation for ingrowing toenail
radicotomy
radicular compression
radicular neural deficits
radicular neuropathy, familial sensory
radicular pain
radicular symptom
radicular syndrome
radiculectomy
radiculitis
  cervical
  manual traction test for cervical
radiculomedullary artery

radiculoneuritis
radiculopathy
  compressive cervical
  lumbar
  lumbosacral
  radiation-induced
  S1
  spondylitic caudal
  spondylotic
radiculospinal artery
radioactive xenon clearance
radiocapitellar joint
radiocarpal angle
radiocarpal joint
radiocarpal portal
radiofrequency (RF)
radiofrequency coil
radiofrequency pulse
radiogram, radiograph
  oblique
  plain film
  soft tissue
  stress
  weightbearing
radiographically firm synostosis
radiography, high-resolution, low-speed
radiohumeral articulation
radioimmunoassay of cerebrospinal fluid
radioiodinated serum albumin (RISA)
radioisotope cisternography
radioisotope clearance assay
radioisotope (static) scanning
radioisotope uptake in bone
radioisotope uptake in vascular brain tumors
radiologic protection
  adequate collimation
  filtration
  gonadal shielding
radiolucency
radiolucent area
radiolunotriquetral ligament
radionecrosis, cerebral
Radionics CRW stereotactic head frame
Radionics fiducial localizer
Radionics stereotactic frame
radionuclide blood flow (dynamic) studies
radionuclide cisternography, Katzman infusion of
radionuclide flow scan
radionuclide, HMPAO (hexamethyl propylene amine oxime)
radiopaque
radioresistant
radioscaphocapitate ligament
radioscaphoid ligament
radioscapholunate ligament
radiosensitive
radiosensitivity
radiostyloid process
radiosurgery
  Bragg-peak
  charged-particle
  dynamic stereotactic
  Gamma knife
  heavy-charged particle Bragg peak
  interstitial
  LINAC (linear accelerator)
  linear accelerator
  multiarc LINAC
  stereotactic or stereotaxic
radiosurgically
radiosynovectomy
radiotelemetry EEG
radiotherapy
  fractionated
  fractionated external beam
  hyperfractionated
  neuroaxis
  palliative
radioulnar articulation
radioulnar joint

radioulnar subluxation
radioulnar surface
Radley-Liebig-Brown resection
Radolf nail pulling forceps
Raeder paratrigeminal syndrome
RA factor (rheumatoid arthritis)
ragged-red fibers on biopsy in Kearns-Sayre syndrome
Ragnell hand-held retractor
RAI (Rivermead ADL Index)
railroad track pattern on x-ray in Sturge-Weber syndrome
railway (physiological) nystagmus
Raimiste sign
Raimondi infant scalp hemostatic forceps
Raimondi spring peritoneal catheter
Raimondi ventricular catheter
Rainbow cast sandal
Rainin clip-bending spatula
raised and padded toilet seat
raising
  crossed straight leg
  straight leg (SLR)
rake, Israel
rales and rhonchi
Ralk hand drill
Ralks mallet
Ralston-Thompson pseudarthrosis technique
RAM (rapid-alternating movements)
RAM knee prostheses
rami of lateral sulcus
Ramsay Hunt cerebellar myoclonic dyssynergia
Ramsay Hunt dyssynergia cerebellaris myocloniam 8
Ramsay Hunt progressive cerebellar tremor
Ramsay Hunt syndrome
Ramsay Hunt type of inherited dentatorubral degeneration
ramus (pl. rami)
Ranawat-Burstein hip prosthesis
Ranawat-DeFiore-Straub technique
Rancho cube
Rancho mounting technique for Ilizarov apparatus
Rancho pin gripper cube
Rancho swivel hinge
Rancho system modification of Ilizarov external fixation
Rancho trocar-drill sleeve
Rancho-type anklet foot control device
Rand Functional Limitations Battery
Rand microballoon
Rand Physical Capacities Battery
Rand Social Health Battery
random letter test
Raney clip-applying forceps
Raney coagulating forceps
Raney cranial drill
Raney-Crutchfield drill points
Raney-Crutchfield skull tongs
Raney forceps
Raney hemostatic clip
Raney laminectomy punch
Raney laminectomy rongeur
Raney perforator drills
Raney rongeur forceps
Raney saw guide
Raney scalp clip-applying forceps
Raney stirrup-loop curet
range
  alpha frequency
  delta frequency
  frequency
  theta frequency
range of excursion
range of flexion and extension
range of motion (ROM)
  active (AROM)
  active and passive
  active-assisted
  passive
  restricted
range of motion therapy
Rankin Scale

Ranvier groove
Ranvier node
Ranvier segment
raphe nucleus of midbrain
raphe, ventral median
rapid-alternating movements (RAM)
rapid eye movement (REM) sleep
rapid saccades (corrective)
Rappaport Disability Rating Scale
raptus of attention
rarefaction, fluffy (of Paget disease on x-ray)
rarefaction of cortex, on x-ray
RAS (reticular activating system)
rash
  dermatomal
  heliotrope, in polymyositis or dermatomyositis
Rasmussen encephalitis
Rasmussen syndrome
rasp, raspatory
  Acufex
  Acufex convex
  Alexander
  Alexander-Farabeuf
  angled
  Aufricht glabellar
  Austin Moore
  Bacon
  Bardeleben
  Black
  Bristow
  Brown
  carbon-tungsten
  Charnley
  convex
  Coryllos
  costal
  Cottle-MacKenty
  DePuy
  diamond
  Doyen costal
  Doyen rib
  Epstein bone

rasp *(cont.)*
  Farabeuf
  Farabeuf bone
  Farabeuf-Collin
  Farabeau-Lambotte
  Filtzer interbody
  Fisher
  Fomon
  Gallaher
  glabellar
  Good
  Herczel
  Herczel rib
  Hylin
  interbody
  intramedullary
  Israel
  Jansen
  Key
  Kirmission periosteal
  Kleinert-Kutz
  Koenig
  Lambotte
  Langenbeck
  Lewis
  Lewis periosteal
  Mallory-Head
  Maltz
  Mathieu
  McCabe-Farrior
  McKenty
  micro
  Miller
  Nicoll
  Nicola
  Olivecrona
  Phemister
  Plenk-Matson
  power
  Putti bone
  rib
  Rubin
  Schneider
  Schneider-Sauerbruch

rasp *(cont.)*
  Seawell
  Semb rib
  Thompson
  Yasargil micro
  Zoellner
rasped, rasping
RAT (right anterior temporal) EEG lead
ratchet spanner
ratchet syndrome
rate
  alternating motion (AMR)
  click stimulus
  sed (sedimentation)
Rathke pouch (in the brain)
rating scale
rating system, Iowa hip status
ratio
  ankle-brachial pressure
  Holdaway
  Insall ratio in patella alta
  Insall-Salvati
  metatarsal length
  P:A (peroneal to anterior compartment)
  patellar ligament-patellar
  Poisson
  recruitment
  serum glucose:CSF glucose
  signal-to-noise (on EEG)
  signal-to-noise (on MRI)
  TME (trapezium-metacarpal eburnation)
ratio scales, in rehabilitation testing
Ratliff classification of avascular necrosis
Rauchfuss sling
ray, rays
  central
  digital
  hypermobile first
  long axis
  pollicized
ray amputation
Ray brain spatula spoon
Rayleigh scattering law
Raymond-Céstan syndrome
Raymond shoulder immobilizer
Raynaud disease
Raynaud phenomenon
  bilateral
  unilateral
Raynaud syndrome
Ray-Parsons-Sunday staphylorrhaphy elevator
Ray pituitary curet
Rayport dural dissector and knife
Rayport muscle biopsy clamp
ray resection
Ray-Tec sponge
Ray TFC (threaded fusion cage)
Ray ventricular cannula
RC (rehabilitation counseling)
RCA (*Ricinus communis* agglutinin 1) antibody
RCA lectins
rCBF (regional cerebral blood flow)
rCBV (regional cerebral blood volume)
RCC (Rathke cleft cyst)
rCPP (regional cerebral perfusion pressure)
RCT (retinocortical time)
RDF (registered deafness specialist)
RE (rehabilitation engineering)
re-arthroscoped
reach, of gait
ReAct neuromuscular stimulator
reaction
  acute exogenous
  catastrophic (of a demented person)
  doll's eye
  equilibrium
  groping
  hypersensitivity reaction to anticonvulsants
  hysterical conversion

reaction *(cont.)*
- Jarisch-Herxheimer
- lamellar (on x-ray)
- light
- magnetic (grasp reflex)
- migrainous
- migrainoid
- periosteal (on x-ray)
- pupillary
- pupillary light
- synovial inflammatory (in rheumatoid arthritis
- tonohaptic (of pupil)
- tyramine (cheese, red wine)
- Weil-Felix

reactive pupils
reactivity of pupils
Read gouge
reading comprehension impairment
reading epilepsy
reading impairment
readout delay
real strabismus
realign
realignment, patellofemoral
ream
reamed and rasped
reamed, sequentially
reamer
- acetabular
- Anspach
- Aufranc
- Austin Moore
- ball
- barrel
- blunt tapered T-handled
- bone
- brace-type
- calcar
- Campbell
- cannulated Henderson
- chamfer
- Charnley

reamer *(cont.)*
- Charnley deepening
- Charnley expanding
- Charnley taper
- Charnley trochanter
- Christmas tree
- congruous cup-shaped
- conical
- corrugated
- cup
- deepening
- DePuy
- expanding
- female
- femoral shaft
- fenestrated
- flexible medullary
- grater
- grooving
- Hall Versipower
- handle type
- Harris center-cutting acetabular
- hemispherical
- hollow mill
- Indiana
- Intracone intramedullary
- intramedullary
- Küntscher intramedullary
- male
- Marin
- medullary canal
- Micro-Aire
- Mira
- Moore bone
- multisized
- Norton ball
- Perthes
- power
- power-driven
- progressively larger
- Richards
- rigid
- Rotalink flexible shaft

reamer *(cont.)*
- Rush awl
- self-centering
- Smith-Petersen
- spiral cortical
- spiral trochanteric
- square
- starting
- step-cut
- straight
- Swanson
- T-handled
- tapered
- tapered hand
- triangular bone
- trochanter
- trochanteric
- Wagner acetabular

reaming awl
reanastomosis of blood supply to bone graft
reapproximation
rearfoot eversion
rearfoot pronation
rearfoot striker
rearfoot varus
rebleeding of aneurysm
recalcitrance of syndromes
recalcitrant pain
recall of events
recall of information
recanalization, angiographic
receiver coil
recent memory
receptive aphasia
receptive aphasic disorder, impairment
receptive language
receptor
- acetylcholine
- ACh (acetylcholine)
- dopaminergic
- Krause sensory
- Meissner corpuscle sensory
- Merkel disc sensory

receptor *(cont.)*
- pacinian corpuscle sensory
- postsynaptic
- Ruffini corpuscle sensory

receptor site
recess
- infraglenoid
- popliteal
- pre-styloid
- subscapularis

recheck
recipient team
reciprocal agonist-antagonist relaxation
Reciprocal Coordination Test
reciprocating gait orthosis (RGO)
reciprocating saw
Reci-Vacette
reconstruction (see *operations*)
record, recording
- all-night sleep
- ambulatory EEG
- artifact-free
- bipolar EEG
- cassette EEG
- clinical EEG
- ear reference EEG
- electromyographic (EMG)
- evoked potential
- flat (isoelectric) EEG
- microelectrode
- multichannel EEG
- neonatal EEG
- referential EEG
- scalp EEG
- serial EEG
- waking baseline

recording channel (on EEG)
recovery, functional
Recovery Locus of Control
recrudescence
recruiting response on EEG
recruitment of motor unit potential
recruitment ratio
recruitment spasm in tetanus

rectangle
  Hartshill
  Luque
rectus abdominis musculocutaneous free flap
rectus muscle flap
rectus position
recurrence, local
recurrent artery of Heubner
recurrent dislocation
recurrent meningeal nerve
recurrent torsion spasms
recurvatum during gait
Red Cross freeze-dried allograft
Redi-Around finger splint
Redi-Drap
Redigrip knee pad
Redigrip pressure bandage
Redi head halter
Redi-Trac traction device
Redi-Vac cast cutter
Redi-Vacette
red light neon laser for acupressure points (chiropractic)
red migraine
red nucleus syndromes
reduce, reduction
reduced subluxations (sprains)
reduction (see *operations*)
  anatomic
  closed
  concentric
  congruent
  fracture
  manual
  manual fracture
  open
  stable
  surgical
  trial
re-education, neuromuscular
REE (resting energy expenditure)
Reebok shoes
Reed cast belt
reefing, capsular
reefing of the medial retinaculum of the knee
reefing procedure
Reese dermatome
Reese stimulator
reevaluate
reexploration
reference
  Goldmann-Offner
  Stephenson-Gibbs
reference electrode
reference, sternospinal
referential alternating montage
referential block montage
referential montage
referred neuritic pain
referred pain
refill, capillary
ReFix stereotactic head fixator
ReFix stereotactic head holder
refixation reflexes
refixational shift of gaze
reflect, reflected
reflex, reflexes
  abdominal (superficial)
  absent
  accommodation
  Achilles tendon
  adductor
  anal wink
  ankle jerk
  asymmetric tonic neck
  automatic bladder
  Babinski
  Bekhterev-Mendel
  biceps stretch
  blink reflex to corneal stimulation
  brachioradialis
  brain stem
  brain stem mediated
  brisk
  bulbar
  bulbocavernous

reflex *(cont.)*
- Chaddock
- chewing ("bulldog response")
- ciliary or pupillary-skin
- ciliospinal or pupillary-skin
- consensual light
- contralateral grasp
- corneal
- cough
- cremasteric
- cubital tendon
- deep tendon (DTRs)
- delayed
- deltoid
- depressed
- diminished
- diving
- doll's eye (oculocephalic)
- dorsal
- elbow
- equivocal plantar
- exaggerated deep tendon
- extensor plantar
- facial
- fencing posture
- fixation
- flexion
- frontal lobe
- gag
- gastrocnemius
- glabella
- glabellar
- Golgi
- Gordon
- grasp
- H reflex (Hoffmann monosynaptic)
- hamstring
- Hirschberg
- hung-up (slowed)
- hyperactive deep tendon
- hypoactive deep tendon
- intramuscular recording
- jaw jerk
- Kimura blink

reflex *(cont.)*
- knee jerk
- Landau
- laryngeal-tracheal
- lengthening
- masseter-temporalis stretch
- Mayer
- Mendel-Bekhterev
- monosynaptic
- Moro
- motor
- muscle stretch
- myotatic
- near
- neck righting
- neonatal
- nuchocephalic
- oculocephalic
- oculovestibular (OVR)
- Oppenheim
- optokinetic
- orbicularis pupillary
- palmomental
- parachute
- patellar
- patelloadductor
- pathologic
- pathological
- pectoral
- pectoralis
- pendular
- periosteal
- plantar, equivocal
- polykinetic
- pressor
- primitive
- pseudomyotonic
- psycho-optical
- pupillary light
- pyramidal tract
- quadriceps stretch
- radial
- refixation
- Remak

reflex *(cont.)*
  righting
  rooting
  rotular
  scapular
  scapulohumeral
  snout
  spinal
  spindle system
  stepping
  sternutatory
  Stookey
  stretch
  suck
  sucking
  superficial abdominal
  suprapatellar
  swallow
  tendon
  toe
  tonic neck
  triceps
  triceps surae
  ulnar
  vasovagal
  ventral suspension
  vestibulo-ocular (VOR)
  von Bekhterev
  Wartenberg
  withdrawal
  mass limb
reflex arc, monosynaptic
reflex controls
  psycho-optical
  static
  stato-kinetic
reflex epilepsy
reflex eye movement
reflex inhibition
reflex iridoplegia
reflex neurologic activity
reflex plantar
reflex rebound component of whiplash
reflex relaxation delay
reflex sympathetic dystrophy (RSD)
reflex sympathetic dystrophy
  syndrome (RSDS)
reflexic
reflux, venous
refluxing spastic neurogenic bladder
refractory
refracture
Refsum disease
Refsum syndrome
Regen flexion exercises
regenerating peripheral fibers
regeneration
  axon
  imperfect
  neural
region
  anesthesic
  anterior head
  Broca
  central head
  centroparietal head
  cervical
  cervicothoracic
  clival
  craniofacial
  frontal
  frontocentral head
  frontotemporal
  frontozygomatic
  geniculocalcarine
  hippocampal
  insular
  interseptal
  lumbar
  lumbosacral
  mesiotemporal
  midbrain subthalamic
  midfrontal
  occipital
  orbitofrontal
  paracervical
  parasagittal head
  parasellar

region *(cont.)*
paraspinal
paravermian
paravertebral
patellofemoral
periaqueductal
petroclival
petrous
pineal
pontomedullary
pretectal
pretibial
retrosellar
rolandic head
sacral
septal
subfrontal
subthalamic
supramalleolar
suprasellar
temporal
temporozygomatic
thoracolumbar
Wernicke
regional cerebral perfusion pressure (rCPP)
registered deafness specialist (RDF)
Registry of Interpreters for the Deaf (RID)
Regnauld degeneration of MTP joint
Regnauld modification of Keller arthroplasty
Regnauld-type degeneration of great toe
regressive remodeling
rehabilitation (rehab)
aquatic
community
free weight
muscular
neurological
Office of Vocational (OVR)
swallowing
vocational (VR)
rehabilitation assessment
rehabilitation behaviors
rehabilitation care
rehabilitation counseling (RC)
rehabilitation engineering (RE)
rehabilitation evaluation
rehabilitation interventions
rehabilitation planning
rehabilitation psychiatry (RP)
Rehabilitation Services Administration (RSA)
rehabilitation treatment
Rehbein rib spreader
Reichenheim-King procedure
Reichert-Mundinger biopsy needle
Reichert-Mundinger-Fischer stereotactic frame
Reichert-Mundinger hematoma evacuator
Reichert-Mundinger stereotactic head frame
Reil, island of
reimplantation
Reiner bone rongeur
Reiner plaster knife
reinnervation after nerve injury
reinnervation, motor
Reintegration to Normal Living Index
re-irrigation
Reiter syndrome
relapsing course
relation, phase
relationships, stress-strain
relative elective mutism
relative scotomata
Relax-A-Bac posture support
relaxation rate
relaxation, reciprocal agonist-antagonist
relaxation techniques
relaxation time
Re-Lax-O chiropractic table
release (see also *operations*)
abductor hallucis muscle
adductor tendon and lateral capsular
brevis

release *(cont.)*
 capsular
 carpal tunnel
 clubfoot
 Dupuytren contractor
 fascial
 flexor-pronator origin
 hamstring
 key
 lateral capsular
 lateral retinaculum
 plantar plate
 posteromedial (PMR)
 retinacular
 snapping tendon
 soft tissue
 tendon
 trigger finger
 trigger thumb
 ulnar nerve
reliability of rehabilitation testing
Relton-Hall frame
REM (rapid eye movement) sleep
 bursts of
 periods of
REM onset sleep
remineralization
remitting course
remnants, notochordal
remodeling
 bone
 craniofacial
 para-articular bone
 regressive
remote afterloading brachytherapy (RAB)
remote lower motor neuron lesion
remote memory
removal, subtotal, of tumor
remover
 cast
 Wolfe-Boehler cast
remyelination
renal osteodystrophy
Renee creak sign (friction rub in knee)
Renografin contrast media
Renshaw cell
repair (see *operations*)
repeated FID (free induction decay)
repeated microtraumas
repetition time (TR)
repetitive seizures
repetitive strain (or stress) injury (RSI)
rephasing gradient
replacement (see *operations*)
replantation of amputated digit or extremity
replantation of finger
reprep and drape
Repro head halter
rerotation, varus
reroute
rerupture of aneurysm
resected, surgically
resecting fracture
resection (see *operations*)
 anteromedial temporal lobe (AMTR)
 en bloc
 first rib
 microsurgical
 panmetatarsal head
 ray
 subtotal
 surgical
 temporal bone
 tumor
 volumetric stereotactic surgical
resection arthroplasty
resection of epileptogenic foci
resection of iliopsoas tendon
resection of meniscus
resector
 Accu-Line femoral
 Accu-Line tibial
 femoral
 full radius
 orthotome

resector *(cont.)*
  synovial
  tibial
reservoir
  Accu-Flo CSF
  Braden flushing
  Cordis implantable drug
  CSF (cerebrospinal fluid)
  double bubble flushing
  flush
  flushing
  Foltz flushing
  McKenzie
  Ommaya ventriculostomy
  Rickham intraventricular
  Salmon Rickham ventriculostomy
  Secor implantable drug
  ventricular catheter
residual cement
residual hemiparesis
resin, polyacetal
resistance
  flexion against
  progressive
  strength against
  tensile stretch
resistive exercise table
resistive magnet
resolution, spatial
resonance, nuclear magnetic (NMR)
resonant frequency
resorbable pin
resorbable plate
resorbable rod
resorbable screw
resorption
  bone
  osteoclastic
respiration
  ataxic
  hissing, in uremic coma
respiratory embarrassment
Respond Select neuromuscular
  stimulator
response
  adaptive
  brain stem auditory-evoked
  bulldog (chewing reflex)
  clasp-knife
  corneal
  Cushing
  decremental
  driving
  EEG augmenting
  EEG recruiting
  evoked (ER)
  evoked cortical (ECR)
  extensor plantar
  F wave
  focal epileptiform
  galvanic skin (GSR) on EEG
  ice water caloric
  jittery
  mass motor reflex
  oculocephalic
  on and off
  pattern reversal visual evoked
  photic pattern-evoked
  photoconvulsive
  photomyoclonic
  photoparoxysmal
  placebo
  prominent flash evoked
  psychogalvanic skin
  pupillary
  recruiting
  short-latency somatosensory evoked
  somatosensory evoked (SER)
  triple
  visual evoked (VER)
responsive
responsiveness, reduced
rest
  foot
  Greenberg hand
  hand
  head
  horseshoe head

rest *(cont.)*
  kidney
  Mayfield horseshoe head
  Mayfield tic head
  tic head
rest, ice, compression, elevation
  (RICE)
rest splint
rest tremor
Restcue bed
restiform body
resting ankle/arm Doppler index
resting calcaneal stance position
resting energy expenditure (REE)
resting potential
restive
restless legs syndrome (RLS)
restlessness
Reston dressing
Reston foam-padded headrest
restorator
Restore tools for knee surgery
restraint, Posey
restriction
  activity
  shoe
restrictor
  cement
  plastic marrow canal
retained foreign body
retardation
  mental
  profound mental
  psychomotor
  severe mental
rete (pl. retia)
reticular activating formation (RAF)
reticular activating substance
reticular activating system (RAS)
reticular formation
reticular formation of brain stem
reticular formation of the brain stem
reticulin
reticulocortical pathway
reticulocytosis, cerebroside
reticulospinal tract
reticulum cell sarcoma
reticulum, hematopoietic (of marrow)
retina, angiomatosis of
retinacular disruption
retinacular ligaments
retinaculum
  avulsed
  extensor
  flexor
  patellar
  superior peroneal (SPR)
retinitis pigmentosa
retinoneuropathy, toxic
retraction exercises, prone scapular
retractor
  Adson
  Adson brain
  Adson cerebellar
  Adson hemilaminectomy
  Adson-Anderson cerebellar
  Allport
  Alm wound
  amputation
  Anderson-Adson scalp
  angled
  appendiceal
  Army-Navy
  Aufranc cobra
  Badgley laminectomy
  Ballantine hemilaminectomy
  Bankart shoulder
  Beckman
  Beckman-Adson laminectomy
  Beckman-Eaton laminectomy
  Beckman-Weitlaner laminectomy
  Bennett bone
  Bennett tibial
  blade
  Blount anvil
  Blount hip
  Blount knee

retractor *(cont.)*
Bodnar
bone
brachial plexus root
brain
Budde-Greenberg-Sugita
bunion
Campbell nerve root
carotid
Carroll-Bennett
Carroll hand
cerebellar
cervical disk
Chandler knee
Charnley horizontal
Charnley initial incision
Charnley knee
Charnley pin
Charnley self-retaining
Charnley vertical
Cherry brain
Cherry laminectomy
Cloward blade
Cloward brain
Cloward cervical
Cloward-Cushing vein
Cloward dural
Cloward-Hoen hemilaminectomy
Cloward-Hoen laminectomy
Cloward lumbar lamina
Cloward nerve root
Cloward skin
Cloward small cervical
Cloward tissue
cobra
Collis-Taylor
Cone laminectomy
Cone scalp
Contour scalp
Cooley rib
Crego
curved
Cushing brain
Cushing decompression

retractor *(cont.)*
Cushing nerve
Cushing vein
Davis brain
Davis scalp
Deaver
decompression
D'Errico-Adson
D'Errico nerve root
Doane knee
Dohn-Carton brain
Dott
double-ended right-angle
double-hook Lovejoy
Downey hemilaminectomy
Downing
dural
East-West
Echols
Elite Farley
endaural
Enker brain
Fahey
fat pad
finger
Finochietto laminectomy
Frazier laminectomy
Frazier lighted brain
Fujita snake
Fujita suction
Gelpi
Gifford mastoid
Glaser automatic laminectomy
Goulet
Greenberg Universal
hand
Haverfield-Scoville hemilaminectomy
Hayes
Hays hand
heavy-duty two-tooth
Hedblom rib
Heiss soft tissue
hemilaminectomy
Henley carotid

retractor *(cont.)*
Henning meniscal
Hertzler rib
Hibbs
Hoen hemilaminectomy
Hoen scalp
Hohmann bone
Holscher knee
Holscher nerve root
Holzheimer
horizontal
House-Fisch dura
humeral head
humpback Weitlaner
Inge laminectomy
initial incision
Israel
Jannetta posterior fossa
Jansen mastoid
Jansen scalp
Jansen-Wagner
Johnson
Kasdan
Kennerdell-Maroon orbital
Kleinert-Ragdell
Klemme laminectomy
knee
Knighton hemilaminectomy
Knighton lamincctomy
Kocher
lamina
laminectomy
Lange-Hohmann bone
Langenbeck
lateral collateral ligament
Leyla
Leyla brain
Love nerve root
lower-hand
Lowman hand
lumbar lamina
Luongo hand
Maison
Malis brain

retractor *(cont.)*
Mark II Chandler
Mark II distal femur
Mark II PCL
Mark II S
Mark II Z knee
Markham-Meyerding hemi-
laminectomy
Martin nerve root
mastoid
Mayo-Collins
meniscus
metacarpal
Meyerding finger
Meyerding laminectomy
Miller-Senn
mini-Hohmann
Miskimon cerebellar
Morris
Myers knee
narrow-blade
narrow-neck mini-Hohmann
Nelson rib
nerve root
North-South
Oberhill laminectomy
Oldberg brain
Ollier rake
Omni
orbital
Paulson knee
PCL (posterior collateral ligament)
Percy amputation
pin
pitch-fork
Poppen-Gelpi laminectomy
posterior fossa
Ragnell hand-held
rake
rib
Richardson
right-angle
Robotrac
Roos brachial plexus root

retractor *(cont.)*
- Rosenberg
- Rowe capsular
- Rowe humeral head
- S-shaped brain
- Sachs vein
- Sauerbruch
- scalp
- Schink
- Schwartz laminectomy
- Scoville cervical disk
- Scoville-Haverfield hemilaminectomy
- Scoville hemilaminectomy
- Scoville nerve root
- Scoville-Richter laminectomy
- Seletz-Gelpi laminectomy
- self-retaining
- Senn double-end
- sharp
- Sheldon hemilaminectomy
- Sherwin knee
- Sims
- skid humeral-head
- Smillie knee
- Smith nerve root suction
- snake
- Snitman endaural
- Sofield
- Spurling nerve root
- Stack hand
- staple-shaped
- stiff ribbon
- Stiwer
- straight
- Stuck laminectomy
- suction
- Taylor spinal
- Teflon-coated brain
- Temple-Fay laminectomy
- tibial
- toothed
- tracheal
- trigeminal nerve
- Tuffier laminectomy

retractor *(cont.)*
- Tuffier-Raney
- two-prong rake
- U-shaped
- U.S. Army
- universal
- upper-hand
- Valin hemilaminectomy
- vein
- Verbrugge Hohmann bone
- vertebral body
- vertical
- vessel
- Volkmann rake
- Wagner
- Weary nerve root
- Weitlaner-Beckman
- Wilson gonad
- Wiltse-Bankart
- Wiltse-Gelpi
- Wink
- Zinn

re-treating
retriever, Kleinert-Kutz tendon
retrobulbar hemorrhage
retrobulbar neuritis
retrocalcaneal bursa
retrocalcaneal bursitis, chronic
retrocalcaneal exostosis (pump bump)
retrocalcaneal spur
retrochiasmal lesion
retrochiasmal visual pathway
retroclavicular
retrocollic spasm (back of the neck)
retrograde amnesia
retrograde Beaver blade
retrolisthesis
retromastoid craniectomy
retromedullary arteriovenous malformation
retronuchal muscle
retropulsed bony fragment
retropulsion of gait
retrosellar region

retrotorsion, femoral
retroversion, femoral
Retter aneurysm needles
Retter knot tier and ligature carrier
revascularization
  cerebral
  endosteal
revascularization of foot
revascularization of graft
revascularized tissue
Reverdin epidermal free graft
Reverdin-Green osteotomy
reversal
  instrumental phase
  letter
  phase (on EEG)
  true phase
reversal of cervical lordosis
reversal of fore-aft shear phase of gait
reverse last shoes
reverse Mauck knee procedure
reverse pivot shift test
reverse urea syndrome
reversible (or resolving) ischemic neurologic deficit (RIND)
reversible organic brain syndrome
revision of total hip
revision, stump
revision total hip surgery
Rey Auditory Verbal Learning Test
Rey Osterrieth Complex Figure Test
Reye syndrome, adult
Reynolds skull traction tongs
REZ (root exit zone)
Rezinian external fixation
Rezinian interbody device
RF (radiofrequency) coil
RF (radiofrequency) pulse
RF (rheumatoid factor) test
RF (right frontal) (EEG lead)
RFE (radiofrequency electro-coagulation)
RGO (reciprocating gait orthosis)
rhabdoid suture
rhabdomyolysis
rhabdomyoma
rhabdomyosarcoma, alveolar
rhachotomy
  Capener
  decompression
rheumatic chorea
rheumatism
  palindromic
  psychogenic
rheumatoid arthritis (RA) factor
rheumatoid arthritis agglutinin test
rheumatoid factor (RF)
rheumatoid neuropathy
rheumatoid nodule
rheumatoid spondylitis
rheumatoid synovitis
rheumatoid vasculitis
rheumatologist
Rhinelander pin
Rhinelander wire tightener
rhinencephalic mamillary body
rhinolalia aperta
rhinolalia clausa
rhinophyma
rhinorrhea, CSF (cerebrospinal fluid)
rhizomelic
rhizotomy
rhizotomy (radicotomy)
  chemical
  dorsal root
  glycerol
  percutaneous high-frequency
  selective dorsal (SDR)
  surgical
  thermal
rhombencephalon
rhomboid fossa
rhonchus (pl. rhonchi)
Rhoton ball dissector
Rhoton bayonet scissors
Rhoton bipolar forceps

Rhoton cup forceps
Rhoton curet
Rhoton-Cushing forceps
Rhoton dissecting forceps
Rhoton elevator
Rhoton enucleator
Rhoton forceps
Rhoton fork
Rhoton hook
Rhoton loop curet
Rhoton-Merz suction tube
Rhoton micro curet
Rhoton needle holder
Rhoton osteotome
Rhoton pituitary curet
Rhoton punch
Rhoton scissors
Rhoton sellar punch
Rhoton spatula dissector
Rhoton spoon curet
Rhoton suction tip
Rhoton-Tew bipolar forceps
rhythm
  alpha
  alpha variant
  alphoid
  arceau
  attenuation of alpha
  attenuation of background
  Berger (on EEG)
  beta
  comb
  fast alpha variant
  focal parietal theta
  frontal beta
  gamma
  kappa
  M-type (minimal) alpha
  midline theta
  monorhythmic occipital
  mu (μ)
  occipital
  P-type (persistent) alpha
  paradoxical alpha

rhythm *(cont.)*
  paradoxical mu (μ)
  persistent slowing of alpha
  posterior beta
  posterior theta
  postictal slowing of alpha
  projected EEG
  R-type (reactive) alpha
  regular sinus
  sigma
  slow alpha variant
  spike-and-slow-wave
  theta
  trains of mu (μ)
  wicket
  widespread beta
rhythm on EEG
rhythmic (jerk) nystagmus
rhythmical spindle-shaped activity (on EEG)
rhythmicity of wave on EEG
rib
  bed of
  bicipital
  cervical
  false
  floating
  minced
  rudimentary
  slipping
  sternal
  true
  vertebral
rib belt orthosis
rib belt, Zim-Zap
Ribble bandage
rib contusion
rib fracture from cough
rice bodies
RICE (rest, ice, compression, elevation)
Rich theory of tuberculous meningitis
Richards angle guide
Richards compression screw

Richards curet
Richards hip prosthesis
Richards-Hirschhorn plate
Richards hydroxyapatite PORP
Richards mallet
Richards modular hip system (RMHS)
Richards reamer
Richards reconstruction nail
Richards self-tapping screw
Richards Solcotrans Plus
Richards Spectron metal-backed
  acetabular prosthesis
Richards Zirconia femoral head
  prosthesis
Richardson retractor
Richardson rod
Riche-Cannieu anastomosis
Riches artery forceps
Richet bandage
Richet, tibio-astragalocalcaneal
  canal of
Richmond subarachnoid screw
  instruments
Richter laminectomy punch forceps
Ricinus communis agglutinin 1 (RCA)
  antibody
rickets
rickettsial infections of the central
    nervous system
  murine typhus
  Rocky Mountain spotted fever
  scrub typhus (tsutsugamushi)
Rickham reservoir
RID (Registry of Interpreters for the
  Deaf)
ridge, ridging
  apical ectodermal (AER)
  bisagittal
  cranial
  dorsal
  fibrocartilaginous
  greater multangular
  Outerbridge
  petrous
ridge *(cont.)*
  sagittal
  sphenoid
  supraorbital
  vastus lateralis
Ridley sinus
Ridlon hip reduction
Ridlon plaster knife
Rienhoff rib spreader
right and left respiratory nerves
  (phrenic nerve)
right anterior temporal (RAT)
  (EEG lead)
right-bearing nystagmus
right frontal (RF) (EEG lead)
right-hand dominant
right-handed patient
right hemiplegia
right-left disorientation
right motor (RM) (EEG lead)
right occipital (RO) (EEG lead)
right parietal (RP) (EEG lead)
right posterior temporal (RPT)
  (EEG lead)
right respiratory nerve (phrenic nerve)
right-sided weakness
righting reflex
rigid bars
rigid flatfoot
rigid internal fixation
rigidity
  axial
  clasp-knife
  cogwheel rigidity in parkinsonism
  cogwheel-type
  decerebrate
  decorticate
  lead-pipe
  nuchal
  ratchet
  reflex
Riley-Day syndrome
rim, glenoid
rim of capsule

rim of dark signal intensity
rim of signal enhancement
riMLF (rostral interstitial nucleus of medial longitudinal fasciculus)
rims in gout, sclerotic (on x-ray)
RIND (reversible or resolving ischemic neurologic deficit)
ring, rings
  Ace-Colles half
  arc
  BRW (Brown-Roberts-Wells) head
  CBI stereotactic
  centering
  Charnley centering
  constriction
  doughnut
  drop-lock
  femoral
  fibrous
  Fischer
  half
  halo
  Ilizarov
  ischial weightbearing
  Kayser-Fleischer in the cornea
  K-F (Kayser-Fleischer)
  Mose concentric
  olive
  orthosis drop-lock
  pelvic
  perichondral
  proximal-to-distal
  stereotactic or stereotaxic
  vertebral
ring blush on cerebral arteriography
ring curet, Cloward-Cone
ring fracture
ring man shoulder, in gymnasts
Ring total hip prosthesis
Ring UPM total hip replacement
Ring UPM total knee replacement
Rinne hearing conduction test
Riordan classification of club hand
Riordan finger flexion
Riordan finger opponensplasty
Riordan finger pollicization
Riordan tendon transfer technique
RISA (radioiodinated serum albumin)
Riseborough-Radin classification of intercondylar fracture
Rish osteotome
Risser-Ferguson scoliosis measuring technique
Risser localizer scoliosis cast
Risser sign
risus sardonicus
Ritcher screwdriver
Ritchie index, for RA
Ritchie nail starter
Rivermead ADL Index (RAI)
Rivermead Mobility Index (RMI)
Rivermead Motor Assessment
Rivermead Perceptual Assessment Battery (RPAB)
RLE (right lower extremity)
RLS (restless legs syndrome)
RM (right motor) (EEG lead)
RM isoelastic hip prosthesis
RM stereotaxic system
RMC knee replacement device
RMHS (Richards modular hip system)
RMI (Rivermead Mobility Index)
RMTD (rhythmical midtemporal discharge)
RO (right occipital) (EEG lead)
R/O (rule out)
Robert Brigham total knee prosthesis
Robert Jones dressing
Roberts-Gill periosteal elevator
Roberts rib shears
Roberts technique
Robin Hood phenomenon (steal syndrome)
Robinson anterior cervical discectomy
Robinson arthrometer
Robinson cervical spine fusion
Robinson-Chung-Farahvar clavicular morcellation

Robinson-Riley cervical arthrodesis
Robinson-Riley spinal fusion
Robinson-Southwick fusion
Robodoc instrument holder
robot
  Grenoble stereotactic
  Kwoh-Young stereotactic
  Lausanne stereotactic
  Long Beach stereotactic
  Mayo Clinic stereotactic
  neurosurgical stereotactic
  stereotactic
Robotrac passive retraction system
Rochester bone trephine
Rochester-Carmalt forceps
Rochester compression system
Rochester harvest bone cutter
Rochester hip-knee-ankle-foot orthosis
Rochester HKAFO (hip-knee-ankle-foot orthosis)
Rochester lamina dissector
Rochester lamina elevator
Rochester-Ochsner forceps
Rochester-Pean forceps
Rochester recipient bone cutter
Rochester spinal elevator
rocker, Carolina
rocker foot
rockerbottom flatfoot
rockerbottom foot
RocketSoc
Rockwood classification of acromioclavicular injury
Rockwood-Green technique
Rocky Mountain spotted fever meningoencephalitis
rod
  absorbable
  acetabular cup detaching
  acetabular cup push (pushing)
  alignment
  Alta tibial/humeral
  Amset R-F
  auto-reinforced polyglycolide

rod *(cont.)*
  Bickel intramedullary
  biodegradable
  C-D or CD (Cotrel-Dubousset)
  compression
  Dacron-impregnated silicone
  degradable polyglycolide
  distraction
  Edwards-Levine
  Edwards reverse ratchet
  Ender
  Fixateur Interne
  fluted medullary
  Hall
  Harrington compression
  Harrington distraction
  Harris condylocephalic
  hinge
  humeral
  Hunter Silastic
  Hunter tendon
  IM (intramedullary)
  impactor
  Isola
  Jacobs distraction
  Kaneda
  Knodt compression
  knurled
  Kostuik
  Küntscher condylocephalic
  Luque
  Moe distraction
  Moe-modified Harrington
  Moss
  Mouradian
  Olerud PSF
  partially threaded
  pedicular
  polyglactin
  polyglycolide, self-reinforced
  PWB (Puno-Winter-Byrd)
  rectangular
  resorbable
  Richardson

rod *(cont.)*
  Rogozinski spinal
  Rush
  Russell-Taylor reconstruction
  Sage
  Schanz
  Schmidt
  Schneider
  Seidel humeral
  Seidel intramedullary
  Selby I and II
  Serrato forearm
  Silastic
  silicone flexor
  Smith & Nephew Richards
  spinal
  Steffee pedicular
  Stenzel
  straight threaded
  Synthes
  telescopic
  telescoping medullary
  tendon
  threaded
  titanium alloy
  TSRH
  V-A alignment
  VDS (ventral derotating spinal) compression
  VSF (Vermont spinal fixator)
  Wiltse
  Wissinger
  Zickel
  Zielke
roentgen knife
roentgenogram, two-plane
Roger Anderson compression device
Roger Anderson external fixation apparatus
Rogers cervical fusion technique
Rogers wire-cutting scissors
Rogozinski hook
Rogozinski screw
Rogozinski spinal fixation system
Roho cushion
Roland index of low back pain
rolandic cortex
rolandic dip transient on EEG
rolandic epilepsy
rolandic epileptiform discharges on EEG
rolandic fissure
rolandic seizure
rolandic sharp transient on EEG
rolandic spike
rolandic sulcus
rolandic vein syndrome
rolandi, substantia gelatinosa
Rolando angle
Rolando area
Rolando cell
Rolando fissure
Rolando fracture
Rolando line
Rolando point
Rolando tubercle
Rolando zone
rolandoparietal glioma
Rolator walker
rolfing (massage)
roll
  axillary
  chest
  cotton
  hand
  hip
  iliac crest
  palmar
  positioning
  radiolucent
  towel
rollback, femoral
roller
  cranioplastic
  Spence cranioplastic
Rolyan tibial fracture brace
ROM (range of motion)
Romberg sign

Romberg station
Romberg syndrome
Romberg tandem
Romberg test
Rome criteria for rheumatoid arthritis
rongeur (see also *forceps*)
  Adson cranial
  angled jaw
  angled pituitary
  angular bone
  Bacon bone
  Bacon cranial
  Baer bone
  Bane-Hartmann bone
  basket
  bayonet
  Beyer-Stille bone
  Blumenthal bone
  Boehler bone (Böhler)
  bone-nibbling
  Bruening-Citelli
  Bucy laminectomy
  Campbell
  cervical laminectomy
  Cherry-Kerrison laminectomy
  Cicherelli bone
  Cintor bone
  Cleveland bone
  Cloward intervertebral disk
  Cloward large cervical
  Cloward-English laminectomy
  Cloward-Harper laminectomy
  Codman-Harper laminectomy
  Codman-Kerrison laminectomy
  Codman-Leksell laminectomy
  Codman-Schlesinger cervical laminectomy
  Cohen
  Colclough-Scheicher laminectomy
  Corbett bone
  cranial
  curved bone
  Cushing cranial
  Cushing intervertebral disk

rongeur *(cont.)*
  Dahlgren cranial
  Dale first rib
  Dean bone
  Decker microsurgical
  Decker pituitary
  Defourmentel bone
  DeVilbiss cranial
  disk
  double-action
  downbiting
  duckbill
  Echlin bone
  Echlin duckbill
  Echlin laminectomy
  Echlin-Luer
  Ferris Smith intervertebral disk
  Ferris Smith laminectomy
  Ferris Smith-Kerrison laminectomy
  Ferris Smith-Spurling disk
  first rib
  Fisch bone
  Friedman bone
  Frykholm bone
  Fulton laminectomy
  Geiger
  gooseneck
  Gruenwald neurosurgical
  Guleke bone
  Hajek-Koffler laminectomy
  Hakansson bone
  Hartmann bone
  Hein
  Hoen intervertebral disk
  Hoen laminectomy
  Horsley bone
  Hudson cranial
  Husk bone
  intervertebral disk
  Jackson intervertebral disk
  Jansen
  Jarit-Kerrison laminectomy
  Jarit-Liston bone
  Jarit-Ruskin bone

rongeur *(cont.)*
- Kerrison down-biting
- Kerrison laminectomy
- Kleinert-Kutz bone
- Kleinert-Kutz synovectomy
- laminectomy
- Lebsche
- Leksell laminectomy
- Leksell-Stille thoracic
- Lempert bone
- Liston bone
- Liston-Littauer bone
- Littauer-West
- Love-Gruenwald intervertebral disk
- Love-Gruenwald pituitary
- Love-Kerrison laminectomy
- Luer bone
- Luer-Friedman bone
- Luer-Hartmann
- Markwalder bone
- Marquardt bone
- Mayfield
- McIndoe bone
- Mead bone
- micro-Kerrison
- microlaminectomy
- mini-Ruskin
- Montenovesi
- Mount laminectomy
- Mueller (Müller)
- Nicola pituitary
- Oldberg intervertebral disk
- Oldberg pituitary
- Olivecrona
- osteophyte nipper
- peapod intervertebral disk
- Peiper-Beyer laminectomy
- Pilling-Liston
- pituitary
- Poppen intervertebral disk
- Raney laminectomy
- Reiner bone
- Rottgen-Ruskin bone
- Ruskin-Jansen bone

rongeur *(cont.)*
- Ruskin-Jay
- Ruskin-Liston bone
- Ruskin-Rowland bone
- Rust
- Sauerbruch-Coryllos
- Sauerbruch-Stille
- Sauerbruch rib
- Schell bone
- Schlesinger cervical
- Schlesinger intervertebral disk
- Schlesinger laminectomy
- Selverstone intervertebral disk
- Semb-Stille bone
- Shearer
- single action
- Smith-Petersen laminectomy
- Spence intervertebral disk
- Spurling intervertebral disk
- Spurling pituitary
- Spurling-Kerrison laminectomy
- Spurling-Kerrison up-biting and down-biting
- Stellbrink synovectomy
- Stille-Horsley bone
- Stille-Leksell
- Stille-Liston bone
- Stille-Luer bone
- Stille-Luer-Echlin
- Stille-Ruskin bone
- Stookey cranial
- straight bone
- straight pituitary
- Strully-Gigli
- Strully-Kerrison
- synovectomy
- Takahashi
- thoracic
- upbiting
- Urschel first rib
- Walton-Liston bone
- Walton-Ruskin bone
- Watson-Williams intervertebral disk
- Weil-Blakesley intervertebral disk

rongeur *(cont.)*
  Whitcomb-Kerrison laminectomy
  Wilde intervertebral disk
  Yasargil pituitary
  Zaufel-Jansen bone
rongeur forceps
roof, intercondylar
roof of insula
roof of ventricle
room
  Allender vertical laminar flow
  Charnley laminar flow
Roos approach
Roos brachial plexus root retractor
Roos first rib shears
root, roots
  cervical nerve
  compression of nerve
  extrathecal nerve
  fila of nerve
  impingement on nerve
  injury to nerve
  intradural nerve
  intrathecal
  neoplastic invasion of
  nerve
  posterior
  somatosympathetic fibers of nerve
  ventral nerve
root compression syndrome
root exit zone (REZ)
root fiber
root irritation
root lesion
root level motor impairment
Root-Siegal osteotomy
rooting reflex (primitive)
rootlets of nerve
rosary, rachitic
Rose foot procedure
Rose, lateral mamillary nucleus of
Rose-Waaler test
Rosen bur
Rosen elevator
Rosenberg retractor
Rosenfeld hip prosthesis
Rosenmüller, fossa of
Rosenthal, basal vein of (BVR)
Rosenthal fiber formation in leukodystrophy
Rosenthal vein (basal vein)
rosette Beaver blade
Rosser classification of illness states
Rosser crypt hook
Rossolimo contraction
rostral brain stem
rostral brain stem ischemia
rostral cervical nerve
rostral connection
rostral hypothalamus
rostral medulla
rostral pons
rostral spinal cord
rostral terminus
rostrally
rostrum of corpus callosum
Rotablator rotating bur
rotary instability
rotary scoliosis
rotary subluxation
rotating frame of reference
rotation
  axis of
  eccentric axis of (of ankle)
  external
  hip lateral
  hip medial
  internal
  internal femoral
  inward
  lateral
  medial
  neutral
  outward
  passive head
  pelvic
  tibiofibular
  transverse (of lower extremity)

rotational alignment
rotational flaps
rotational force
rotational scarf bunionectomy
rotationplasty
rotator
  external
  internal
  Jarit
  long external
  short external
rotator cuff calcific tendinitis
rotator cuff impingement syndrome
rotator cuff tear
rotator cuff tendon
rotatory loads on spine
rotatory nystagmus
Rothman Institute femoral prosthesis
RotoRest bed
rotoscoliosis
Rottgen-Ruskin bone rongeur
roughened surface
roughening
rouleaux formation
round back posture
round cell tumors
round pronator (pronator radii teres)
Rousek extraction set
Rousek extractor
Roussy-Dejerine thalamic pain syndrome
Roussy-Lévy disease
Roussy-Lévy hereditary areflexic dystasia
Roussy-Lévy syndrome
Rouviere, ligament of
Roux-duToit staple capsulorrhaphy
Roux-Goldthwait procedure
roving eye movements
roving ocular movements
row
  carpal
  proximal carpal
row of sutures
Rowe calcaneal fracture classification
Rowe capsular retractor
Rowe disimpaction forceps
Rowe fusion
Rowe glenoid punch
Rowe glenoid-reaming forceps
Rowe-Harrison bone-holding forceps
Rowe humeral head retractor
Rowe-Lowell fracture-dislocation classification system
Rowe modified-Harrison forceps
Rowe-Zarins shoulder immobilization technique
Rowland-Hughes splint
Roy-Camille cervical plate
Roy-Camille occipitocervical plate
Roy-Camille pedicle plate
Roy-Camille screw placement technique
Royalite body jacket
Royle-Thompson transfer technique
RP (rehabilitation psychiatry)
RP (right parietal) (EEG lead)
RPAB (Rivermead Perceptual Assessment Battery)
RPS (reverse pivot shift) test
RPT (right posterior temporal) (EEG lead)
RSA (Rehabilitation Services Administration)
RSD (reflex sympathetic dystrophy)
RSDS (reflex sympathetic dystrophy syndrome)
RSI (repetitive strain injury)
RSI (repetitive stress injury)
R-type (reactive) alpha rhythm
rub, friction (in knee) (Renee creak sign)
rubber-shod (protected) clamp
rubella, congenital
Rubin bone planer
Rubin cartilage planer
Rubin gouge
Rubin rasp
Rubinstein-Taybi syndrome

rubor
rubral tremor
rubrospinal tract
rubrum, Tricophyton
rucksack paralysis
Rud syndrome
rudimentary ribs
RUE (right upper extremity)
Ruedi-Allgower tibial plafond fracture
  classification
Ruffini corpuscle sensory receptor
Ruffini mechanoreceptor
rugger jersey spine
Ruiz-Mora procedure
rule of squares to plot scotomas
ruler
  Berndt hip
  stainless steel
Rumel aluminum splint
runner, runners
  extrinsic-dominant
  heel-toe
  intrinsic-negative
  intrinsic-positive
runner's bump
runner's knee
running epilepsy
running-related injury
running seizures
rupture
  attrition (of tendon)
  buttonhole
  complete Achilles tendon
  plantaris (tennis leg)
ruptured Achilles tendon
  complete
  partial
ruptured disk
ruptured intracranial aneurysm
Rush awl
Rush driver-bender-extractor
Rush mallet
Rush pin
Rush rod
Ruskin bone-cutting forceps
Ruskin bone-splitting forceps
Ruskin-Jansen bone rongeur
Ruskin-Liston bone-cutting forceps
Ruskin-Liston rongeur
Ruskin-Rowland bone-cutting forceps
Russe approach
Russe bone graft
Russell-Taylor interlocking nail
Russell-Taylor reconstruction rod
Russell traction for femoral fracture
Russell-Rubinstein classification of
  cerebrovascular malformation
Russian forceps
Rust amputation saw
Rust rongeur
Rust saw
Rust sign
RVAF (reversed vertebral blood flow)
Rydell nail
Ryder needle holder
Ryder test
Ryerson graft
Ryerson tenotome
Ryerson triple arthrodesis

S, s

SAB (short-acting block) anesthesia
Sabel cast walker
saber shin
Sabin-Feldman dye test for congenital toxoplasmosis
sac
  bursal
  common dural
  cystic
  dural
  effacement of dural
  narrowing of thecal
  spinal
  thecal
  tight dural
SAC (short arm cast)
saccade, saccades
  adduction
  back-to-back
  contralateral
  corrective
  dysmetric
  optic dysmetric
  rapid (corrective)
  rapid lateral
  volitional
saccade velocity (on EMG)
saccadic blur
saccadic corrections
saccadic eye movements
saccadic oscillations
saccadic palsy
saccadic slowing
saccadic snap
saccharopinuria
saccular aneurysm
SACH (solid-ankle, cushioned heel) foot prosthesis
SACH heels
Sachs brain suction tip
Sachs dural hook
Sachs dural separator
Sachs nerve separator-spatula
Sachs suction tube
Sachs vein retractor
sacral ala
sacral cyst
sacral dermatomes
sacral gutter
sacral sparing, in sensory loss
sacralgia
sacralization of transverse process of vertebra
sacralization of vertebrae
sacralized transverse process
Sacro-ease pillow
Sacro-Eze lumbar support
sacrococcygeal chordomas
sacrococcygeal remnant tumor
sacrococcyx
sacroiliac (SI) joint
sacroiliac joint syndrome
sacroiliac resisted abduction test
sacroiliac sprain
sacroiliac stretch test
sacroiliac subluxation
sacroiliac syndrome
sacroiliitis

sacrotuberous ligament
sacrovertebral angle
sacrum (sacral spine)
saddle anesthesia
saddle-area anesthesia
saddle-area sensory loss
saddle clamp
saddle coil
saddle distribution of sensory loss
saddle hypesthesia
saddle joint
saddle, trapezial
SADIA (small angle double incidence angiograms)
Sadowsky Breast Marking System (SBS)
SADS (seasonal affective disorder syndrome)
Saethre-Chotzen syndrome
SAFE foot (stationary attachment flexible endoskeletal)
SAF hip replacement (self-articulating femoral)
Sage-Clark technique
Sage radial nail
Sage-Salvatore classification of acromioclavicular joint injury
Sager traction splint
sagittal orientation
sagittal plane faults
sagittal roll spondylolisthesis
sagittal sinus
SAH (subarachnoid hemorrhage)
Saha transfer technique
SAID (specific adaptation to imposed demands) of disability
sail sign
Saint (see *St.*)
Sakellarides classification of calcaneal fracture
salaam attack
salaam seizures
Salenius meniscus knife
Salibi carotid artery clamp
salicylic acid plaster for plantar warts
salicylic acid tape
salient antecedents to injury
saline
  heparinized
  sterile
saline flush
saline torch
Salmon Rickham ventriculostomy reservoir
Salmonella arthritis
Salmonella osteomyelitis
salt bridges connecting EEG electrodes
salt wasting, cerebral
saltans, coxa
saltatory nerve conduction
saltatory spasm
Salter fracture (I-VI)
Salter-Harris classification of epiphyseal fracture
Salter-Harris classification of tibial-fibular injury
Salter-Harris-Rang classification of epiphyseal fracture
Salter innominate osteotomy
Saltiel brace
salts, gold
salvage, limb
salvage procedure
salvage reconstruction
salvo (pl. salvos)
Salzer prosthesis
Salzer resurfacing procedure
Sam splint
Samilson osteotomy
sample, Pennsylvania bimanual work
sampling rate on EEG
Sampson medullary nail
Samuels forceps
sandal, Rainbow cast
sandbagging fracture of long bones
Sanfilippo syndrome
sanguineous
Santa Casa distractor

Santavuori-Haltia-Hagberg disease
Sarbo sign
sarcoid, Boeck
sarcoidosis, spinal cord
sarcoma
  alveolar soft part
  botryoid
  classic Kaposi
  clear cell
  epidemic Kaposi
  epithelioid
  Ewing
  extraosseous Ewing
  high-grade surface osteogenic
  intracortical osteogenic
  juxtacortical
  Kaposi
  low-grade central osteogenic
  malignant myeloid
  multicentric osteogenic
  osteogenic
  Paget associated osteogenic
  parosteal osteogenic
  postirradiation osteogenic
  primary
  reticulum cell
  small cell osteogenic
  spindle cell
  synovial
sarcotubular myopathy
sardonicus, risus
Sargent knee procedure
Sarmiento (STH-2) hip prosthesis
Sarmiento short leg patellar tendon-bearing cast
sartorius tendon
SAS II (shoulder arm system) brace
S.A.S. shoes
Sassouni analysis
Sat-A-Lite seat cushion
Satalite cushion (by Bodyline)
Sateen knee immobilizer
satellite plantar wart
Satterlee amputating saw
Satterlee bone saw
saturation, jugular venous oxygen
saturation recovery
saturation transfer
Saturday night palsy
Saturday night radial palsy
saucerization
saucerize
Sauerbruch-Britsch rib shears
Sauerbruch-Coryllos rongeur
Sauerbruch-Frey bone punch
Sauerbruch-Frey rib shears
Sauerbruch rib elevator
Sauerbruch rib forceps
Sauerbruch rib rongeur
Sauerbruch rib shears
Sauerbruch-Stille rongeur
sausage finger, in syringomyelia
Savastano Hemi-Knee prosthesis
Saver, Haemonetics Cell
saw
  Adams
  Adson wire
  Aesculap
  air-powered
  amputating
  Bailey-Gigli
  Bailey wire
  bayonet
  Beaver
  Bier amputation
  Bishop
  bow-type
  cast
  Charriere amputating
  Charriere bone
  circular
  Cottle
  counter rotating
  craniotomy
  crosscut
  Cushing
  Davis
  DeMartel wire

saw *(cont.)*
- electric cast
- end-cutting reciprocating
- Engel plaster
- fenestration
- Gigli wire
- Hall air-driven oscillating
- Hall Micro E oscillating
- Hall Micro E reciprocating
- Hall Micro E sagittal
- Hall Versipower oscillating
- Hall Versipower reciprocating
- Herbert
- Langenbeck metacarpal
- Lebsche wire
- Luck-Bishop bone
- metacarpal
- micro sagittal
- Micro-Aire oscillating
- micro-oscillating
- Midas Rex craniotomy
- Mueller (Müller)
- Olivecrona-Gigli
- Orthair oscillating
- oscillating
- Oscillo III plaster
- Percy amputating
- plaster
- Poppen
- power oscillating
- power-driven
- Raney
- reciprocating motor
- Rust amputation
- sagittal surgical
- Satterlee amputating
- single-blade
- straight oscillating
- Strully-Gigli
- twin-blade oscillating
- Tyler-Gigli
- Weiss amputation
- Wigmore plaster
- wire
- Zimmer oscillating

SAWA shoulder brace

sawcut

saw guide
- Bailey Gigli
- Poppen Gigli

saw handles, Strully Gigli

Sayk preparation of CSF cells

Sayre periosteal elevator

Sayre splint

Sayre traction

Sbarbaro tibial plateau prosthesis

SBO (spina bifida occulta)

SBRN (sensory branch of the radial nerve)

SCA (superior cerebellar artery)

Scaglietti closed reduction technique

scale, Scale
- Abnormal Involuntary Movement (AIMS)
- ADAS noncognitive subscale
- American Musculoskeletal Tumor Society rating
- Arthritis Impact Measurement (AIMS)
- Ashworth
- Blessed Behavior Scale
- Blessed Dementia Rating (BDRS)
- Blessed-Roth Dementia Scale (BRDS)
- Bonney hallux valgus outcome
- Brief Cognitive Rating Scale (BCRS)
- Canadian Neurological Scale
- Charnley-Merle D'Aubigné disability grading
- Charnley pain and function grading
- Clinical Dementia Rating (CDR)
- Comprehensive Level of Consciousness (CLCS)
- Cornell Scale for Depression, Dementia (CSDD)
- Dementia Behavior Disturbance (DBD)
- Dementia Mood Assessment (DMAS)

scale *(cont.)*
- Edinburgh Rehabilitation Status
- Ficat grading
- Gait Abnormality Rating (GARS)
- Glasgow Coma (GCS)
- Glasgow Outcome
- Guttman
- Hamilton Rating Scale for Depression
- Harris hip
- hierarchical scale of ADLs
- Hospital Anxiety and Depression
- HSS (Hospital for Special Surgery) ligament rating
- Hunt-Hess subarachnoid hemorrhage
- interval scale in rehabilitation testing
- Johnson-Boseker
- ligament sizing
- linear analog pain
- linear analog self-assessment
- Lovett's clinical scale of strength
- Lysholm knee function
- MAS (Motor Assessment)
- Merle D'Aubigné pain and mobility rating
- modified Ashworth scale for grading spasticity
- Motor Assessment (MAS)
- Neurobehavioral Rating
- NIH (National Institutes of Health) Stroke
- Nottingham Ten-Point ADL Scale
- Noyes knee rating
- Outerbridge
- Oxford scale, measuring muscle strength
- Prosthetic Problem Inventory
- Quality of Well-Being
- Rankin
- Rankin Scale
- Rappaport Disability Rating
- Tegner activity level
- Zung Self-Rating Depression

scalene block
scalene fat pad
scalene musculature
scalenus anticus muscle
scalenus anticus syndrome
scalenus anticus test
scalloping of margin of vertebral body
scalloping of vertebrae
scalp clip applicator
scalp clips
- Children's Hospital
- Raney

scalp edema
scalp EEG (SEEG)
scalp electrode
scalp-electrode interface
scalp hematoma
scalp inclusion cyst
scalp recording of EEG
scalp slips, LeRoy
scalp vein
scalpel
scan, scanning
- bone
- brain
- CAT (computerized axial tomographic)
- contrast material enhanced
- CT (computed tomography)
- CT (computerized tomography)
- CTAT (computerized transverse axial tomography)
- duplex
- duplex carotid
- gallium
- gallium-67 bone
- high-resolution ultrasound scan for foreign bodies
- indium-111-labeled leukocyte bone
- isotope
- isotope bone
- isotope shunt
- linear
- MRI (magnetic resonance imaging)
- nuclear bone

scan *(cont.)*
  PET (positron emission tomography)
  positron emission transaxial tomography
  postmetrizamide CT
  radioisotope gallium
  radioisotope indium-labeled white blood cell
  radioisotope (static)
  radioisotope technetium
  radionuclide
  radionuclide brain
  rectilinear bone
  sector
  serial
  SPECT (single photon emission CT)
  stacked
  technetium
  technetium-99m diphosphonate
  technetium-99m MDP bone
  technetium-99m pyrophosphate
  technetium-99m sulfur colloid
  three-phase bone
  total body
  triple-phase bone
  TSPP rectilinear bone
  unenhanced
scan with contrast, CT
scanner, ATL real-time Neurosector
scanning speech
scanogram, extremity
scanography
scapho-trapezium-trapezoid (STT) joint
scaphocapitate joint
scaphocephalic head shape
scaphocephaly
scaphoid bone (navicular)
  pole of
  waist of
scaphoid cookie in shoe
Scaphoid-Microstaple system
scaphoiditis
scapholunate (SL) joint
scapholunate arthritic collapse (SLAC) wrist
scapholunate dissociation
scapholunate joint
scapholunate ligament
scapholunate space
scaphotrapezoid-trapezial (STT) joint
scapula
  body of
  margin of
  high-riding
  winged
  winging of the
scapular flap
scapular winging
scapulectomy
  Das Gupta
  Phelps
scapuloclavicular
scapulocostal syndrome
scapuloperoneal dystrophy
scapuloperoneal muscular atrophy
scapulothoracic motion
scapulovertebral border
scar
  dural
  incisional
  retractile
  scarring
Scarborough total hip replacement
scar contracture
scarf bunionectomy, rotational
scarified
Scarpa fascia
Scarpa ganglion
scarred
scarring
scattered dysrhythmic slow activity (on EEG)
Scerratti goniometer
SCFE (slipped capital femoral epiphysis)
Schaberg-Harper-Allen technique
Schaltenbrand atlas of stereotaxy for neurosurgery
Schanz angulation osteotomy
Schanz brace

Schanz collar
Schanz metaphyseal screws
Schanz rod
Scharff microbipolar and suction forceps
Schatzker fracture classification system
Schauwecker patellar wiring technique
Schede bone curet
Schede hip osteotomy
Schedule
  General Well-Being
  Glasgow Assessment
Scheicker laminectomy punch forceps
Scheie syndrome
Schell bone rongeur
Scheuermann disease
Scheuermann juvenile kyphosis
Schiefferdecker disk
Schiff-Sherrington phenomenon
Schilder disease
Schilder encephalitis
Schink retractor
Schirmer test
schistosomiasis, spinal
schizencephaly
Schlein clamp
Schlein elbow arthroplasty
Schlein prosthesis
Schlesinger cervical punch forceps
Schlesinger cervical rongeur
Schlesinger intervertebral disk rongeur
Schlesinger laminectomy rongeur
Schlesinger rongeur forceps
Schlesinger sign
Schlesinger, vein of
Schmeisser spica
Schmidt rod holder
Schmidt syndrome
Schmieden dural scissors
Schmieden-Taylor dissector
Schmitt disease
Schmorl node
Schmorl nodule
Schneider arthrodesis
Schneider driver-extractor
Schneider nail
Schneider rasp
Schneider rod
Schneider-Sauerbruch rasp
Schnute wedge resection technique
Schober test of lumbar flexion
Schoeber sign
Schoemaker-Burkart marker
Scholl's pads
school
  back
  neck
school performance, deterioration in
Schrötter chorea
Schreiber maneuver
Schrock procedure
Schuchart rib shears
Schuknecht wire-cutting scissors
Schuller view (on x-ray)
Schultze bundle
Schumacher criteria for diagnosis of multiple sclerosis
Schumacher rib shears
Schutte basket, shovel-nose
Schwalbe nucleus of cerebellum
Schwann cell body
Schwann cell of myelin sheath
Schwann cell tube
Schwann cells, proliferation of
Schwann tumor
schwannoma
  orbital
  vestibular
Schwartz aneurysm clip
Schwartz clip-applying forceps
Schwartz intracranial clamp
Schwartz-Jampel syndrome (SJS)
Schwartz laminectomy retractor
Schwartz temporary clamp applying forceps
Schwartz temporary intracranial artery clamps
Schwartze chisel

Schwarz finger extension bow
Schweitzer spring plate
SCI (spinal cord injury)
sciatic nerve irritation
sciatic notch
sciatic plexus
sciatic stretch test
sciatica
scimitar sign on x-ray
scintigraphy
  bone
  indium-111
  indium scintigraphy with ^{111}In white blood cells (^{111}In-WBC)
  three-phase bone (TPBS)
  white blood cell scintigraphy (WBCS) with indium-111
scintilla
scintillating scotoma (pl. scotomata)
scissor gait
scissoring of legs
scissors
  Acufex
  Adson ganglion
  alligator
  arthroscopic
  Babcock wire-cutting
  bandage
  Bantam wire-cutting
  bayonet-shaped
  Beebe wire-cutting
  Bellucci alligator
  Bergmann plaster
  bipolar cautery
  blunt-tipped iris
  brain
  cartilage
  circumflex
  Crafoord thoracic
  crown and collar
  curved Mayo
  Dandy neurosurgical
  Dandy trigeminal nerve
  Dean

scissors *(cont.)*
  DeBakey endarterectomy
  Decker alligator
  Decker micro
  Decker microsurgical
  DeMartel neurosurgical
  dissecting
  dural
  ear, nose and throat (ENT)
  endarterectomy
  ENT (ear, nose, and throat)
  Esmarch plaster
  face-lift
  Frazier dural
  Giertz-Stille
  Halsey nail
  Harvey wire-cutting
  hook
  iris
  Jacobson microneurosurgical
  Jannetta-Kurze dissecting
  Koenig nail splitting
  Kreuscher
  Kurze dissecting
  Lister
  Malis bipolar cautery
  Malis neurological
  Martin cartilage
  Mayo
  McCain TMJ
  McIndoe
  Medi plaster
  meniscectomy
  meniscus
  Metzenbaum
  micro
  microneurosurgical
  Micro-One
  microsurgery or microsurgical
  Micro-Two
  moleskin
  nail
  nail splitting
  Nelson

scissors *(cont.)*
    neurological
    neurosurgical
    Nicola
    Olivecrona dural
    Olivecrona trigeminal
    operating
    Penn wire-cutting
    pituitary
    plaster
    Potts-Smith
    Potts tenotomy
    Potts-Yasargil
    Rhoton bayonet
    Rogers wire-cutting
    Schmieden dural
    Schuknecht wire-cutting
    Seutin plaster
    Slip-N-Slip
    Smillie meniscus
    Smith wire-cutting
    spring-handled
    Stiwer
    strabismus
    Strully
    Strully dissecting
    Strully dural
    Strully neurological
    suture
    Sweet pituitary
    Take-apart
    Taylor brain
    Taylor dural
    tenotomy
    thoracic
    Tindall
    Toennis dissecting
    trigeminal
    Walton
    Webster meniscectomy
    Weller cartilage
    Wiet otologic
    wire
    wire-cutting

scissors *(cont.)*
    Yasargil bayonet
    Yasargil micro
scleroderma
sclerosant
sclerosing nonsuppurative osteitis
sclerosis
    Ammon horn (mesial temporal)
    amyotrophic lateral (ALS)
        (Lou Gehrig disease)
    Baló
    congenital hippocampal
    diffuse
    disseminated
    familial amyotrophic lateral
    incisural
    Krabbe diffuse
    lobar
    mesial temporal
    Mönckeberg
    multiple (MS)
    pedicle (on x-ray)
    posterolateral (of the spinal cord)
    subchondral
    tuberous
sclerotherapy
sclerotic area
sclerotic rims in gout (on x-ray)
sclerotomal diagram of pain
sclerotomal pain
sclerotome area
scoliorachitis
scoliosis
    adolescent idiopathic (AIS)
    Aussies-Isseis unstable
    Cobb measurement of
    dextrorotary
    Dwyer correction of
    Fergusson method for measuring
    fixation of a
    functional
    idiopathic
    King classification of thoracic
    King-Moe

scoliosis *(cont.)*
  levorotary
  levoscoliosis
  lumbar component of
  Moe and Kettleson distribution of curves in
  rotary
  S-shaped
  thoracic component of
  thoracolumbar
  uncompensated rotary
  Winter-King-Moe
scoliosis correction with Dwyer cable
scoliotic spine
scoop
  bone
  Cushing pituitary
  intervertebral disk
  Scoville intervertebral disk
  Yasargil
scope
  Doppler
  Harris
  Hughston knee
  Lysholm knee joint instability
  Lysholm knee stability
score, Score
  Ashworth muscle spasticity
  Champion Trauma (CTS)
  Children's Coma (CCS)
  GCS (Glasgow Coma Scale)
  Hachinski ischemia
  Hannover Polytrauma
  HSS (Hospital for Special Surgery) knee
  Hughston knee
  injury-severity
  Karnofsky performance (KPS)
  Kurtzke disability
  Lysholm knee joint instability
  Lysholm knee stability
  Lysholm-Gillquist
  Mangled Extremity Severity (MESS)

score *(cont.)*
  Rankin
  skeletal-injury
scorings on bone on x-ray
Scotchcast 2 casting tape
Scotchcast splint
scotoma (pl. scotomata)
  absolute
  bilateral
  cecocentral
  central
  dense
  fortification
  homonymous scintillating
  march of
  mental
  negative
  paracentral
  relative
  scintillating
scotomata of action
scotometry
scotomization
Scott glenoplasty technique
Scott-McCracken periosteal elevator
Scott silicone ventricular catheter
Scott ventricular cannula
Scottish Rite hip orthosis
scout film (x-ray)
ScoutView targeting
Scoville blade
Scoville brain clip-applying forceps
Scoville brain spatula forceps
Scoville cervical disk retractor
Scoville clip-applying forceps
Scoville disk curet
Scoville dissector
Scoville-Haverfield hemilaminectomy retractor
Scoville intervertebral disk scoop
Scoville nerve root hook
Scoville nerve root retractor
Scoville-Richter laminectomy retractor
Scoville ruptured disk curet

Scoville skull trephine
Scoville spatula forceps
Scoville ventricular needles
scraping toe gait
scratching automatism
  blood
  drug
  Lanex
Screening Test, Halstead-Wepman
  Aphasia
screw
  Ace
  AcroMed VSP
  Aesculap
  AMBI hip
  Amset R-F
  AO cancellous
  AO cortical
  AO lag
  AO spongiosa
  AO-ASIF
  arthrodesis
  ASIF cancellous
  ASIF cortical
  Asnis 2 guided
  Asnis cannulated
  Aten olecranon
  Barouk cannulated bone
  Barouk micro
  Basile
  Bechtol
  bicortical
  biodegradable
  Bosworth
  breakout of
  buttress
  C-D (Cotrel-Dubousset)
  Calandruccio compression
  Campbell cannulated
  cancellous bone
  cannulated
  Carrell-Girard
  Caspar cervical
  chrome cobalt
  Collison

screw *(cont.)*
  compression hip
  compression lag
  Concept cannulated
  cortex
  cortical bone
  cortical cancellous
  Cotrel-Dubosset vertebral
  Coventry
  cross-slot
  cruciate head
  cruciform-head
  Cubbins
  DDT (device for transverse traction)
  DeMuth
  double-fluted tip
  double-threaded Herbert
  Duo-Driv
  DuVal
  Dwyer cable and
  ECT (European compression technique) bone
  Edwards
  Eggers
  epidural
  Fixateur Interne
  fretted
  fully threaded
  Geckler
  Glasgow
  Glass-Bessen transfixion
  Hahn
  Hamilton
  Henderson lag
  Herbert bone
  Herbert-Whipple bone
  hex (hexagonal)
  hex head
  hexagon
  hexagonal slot-cap
  hollow mill Asnis cannulated
  home run
  Howmedica ICS

screw *(cont.)*
- Howmedica VSF
- Ilizarov
- interference
- interfragmentary
- Isola vertebral
- Johansson lag
- Jones
- Kaessmann
- Knöringer
- Kostuik
- Kristiansen eyelet lag
- Kurosaka fixation
- lag
- Lane bone
- large-headed
- Leibinger Micro Plus
- Leibinger mini-Wurzburg
- Leinbach
- Lorenz cranial
- Lorenzo
- Luhr
- Lundholm
- Luque II
- Maconor
- Magerl transarticular
- malleolar
- Marion
- Martin
- McLaughlin
- metallic
- micro self-tapping
- Mille Pattes
- mini AO
- Morris biphase
- Morris biplane
- Moss
- Mouradian
- navicular
- Neufeld
- NoLok
- Olerud PSF
- Orthofix
- pedicle

screw *(cont.)*
- Phillips
- Phillips recessed head
- pitch of threads on
- PWB (Puno-Winter-Byrd)
- resorbable
- Richards compression
- Richards self-tapping
- Rockwood
- Rogozinski
- Salzburg
- Schanz metaphyseal
- Selby I and II
- self-tapping bone
- Shelton bone
- Sherman bone
- Simmons
- sliding compression hip
- small-fragment
- small-headed
- stainless steel
- Steffee pedicle
- Steffee plate and
- Steinhauser cranial
- Storz
- stripout of
- Stryker
- subarachnoid
- subdural pressure
- suprasyndesmotic
- Swiss cancellous
- syndesmosis
- syndesmotic
- Synthes compression hip
- tension
- Thornton
- threaded cancellous
- thumb
- tibial head
- tip of
- titanium lag
- Townley
- Townsend-Gilfillan
- transarticular

screw *(cont.)*
- transfixing
- transfixion
- transpedicular
- transsyndesmosis
- transsyndesmotic
- triangulated
- Tronzo VLC cannulated compression
- TSRH vertebral
- unicortical
- varus-valgus adjustment
- VDS (ventral derotating spinal)
- Venable-Stuck
- Vitallium
- von Bahr
- VSF (Vermont spinal fixator)
- VSP (variable screw placement)
- Wagner-Schanz
- Wurzburg
- Wiltse
- wood
- Woodruff
- Zimmer compression hip
- Zuelzer

screwdriver
- automatic
- Becker
- Bosworth
- cannulated
- Cardan
- collet adapter
- Collison
- cross-slot
- cruciform
- Flatt self-retaining
- Ken
- Phillips head
- Ritcher
- self-retaining
- single-slot
- torque
- VDS (ventral derotating spinal)
- Williams

screw and plate (screw-plate)
screw fixation
screw head
- countersink
- Phillips

screwhome mechanism
screw-in ceramic acetabular cup
screw placement, variable (VSP)
screw-plate
- Calandruccio impaction
- pedicle
- Zimmer impaction

screw pull-out
screw-rod
- Edwards D-L modular
- Wiltse

screw tap
screw toggle
scriptorius, calamus
scrub
- Betadine
- Hibiclens

scrum ear (in rugby players)
SCT (spinal cord tether)
SCT (star-cancellation test)
Scuderi technique
scultetus bandage
SDAT (senile dementia, Alzheimer type)
SDEEG (stereotaxic depth electroencephalogram)
SDH (subdural hemorrhage)
SDRI (small, deep, recent infarct)
SEA (spinal epidural abscess)
seat
- Heffington lumbar surgical
- ischial-bearing
- LiteNest portable
- Wayne laminectomy

seat belt fracture
seat belt injury
seat belt sign
seat surface
seated prosthesis

seating of the prosthesis
  adaptive
  proper
Seattle foot prosthesis
Seattle orthosis
Seawell rasp
sebaceum, adenoma (in tuberous sclerosis)
Sebileau periosteal elevator
Seckel syndrome
second compartment
second cranial nerve (optic)
second double support, of gait
secondary brain tumor
secondary closure
secondary contractures
secondary fracture
secondary gain
secondary intention, healing by
secondary metatarsalgia
secondary or acute hematogenous osteomyelitis
secondary suture of ruptured tendons
secondary union
Secor drug pump (I and II)
Secor implantable drug reservoir
secretomotor (parasympathetic) fibers
section, permanent
sector
  lower field visual
  Sommer sector of the hippocampus
sed (sedimentation) rate
Sedan goniometer
Sedan-Vallicioni cannula
Seddon classification of nerve injuries
Seddon technique
sedentary lifestyle
Sedillot periosteal elevator
seeding, intracranial
seeding of tumor
SEEG (scalp EEG)
SEEG (stereotactic electroencephalogram)
seesaw nystagmus
segment, transected
segment distraction
segment fixation
segmental bone loss
segmental branch of vertebral artery
segmental distribution of syringomyelia
segmental epidural nerve block with local anesthesia
segmental narrowing
segmental sign
segmental spinal instrumentation (SSI)
segmental symptoms
segmental tract of trigeminal
Segond fracture
Seguin sign
SEH (spinal epidural hemorrhage)
Seidel humeral locking nail
Seidel intramedullary fixation
Seidel intramedullary rod
Seinsheimer classification of femoral fracture
Seitelberger disease
seizure (see also *epilepsy*)
  absence
  acute
  adversive motor
  akinetic
  alcohol as cause of
  alcohol-related
  alcohol-withdrawal
  alimentary
  aphasic
  apneic
  astatic
  asymptomatic
  atonic absence
  atypical absence
  audiogenic
  auditory
  benign neonatal familial
  bilateral myoclonic
  cardiovascular
  centrencephalic

seizure *(cont.)*
cephalgic
cerebellar fits
cerebral
cessation of
chewing automatism during
chewing during
clonic
clonic-tonic-clonic
complex partial (CPS)
continuing petit mal
contraversive
convulsive
cryptogenic
diencephalic
drug-induced
drug-withdrawal
ectopic foci of
electrodecremental
electrographic
emotion as cause of
epigastric sensation prior to
epileptic
epilepsia partialis continua
extratemporal origin of
eye movements during
facial expression automatism during
fatigue as cause of
febrile
fecal incontinence during
foaming at the mouth during
focal
focal cerebral
focal motor with march
focal sensory
focus of
generalized convulsive with focal onset
generalized convulsive without focal onset
generalized nonconvulsive
generalized symmetrical and without focal onset
generalized tonic-clonic (GTC)

seizure *(cont.)*
gestural automatism during
grand mal (tonic-clonic)
gustatory
hippocampal
history of
hybrid
hysterical
iatrogenic
ictal confusional
idiopathic primarily generalized
infantile spasms
inhibitory motor
intractable
jackknife
jacksonian
Janz juvenile myoclonic
laughing (gelastic epilepsy)
lip smacking automatism during
long-lasting
major motor
menstrual cycle and occurrence of
minor motor
multifocal
mumbling automatism during
myoclonic
myoclonic jerks
myoclonic-astatic
neonatal
neonatal withdrawal
new-onset
nonmotor somatosensory
occult
olfactory
olfactory psychomotor
parietal
paroxysmal choreoathetosis
partial complex
partial elementary with motor symptoms
partial sensory
partial tonic
patting automatism during
petit mal (typical absence)

seizure *(cont.)*
petit mal variant
phonatory
photogenic
piloerection prior to
post-traumatic
postdialysis
postdiuresis
posthypoxic myoclonic
postictal depressive phase of
postural
precentral
precipitation of
premonition of
primary
psychic
psychogenic
psychomotor
recurring
reflex
repetitive
repetitive partial
retropulsive absence
rolandic
running
salaam
scratching automatism during
secondary generalization with
secondary spread from focus of
sensory-evoked
simple partial
single partial
situation-related
sleep-waking cycle and occurrence of
somatosensory
subclinical
swallowing automatism during
swimming movements during
sylvian
symptomatic
temporal lobe
tonal axial
tongue biting during

seizure *(cont.)*
tonic
tonic-clonic (grand mal)
traumatic
typical
typical absence (petit mal)
uncinate
unilateral
unilateral onset of
urinary incontinence during
versive
vertiginous
visual
withdrawal
seizure disorder
seizure focus
seizure localization
seizure manifestations
seizure pattern
seizure phenomenon
seizure propagation
seizure threshold
Selby I (or II) fixation system
Selby I (or II) hook
Selby I (or II) rod
Selby I (or II) screw
Seldinder-technique angiography
Select ankle prosthesis
Select joint orthosis
Select shoulder prosthesis
selective excitation
selective irradiation
Seletz-Gelpi laminectomy retractor
Seletz nonrigid ventricular catheter
self-articulating femoral (SAF) hip replacement
self-bearing ceramic total hip replacement
self-care activity
self-inflicted gunshot wound
self-reinforced polyglycolide
self-retaining screwdriver
Selig hip procedure

sella
  ballooned
  ballooning of
  empty
  pressure
  atrophy of the dorsum
  decalcified dorsum
  dorsum
  tuberculum
sella-nasion plane
sellar tomography
sella turcica
Sell-Frank-Johnson extensor shift technique
Sellors rib contractor
Selverstone carotid artery clamp
Selverstone cordotomy hook
Selverstone intervertebral disk rongeur
Selverstone rongeur forceps
semantic (or verbal) paraphasia
Semb bone forceps
Semb bone rongeur
Semb rib forceps
Semb rib rasp
Semb rib shears
Semb-Stille rongeur
semi-Fowler position
semicircular canals, hydrops of the
semicoma
semicomatose
semiconscious
semiconsciousness
semidynamic splint
semilunar bone
semilunar cartilages
semiovale, centrum
semipurposeful behavior in petit mal seizures
semirigid, carbon fiber-reinforced plastic plates
semirigid polypropylene ankle-foot orthosis
semisitting position
semitendinosus tendon
Semkin tissue forceps
Semmes spinal fusion curet
Semmes-Weinstein esthesiometer
Semmes-Weinstein monofilament hair test of sensory loss
Semon law
SEMs (slow lateral eye movements)
Senegas approach to hips
senile chorea
senile dementia, Alzheimer type (SDAT)
senile osteoporosis
senile tremor
senilis, coxa
Senn double-end retractor
sensation
  altered
  buzzing
  catching
  deep
  diminished
  dysesthesic
  epigastric (prior to seizure)
  facial
  fine tactile
  impaired
  light touch
  pain
  phantom
  pinprick
  pins and needles
  pins sticking
  popping
  return of
  superficial
  temperature
  tingling
  touch
  vibration
  vibratory
sensation of heat; warmth
sense
  joint position (JPS)
  position
  proprioceptive sense of muscles and ligaments
  vibration
  vibratory (pallesthesia)

sense of time
sensitive plane
sensitive point
sensitive volume
sensitivity of rehabilitation testing
sensitivity, vibration
sensorial epilepsy
sensorimotor cortex
sensorimotor neuropathy
sensorimotor polyneuropathy
sensorimotor skills
sensorimotor stroke
sensorimotor syndrome
sensorimotor system
sensorineural
sensorium
  altered
  changes in
  clouded
  depressed
sensory apraxia
sensory branch of the radial nerve (SBRN)
sensory deficit
  central
  peripheral
sensory-deprivation nystagmus
sensory dermatome
sensory disassociation
sensory discrimination
sensory dysphasia
sensory evoked potential (SEP)
sensory evoked seizures
sensory extinction test
sensory input
sensory jacksonian attack
sensory level
sensory long tract
sensory loss
  cortical
  dense
  level of
  saddle area
  stocking-glove
  tactile
sensory manifestation
sensory modality
sensory nerve action potential (SNAP)
sensory nerve conduction study
sensory nerve fiber
sensory neuropathy
sensory or motor deficit
sensory paralytic bladder
sensory shocks of predormitum
sensory stimulation, double simultaneous
sensory stroke, pure
sensory symptoms
sensory transcortical aphasia
sentence closure tasks
sentence closure test
Sentence Repetition Test
sentences, Babcock
SEP (sensory evoked potential)
SEP (somatosensory evoked potential)
separation
  AC (acromioclavicular)
  atlantoaxial
  atlanto-occipital
  costochondral junction
  shoulder
separator
  Davis nerve
  Dorsey dural
  dural
  Frazier dural
  Hoen dural
  Horsley dural
  Hunter dural
  nerve
  Sachs dural
  Sachs nerve
  toe
  Woodson dural
separator-spatula
  Sachs nerve
  Woodson dural
sepsis, pin-tract
septal area
septal region
septic arthritis

septum
  intermuscular
  internal intermuscular
  posterior median (of cord)
septum hematoma, nasal
septum pellucidum
sequela, sequelae
sequence memory
sequence time
sequential plane imaging
sequential point imaging
sequentially reamed
sequester, sequestered,
sequestra (pl. of sequestrum)
sequestration
sequestrectomy
sequestrotomy
sequestrum (pl. sequestra)
  bone
  bony
  necrotic
  primary
  secondary
  tertiary
sequestrum forceps
SER (somatosensory evoked response)
SER-IV (supination, external rotation-type IV fracture)
serendipity view
serial casts
serial EEG recording
serial sevens test
serial splinting
serial subtractions
serial threes test
seriation tests
series, Valpar component work sample
Series-II humeral head
seropositive rheumatoid arthritis
serosanguineous
serotonergic activity
serotonin (5-HIAA)
serration
Serrato forearm pin
Serrato forearm rod
Serter, C-wire
Servo pump
Servox device
sesamoid bones of foot
  accessory
  bipartite
  entrapped plantar
  fibular
  great toe
  hallux
  Hardy-Clapham classification of
  lateral
  medial
  quadripartite
  tibial
  tripartite
  symptomatic bipartite
sesamoid complex
sesamoidectomy dissector
sesamoiditis
sesamoid ligament
sesamoid migration
sesamoidometatarsal joint
sesamophalangeal ligament
sessile
set, sets
  acetabular trial
  AO minifragment
  Hollywood bed extension hook
  Mira Mark V craniotome
  Moore nail
  nail
  quad
  Rousek extraction
  spondylophyte impaction
set angle of toes
Seton hip brace
setter, bone plug
setting-sun phenomenon
Seutin plaster shears
sevens test, serial
seventh cranial nerve (facial nerve)
Sever disease

Sever-L'Episcopo repair of shoulder
Sever modification of Fairbank
 technique
severe ataxia
severe diffuse brain dysfunction
severe dysarthria
Sewall brain clip-applying forceps
SEWHO (shoulder-elbow-wrist-hand
 orthosis)
SFEMG (single-fiber electromyography)
shadowing
 acoustical
 paraspinal soft tissue (on x-ray)
Shaeffer rigid orthosis
shaft
 distal third
 femoral
 middle third
 ministem
 proximal third
shaft fracture
shaft of bone
shagreen patches in tuberous sclerosis
shakes, morning
shank of shoe
shank, steel
Shannon 44 bur
Shanz dressing
Shanz pin
Shanz screw
shape
 brachycephalic head
 head
 mesocephalic head
 scaphocephalic head
shaper, interbody
shark mouth of myotonic dystrophy
sharp trocar
sharp waves on EEG, interictal
 paroxysmal
Sharpey fibers
Sharp-Purser test
Sharplan ultrasonic aspirator
Sharrard transfer technique
Sharrard-Trentani prosthesis
Sharrard-type kyphectomy
shaver
 automated
 Concept
 Dyonics
 intra-articular (IAS)
 motorized meniscus
 motorized suction
 patellar
 powered
 sucker
 synovial
 whisker
shaving
 arthroscopic
 femoral condylar
 patellar
shaving of patella
Shaw aneurysm needle
Shaw catheter
shear
 anterior
 transitional
shear motion
shear stress
Shearer rongeur
shearing forces on the sacroiliac joints
 in runners
shearing of white matter in head
 injury
shears
 Bacon thoracic
 Baer rib
 Bethune-Coryllos rib
 Bethune rib
 Brunner rib
 Bruns plaster
 Collins rib
 Cooley rib
 Coryllos rib
 Esmarch plaster
 first rib
 Giertz-Shoemaker rib

shears *(cont.)*
- Gluck rib
- Hercules plaster
- Horsley-Stille rib
- Lefferts rib
- Liston-Key-Horsley rib
- plaster
- Potts rib
- rib
- Roberts rib
- Roos first rib
- Sauerbruch-Britsch rib
- Sauerbruch-Frey rib
- Schuchart rib
- Schumacher rib
- Semb rib
- Seutin plaster
- Shoemaker rib
- Stille-Giertz rib
- Stille plaster
- Stille rib

sheath, sheaths
- arthroscope
- carotid
- flexor tendon
- ganglionic cyst in synovial tendon
- intratendon
- muscle
- myelin
- nerve root
- neural
- periradicular
- plicated dural
- Schwann cell of myelin
- synovial
- tendon
- unplicated

sheath of muscle
Sheehan chisel
Sheehan gouge
Sheehan knee prosthesis
Sheehan osteotome
Sheehy incus replacement prosthesis
sheet, sheeting
- cranial incise
- fenestrated
- head
- laparotomy
- Silastic
- Silastic gel
- split
- sterile
- tantalum

Sheffield collimator helmet
Sheffield gamma knife unit
Sheffield hand elevator
Sheldon hemilaminectomy retractor
Sheldon-Spatz vertebral arteriogram needle
shelf
- Blumer
- lateral
- Mayeda
- medial
- patellar

shelf procedure
shell, acetabular
shelling off of cartilage
Shelton femur fracture classification
shelving
Shenton line
Shepherd fracture
shepherd's crook deformity
Sherfee prosthesis
Sherk-Probst technique
Sherman block test
Sherman bone plate
Sherman bone screw
Sherwin knee retractor
shield
- AME PinSite
- arthroscopic
- Faraday
- splash

Shier total knee prosthesis
Shifrin wire twister

shift
  anterior capsular
  intracranial
  midline (on x-ray)
  pivot
  plantar
  reverse pivot (RPS)
  ventricular
  weight
shift of midline structures (of the midbrain) (on x-ray)
shift of pineal gland (on x-ray)
shift of ventricle
shift to the left on white count
shift to the right on white count
shill, protrusio
shim coil
shimmering, visual
shin, saber
shin soreness
shin splints
shingles (herpes zoster)
Ship hammertoe implant
Shirley drain
shock
  neurogenic
  spinal
  sensory
shock-absorbent heel pad
shod, rubber
shoe, shoes
  accommodative
  Acor Quikform I or II
  Ambulators
  Anti-Shox cushion for
  balmoral laced
  balmoral throat opening of
  Bebax (for forefoot deformity)
  Bevin
  blucher laced
  blucher throat opening of
  broad-toed
  Comed postoperative
  corrective

shoe *(cont.)*
  counter of
  custom-made
  custom-made insert for
  custom-molded
  cut-out
  Darco surgical
  dress
  extended-counter
  extra-depth
  heel lift with
  high heel
  high heeled
  ill-fitting
  infant clown cast
  low-heeled
  Markell Mobility
  Markell open-toe
  Markell tarso medius straight
  Markell tarso pronator outflare
  metatarsal bar for
  Moon Boot
  narrow toebox
  normal last
  open-toe
  orthopedic
  orthopedic oxford
  oversize tennis
  oxford
  Pelite liner for
  plaster sole of
  Plastizote/PTT insert for
  pointed toe
  postoperative
  PRN
  Reece postoperative
  reverse last
  ribbed sole
  rocker
  rockerbottom sole of
  S.A.S.
  shank of
  soft sole or solft-soled
  soft-vamp

shoe *(cont.)*
  space
  Spenco insert for
  standard shell orthopedic
  stiff-soled
  straight last
  tarsal pronator
  therapeutic
  throat of
  toe box of
  torque heel
  vamp of
  Vibram rockerbottom
  Viking postoperative
  Viva
  WACH (wedge adjustable cushioned heel)
  wedged
  wide toebox
  wooden
  wooden-soled
  Zimmer postoperative
shoe cookie
shoe extension, Lee-Perthes
shoe filler
shoe heel height
shoe insert
  cushioned
  UCB
Shoemaker rib shears
shoemaker's swan
shoe modification
shoe restriction
shoe sandal
shoe size
shoe wear, abnormal
shoe width
short arm cast
short arm splint
shortening
  Achilles tendon
  Hoffa tendon
  leg
  suboccipital
shortening collectomy
short head of biceps
short increments sensitivity index (SISI) measurement
short leg brace
short leg cast (SLC)
short leg polypropylene splint
short leg walking cast
short orientation-memory-concentration (OMC) test
short-term memory
short-wave diathermy
"shot, hot" (cervical or brachial plexus injury)
shot, tetanus booster
shoulder
  apprehension
  baseball
  drop
  flail
  frozen
  knocked-down
  Little Leaguer
  loose
  Neviaser classification of frozen
  ring man (in gymnasts)
  sprained
  swimmer's
  tennis
shoulder arthroplasty, UCLA anatomic
shoulder compression test
shoulder depression test
shoulder-hand-finger syndrome
shoulder immobilizer
shoulder pointer
shoulder prosthesis
shoulder repair
shoulder rock test
shoulder separation
shoulder shrugs, repetitive
shoulder spica cast
shoulder-upper extremity-thoracic outlet syndrome
Shriner pin

shrinkage of ganglion cells
shrinker, stump
Shriver-Johnson interphalangeal
  arthrodesis
shrugging sign
shucking
shunt
  barium-sulfate impregnated
  CSF (cerebrospinal fluid)
  cysto-atrial
  Denver hydrocephalus
  DVP flush
  endarterectomy
  Hakim-Cortis ventriculoperitoneal
  hermetic external
  Heyer-Schulte neurosurgical
  high-pressure
  infant
  Javid
  low-pressure
  lumbar arachnoid peritoneal
  lumboperitoneal (LP)
  medium-pressure
  migration of
  Ommaya ventriculoperitoneal
  one-piece
  posterior fossa-atrial
  Pruitt-Inahara
  Pudenz
  Spetzler lumboperitoneal
  subdural to peritoneal
  Sundt loop
  T-tube
  thecoperitoneal
  UNI-SHUNT hydrocephalus
  ventriculoatrial (VA)
  ventriculojugular (VJ)
  ventriculoperitoneal (VP)
  ventriculovenous
shunting of cerebrospinal fluid
shunting procedure
shunt syndrome, lumbar theco-
  peritoneal
shunt valve
Shutrack carbon paper
Shutt Mantis retrograde forceps
Shy-Drager atrophy
Shy-Drager neuropathy
Shy-Drager syndrome
SI (sacroiliac) joint
SIADH (syndrome of inappropriate
  antidiuretic hormone) excretion
sialidosis
sialorrhea
Sibson fascia
Sicard test
sick headache (migraine)
sickle cell anemia
sickle-shape Beaver blade
"sickling in," peroneal tendinitis (in
  dancer's terminology)
sickness
  decompression
  sleeping
Sickness Impact Profile (SIP)
siderosis
sideswipe elbow fracture
sidewall
Siebenmann syndrome
Siemens LINAC (linear accelerator)
Siffert-Forster-Nachamie arthrodesis
Siffert-Storen intraepiphyseal
sigma rhythm on EEG
sigmoid cavity of radius
sigmoid cavity of ulna
sigmoid sinus
sign (see also *syndrome*; *test*)
  Achilles bulge
  Adson
  alien hand
  Allen
  Allis
  Amoss
  Anghelescu
  antecedent
  anterior drawer
  anterior foot drawer
  anterior tibial

sign *(cont.)*
- anvil
- Apley
- apprehension
- Ashhurst
- Babinski
- ball-bearing eye
- Bancroft
- barber's chair
- Barlow
- Battle
- bayonet
- Beevor
- bilateral Babinksi
- bilateral pyramidal
- bow-tie
- bowstring
- Bragard
- brain stem
- brim
- Brudzinski
- Bryant
- Burton
- buttock
- camelback
- Cantelli
- cerebellar eye
- cerebral
- Chaddock
- choppy sea
- Chvostek-Weiss
- Cleeman
- Codman
- Cogan lid twitch
- cogwheel
- Collier
- commemorative
- Comolli
- contralateral
- Coopernail
- cord
- corticospinal tract
- cranial nerve
- crescent

sign *(cont.)*
- cross-chest impingement
- crossed sciatica
- Dawbarn
- Dejerine
- delta
- Demianoff
- dense sigmoid-sinus
- dense vein
- Desault
- Deyerle
- dimple
- doll's eyes
- door-bell
- dorsal column
- double camelback
- drawer (ankle or knee)
- drop Lasègue
- Duchenne
- Dupuytren
- Egawa
- empty delta
- Erb
- Erichsen
- extrapyramidal tract
- fabere (flexion, abduction, external rotation, extension)
- fadir (flexion, adduction, internal rotation)
- Fajersztajn crossed sciatic
- false localizing
- fan
- fat pad (on x-ray)
- Finkelstein
- Fleck
- focal
- focal motor
- focal neurologic
- Forestier bowstring
- Fränkel (Fraenkel)
- Friedreich
- Froment paper
- frontal lobe
- frontal release

sign *(cont.)*
Gaenslen
Gage
Galant
Galeazzi
Goldthwait
Gordon
Gowers
Green-Joynt
Griesinger
Guilland
Hamman
harlequin eye
Hart
Hawkins impingement
head-at-risk
Helbing
Hirschberg
Hoffmann
Homans'
Hoover
hot-cross-bun skull
Hueter fracture
Huntington
J
Jenet
jump
Kanavel
Kaplan
Keen
Kehr
Kellgren
Kernig
Kerr
knee jerk
Kocher-Cushing
Lachman
Langoria
Lasègue
lateralizing
Laugier
Lazarus
Leichtenstern
Leri

sign *(cont.)*
Lhermitte
Linder
localizing
localizing neurological
long-tract
Lorenz
Lowenberg
lower motor neuron
Ludloff
Macewen
Maisonneuve
Marie
Marie-Foix
McMurray
Mendel-Bekhterev
meningeal
meningeal irritation
meningoencephalitic
Mennell
Minor
Morquio
Morton-Horwitz nerve cross-over
motor
movie
Mulder
mute toe
Myerson
Naffziger
Neer impingement
negative delta (on CT)
Negro
Nelson
Neri bowing
neurologic soft
obturator
oculomotor
Oppenheim
orbicularis
organic (of brain damage)
Ortolani
parietal
parietal lobe
Parrot

sign *(cont.)*
- pathognomonic
- pathologic lid retraction
- Patrick fabere
- Payr
- percussion
- peroneal
- Phalen
- phonatory
- piano key
- Piotrowski
- piston (on x-ray)
- pivot-shift
- plane
- Plummer
- positive bottle
- postural motor
- precursor
- premonitory
- Prévost
- pronation
- pronator
- pseudobulbar
- pseudo-Babinski
- pseudo-Foster-Kennedy
- pseudo-Romberg
- pupillary
- pyramidal
- Queckenstedt
- raccoon eyes
- rachitic rosary
- radialis
- Raimiste
- release
- Renee creak
- ring sign of cribriform plate fracture
- Rinne
- Riordan
- Risser
- Romberg
- Rust
- sail
- Sarbo

sign *(cont.)*
- Schlesinger
- Schoeber
- scimitar
- seat belt
- segmental
- Seguin
- setting-sun
- shrugging
- soft neurologic
- somatic
- Soto-Hall
- Spalding
- Speed
- spine
- spread suture
- Spurling
- stairs
- Steinberg thumb
- Steinmann
- Sterling-Okuniewski
- Stewart-Holmes
- Strunsky
- Strümpell (Struempell)
- tandem Romberg
- Terry fingernail
- theater
- Thomas
- thorn
- Thurston-Holland
- tibialis (of Strümpell)
- Tinel percussion
- toe
- toe spread
- tripod
- tripoding
- Trömner (Troemner)
- Trousseau
- Turyn
- Uhthoff
- unilateral Babinski
- upper motor neuron
- VAD (voluntary anterior drawer)
- Vanzetti

sign *(cont.)*
- versive motor
- voluntary posterior drawer (VPD)
- Voshell
- VPD (voluntary posterior drawer)
- Waddell
- Walter-Murdoch wrist
- Wartenberg
- Weber
- Weiss
- wet leather
- white matter
- Wilson
- windshield wiper (on x-ray)
- winking owl spinal (on x-ray)
- Yergason

signal
- antiphase EEG
- differential
- disk water (on MRI)
- out-of-phase EEG
- random (on EEG)
- water (on MRI)

signal characteristics of lesion
signal intensity curve
signal-to-noise ratio (SNR or S/N ratio) on MRI
Sigvaris stocking
Silastic ball spacer prosthesis
Silastic ball therapy
Silastic button
Silastic finger joint
Silastic gel sheeting
Silastic radial head prosthesis
Silastic rod
Silastic sheeting
Silastic sleeve
silence, electrocerebral (ECS)
silent areas of the brain
Silesian bandage prosthetic support
Silflex intramedullary prosthesis
Silfverskiöld Achilles tendon reconstruction
silicone elastomer rubber ball implant
silicone flexor rod
silicone gel
silicone gel pocket insert
silicone synovitis
silicone trapezium prosthesis
Silipos Distal Dip prosthetic sheath/liner
silk suture
Silopad friction pad
silver-fork deformity
Silver bunionectomy
Silver osteotome
Silverman placement of electrodes
simian griffe (ape hand)
similarities mental status testing
Simmonds-Menelaus metatarsal osteotomy
Simmonds test
Simmons fixation system
Simmons plate
Simmons screw
Simmons Vari-Hite orthopedic bed
Simon curet
Simons subtalar clubfoot release
simple dislocation
simple skull fracture
Simplex adhesive
Simplex cement
Simplex P bone cement
Simpson catheter
Simpson sugar-tong splint
Simpulse S/I pulsing lavage system
Simpulse suction irrigator
Simpulse system
Sims retractor
simulator
- BTE Work (Baltimore Therapeutic Equipment)
- Work Seat driving

simultagnosia
simultanagnosia
simultaneous volume imaging

Sinding Larsen-Johansson disease (SLJD)
Singh index of osteoporosis
single-axis foot
single axis on knee prosthesis
single-contrast arthrography
single-level decompressive laminectomy
single-limb stance of gait
single plantar verruca
single plantar wart
sinogenic meningitis
sinogram
sintering
Sinterlock CSTi bonding process
Sinterlock implant metal
sinus
  atlas articular
  Breschet
  cavernous
  cerebral
  cerebral venous
  circular
  coccygeal
  cranial
  dura mater venous
  dural venous
  inferior sagittal (ISS)
  lateral
  lumbosacral dermal
  osteomyelitic
  petrosal
  pilonidal
  precoronal sagittal
  Ridley
  sagittal
  sigmoid
  sphenoparietal
  superior sagittal (SSS)
  transverse
  venous
  vertebral articular
sinus lesion, cavernous
sinus tarsi syndrome
sinus thrombosis
sinus *(cont.)*
  cavernous
  intracranial
sinus tract
sinuvertebral nerve (of Luschka)
SIP (Sickness Impact Profile)
siphon, carotid
Siri formula for percentage of body fat
SISI (short increments sensitivity index) measurement
Sisson fracture reducing elevator
site
  donor
  fracture
  nociceptor
  nonunion of fracture
  operative
  pin
  previous surgical
  recipient
  surgical
  nociceptor
sitting balance
  reclined
  supported
sitting SLR test (straight leg raising)
Sivash hip prosthesis
Sivash stem
sixth compartment
sixth cranial nerve (abducens nerve)
sixth nerve palsy
size
  increased head circumference
  ventricular
sizer
SJO_2 (jugular bulb venous oxygen saturation)
Sjögren-Larsson syndrome
Sjögren syndrome
SJS (Schwartz-Jampel syndrome)
skateboarding accident
skeletal amyloidosis
skeletal bed
skeletal defects

skeletal growth factor
skeletal hyperostosis
skeletal traction
skeletally immature
skeletally mature
skeleton, bony
skeletonize
skeletonizing
skew deviation of eyes
skew, ocular
skewer, skewering
SKI knee prostheses
skid
  bone
  hip
  Meyerding bone
  Murphy-Lane bone
skier's fracture
skier's injury
skier's thumb
Skil Saw
skill, skills
  articulatory
  ambulation
  bed mobility
  motor
  physical daily living (PDLs)
  sensorimotor
  transfer
  transfers
  word-finding
skilled nursing facility (SNF)
Skillern fracture
skin blade knife
skin blood flow determination
skin bridge
skin depth
skin-rolling scapular tenderness
skinfold thickness monitoring
skive (shave), skived
Skoog release of Dupuytren contracture
skull
  asymmetry of the
  base of

skull *(cont.)*
  beaten silver appearance of
  foramen magnum of
  hammer-marked, secondary to thinning
  hot cross bun
  lytic lesion of the
  molding of
  sonolucent
skull asymmetry
skull base
skull clamp
skull clamp pin
skull defect, postoperative
skull fracture
  basilar
  compound
  depressed and compound
  linear
  simple
  stellate, undepressed
skull hyperostosis
skull plate
  stainless steel preformed
  tantalum preformed
skull plate anvil
skull tongs
  Gardner-Wells
  Raney-Crutchfield
skull trephine
  D'Errico
  Scoville
skullcap
skyline view of patella
Skytron bed
Skytron operating room table
SL (scapholunate) joint
Slatis pelvic fracture frame
slab, plaster
SLAC wrist (scapholunate arthritic collapse)
slap foot gait
SLAP lesion (superior labrum anterior posterior)
SLC (short leg cast)

SLE (systemic lupus erythematosus)
sleep
  active
  arousal from
  arousing from
  benign epileptiform transients of (BETS)
  deep
  depth of
  descending into
  descent through non-REM to REM
  disorder of initiating and maintaining (DIMS)
  disturbed
  dreamless
  indeterminate
  non-REM (non-rapid eye movements)
  NREM (non-rapid eye movement)
  onset of
  paradoxical (REM sleep)
  quiet
  rapid eye movement (REM)
  REM (rapid eye movement)
  REM onset
  slow wave
  stage I (drowsiness)
  stage I of non-REM (drowsiness)
  stage II of non-REM (light sleep)
  stage III of non-REM (deep sleep)
  stage IV of non-REM (very deep)
  stage of REM
  stage W (wakefulness)
  transiting through
  transitional
  very deep
  very light
sleep apnea
sleep arousal disorder
sleep attacks (epilepsy)
sleep cycle
sleep deprivation
sleep disorder
sleep onset episode
sleep onset REM period (SOREMP)
sleep paralysis
  postdormital
  predormital
sleep pattern
sleep spindle on EEG
sleep state
sleep-wake cycle
sleep-wakefulness cycle
sleep-waking cycle
Sleeper II sleep support, by Bodyline
sleepiness, daytime
sleeping sickness
sleeplessness
sleeptalking
sleepwalking
sleeve
  alignment
  circumferential ligamentous
  distal
  drill
  dural root
  Edwards-Levine
  guide
  metaphyseal
  nerve root
  obturator
  periosteal
  polyethylene
  Rancho trocar-drill
  Silastic
  taper
  2T
sleeve fracture
sleeve of drillbit
slide, vastus
sling
  arm elevator
  Barton
  buckle
  collar-and-cuff
  cradle arm
  envelope
  envelope-type arm

sling *(cont.)*
- extra-articular lateral
- felt
- foam
- foot
- Glisson
- Haacker
- immobilizer
- Kenny Howard shoulder
- knee
- Kodel knee
- Legg-Perthes
- muslin
- Pavlik
- pelvic
- Rauchfuss
- rubber
- shoulder
- sleeve
- Slingers arm
- stockinette
- strap
- Teare
- tendon
- thigh
- Thomas
- Thomas buckle
- tibialis anterior tendon
- triangle
- triangular
- Velpeau
- Velpeau shoulder
- Vogue arm
- volar
- volar ulnar
- Weil pelvic
- Westfield envelope

sling-and-swathe bandage
Slingers arm sling
slip angle
slip of tendon
slip-on finger splint
Slip-N-Snip scissors
slipped capital femoral epiphysis
slipped disk
slipper-type cast
- kite
- plaster-of-Paris

slit-catheter system for compartment syndrome of foot
sliver of bone
SLJD (Sinding-Larsen-Johansson disease)
Slocum lateral pivot-shift test
Slocum meniscal clamp
Slocum knee procedure
Slot distraction device
slough, skin
slowing (on EEG)
- bilateral theta
- delta
- diffuse delta
- generalized background
- monorhythmic frontal
- postictal
- psychomotor
- saccadic
- scattered

slow spike and wave EEG pattern
slow virus infection of the nervous system
slow wave activity, on EEG
slow wave, phase reversing (on EEG)
SLR (straight leg raising) test
SLRT (straight leg raising test)
Sluder neuralgia
Sluder sphenopalatine syndrome
Sluder syndrome
slurred speech
Sluyter-Mehta thermocouple electrode
SLWC (short leg walking cast)
SMA (spinal muscular atrophy)
SMA (supplementary motor area)
SMA prosthesis
small-vessel disease of the diabetic foot
small-vessel stroke

smear for parasites and fungi, wet, (in meningitis)
Smedberg hand drill
Smedberg twist drill
SMI 3000 bed
SMI 5000 bed
Smiley-Williams arteriogram needle
Smillie-Beaver blade
Smillie cartilage knife
Smillie knee retractor
Smillie meniscotomy chisel
Smillie meniscus knife
Smillie nail
Smillie retractor
Smith & Nephew Richards rod
Smith air craniotomes
Smith ankle prosthesis
Smith ankle fracture
Smith automatic perforator drills
Smith bone clamp
Smith cartilage knife
Smith classification of sesamoid position
Smith cranial drill
Smith-Davis Converta-Hite orthopedic bed
Smith-Lemli-Opitz syndrome
Smith nerve root suction retractor
Smith-Petersen chisel
Smith-Petersen femoral neck nail
Smith-Petersen gouge
Smith-Petersen impactor
Smith-Petersen intertrochanteric plate
Smith-Petersen laminectomy rongeur
Smith-Petersen nail with Lloyd adapter
Smith-Petersen osteotome
Smith-Petersen rongeur
Smith-Petersen test
Smith physical capacities evaluation (PCE)
Smith-Robinson diskectomy
Smith-Robinson interbody fusion
Smithwick button hook
Smithwick clip-applying forceps
Smithwick dissector
Smithwick nerve hook
Smithwick sympathectomy hook
Smith wire-cutting scissors
SMo (stainless steel and molybdenum)
SMO (supramalleolar orthosis)
SMON (subacute myelo-optico–neuropathy)
smoother, Gore
smooth pursuit eye movements
SNA cephalometric measurement
snap, saccadic
SNAP (sensory nerve action potential) amplitude
snapping hip
snapping of tendons, in hand
snapping tendon release
snapping thumb flexor
SNB cephalometric measurement
SNCV (sensory nerve conduction velocity)
Sneppen fracture of the talus
SNF (skilled nursing facility)
Snitman endaural retractor
SN-MPA cephalometric measurement
Sno-Traks wheelchair chains
snout reflex
SNR (signal-to-noise ratio)
SNSF (second neuroma, same foot)
snuffbox, anatomical
snug, snugged, snugging
soap, Betadine
soap bubble appearance
Social Security Disability Insurance (SSDI)
socialization skills
Society for the Prevention of Blindness, National
Society, National Multiple Sclerosis (NMSS)
sock
  cast
  Orlon with Lycra stump
  Spandex Lycra three-ply stump
  stump

socket
  check
  Poly-Dial
  quadrilateral
  threaded
  total contact
socket wrenches
sodium urate crystals
Sofamor spinal instrumentation device
Sof-Rol cast padding
Sof-Rol dressing
Sofield osteotomy
Sofield retractor
Sofsponge material
soft clavus
soft corn
soft disk herniation
softening of brain
soft neurologic sign
soft opposition, of thumb muscles
soft tissue abnormality
soft tissue ankle injuries
soft tissue contracture
soft tissue contusion
soft tissue defect
soft tissue entrapment
soft tissue infection
soft-tissue mass
soft tissue mobilization
soft tissue necrosis
soft tissue osteochondroma
soft tissue plication
soft tissue radiograph
soft tissue realignment
soft tissue reconstruction
soft tissue swelling
Solcotrans drainage/reinfusion system
Solcotrans Plus autotransfusion system
sole
  shock-absorbent
  shoe
soleal line
solenoid coil
sole of foot
solid ankle, cushioned heel (SACH)
solitary neurofibroma
solitary plasmatoma
solution
  antibiotic
  Betadine Helafoam
  dilute heparin
  hypo-osmolar glucose
Somanetics INVOS cerebral oximeter
SomaSensor
somatagnosia (corporal agnosia)
somatectomy
somatesthetic fiber
somatic alpha fiber
somatic denervation
somatic nerve fiber
somatic sensory seizures
somatic sign
somatization disorder
somatosensory evoked potential (SEP or SSEP)
somatosensory evoked response (SER)
somatosensory seizure
somatosensory symptoms
somatosympathetic fibers of nerve root
Somerville procedure
SOMI orthosis (sternal occipital mandibular immobilization)
Sommer sector of hippocampus
somnambulism
somniloquy
somnolence, excessive
somnolent
sonicated tendon
Sonicator portable ultrasound
Songer spinal cable system
Sonocut ultrasonic aspirator
sonography, transcranial Doppler
Sophy programmable pressure valve
Sorbie calcaneal fracture
Sorbothane heel cushions
Sorbothane II heel cup
sore, pressure
SOREMP (sleep onset REM period)

soreness, delayed-onset muscle
 (DOMS)
Soto-Hall bone graft
Soto-Hall sign
sound
 cracked pot
 tearing
Souter hip procedure
Souter unconstrained elbow prosthesis
southern access to the hip joint in
 surgery
Southwick biplane osteotomy
Southwick-Robinson anterior cervical
 approach
SPA (speech pathology/audiology)
space
 dead
 disk
 dorsal subaponeurotic
 dorsal subcutaneous
 epidural
 extradural
 first web
 foraminal
 hyperintense marrow
 increased lateral joint
 intercondylar (ICS) joint
 intermetatarsal
 interpeduncular
 intrathecal
 joint
 lateral joint
 medial joint
 midpalmar
 narrowing of joint
 Parona (subtendinous)
 patellofemoral joint
 popliteal
 pulp
 retroparotid
 retrosphenoidal
 scapholunate
 subarachnoid
 subdural
space *(cont.)*
 subtendinous
 syndesmotic clear
 thenar
 tibiocalcaneal
 ventricular
 Virchow-Robin space of the brain
 web
space deficits
space-occupying lesion
space of Poirier
spacer
 acetabular
 Barouk
 cement
 GAIT (great toe arthroplasty
  implant technique)
 joint
 PMMA
 tibial
spacer between toes
spacer-tensor jig IV
space shoes
Spalding sign
span
 attention
 ventricular
Spandex Lycra three-ply stump sock
spanner, socket
sparing, sacral (in sensory loss)
spasm
 carpopedal
 cerebrovascular
 convergence
 dystonic
 facial
 flexion
 habit
 hamstring
 hemifacial
 infantile massive
 intercostal
 intrinsic muscles
 involuntary flexor

spasm *(cont.)*
- lightning-like flexion (of the head in infant)
- medial facial (of Meige)
- mobile
- muscle
- nodding
- paraspinal muscle
- paravertebral muscle
- peripheral facial
- protective
- recruitment (in tetanus)
- recurrent torsion
- saltatory
- torsion

spasmodic flexion
spasmodic torticollis
spasmus nutans
spastic ataxia, familial
spastic diparesis
spastic diplegia
spastic equinovarus deformity
spastic gait
spastic hand
spastic hemiparesis
spastic hemiplegia, Wernicke-Mann
spastic hindfoot valgus deformity
spasticity
- limb
- nocturnal leg muscle
- spinal

spastic neurogenic bladder, refluxing
spastic palsy, pure
spastic paralysis
spastic paraparesis
spastic paraplegia and distal muscle wasting
spastic paraplegia, familial
spastic paresis
spastic pseudosclerosis
spastic state
spatial disorganization
spatial disorientation
spatial distortion
spatial neglect
spatial orientation
spatial resolution
spatium subdurale
spatula
- brain
- cement
- Children's Hospital brain
- clip bending
- Cushing brain
- D'Errico brain
- Davis brain
- Davis nerve
- dura
- endarterectomy
- House-Fisch dura
- Jacobson endarterectomy
- malleable
- Mayfield brain
- nerve
- nerve separator
- Olivecrona brain
- Peyton brain
- Rainin clip-bending
- Ray brain
- Rhoton
- S-shaped brain
- Sachs nerve
- Scoville brain
- Weary brain

spatula spoon
- Cushing brain
- Ray brain

Speare dural hook
special leads, on EEG
Special Olympics, National
specialist, registered deafness (RDF)
specific thalamic nuclei
specimen
- biopsy
- grossly resected

specious finding
SPECT (single photon emission computed tomography)

SPECT determination of cerebral
  blood flow
spectra (see *spectrum*)
spectral analysis of EEG
spectral array, compressed
spectral averaging on EEG
spectral peak frequency of activity
spectral plot
spectrometer
Spectron hip prosthesis
spectrum (pl. spectra)
  fortification
  migraine
speculum
  bivalve
  Cushing-Landolt transsphenoidal
  forceps
  Halle nasal
  Hardy
  Killian septum
  Landolt pituitary
  transsphenoidal
speech
  agrammatic
  arrest of
  articulate
  articulation of
  ataxic
  cerebellar scanning quality of
  cerebellar scanning type of
  circumlocution of
  circumstantial
  confabulation of
  dysarthric
  dysrhythmic
  emotive
  executive
  festinant quality in parkinsonian
  flaccid
  fluent aphasic
  fluent paraphasic
  halting
  hyperkinetic
  hypokinetic
speech *(cont.)*
  impaired
  incoherent
  incomprehensible
  internal
  irrelevant
  labored
  monosyllabic
  nonelaborative
  nonfluent aphasic
  nonsensical
  paraphasic
  rambling
  rhythm of
  scanning
  slurred
  spontaneous
  staccato
  tangential
  telegraphic
  unintelligible
  unvoiced
speech mannerisms
speech pathologist
speech pathology/audiology (SPA)
Speech Questionnaire
Speed-Boyd radial-ulnar technique
Speed hand splint
speed of gait
Speed V-Y muscle-plasty
spell, spells
  akinetic
  breathholding
  fainting
  myoclonic
  staring
Spence cranioplastic roller
Spence intervertebral disk rongeur
Spence rongeur forceps
Spencer tendon lengthening operation
Spenco liners
Spenco shoe insert
Spetzler lumboperitoneal shunt

Spetzler-Martin classification of arteriovenous malformation
SpF Spinal Fusion Stimulator
sphenoethmoidal encephalocele
sphenoethmoidal suture
sphenoidal electrode
sphenoidal fissure syndrome
sphenoidal fossae EEG leads
sphenoidal wing
sphenoid ridge tumors
sphenoid wing
spheno-occipital suture
spheno-orbital encephalocele
spheno-orbital suture
sphenopalatine ganglion
sphenopalatine neuralgia
sphenoparietal suture
sphenopetrosal suture
sphenopharyngeal meningo-encephalocele
sphenosquamous suture
sphenotemporal suture
sphenovomerine suture
spheres, oriented in all
Spherocentric fully constrained tricompartmental knee prosthesis
sphincter control, loss of
sphincter disturbance
sphincter incompetence
sphincter pupillae
sphingomyelin lipidosis
sphingomyelinase
spica bandage
spica cast
spica splint
spicular density on x-ray
spicules on EEG
spider-web circulation on angiography of glioblastomas
Spiegelberg epidural balloon
Spiegleman acromioclavicular splint
Spielmeyer-Vogt disease
Spielmeyer-Vogt-Sjögren disease
Spier elbow arthrodesis
spike
  benign small sharp (BSSS)
  blind person's occipital
  centromidtemporal
  centrotemporal
  cortical
  epileptiform EEG
  focal interictal
  frontal
  generalized
  Gissane
  high-amplitude
  infantile pattern of
  interictal continuous
  interictal temporal lobe
  intermittent focal
  juvenile pattern of
  lateral rectus
  low-amplitude
  multifocal independent
  negative vertex
  occipital
  polyphasic
  positive
  repetitive
  rolandic
  small sharp (SSS)
  slow waves interrupted by
  stereotyped
  temporal
  temperature
  unilateral
  wicket
spike-and-dome complex
spike and slow wave bursts
spike-and-wave complex on EEG
spike-and-wave discharge
spike and wave forms on EEG
spike averaging
spike discharges on EEG
spike of bone
spike on EEG
spike osteotomy
spike waves, interictal paroxysmal

Spiller-Frazier neurotomy
spin density
spin echo
spin-echo imaging
spin-echo technique, on MRI
spin-lattice relaxation time
spin-spin relaxation time
spin-warp imaging
spina bifida
spina bifida anterior
spina bifida aperta
spina bifida cystica
spina bifida manifesta
spina bifida occulta (SBO)
spina bifida posterior
spinal abscess, epidural
spinal accessory nerve (eleventh cranial nerve)
spinal angiogram
spinal arthritis
spinal axial loading
spinal axis
spinal block by cord compression
spinal canal
spinal canal narrowing
spinal column
spinal cord
  caliber of
  compression of
  hemisection of
  infarction of the
  laceration of the
  multiple focal lesions of the (as in multiple sclerosis)
  myelopathy of the
  posterolateral sclerosis of the
  size of
  tethered
  transection of
spinal cord compression by lymphoma
spinal cord diameter
spinal cord-injured patient
spinal cord injury (SCI)
spinal cord lesion
Spinal Cord Motor Injury and Sensory Indices
spinal cord neoplasm
spinal cord parenchyma
spinal cord stroke
spinal cord tumor
  intradural but extramedullary
  intramedullary
spinal dysraphism, occult
spinal elements, neoplastic destruction of
spinal epidural abscess
spinal epidural hematoma
spinal fixation
spinal fluid cytology
spinal fluid, xanthochromic
spinal fusion
spinal hemiplegia
spinal instability
spinal integrity
spinal manipulative therapy
spinal needle
spinal nerve level motor impairment
spinal neural deficits
spinal neuraxis
spinal osteomyelitis, *Staphylococcus aureus*
spinal paraplegia
spinal retractor
spinal roots
  C1-7 (cervical)
  Co. 1 (coccygeal)
  L1-5 (lumbar)
  S1-5 (sacral)
  T1-12 (thoracic)
spinal shock
Spinal-Stim
spinal subarachnoid hemorrhage
spinal subdural hematoma
spinal sympathetic fibers
spinal tap, traumatic
spinal tract of trigeminal
spinal tuberculosis
spinal videofluoroscopy

spindle
  asynchronous sleep
  muscle
  sinusoidal appearing sleep
  sleep (on EEG)
  unilateral sleep
spindle burst
spindle cell carcinoma
spindle coma pattern
spindle system reflexes
spine
  angulation of
  anterior column of
  cervical (C)
  Charcot
  coccygeal (coccyx)
  dendritic
  dorsal (D)
  functional units of
  iliac
  ischial
  kinetic cervical
  kissing
  lateral bending views of the
  lumbar (L)
  lumbarized
  lumbosacral (LS)
  mandibular
  maxillary
  nasal
  poker
  posterior column of
  posterior-inferior
  rotatory loads on
  rugger jersey
  sacral (S)
  static cervical
  thoracic (T)
  thoracolumbar
  trochanteric
spine board
spine strain, lumbosacral
spino-olivary tract
spinocerebellar degeneration
spinocerebellar disease
spinocerebellar tract
spinocerebellopathy
spinoglenoid notch
spinographic angle
spinographic lines
spinography, digitized
spinoreticular tract
spinotectal tract
spinothalamic tract
  anterior
  lateral
Spira procedure
spiral band of Gosset
spiral fracture
spirochete
Spittler procedure
splash shield
SPLATT (split anterior tibial tendon transfer)
splayfoot deformity
splaying of forefoot
splaying of frontal horns
splaying of toes
splenium of corpus callosum
spline
  Blount
  Bosworth
  flat
  Rowland-Hughes
splint, splinting
  Abbott
  abduction
  abduction humeral
  acrylic template
  Adam and Eve
  Adams
  adjustable
  aeroplane (also airplane)
  Agnew
  air
  airplane
  air pressure
  airfoam

splint *(cont.)*
- airplane (also aeroplane)
- Alumafoam
- aluminum bridge
- aluminum fence
- aluminum foam
- anchor
- Anderson
- angle
- anterior shin
- any-angle
- Aquaplast
- Asch
- Ashhurst
- balanced
- Balkan
- ball-peen
- banjo
- Barlow cruciform infant
- baseball
- baseball finger
- basswood
- Bavarian
- Baylor
- Bennett basic hand
- birdcage
- Bloom
- Boehler (Böhler)
- Böhler-Braun
- Bond
- Boston thoracic
- boutonnière
- Bowlby
- boxing glove
- bracketed
- Brady leg
- Brant aluminum
- Buck
- buddy finger
- Budin hammertoe
- bunion
- Bunnell active hand and finger
- Bunnell finger extension
- Bunnell knuckle-bender

splint *(cont.)*
- Bunnell outrigger
- Bunnell reverse knuckle-bender
- Bunnell safety-pin
- Bunny Boot
- Burnham thumb and finger
- Cabot posterior
- Campbell
- cap
- Capner
- Carl P. Jones traction
- Carter
- Chandler felt collar
- Chatfield-Girdlestone
- clavicle
- clavicular cross
- Clayton greenstick
- clubfoot
- coaptation
- cock-up
- cock-up hand
- Colles
- Comforfoam
- composite spring
- conforming
- constant tension
- Cosmolon closure for
- countertraction
- Craig
- Cramer wire
- Culley
- Curry
- Darco foot
- Darco medical-surgical shoe and toe alignment
- Darco toe alignment
- Davis
- Delbet
- Denis Browne clubfoot
- Denis Browne talipes hobble
- DePuy open spindle
- derotator
- Digit-Aid fifth toe
- DonJoy knee

splint *(cont.)*
DonJoy wrist
dorsal wrist
drop foot
dropout
Dupuytren
Duran-Houser wrist
Dyna knee
Dyna leg
dynamic extensor
dynamic flexor
Eaton
Eggers
elastic
Elastomull
elbow
elephant-ear clavicle
Engelmann
Engen palmar wrist
Erich
extension block(ing)
extrinsically-powered
felt collar
fence
Ferciot tiptoe
fiberglass
figure-of-8
Fillauer night
finger
finger cot
finger extension
finger knuckle-bender
flexor hinge
foot
footdrop
forearm
Forrester
Foster
Fox
Frac-Sur
Framer
Frejka pillow
frog
Fruehevald

splint *(cont.)*
full-ring leg
functional
Funsten
Futura cock-up
Futura wrist
Gagnon
gauntlet
Gibson
Gilmer
Gooch
Gordon
Granberry
Gunning
gutter
half-ring leg
half-shell
hallux valgus night
hammertoe
Hammond
hand
Hanna night
Hare traction
Harrington outrigger
Hart
Haynes-Griffin
hinged cylinder
Hirschtick
Hodgen
Ilfield
Ilfield-Gustafson
inflatable
isoprene plastic
Jacoby bunion
Jelanko
Joint-Jack finger
Jonell
Jones
Joseph
Kanavel cock-up
Karfoil
Kazanjian
Keller-Blake half ring
Kerr

splint *(cont.)*
- Keystone
- kinetic
- Kleinert
- knee
- knuckle-bender
- Lambrinudi
- lead hand
- leg
- Levis
- Lewin baseball finger
- Lewin finger
- Lewin-Stern thumb
- Link Stack Split
- Liston
- live
- long arm
- long leg
- long opponens
- loop-lock cock-up
- Love
- Lytle
- Magnuson
- malleable metal finger
- Malmö hip
- Mason-Allen universal
- Mayer
- McGee
- McIntire
- McLeod
- metacarpal
- Middeldorpf
- MindSet toe
- modified Oppenheimer
- modified safety-pin
- Mohr
- moldable
- molded posterior plaster
- munster
- Murray-Jones
- Murray-Thomas
- Neubeiser
- New Mind Set toe
- night

splint *(cont.)*
- O'Donoghue
- OEC
- Oppenheimer spring wire
- Oppenheimer with knuckle-bender
- Oppenheimer with reverse knuckle-bender
- opponens
- Orfit
- Ortho-last
- Orthoplast
- orthoplastic
- outrigger with
- padded
- padded tongue blade
- palmar
- Pavlik
- Peabody
- Pearson attachment to Thomas
- pelvic
- PF Night
- Phelps
- pillow
- Plastalume finger
- plaster
- plaster slab
- platform
- Plexiglas
- Polysar
- Polysplint A
- polyvinylalcohol
- Pond adjustable
- Ponseti
- posterior
- posterior shin
- Potts
- protective
- Protecto
- Putti
- quick
- Redi-Around finger
- rest
- reverse finger knuckle-bender
- reverse knuckle-bender

splint *(cont.)*
Roger Anderson
Rowland-Hughes
Rumel aluminum
safety-pin
Sager traction
Sam
Sayre
Scotchcast
Scott
semidynamic
serial
shin
short opponens
short arm
short leg polypropylene
shoulder spica
Simpson sugar-tong
slip-on finger
Slocum
Speed hand
spica
Spiegleman acromioclavicular
spreading hand
spring cock-up
spring wire safety-pin
Stack
Stader
static
Stax finger
stirrup plaster
Strampelli
Stromeyer
Stuart Gordon
sugar-tong plaster
suspension
Swanson hand
Synergy
talipes hobble
Tauranga
Taylor
Thomas half-ring
Thomas hinged
Thomas leg

splint *(cont.)*
Thomas suspension
Thompson
thumb
thumb abduction
thumb web
Tobruk
toe
Toronto
traction
triangular pillow
universal gutter
vacuum
Valentine
Velcro
VersaWrist wrist
Vesely-Street
volar cock-up
volar plaster
Volkmann
von Rosen cruciform
Weil
well leg
Wertheim
Wilson
wire grip finger
wire grip toe
wraparound
wrist cock-up
wrist extension
wrist rest
wrist-driven
yucca wood
Zimfoam
Zimmer
Zucker

splint attachment, Pearson
splinted in position of function
splinter
splinter hemorrhage
splinting material
splint-like pain
splint with outriggers
splint with wrist support

split-brain studies
split posterior tibial tendon transfer
split Russell skeletal traction
split stirrup
splitter, nail
split-thickness skin excision (STSE)
split-thickness skin graft
Sponastrine dysplasia
spondylalgia
spondylarthritis
spondylarthrocace
spondylectomy
spondylexarthrosis
spondylitic change
spondylitis
  ankylosing
  rheumatoid
spondylitis deformans
spondylizema
spondyloarthropathy
spondylodynia
spondylolisthesis
  sagittal roll
  slip angle
  traumatic (grades 1-4)
spondylolisthetic crisis
spondylolisthetic habitus
spondylolysis
spondylomalacia
spondylopathy
spondylophyte impaction set
spondylopyosis
spondyloschisis
spondylosis
  cervical
  degenerative
  diffuse
  Nurick classification of
spondylosyndesis
spondylotic bar
spondylotic myelopathy
spondylotic radiculopathy
spondylotomy
sponge
  Adaptic
  cellulose
  collagen
  gauze
  lap (laparotomy)
  Mikulicz
  Ray-Tec
  Taka microneurosurgical
  Telfa
  Vistec
sponge test
spongiform encephalopathy
  amyotrophic type
  classic type (Jakob-Creutzfeldt type)
  optic type (Heidenhain type)
  subacute type (Nevin-Jones type)
spongioblast
spongioblastoma multiforme
spongioblastoma, unipolar
spongiocyte
spongiocytoma
spongy appearance
spongy degeneration leukodystrophy
Sponsel oblique osteotomy
spontaneity
  loss of
  reduction in
spontaneous autosympathectomization
spontaneous rupture of Achilles tendon
spontaneous speech
Spontastrine dysplasia
spoon
  Cushing brain spatula
  Cushing pituitary
  Hardy pituitary
  pituitary
  Ray brain spatula
  spatula
sponge and needle count
Spork utensil
Sports Brace, by Bodyline
Sports-Caster I and II knee braces

- sports chiropractic
- sports, lateral motion racket
- spot
  - capitate soft
  - café au lait
- SPR (superior peroneal retinaculum)
- sprain
  - ankle
  - chronic
  - chronic ankle
  - eversion spain of the ankle
  - inversion
  - lateral ligamentous
  - major
  - minor
  - muscle
  - sacroiliac
  - syndesmosis sprain of the ankle
- sprain-strain
- Spratt bone curet
- Spratt mastoid curet
- spray-stretch technique
- sprays, vasocoolant
- spreader
  - Bailey rib
  - Beeson cast
  - Beeson plaster
  - Blount lamina
  - Bobechko
  - Burford-Finochietto rib
  - cast
  - cervical lamina
  - cervical vertebrae
  - Cloward cervical vertebra
  - Cloward lamina
  - Davis rib
  - DeBakey rib
  - Favoloro-Morse sternal
  - Finochietto rib
  - Gerbode-Burford rib
  - Haglund-Stille plaster
  - Haight-Finochietto rib
  - Haight rib
- spreader *(cont.)*
  - Harken rib
  - Harrington
  - Henning cast
  - Henning meniscal retractor
  - Henning plaster
  - Hoffer-Daimler cast
  - Inge cervical lamina
  - Inge laminectomy
  - intervertebral
  - lamina
  - Landolt
  - Lemmon sternal
  - Lilienthal rib
  - Miltex rib
  - Morse sternal
  - Nelson rib
  - plaster
  - Rehbein rib
  - rib
  - Rienhoff-Finochietto rib
  - Rienhoff rib
  - spinous process
  - sternal
  - Tuffier rib
  - vertebrae
  - Weinberg rib
  - Wilson rib
  - Wiltberger spinous process
- spreader bar of Denis Browne splint
- spread of tumor
- Sprengel deformity
- Spri Xercise board
- spring fixation
- spring-loaded lock on orthosis
- spring swivel thumb
- spring, Weiss
- Springer fracture
- sprinter's fracture
- sprouting
  - axonal
  - collateral
- sprouting with axonal neuropathy

spur, spurring
  acromial
  anterior
  bone
  bony
  calcaneal
  degenerative
  heel
  impingement
  inferior
  marginal
  osteoarthritic
  plantar
  prominent
  retrocalcaneal
  traction
  uncovertebral
spurious ankylosis
Spurling intervertebral disk rongeur
Spurling-Kerrison laminectomy rongeur
Spurling-Kerrison up-biting and down-biting rongeurs
Spurling neck compression test
Spurling nerve root retractor
Spurling pituitary rongeur
Spurling rongeur forceps
Spurling sign
spurt, growth
squamosomastoid suture
squamosoparietal suture
squamososphenoid suture
square pronator
squat, half
squatting ability
squeak phenomenon on EEG
squeeze test in syndesmosis ankle sprain
SREDA (subclinical rhythmic discharges of adults) on EEG
SROM cup
SSDI (Social Security Disability Insurance)
SSEP (somatosensory evoked potential)
SSFP (steady state free precession)
SSH (spinal subdural hemorrhage)
SSI (segmental spinal instrumentation)
SSI (Supplemental Security Income)
SSI (segmental spinal instrumentation) in scoliosis treatment
SSP (subclavian steal phenomenon)
SSPE (subacute sclerosing panencephalitis)
SSPE viral encephalitis
SSS (small sharp spike) on EEG
SSS (subclavian steal syndrome)
SSS (superior sagittal sinus)
stability
  lateral
  ligamentous
  subtalar joint
  varus-valgus
  viscoelastic
stabilization
  atlantoaxial
  bony
  subtalar
  surgical
stabilize, stabilized, stabilization
stabilizer
  first ray (muscles)
  forearm
  patellar
stable hinge joint
stable to motion
stab wound
stab wound arthroscopy entry portal
Stack hand retractor
Stack shoulder procedure
Stack splint
Stader pin
Stader splint
stage, staging
  Berndt-Harty talar lesion
  distraction-flexion (DFS)
  FAST (Functional Assessment Staging) for Alzheimer's disease
  Ficat avascular necrosis
  Outerbridge degenerative arthritis

stage *(cont.)*
  pre-slip
  W (wakefulness) of sleep
Stagnara wake-up test
Staheli rotational profile
Staheli shelf procedure
stain, staining
  Gomori
  Grimelius
  hamstring
  Masson-Fontana
  periodic acid-Schiff
  tumor (on cerebral angiography)
stainless steel preformed skull plates
StairClimber assist device
stairs sign
stairstep-type fracture
stairs, ascending and descending
stalk
  infundibular
  pituitary
stalk of meningoencephalocele
stalk of tumor
STA-MCA anastomosis (superficial
  temporal artery to middle cerebral
  artery)
Stamm intra-articular hip fusion
stammering of the bladder
stamps, Gelfoam
stance (of gait)
  single-limb
  terminal
stance-phase of gait cycle
stance-phase periods of gait
  initial contact
  loading response
  midstance
  preswing
  terminal
Stand, IMP-Turnstile Casting
standard shell orthopedic shoe
standardized growth curves
standby assist
standing balance test
standing frame orthosis
Stanmore elbow prosthesis
Stanmore knee replacement
Stanmore shoulder arthroplasty
Stanmore total hip replacement
STA-PCA bypass (superficial
  temporal artery-posterior cerebral
  artery)
Staphylococcus aureus spinal
  osteomyelitis
staphylorrhaphy elevator
staple
  automatic
  barb
  barbed
  Blount
  bone
  Coventry
  Day
  Downing
  duToit
  epiphyseal
  Hernandez-Ros bone
  Howmedica Vitallium
  Johannesberg
  metallic
  Mitek
  O'Brien
  osteoclast tension
  Owestry
  power-drive
  scalp marker
  skin
  stabilizing
  Stone four-point
  tabletop Stone
  titanium
  Vitallium
  Wilberg bone
  Zimaloy
staple arthroereisis
staple fixation
staple gun
staple migration

stapler
  EEA (end-to-end anastomosis)
  Powered Metaphyseal
  TA-55
Staples-Black-Brostrom ligament repair
Staples elbow arthrodesis
stapling
  Blount
  epiphyseal
star-cancellation test (SCT)
star, macular
starch bandage
stare
  empty
  glassy-eyed
  glassy stare of petit mal epilepsy
  post-basic
  posterior fossa
Stark-Moore-Ashworth-Boyes technique
Starr-Edwards aortic valve prosthesis
Starr-Edwards Silastic ball valve prosthesis
stars, seeing
starter, Ritchie nail
start hesitation
startle myoclonus
startle reflex
startling noise on EEG
Statak device
state, states
  acute confusional
  alpha
  amnestic
  apallic
  central excitatory
  confusional
  crepuscular (twilight)
  delirium-like
  disequilibrium
  dissociative
  dreamy
  epileptic fugue
  fugue

state *(cont.)*
  hyperdopaminergic
  hypnagogic
  hysteric coma-like
  hysterical fugue
  lacunar
  locked-in
  marble
  moribund
  nonresponsive
  acute confusional
  parasomniac conscious
  persistent vegetative (PVS)
  postictal
  sleep
  spastic
  toxic-confusional
  trance
  transient state of depersonalization in migraine
  twilight
  unresponsive
  vegetative
  wakeful
state of alertness
state of consciousness
state of heightened attention
state of heightened awareness
static cervical spine
static fixation
static foot deformity
static foot pain (when standing)
static friction
static locking nail
static reflex controls
static splint
static standing balance
static torticollis
static wryneck
station
  gait and
  gait, station, and base
  Romberg
  unsteadiness of gait and

station and gait
station test
stato-kinetic reflex controls
status
  absence
  altered mental
  ambulatory
  deterioration of
  intact neurovascular
  mental
  neurocirculatory
  neurologic
  off work
  permanent and stationary
  petit mal
status aura
status dysgraphicus
status dysmyelinatus
status epilepticus
  convulsive
  nonconvulsive
  subclinical
status marmoratus
status post
status spongiosus
Stax finger splint
Stayoden 9000F TENS
STD hip prosthesis
steady state free precession (SSFP)
steal phenomenon in diabetic microvasculature of lower extremities
steal syndrome, subclavian
Stecher arachnoid knife
steel shank
steel sole plate
Steel shelf procedure
Steel triple innominate osteotomy
Steele-Richardson-Olszewski disease
Steele-Richardson-Olszewski syndrome
Steffee pedicle plate
Steffee pedicular rod
Steffee plates and screws for lumbar fusion
Steinbach mallet
Steinberg thumb sign
Steinbrocker classification of rheumatoid arthritis
Steindler flexorplasty
Steindler stripping operation
Steinert classification of epiphyseal fracture
Steinhauser bone clamp
Steinhauser cranial screw
Steinmann extension nail
Steinmann pin with Crowe pilot point
Steinmann sign
Steinmann tendon forceps
stellate chemicals
stellate fracture
stellate sympathetic ganglion block
stellate undepressed fracture
Stellbrink synovectomy rongeur
stem
  Aufranc-Turner
  brain
  fenestrated
  fin of prosthetic
  Harris-Galante
  infundibular
  Kirschner
  Mallory-Head femoral
  Moore
  nonfenestrated
  Omnifit HA hip
  Press-Fit
  regular
  reticular formation of the brain
  roundback
  Sivash
  straight
  trial
  Zimmer bone
stem base plate
stem envelope
stem extender
stemmed tibial prosthesis
Stener-Gunterberg hip procedure
Stener lesion

stenosing tendovaginitis
stenosing tenosynovitis (tendosynovitis)
stenosis
  aqueductal
  bilateral carotid
  carotid artery
  central canal
  central spinal
  cerebral artery
  congenital aqueductal
  congenital spinal
  hemodynamically significant
  spinal
  subclavian artery
  unilateral carotid
  vertebral artery
stent dressing
Stenver view (on x-ray)
Stenzel rod
step-cut osteotomy
step-cut transection
step-down deformity of the shoulder
step-down osteotomy
step-off fracture
step-off in facial fracture diagnosis
step-off, orbital rim
step-osteotomy
step-second test
step-up in the spinous processes in spondylolisthesis
Stephenson-Gibbs reference electrode
steppage gait due to footdrop
stepped flash photic stimulation
stepwise increase in drug dosage
stereoanesthesia
stereognosis
stereotactic or stereotaxic
stereotactic ablation
stereotactic atlas
stereotactic bag
stereotactic biopsy
stereotactic carrier
stereotactic coordinates
stereotactic craniotomy
stereotactic depth electroencephalogram
stereotactic endoscopy
stereotactic frame
stereotactic head frame
stereotactic neurosurgery
stereotactic operating microscope
stereotactic placement of depth electrodes
stereotactic puncture
stereotactic radiosurgery
stereotactic ring
stereotactic robot
stereotactic surgery
stereotactic target
stereotactic thalamectomy
stereotactic thalamotomy
stereotactically guided
stereotaxis, computer-assisted volumetric
stereotaxy
stereotypic behavior
Steri-Strips
sterile 4 x 4's
sterile saline solution
sternal occipital mandibular immobilization (SOMI)
sternobrachial reflex
sternoclavicular joint
sternocleidomastoid, clavicular head of
sternocleidomastoid muscle weakness
sternomastoid
sternospinal reference electrode
steroid block, epidural
steroid injection
steroid myopathy
steroids
  tapering dose
  tapering regimen of
steroid therapy
stertorous hyperventilation
Stevens-Street elbow prosthesis
Stevenson alligator forceps
Stevenson grasping forceps
Steward-Milford fracture classification

Stewart-Harley ankle arthrodesis
Stewart-Holmes sign
Stewart-Morel syndrome
Stewart arm procedure
St. George-Buchholz ankle prosthesis
St. George total elbow prosthesis
St. Louis encephalitis
St. Louis encephalitis antibody
St. Louis viral encephalitis
St. Vitus dance
STH-2 (Sarmiento) hip prosthesis
stick, switching
Stickler syndrome
Stieda fracture
stiff-man syndrome
stiffness
  joint
  neck
stiffness coefficient
Stiles-Bunnell transfer technique
Still-Chauffard polyarthritis syndrome
Still disease (juvenile rheumatoid arthritis)
Stille bone biter
Stille bone chisel
Stille bone drill
Stille bone gouge
Stille-Broback retractor
Stille bur
Stille chisel
Stille cranial drill
Stille drill points, burs, and trephine
Stille-Giertz rib shears
Stille gouge
Stille hand drill
Stille-Horsley bone forceps
Stille-Horsley rongeur
Stille-Lauer bone rongeur
Stille-Leksell rongeur
Stille-Liston bone-cutting forceps
Stille-Liston bone rongeur
Stille-Luer bone rongeur
Stille-Luer-Echlin rongeur
Stille-Luer rongeur forceps
Stille osteotome
Stille plaster shears
Stille probe
Stille rib shears
Stille rongeur forceps
Stille-Ruskin bone rongeur
Stille-Sherman bone drill
Stille tourniquet
Stille trephine
Stimson dressing
Stimson maneuver
stimulation, stimulator
  AME bone growth
  Amrex muscle
  auditory
  Axostim nerve
  battery pack
  blink reflex to corneal
  capacitor plate for electrical
  constant direct current
  diffuse photic
  digital
  dorsal column (DCS)
  double simultaneous
  double simultaneous sensory
  EBI SpF-2 implantable bone
  EBI SpF-T bone
  EBI spinal fusion
  electrical (of bone)
  electrical surface
  electrogalvanic
  epidural spinal cord (ESCS)
  epileptogenic
  facial nerve
  faradic current (electrical)
  flash
  flashes of light
  flashes per second of photic
  galvanic
  glissando photic
  high-volt biphasic
  high-volt inferential
  Hilger facial nerve
  intermittent flashes of light

stimulation *(cont.)*
intraoperative nerve
Intrel II spinal cord
JACE-STIM electrotherapy
Jako
magnetic
Medtronic neuromuscular
Medtronic spinal cord
nerve
Neuromed
neuromuscular
neuromuscular electrical (NMES)
OrthoPak bone growth
OrthoPak II bone
OsteoGen bone growth
Osteo Stim bone
Osteo Stim implantable bone growth
patterned light
patterned photic
photic (during EEG recording with a stroboscopic light)
Pisces spinal cord stimulation system
ReAct neuromuscular
Reese
repetitive clicking
repetitive flashes of light
repetitive nerve
repetitive photic
Respond Select neuromuscular
sensory
somatosensory
SpF Spinal Fusion Stimulator
spinal cord
startling noise
stepped flash photic stimulation
stepwise photic
stimulator
stroboscopic
stroboscopic light
tactile
TENS (transcutaneous electrical nerve)
touch and tickle

stimulation *(cont.)*
transcranial magnetic (MAG)
transcutaneous electrical nerve (TENS)
VIM (ventral intermedius nucleus)
visual
WR nerve
stimulus (pl. stimuli)
alerting
auditory
checkerboard pattern-reversal
click
double simultaneous
environmental
epileptogenic
external
extinction of
flickering
full-field monocular
insensitivity to painful
matching
musical
noxious
outside
painful
psychosensory
responded purposefully to
sensory
startling
stimuli
supramaximal
tactile
thermal
threshold of
train of repetitive
triggering
visual
stimulus artifact
stimulus bound
stimulus rate, click
stinger (nerve pain from cervical or brachial plexus injury)
stippled epiphysis
stippling

stirrup, stirrups
  Aircast pneumatic air
  Allen
  ankle air
  high
  split
  traction
  walking
stitch (see *suture*)
stitch, Frost
Stiwer forceps
Stiwer retractor
Stiwer scissors
stock, poor bone
stockinette
  basket
  bias
  bias-cut
  Buck traction
  sling-and-swathe
  tubular
stockinette cut on the bias
stockings (also called *hose*)
  antiembolic
  antiembolism
  antithrombotic
  compression
  Jobst
  long leg
  Orthawear antiembolism
  Sigvaris compression
  stockings
  TED (thromboembolic disease)
  thigh-high antiembolic
  Vairox high compression vascular
stocking distribution
stocking-glove distribution
stocking-glove sensory loss
Stokes-Adams attack
Stone and Neale Daily Coping Assessment
Stone arthrodesis
Stone bunionectomy
Stone four-point staple
stone, Whitfield ointment and pumice
Stookey cranial rongeur
stop action brace
stopcock
storiform pattern
stork's legs in Charcot-Marie-Tooth disease
Storz arthroscope
Storz meniscotome
Storz Microsystems cranial fixation plate
Storz Microsystems drill bit
Storz Microsystems microplate
Storz Microsystems miniplate
Storz Microsystems plate cutters
Storz Microsystems plate-holding forceps
Storz Microsystems pliers
Storz screw
Storz telescope
Strümpell-Leichtenstern encephalitis
Strümpell sign
strabismus
  illusory
  kinetic
  real
straddle fracture
straddle injury
straight last shoes
straight leg raising test
straight stem femoral components
strain
  Brunhilde (type I poliomyelitis virus)
  foot (acute, chronic)
  hamstring
  Lansing (type II poliomyelitis virus)
  Leon (type III poliomyelitis virus)
  ligamentous
  lumbosacral spine
  muscle

strain energy
strain fracture
strain gauge evaluation
strain-sprain injury
Strampelli splint
strap
  capsular
  Cho-Pat (**cho**ndromalacia **pat**ellae)
    knee
  Chopart patellar
  clavicular
  crotch
  Meek clavicle
  PTB (patellar tendon-bearing)
  suspension
  touch-fastener
  Velcro
strap muscles
stratigraphy
Strayer tendon technique
streak, meningeal
stream of thought
Street medullary pin
Street-Stevens humeral prosthesis
Streeter dysplasia
strength
  BUE
  extrinsic muscle
  fatigue
  5/5 (five over five)
  foot intrinsic muscle
  grip
  hand grasp
  hand grip
  intrinsic muscle
  isometric muscle
  Lovett clinical scale of
  motor
  tensile
  yield
strength against resistance
Streptococcus pneumoniae meningitis
stress
  adduction (to fingers)
  biomechanical

stress *(cont.)*
  hyperextension
  mediolateral
  shear
  torque
  valgus
  varus
stress films
stress fracture
stress radiograph
stress-strain relationships
stretch
  intermittent passive muscle
  muscle stretch
stretch reflex
stretch reflex pathways
stretch test, sciatic
stretcher, field
stretches (see *exercises*)
stria
  habenular
  longitudinal
  medullary
  meningitic
stria fornicis
stria kaesbekhterevi
stria medullaris thalami
stria pinealis
stria terminalis
stria ventriculi tertii
stria terminalis
striae of Baillarger
striae of floor of ventricle
striatal
striatal lesion
striatal neuron
striatal nigral degeneration
striatal toe
striate cortex
striate hemorrhages in intracranial
  hypertension
striatocerebellar tremor
striatonigral degeneration
striatum, corpus
Strickland tendon repair

stride characteristics
stride length of gait
strike phase of gait
striker
  forefoot
  rearfoot
string of pearls nuclear arrangement, seen in myopathies
strionigral
strip, strips
  AdTech electrode
  epidural electrode
  Fas-Trac
  4-contact electrode sentinel
  moleskin
  motor
  PVA
  subdural electrode
stripe of Baillarger
stripe of Gennari
stripe of Vicq d'Azyr
stripper
  Brand palmaris tendon
  Bunnell tendon
  cartilage
  endarterectomy
  fascia
  Fischer tendon
  Furlong tendon
  Grierson tendon
  IM tendon
  malleable
  New Orleans endarterectomy
  palmaris tendon
  plantaris
  rib
  tendon
stripping, periosteal
stroboscope
stroboscopic flashes of light in EEG
stroboscopic lamp
stroboscopic stimulation
stroke (cerebrovascular accident, CVA)
  acute
  anterior circulation

stroke *(cont.)*
  brain stem
  completed
  cryptogenic
  embolic
  evolving
  hemispheric
  hemorrhagic
  hypertensive
  incomplete
  ischemic
  lacunar
  midbrain
  middle cerebral artery territory
  migrainous
  nonhemorrhagic
  posterior circulation
  progressing
  pure hemisensory
  pure motor
  pure sensory
  sensorimotor
  sensory
  small-vessel
  spinal
  spinal cord
  thalamocapsular
  thromboembolic
  thrombotic
stroke in evolution
strokes, multiple small (état lacunaire)
stroke syndrome
stroma
stromal cells
Stromeyer splint
Stromgren ankle brace
structural epileptogenic lesion
  arteriovenous malformations
  cysts
  neoplasms
structure, structures
  bony
  cordlike
  extrapyramidal
  lateral supporting

structure *(cont.)*
  shift of midline (of midbrain)
  subcortical
Strully dissecting scissors
Strully dural hook
Strully dural scissors
Strully-Gigli rongeur
Strully-Gigli saw handles
Strully-Kerrison rongeur
Strully neurological scissors
Strümpell-Lorrain disease
Strümpell, tibialis sign of
Strunsky sign
strut bone graft
strut, corticocancellous
strut-type pin
Struthers
  arcade of
  ligament of
Stryker bed
Stryker cartilage knife
Stryker CPM exerciser
Stryker fracture frame
Stryker knee joint laxity machine
Stryker knee laxity arthrometer
Stryker leg exerciser
Stryker microsurgery drill
Stryker Quick Pressure Monitor Set, for compartment syndromes
Stryker Surgilav machine
Stryker table
STSE (split-thickness skin excision)
STSG (split-thickness skin graft)
STT (scapho-trapezium-trapezoid) joint
STT (scaphotrapezoid-trapezial) joint
Stuart Gordon splint
Stuck laminectomy retractor
stud, fixation
study, studies
  air contrast
  antidromic (sensory) conduction
  bone age (as indicator of biologic age)
  brachial plexus motor

study *(cont.)*
  continuous wave Doppler
  Doppler
  electrodiagnostic
  electromyographic
  electrophysiologic nerve
  kinematic
  mixed nerve conduction
  motor nerve conduction
  musculocutaneous nerve sensory
  nerve conduction
  orthodromic sensory
  radial nerve motor/sensory
  sensory nerve conduction
  split-brain
  tenographic
  tension-to-failure
  ulnar nerve motor/sensory
Stulberg hip positioner
Stulberg Mark II leg positioner
Stulberg method, in Perthes disease
stump
  bulbous
  distal
  edematous
  hypersensitive
  midfoot
  tendon
stump of bone
stump shrinker, elastic
stump sock
stupor
  alcoholic
  catatonic
stuporous patient
Sturge-Weber syndrome
Sturge-Weber telangiectasia
stuttering gait in parkinsonism
styloid
  radial
  ulnar
styloidectomy, Stewart
stylomastoid foramen
stylus, marking

Styrofoam filler block
sub-falcine (subfalcial) herniation
subacromial bursal adhesion
subacromial bursitis
subacute combined degeneration of the cord
subacute granulomatous meningitis
subacute necrotizing myelitis (Foix-Alajouanine)
subacute sclerosing panencephalitis (SSPE) viral encephalitis
subacute spongiform encephalopathy
subacute type (Nevin-Jones type) spongiform encephalopathy
subarachnoid block
subarachnoid cavity
subarachnoid hemorrhage (SAH)
subarachnoid hemorrhage from rupture of mycotic aneurysm
subarachnoid screw instruments
subarachnoid space
subarticular cyst
subcallosal gyrus
subcapital fracture
subchondral bone cyst
subchondral bone plate
subchondral microfractures
subchondral plate
subchondral sclerosis
subclavian artery occlusion
subclavian artery stenosis
subclavian bruit
subclavian steal phenomenon (SSP)
subclinical EEG discharges
subclinical neuropathy
subclinical seizure activity
subclinical status epilepticus
subcollateral gyrus
subcoracoid shoulder dislocation
subcortical aphasia
subcortical atrophy
subcortical lesion
subcortical neuronal dysfunction
subcortical pacemaker
subcortical pathway
subcortical structures
subcutaneous fibroma
subcutaneous fracture
subcutaneous palmar fasciotomy
subcutaneous tissue gas
subcuticular closure
subdeltoid bursal adhesion
subdeltoid bursitis
subdural abscess
subdural blood
subdural cavity
subdural clot
subdural effusion
subdural electrode
subdural empyema
subdural hematoma
subdural hemorrhage
subdural hygroma
subdural pressure monitor
subdural space
subdural tap
subependymoma
subfalcine (subfalcial) herniation
subfascial transposition
subfrontal meningioma
subfrontal meningioma tumor
subgaleal abscess
subgaleal CSF (cerebrospinal fluid)
subgaleal hematoma
subglenoid shoulder dislocation
subharmonic of rhythm on EEG
subhyaloid retinal hemorrhage(s)
subjective cosmesis
subjective impairment
subjective limited movement
subjective symptoms of impairment
subjective vertigo
sublamina wiring
sublux, subluxed
subluxation
  atlanto-axial
  occult
  patellar

subluxation *(cont.)*
  posterior
  radial head
  reduced (sprains)
  rotary
  tendon
subluxation complex
subluxation correction
subluxing patella
subluxing tendon
submandibular ganglion
suboccipital headache
suboccipital shortening
subperiosteal fracture
subperiosteal new bone
subperiosteally
subpial resection
subsartorial tunnel
subscapular tendon
subscapularis muscle
subscapularis recess
subscapularis tendon
substance
  anterior perforated
  posterior perforated
substantia gelatinosa of spinal cord
substantia gelatinosa rolandi
substantia nigra
substantia perforata rostralis
subsultus tendinum
subtalar arthralgia
subtalar arthrodesis
subtalar arthrotomy
subtalar articulation
subtalar axis
subtalar instability
subtalar joint as torque converter
subtalar joint pronation
subtalar joint space
subtalar joint stability
subtalar posterior displacement
  osteotomy of the calcaneus
subtalar stabilization
subtemporal approach
subtendinous space
subtentorial lesions
subthalamic nucleus of Luys
subthalamic region, midbrain
subthalamus, zona incerta of
subtotal meniscectomy
subtotal removal of tumor
subtractions, serial
subtrochanteric fracture
subungual abscess
subungual amelanotic melanoma
subungual hematoma
subungual tumor (glomus tumor)
suck reflex
sucker shaver
sucker tip
Sucker, KAM Super
sucking reflex (primitive)
suction-irrigation system
suction-irrigator
  House
  Kurze
suction tip
  Frazier
  neurosurgical
suction tube
  Adson
  New York Glass
  Pribham
  wall
suction via trap-bottle system
sudanophilic leukodystrophies
Sudeck atrophy
Sudeck disease
sudomotor autonomic hyperactivity
  (not pseudo)
sugar-tong cast
sugar-tong plaster splint
Sugioka transtrochanteric osteotomy
Sugita aneurysm clip
Sugita head frame
Sugita table
suit, isolation
Sukhtian-Hughes fixation devices

sulcal atrophy
sulcal obliteration
sulcus (pl. sulci)
    calcarine
    callosal
    central
    cingulate
    collateral
    dilatation of the
    effacement of
    frontal
    hypothalmic
    lateral
    lateral occipital
    lips of lateral
    occipitotemporal
    olfactory
    parieto-occipital
    pontomedullary
    postcentral sulcus
    precentral
    rami of lateral
    rolandic
    supracallosal
    temporal
    ulnar
    widened, on scan
sulcus angle
sulcus calcaneus
sulcus lunatus
sulcus nail
sulcus of metatarsus
sulcus talus
sulfite oxidase deficiency
sulfur bath, hot
sunburst pattern on x-ray
Sundaresan approach
Sunday staphylorrhaphy elevator
Sunderland classification of nerve injury
Sunderland five-degree system
sun-downing
Sundt classification of carotid ulceration
Sundt-Kees aneurysm window clips
Sundt loop endarterectomy shunt
Sundt shunt
sunrise view
sunset eyes
sunset view
Superblade
superciliary arch
superconducting magnet
SuperCup acetabular cup prosthesis
superficial (abdominal) reflexes
superficial palmar arterial arch
superficial sensation
Superfoam II material
Superglue (cyanoacrylate) adhesive
superimposed on EEG
superincumbent spinal curves
superior colliculus
superior frontal gyrus
superior olive in brain
superior parietal lobule gyrus
superior peroneal retinaculum
superior quadriceps retinaculum
superior temporal gyrus
Superior Sleeprite Hi-Lo orthopedic bed
supernumerary sesamoid bones
superolaterally
superomedial portal
supersaturation, muscle glycogen
superselective catheterization
superselective embolization
superselectively introduced
supination-adduction fracture
supination deformity
supination-eversion fracture
supination, external rotation-type IV fracture (SER-IV)
supinator, assistant
supinator canal syndrome
supinator jerks
supine cervical traction
Suppan foot procedure
Supplemental Security Income (SSI)

support (see also *orthosis*; *prosthesis*)
  Accommodator arch
  AliMed wrist/thumb
  alternating single-leg (running gait)
  ankle
  arch
  Arizona leg
  back
  bed cradle
  billet prosthetic
  Body Gard neoprene
  canvas
  cervical
  cock-up hand
  cock-up wrist
  condylar cuff prosthetic
  cutout knee
  elbow
  Epitrain knitted elbow
  foam
  fork strap prosthetic
  Freedom arthritis (for hand)
  Friedman elbow
  Fromison elbow
  hand
  hinged knee
  Houston halo cervical
  initial double (of gait)
  Kerr-Lagen abdominal
  knee
  ligamentous
  Lo Bak spinal
  lumbosacral
  medial arch
  metatarsal
  MKG knee
  Neck-Huggar cervical
  neoprene
  OEC wrist/forearm
  open patella knee
  Philadelphia collar cervical
  Relax-A-Bac posture
  rib
  Sacro-Eze lumbar support

support *(cont.)*
  second double (of gait)
  Sheffield hand
  shoe
  Silesian bandage prosthetic
  Sleeper II sleep (by Bodyline)
  standard U patellar
  tennis elbow
  Thera-Back back
  waist belt prosthetic
  walk with
  walk without
  wrist
  OSI Well Leg
supporter, Malis vessel
supporting foot
suppression, burst (on EEG in diffuse severe encephalopathies)
suppuration
suppurative periostitis
suppurative tenosynovitis
supracallosal gyrus
supracallosal sulcus
supraclavicular region
supracollicular spike of cortical bone
supracondylar femoral derotational osteotomy
supracondylar fracture
supracondylar varus osteotomy
supramalleolar orthosis (SMO)
supramalleolar osteotomy
supramalleolar region
supramarginal gyrus
supranuclear (bilateral upper motor neuron)
supranuclear disorders of ocular movement
supranuclear dysfunction
supranuclear lesion
supranuclear ophthalmoplegias
supranuclear palsy, progressive
supranuclear paralysis
supranuclear weakness
supraorbital bar

supraorbital fissure
supraorbital ridges
suprapatellar bursa
suprapatellar plica
suprapatellar pouch
suprascapular nerve entrapment
suprasellar adenoma
suprasellar aneurysm
suprasellar extension of tumor
suprasellar lesion
suprasellar mass
suprasellar meningioma
suprasellar Rathke cleft cyst (RCC)
suprasellar region
suprasellar tumor
supraspinatus nerve
supraspinatus tendon
supraspinous ligaments
suprasyndesmotic fixation
supratentorial approach
supratentorial arteriovenous malformation
supratentorial astrocytoma
supratentorial brain tumor
supratentorial glioma
supratentorial lesion
supratentorial mass
supratentorial symptoms (euphemism for hypochondriasis)
supratentorial tumor
supratubercular wedge osteotomy
sural nerve
Surbaugh leg holder
surcingle, Von Lackum
Suretac bioabsorbable shoulder fixation device
Suretac biofixation device
surface
    acetabular weightbearing
    apposing articular
    articular
    bleeding bone
    bone
    bosselated
surface *(cont.)*
    cartilaginous joint
    contiguous articular
    endosteal
    grooving of articular
    joint articular
    parallelism of articular
    radioulnar
    roughened articular
    weightbearing
surface coil MR
surface method of Hodes
surface-shoe interaction
surfer's knots
Surfit adhesive
Surg-Assist leg holder
Surg-Assist leg positioner
Surgairtome
surgeon's tarsal joint
surgery (see *operations*)
    aesthetic
    bur
    high-torque burr
    neuro-otologic
    outpatient ambulatory
    salvage
    southern access to the hip joint in
    stereotactic
surgibone
    Boplant
    Unilab
surgical ablation
surgical approach
surgical decompression
surgical neck fracture
Surgical No Bounce Mallet
surgical rhizotomy
surgical site
surgical stabilization
Surgical Dynamics aspiration probe
Surgical Simplex P radiopaque bone cement
surgically resected
Surgilase CO_2 laser

Surgilav machine
Surgilift transportation system
Surgitek prosthesis
Surgi-Tron instruments
Surgivac drain
survey
  four-view wrist
  metastatic bone
survival roles of ICIDH (International Classification of Impairments, Disabilities, Handicaps)
  economic self-sufficiency
  mobility
  occupation of time
  orientation
  physical independence
  social integration
suspended animation
suspension
  adjustable Thomas splint
  balanced
  finger-trap
  half-ring Thomas splint
  overhead
  sling
  Thomas splint
sustentaculum, talar
Sutherland-Greenfield double innominate osteotomy
Sutherland hip procedure
Sutherland tendon transfer
Sutter-CPM knee device
Sutter double-stem silicone implant
Sutter MCP joint prosthesis
Sutter-Smeloff heart valve prosthesis
sutura coronalis
sutura frontalis
sutura lambdoidea
sutura occipitomastoidea
sutura parietomastoidea
sutura plana
sutura sagittalis
sutura serrata
sutura sphenoparietalis
sutura sphenosquamosa
suture, sutures (also called *stitch*)
  absorbable
  apical
  basilar
  Bell
  biparietal
  braided
  bregmatomastoid
  bridging
  bundle
  Bunnell crisscross
  Bunnell wire pull-out
  buried interrupted
  catgut
  cerclage
  chromic catgut
  chromic interrupted
  circular wire
  clove-hitch
  coapting
  compression stay
  coronal
  cotton
  cranial
  crisscross
  Czerny
  Dacron
  delayed closure of
  dentate
  Dermalon
  Dexon
  diastasis of the
  Donati
  double-armed (DAS)
  dural tack-up
  dural traction
  Ethibond
  Ethiflex
  Ethilon
  figure-of-8
  fish-mouth
  flat
  frontal

suture *(cont.)*
- fronto-ethmoidal
- frontoparietal
- frontosphenoid
- Gillies
- Gruber
- guy
- Hawkeye
- heavy silk
- horizontal mattress
- interparietal
- interrupted
- intracuticular
- intradermal
- inverted
- jugal
- Kessler
- Krause
- lambdoid
- lambdoidal cranial
- lashing
- Le Dentu
- leg of
- longitudinal
- loop mattress
- mamillary
- mattress
- Maxon
- McLaughlin modification of Bunnell pull-out
- Mersilene
- metopic cranial
- modified Kessler
- monofilament
- monofilament nylon
- muscle-to-bone
- myodesis
- near-far
- nerve
- nonabsorbable
- nonfusion of cranial
- Nurolon
- nylon
- occipital

suture *(cont.)*
- occipitomastoid
- occipitoparietal
- occipitosphenoid
- Owen silk
- P-3
- parietal
- parietomastoid
- parietooccipital
- Perma-Hand braided silk
- petrobasilar
- petrosphenobasilar
- petrospheno-occipital
- petrosquamous
- plain catgut
- plain gut
- plastic
- Polydek
- polyester
- polyglactin 910
- polyglyconate
- polypropylene
- PRE 2
- prematurely closed
- primary
- primary (of ruptured tendons)
- Prolene
- pull-out
- pull-out wire
- Pulver-Taft fish-mouth
- rhabdoid
- running
- sagittal cranial
- secondary (of ruptured tendons)
- serrated
- silk
- simple
- skin
- sphenoethmoidal
- spheno-occipital
- spheno-orbital
- sphenoparietal
- sphenopetrosal
- sphenosquamous

suture *(cont.)*
- sphenotemporal
- sphenovomerine
- splayed cranial
- spread (cranial sign)
- squamosomastoid
- squamosoparietal
- squamososphenoid
- squamous
- stainless steel
- subcutaneous
- subcuticular
- swaged-on
- tack
- temporal
- Tevdek
- Ticron
- transfixion
- transverse
- twisted
- Tycron
- undyed
- vertical mattress
- Vicryl
- wire
- wire pull-out

suture abscess
suture button
suture line
suture passer
SV-40 virus
Sven-Johansson driver
Sven-Johansson extractor
Sven-Johansson femoral neck nail
Sven-Johansson finisher
swaged-on needle with suture
swaged-on suture
swallow reflex
swallowing automatism
swallowing dysfunction
swallowing mechanism, video fluoroscopy of
swallowing rehabilitation
swan neck
swan-neck deformity
swan, shoemaker's
Swann-Morton surgical blade
Swanson awl
Swanson Convex condylar arthroplasty
Swanson elevator
Swanson finger joint
Swanson great toe prosthesis
Swanson interpositional wrist arthroplasty
Swanson intramedullary broach
Swanson lunate awl
Swanson mallet
Swanson metacarpal prosthesis
Swanson metacarpophalangeal implant
Swanson metatarsal prosthesis
Swanson metatarsophalangeal joint arthroplasty
Swanson osteotome
Swanson osteotomy
Swanson PIP joint arthroplasty
Swanson reamer
Swanson scaphoid awl
Swanson Silastic prosthesis
Swanson T-shaped great toe Silastic prosthesis
Swanson wrist implant
Swanson wrist prosthesis
swathe *or* swath
swathe, sling and (bandage)
SWD (short wave diathermy)
sweat test for thoracic outlet syndrome
sweating of the face, thermoregulatory
Swede-O brace
Swede-O-Universal braces
Swedish knee cage orthosis
sweeny (shoulder slip)
Sweet pituitary scissors
Sweet two-point discriminator
swelling
- blennorrhagic
- boggy
- brain

swelling *(cont.)*
  fusiform
  joint
  postfracture
  posttraumatic
  soft tissue
swimmer's ear
swimmer's shoulder
swimmer's view on x-ray examination
swing-phase control
swing-phase periods of gait
  initial swing
  midswing
  terminal swing
swing through of extremity
swinging flashlight test
swings, mood
Swiss cancellous screw
switch-stick
swivel dislocation (of midfoot)
Swivel-Strap brace
swollen, markedly
Sydenham chorea
sylvian aqueduct syndrome
sylvian candelabra
sylvian fissure
sylvian operculum
sylvian/rolandic junction
sylvian system
Sylvius
  aqueduct of
  cistern of fossa of
  fossa of
Syme amputation, Wagner modification
Syme ankle disarticulation amputation
symmetrical diffuse neuropathy
symmetry of limb movements in infants
Symonds headache
sympathectomy
  cervical
  chemical
sympathetic chain
sympathetic denervation
sympathetic dyspraxia
sympathetic innervation
sympathetic nervous system
sympathetic overactivity
sympathetic reflex dystrophy
sympathetic vascular instability
sympatheticoblastoma
symphalangism, multiple
symphysis
symphysis pubis
symptom, symptoms
  affective (of seizures)
  auditory
  brain stem
  Buerger
  conversion
  functionally debilitating
  gustatory
  insidious onset of
  Kanavel four cardinal
  localizing neurologic
  migrainous
  motor
  myasthenic
  neurologic
  olfactory
  parkinsonian
  premonitory (of seizures)
  prodromal
  pseudomyasthenic
  psychomotor
  psychosensory
  radicular
  segmental
  sensory
  supratentorial (euphemism for hypochondriasis)
  theater
  upper motor neuron
  visual
symptom complex
symptomatic bipartite sesamoids
symptomatic epilepsy
symptomatology

synapse
  abnormal axodendritic
  axodendritic
  excitatory
synaptic cleft
synaptic pathways
synarthrosis
synathresis
Synatomic knee prosthesis
synchondrosis petro-occipitalis
synchondrotomy
Synchromed programmable drug pump
synchronous lesions
synchronous nerve impulse
synchronous wave
synchrony
  bilateral EEG
  interhemispheric
  secondary bilateral
syncopal episode
syncope
  cough
  defecation
  hyperventilation
  micturition
  migrainous
  neck extension precipitating
  orthostatic
  sneeze
  tussive
  vasodepressor
  vasovagal
syndactylization of digits
syndactyly
  complex-complete
  cutaneous
  soft tissue
syndesmectomy
syndesmopexy
syndesmoplasty
syndesmorrhaphy
syndesmosis
  disrupted
  tibiofibular
syndesmosis screw
syndesmosis sprain of the ankle
syndesmotic clear space
syndesmotic diastasis
syndesmotic ligament complex
syndesmotic screw
syndesmotomy
syndrome
  dancing bear
  acute cerebellar
  acute organic brain
  Adie
  adrenogenital
  adult Reye
  Aicardi
  akinetic-rigid
  Albright-McCune-Sternberg
  alcohol withdrawal
  Alpers
  ALS-like (amyotrophic lateral sclerosis)
  amnesic
  amnestic-confabulatory
  amotivational
  amyostatic
  angular gyrus
  anterior cerebellar artery
  anterior cervical cord
  anterior compartment
  anterior cord
  anterior impingement
  anterior spinal artery
  anterior tibial
  anterior tibial compartment
  Anton
  apallic
  Apert
  Arnold-Chiari
  Avellis
  axonopathic neurogenic thoracic outlet
  Baastrupi
  Babinski-Fröhlich
  Babinski-Nageotte
  Balint

syndrome *(cont.)*
- Baltic myoclonus
- Barré-Lieou
- basilar
- Bassen-Kornzweig
- Basser
- Behr
- Benedikt
- benign pain
- Bernard-Horner
- bicipital
- Bing-Horton
- black heel
- Block-Sulzberger
- blue toe
- body cast
- brain death
- brain stem
- Brissaud
- broad thumb-big toe
- Broca
- Brown-Séquard
- burning-feet
- carpal tunnel (CTS)
- carpal tunnel wrist
- Carpenter
- cast
- cauda equina (CES)
- cauda equina compression
- caudal regression
- central cervical cord
- central cord
- central pain (CPS)
- cerebellar hemorrhage
- cerebral steal
- cerebrohepatorenal
- cervical acceleration/deceleration (whiplash)
- cervical dorsal outlet
- Céstan-Chenais
- Charcot-Marie-Tooth
- Chauffard-Still (polyarthritis)
- Chédiak-Higashi
- cherry red spot myoclonus

syndrome *(cont.)*
- Chiari-Foix-Nicolesco
- choreic
- chronic brain (CBS)
- chronic fatigue
- chronic musculoskeletal pain (CMPS)
- chronic pain
- Claude
- clenched fist
- clumsy hand
- Cobb
- Cockayne
- Cogan
- Collet-Sicard
- compartment
- compression
- constriction band
- conus medullaris
- cord traction
- Cornelia de Lange
- Costen
- costoclavicular
- cramp
- cranial nerve vascular compression
- craniofacial
- Creutzfeldt-Jakob
- Crouzon
- crush
- crying face
- cubital tunnel
- Cushing
- dancing-eyes, dancing-feet
- Dandy-Walker
- de Lange
- de-efferented
- dehiscence-disinsertion
- Dejerine anterior bulbar
- Dejerine-Roussy
- Dejerine-Sottas
- Denny-Brown
- depigmentation of the iris with neonatal Horner
- dialysis

syndrome *(cont.)*
- dialysis encephalopathy
- diffuse idiopathic skeletal hyperostosis (DISH)
- DiGeorge
- disconnection
- disinhibitions of a frontal lobe
- dorsal midbrain
- double-crush
- Down
- droopy shoulder (thoracic outlet)
- drug withdrawal
- Duane retraction
- Dudley Morton
- Dyke-Davidoff-Masson
- dysarthria-clumsy hand
- dysequilibrium
- dyssynergia cerebellaris myoclonia
- Eaton-Lambert
- Edwards
- Ehlers-Danlos
- Ekbom restless leg
- empty sella
- entrapment
- eosinophilia-myalgia (EMS)
- epileptic
- facet
- facio-auriculo-vertebral (FAV)
- failed back (FBS)
- failed back surgery (FBSS)
- Fanconi
- Farber
- fat toe
- Fazio-Londe
- Felty
- fetal alcohol (FAS)
- filum terminale
- Fisher
- flat back
- flexor hallucis longus entrapment
- flexor origin
- floppy baby
- floppy-infant
- Foix

syndrome *(cont.)*
- foramen
- foraminal
- Foster-Kennedy
- Foville
- fragile x
- Froin
- frontal lobe
- frozen shoulder
- Funston
- Ganser (syndrome of approximate answers)
- Garcin
- Gerstmann-Straussler
- Gilles de la Tourette
- Gillespie
- Goldenhar
- Gradenigo
- Grisel
- Guillain-Barré (GBS)
- Guillain-Barré-Strohl
- Guillain-Garcin
- Haglund
- half base
- Hallermann-Streiff-François
- hammer digit
- hand-foot
- hand-foot-uterus
- headache
- heel pain
- Heerfort
- hemibasal
- hemichorea-hemiballism
- hemicord
- hemisensory
- hemispheric
- hereditary sensory neuropathy
- HHE (hemiconvulsions, hemiplegia, and epilepsy)
- Hoffmann
- Holt-Oran
- Horner
- Hunter
- Hurler

syndrome *(cont.)*
- hyperactive
- iatrogenic Cushing
- ilioinguinal
- iliotibial band friction
- impingement
- infantile polymyoclonus
- infectious polyneuritis
- infrapatellar contracture (IPSC)
- inguinal ligament
- INO (internuclear ophthalmoplegia)
- insular-opercular
- inverse Marcus Gunn
- Isaacs
- ischemic
- isolation
- Ito hypomelanosis
- Jackson
- Jaccoud (arthritis)
- Jacod (neuralgia) (*not* Jacob)
- Jansky-Bielschowsky
- Jarcho-Levin
- jugular foramen
- Kearns-Sayre (KSS)
- Kernohan notch
- Kiloh-Nevin
- Kinsbourne
- Kleine-Levin
- Klinefelter
- Klippel-Feil
- Klippel-Trenaunay-Weber
- Klüver-Bucy ablation
- Kocher-Debré-Sémélaigne
- Koerber-Salus-Elschnig
- Korsakoff
- Kretschmer
- Kugelberg-Welander
- lacunar
- Lambert-Eaton myasthenic (LEMS)
- Lance-Adams
- Landau-Kleffner
- Landry-Guillain-Barré-Strohl
- Larson
- lateral medullary syndrome

syndrome *(cont.)*
- lateral pontomedullary
- Laurence-Moon-Biedl
- leg-foot-toe
- Leigh
- Lennox
- Lennox-Gastaut
- leprechaun
- Leriche
- Lesch-Nyhan
- Li-Fraumeni (LFS)
- Lindau
- locked-in
- Louis-Bar (ataxia-telangiectasia)
- Lowe
- lower basilar branch
- lumbar facet arthrosis
- Maffucci
- malalignment
- malignant neuroleptic
- Marchand-Waterhouse
- Marchiafava-Bignami
- Marfan
- Marinesco-Sjögren
- Maroteaux-Lamy
- May-White
- McArdle
- McCune-Albright
- medial longitudinal fasciculus
- medial plantar digital proper nerve
- median nerve entrapment
- medicamentosus Cushing
- medulla oblongata
- Meige
- Melkersson-Rosenthal
- Menkes
- metatarsal overload
- Ménière
- midbrain displacement
- middle cerebral artery
- migrainous
- Milch fracture classification
- milk-alkali
- Milkman

syndrome *(cont.)*
- Millard-Gubler
- Miller-Fisher variant of Guillain-Barré
- MLF (medial longitudinal fasciculus)
- Möbius (Moebius)
- Morel
- Morquio
- Morton
- Morvan
- myasthenic
- myofascial pain (MPS)
- myotonic
- Naffziger
- nail-patella
- narcolepsy cataplexy
- naviculocapitate fracture
- neglect
- Nelson
- neonatal neurological
- nerve compression
- nerve entrapment
- nerve root
- neurobehavioral
- neurocutaneous
- neuroleptic malignant
- neuropsychiatric
- Niemann-Pick
- Nievergelt
- Nothnagel
- oculocerebrorenal
- oculosubcutaneous (of Yuge)
- one-and-a-half
- opsoclonus-myoclonus
- orbitofrontal
- organic brain
- organic brain syndrome with psychosis
- organic delusional
- organic mental
- os trigonum
- otopalatodigital
- overuse

syndrome *(cont.)*
- pain
- painful heel
- painful-arc
- Palister-Hall
- pallidal
- Pancoast (thoracic inlet)
- paratrigeminal (of Raeder)
- parietal lobe
- Parinaud
- Parsonage-Turner
- patellar malalignment
- pectoralis minor
- periodic movements of the legs (PMS)
- peroneal palsy footdrop
- Pfeiffer
- PICA (posterior inferior cerebellar artery)
- pickwickian
- PION (posterior interosseous nerve)
- piriformis
- PLED (periodic lateralized epileptiform discharge)
- Poland
- pontotegmental
- postcasting
- postconcussion
- posterior cord
- posterior fossa brain stem compression
- posterior inferior cerebellar artery (PICA)
- posterior interosseous nerve
- posterior joint
- posterior midbrain compression
- posterior spinal artery
- postfracture
- posthemiparesis
- postlaminectomy
- posttraumatic cerebral
- posttraumatic pain
- Pourfour du Petit

syndrome *(cont.)*
- Prader-Willi
- primary fibromyalgia (PFS)
- pronator teres
- Proteus
- pseudocholinesterase
- pseudo-Foster-Kennedy
- pseudoneurasthenic
- punch-drunk (of boxers)
- Putnam-Dana
- rabbit
- radicular
- Raeder paratrigeminal
- Ramsay Hunt
- Rasmussen
- ratchet
- Raymond
- Raymond-Céstan
- recalcitrance of
- red nucleus
- reflex sympathetic dystrophy (RSDS)
- Refsum
- Reiter
- restless legs (RLS)
- reverse urea
- reversible organic brain
- Reye
- Riley-Day
- rolandic vein
- Romberg
- root compression
- rotator cuff impingement
- Roussy-Dejerine thalamic pain
- Roussy-Lévy
- Rubinstein-Taybi
- Rud
- sacroiliac
- sacroiliac joint
- Saethre-Chotzen
- Sanfilippo
- scalenus anterior
- scalenus anticus
- scapulocostal
- Scheie

syndrome *(cont.)*
- Schmidt
- Schwartz-Jampel (SJS)
- seasonal affective disorder (SADS)
- Seckel
- sensorimotor
- shaken baby
- shoulder-hand
- shoulder-hand-finger
- shoulder-upper extremity-thoracic outlet
- shunt, lumbar thecoperitoneal
- Shy-Drager
- Siebenmann
- Sinding-Larsen-Johansson
- sinus tarsi
- Sjögren-Larsson
- sleep apnea
- Sluder sphenopalatine
- Smith-Lemli-Opitz
- spasmus nutans
- sphenoidal fissure
- sphenopalatine, of Sluder
- spinal stenosis
- squat-jump
- steal (Robin Hood phenomenon)
- Steele-Richardson
- Steele-Richardson-Olszewski
- Stewart-Morel
- Stickler
- stiff-man
- Still-Chauffard (polyarthritis)
- stroke
- Sturge-Weber
- subclavian steal (SSS)
- superior mesenteric artery
- supinator canal
- sweat test for thoracic outlet
- sylvian aqueduct
- syringomyelic
- talar compression
- Tapia
- TAR (thrombocytopenia absent radius)

syndrome *(cont.)*
- tardive Tourette
- tarsal tunnel (TTS)
- temporomandibular pain and dysfunction (TMPDS)
- tensor fasciae latae
- Terson
- tethered cord (TCS)
- tethered spinal cord
- thalamic pain
- thoracic inlet (Pancoast)
- thoracic outlet
- Tietze
- tired neck
- Tolosa-Hunt
- top of the basilar
- total cortical blindness
- Tourette
- Treacher Collins
- Troyer
- Turcot
- Turner
- Uhthoff
- ulnar abutment
- ulnar nerve entrapment
- ulnar tunnel
- uncal herniation
- Unverricht
- Unverricht-Lundborg
- useless hand
- uveomeningoencephalic
- VBA (vertebrobasilar artery)
- Vernet
- vertebral steal
- Villaret-Mackenzie
- Vogt-Koyanagi-Harada
- von Hippel-Lindau (VHL)
- von Recklinghausen
- Wallenberg lateral medullary
- Weber
- Werdnig-Hoffmann
- Wernicke-Korsakoff
- West
- whiplash

syndrome *(cont.)*
- withdrawal
- Wolfart-Kugelberg-Welander
- XXX
- XXY
- XYY
- Zellweger

syndrome conus medullaris

syndrome of approximate answers (Ganser syndrome)

syndrome of Harada

syndrome of inappropriate antidiuretic hormone (SIADH) excretion

syndrome of sensory dissociation

syndrome of the great radicular artery of Adamkiewicz

syndrome of the jugular foramen

synergistic contraction

synergistic muscles

Synergy flexible splinting material

synkinesis (pl. synkineses)

synkinetic arm swing

synostosis
- cervical
- congenital radioulnar
- coronal
- lambdoid
- multiple-suture
- premature suture
- radiographically firm
- sagittal
- single suture
- terminal
- tibiofibular

Synovator curved arthroscopic blade

synovectomy
- Albright
- chemical
- open knee
- partial
- total
- wide

synovectomy blade

synovia (see *synovium*)

synovial cavity
synovial chondromatosis
synovial fluid
synovial fringe
synovial frond
synovial frost
synovial hyaluronidase
synovial inflammatory reaction
synovial lining cells
synovial plica
synovial proliferation
synovial surface
synovial thickening
synoviochondromatosis
synoviogram
synovioma
synovitis
  boggy
  disseminated-type pigmented villonodular
  florid
  gonorrheal
  hypertrophic
  intra-articular pigmented villonodular (IPVS)
  parapatellar
  pigmented villonodular (PVS)
  proliferative
  rheumatoid arthritis
  silicone
  toxic
  villonodular
  villous
synovium (pl. synovia)
  boggy
  exuberant
  hyperplastic
  opaque
syntactical disorder
Synthes cervical plate
Synthes compression hip screw
Synthes fixation system
Synthes Microsystem cranial fixation plate
Synthes Microsystem drill bit
Synthes Microsystem microplate
Synthes Microsystem plate cutters
Synthes Microsystem plate-holding forceps
Synthes Microsystem pliers
Synthes minifragment countersink
Synthes modular spine instruments
Synthes I plate
Synthes rod
Synthes screw
Synthes wire guide
synthetic graft bypass to ankle
synthetic polymer, biodegradable
synthetic prosthesis
syphilis
  cerebrospinal
  meningovascular
  parenchymatous
  tertiary
syphilitic amyotrophy
syphilitic meningoencephalitis
syphilitis endarteritis, Heubner
Syracuse I plate
syringe
  bulb
  cement
syringe irrigation with deionized sterile water
syringobulbia
syringocele (or syringocoele)
syringoencephalia
syringoencephalomyelia
syringomeningocele
syringomyelia
  acquired (posttraumatic)
  congenital
  post-traumatic
  segmental distribution of
  traumatic
syringomyelic cavity
syringomyelic syndrome
syringomyelocele
syringomyelus

syringopontia
syrinx cavity
syrinx, traumatic
system
  AcroMed VSP fixation
  American shoulder and elbow (ASES)
  Amset R-F fixation
  Anametric knee
  Andersson hip status
  anterior locking plate (ALPS)
  APR II hip
  APR total hip system
  Ariel computerized exercise
  Arthro-Flo arthroscopic irrigation
  Arthro-Lok
  ArthroProbe laser
  ascending activating
  ascending reticular activating
  Ashhurst fracture classification
  ASIF
  autonomic nervous
  autotransfusion
  axial spinal
  Barouk-Microscrew
  Bassett electrical stimulation
  Biofix
  BIOWARE software for Biodex isokinetic exercise
  Boston Classification
  Bowden cable suspension
  Braille TeleCaption
  Brighton electrical stimulation
  C-D fixation (Cotrel-Dubousset)
  cable suspension
  cannulated guided hip screw
  central nervous (CNS)
  Charnley total hip
  Cordis MPAP
  Cotrel-Dubousset universal instrumentation
  Counter Rotation (CRS), pediatric
  cruciate condylar knee
  Cybex 340 isokinetic rehabilitation and testing

system *(cont.)*
  Cybex I exercise
  Cybex II+ exercise
  D'Aubigné hip status
  Dall-Miles cable grip
  Deknatel orthopedic autotransfusion
  diffuse thalamic projection
  double inflow cannula
  dual-lock total hip replacement
  Duo-Lock
  DUPEL iontophoretic drug delivery
  DuPont Rare Earth Imaging
  Dwyer-Wickham electrical stimulation
  Dyonics shaving
  EBI bone healing
  Ectra
  Edwards fixation
  Electri-Cool cold therapy
  Emed-F foot force measurement
  estimated 10-20
  Evans fracture classification
  Evolution total hip
  Ewald elbow arthroplasty rating
  EX-FI-RE external fixation
  external jugular
  extrapyramidal
  Ficat-Marcus grading
  Fitnet joint testing
  Fixateur Interne fixation
  fixation
  Fowler knee
  Freeman-Swanson knee
  gamma efferent
  gamma loop nervous
  Genesis total knee
  Genucom ACL laxity analysis
  Geomedic
  Global total shoulder arthroplasty
  Golgi
  gray matter of central nervous
  Haid UBP (universal bone plate)
  Halifax interlaminar clamp
  Harris hip status
  haversian

system *(cont.)*
Hemi-Knee
Herbert-Fisher fracture classification
Hexcel total condylar knee
Hoek-Bowen cement removal
Hot/Ice S. III
Howmedica knee
Howmedica VSF fixation
Hunt-Hess aneurysm grading
Ilizarov
Infuse-A-Port drug delivery
Inglis-Pellicci elbow arthroplasty
Insall-Burstein
internal carotid
International 10-20 electrode placement
Intrel II spinal cord stimulation
iontophoretic drug delivery
Iowa hip status
Isola fixation
Judet hip status
kallikrein-kinin (KK)
Kelly-Goerss Compass stereotactic
Kendall A-V Impulse
Kin-Com isokinetic exercise
Kirschner Medical Dimension hip replacement
Kyle fracture classification
Laitinen CT guidance
laminar air flow
Larson hip status
Leksell microstereotactic
Leksell stereotaxic
Lido Active Multijoint
Lido Passive Multijoint
Lidoback isokinetic dynamometry
Life-Port drug delivery
limbic
Luque II fixation
Mason fracture classification
Mazur ankle evaluation or rating
Mazur arthrodesis grading
Micro-Aire pulse lavage

system *(cont.)*
Miniport drug delivery
Mitek anchor
modified 10-20
Monticelli-Spinelli
Morrey arthritis grading
Morrey elbow arthroplasty rating
Moss fixation
MPAP (multipurpose access port)
N fiducial localization stereotactic
NECKSYS home neck care
Neer fracture classification
nigrostriatal
nociceptive afferent
Nucleotome
Olerud PSF fixation
Omega compression hip screw
Orth-evac autotransfusion
PFC total hip
parasympathetic nervous
Patil stereotaxic
PCA primary total knee
PCA universal total knee instrument
Phoresor II iontophoretic drug delivery
Picket Fence fiducial localization stereotactic
picture archive and communication (PACs) (for x-rays)
Pisces spinal cord stimulation
Polycentric and Wide-Track knee
Polysit drug delivery
Postel hip status
posterior cruciate condylar knee
Pro-Trac cruciate reconstruction
Pro-Trac system for knee surgery
Pulse lavage
PWB fixation
reticular activating (RAS)
Richards modular hip (RMHS)
RM stereotaxic
Robotrac passive retraction

system *(cont.)*
  Rochester compression
  Rogozinski spinal fixation
  Rowe-Lowell fracture-dislocation classification
  Russell-Taylor interlocking medullary nail
  S-ROM total hip modular
  Savastano Hemi-Knee
  Scaphoid-Microstaple
  Schatzker fracture classification
  Selby I or II fixation
  sensorimotor
  shaving
  Simmons fixation
  Simpulse lavage
  slit-catheter system for compartment syndrome of foot
  Solcotrans drainage/reinfusion
  Solcotrans Plus autotransfusion
  Songer cable
  Spherocentric knee
  spindle
  Steward-Milford fracture classification
  suction via trap-bottle
  suction-irrigation
  Sunderland five-degree
  sylvian
  sympathetic nervous
  Synthes fixation
  Tarlov neurologic function grading
  TCPM pneumatic tourniquet
  10-20

system *(cont.)*
  Thera-Band Resistive Therapy
  Thera-Ciser Light Exercise
  Ti-Fit modular hip
  Total Condylar Knee
  Total Gym rehabilitation
  Townley anatomic knee
  Trans Q 1 iontophoretic drug delivery
  Trunkey fracture classification
  TSRH fixation
  TSRH universal instrumentation
  UBP (universal bone plate)
  Ultra-Drive bone cement removal
  Ultra-X external fixation
  unicompartmental knee
  Unicondylar Geomedic
  Unidose drug delivery
  Unilink
  variable axis knee
  ventricular
  Versa-Fx femoral fixation
  VICON three-dimensional gait analysis
  VSF fixation
  VSP fixation
  Wiltse fixation
  Wisconsin compression
  Wisconsin spinal fracture
  Zickel fracture classification
  ZMS intramedullary fixation

systemic lupus erythematosus (SLE), arthropathy of hands and feet in

T, u

T (tesla)
tabes, burned-out
tabes dorsalis
tabes spinalis
tabetic crisis
tabetic neurosyphilis
table
  activator
  Adapta physical therapy
  Allen arm/hand surgery
  AM-MI orthopedic
  Andrews SST-3000 spinal surgery
  Back Specialist chiropractic
  Chick CLT operating
  Chick fracture
  Chiro-Manis chiropractic
  DC-101 chiropractic
  fracture
  Gemini chiropractic
  hand surgery
  inner table of skull
  inner iliac crest
  Leander chiropractic
  Leander motorized flexion
  Leander 790 Series distraction
  Lloyd chiropractic
  Mayfield-Larsen
  N-K 330 BRQ exercise
  OrthoVision orthopedic
  passive traction
  pediatric spica
  physical therapy
  Re-Lax-O chiropractic
  resistive exercise
table *(cont.)*
  Skytron operating room
  Stryker
  Sugita
  Zenith chiropractic
table saw injury
taboparesis
Tab-Strap knee immobilizer
Tachdhian orthosis
tackler's arm
tackler's exostosis
tactile agnosia
tactile alexia
tactile sensory loss
tactilegnosis
Taenia solium meningoencephalitis
TA-55 stapler
tag of cartilage
tag, skin
Tai Chi Chuan exercise
tailor's bunion
Tait flaps
Tait graft
Takahashi forceps
Takahashi rongeur
Taka sponge
Takayasu arteritis
Takayasu pulseless disease
Takayasu vasculitis
Take-apart instruments
TAL (tendo Achillis lengthening)
Talairach stereotactic frame
talar compression syndrome
talar dome

talar impingement
talar neck osteotomy
talar osteochondral fractures
talar osteochondritis dissecans
talar osteotomy
talar tilt
talar-tilt angle
talar-tilt test
talectomy
talipes calcaneocavus
talipes calcaneus
talipes cavovalgus
talipes cavovarus
talipes cavus
talipes equinovarus, congenital
talipes hobble splint
talipes planovalgus
talipes planus
talipomanus
talocalcaneal angle
talocalcaneal articulation
talocalcaneal index
talocalcaneal joint
talocalcaneal ligament
talocalcaneal osteotomy, subluxation
talocrural angle
talocrural fusion
talocrural joint
talofibular joint
talofibular ligament
talometatarsal angle
talonavicular angle
talonavicular beaking
talonavicular capsule
talonavicular capsulotomy
talonavicular joint
talonavicular ligament
talus
    congenital vertical
    flat top
    neck of
    Sneppen fracture of the
    sulcus
    vertical (rockerbottom flatfoot)
tamp
    Kiene bone
    wire
tandem walking test
tangential layer of hand
tangential remarks
tangential speech
Tangier disease
tangles, intraneuronal neurofibrillary
tank, Hubbard
tantalum gauze
tantalum preformed skull plates
tantalum sheets
tantalum skull plate
tap
    bloody
    bloody lumbar
    dry lumbar
    glabellar
    reservoir
    screw
    spinal
    subdural
    traumatic (lumbar puncture)
    ventricular
tape
    benzoin adherent
    graded Gore-Tex
    moistened umbilical
    Morse
    OKN (optokinetic nystagmus)
    salicylic acid
    Scotchcast 2 casting
    umbilical
taper sleeve
tapering regimen of steroids
Taperloc femoral prosthesis
tapetum corporis callosi
tapetum ventriculi
Tapia syndrome
taping, basket-weave ankle
tapir's mouth (bouche de tapir) in muscular dystrophy

tapper
  bone
  cervical
  rectangular
  round
tapping, glabellar
tapping tests of arm disability
TARA prosthesis (total articular replacement arthroplasty)
tardive dyskinesia (oral-buccal-lingual)
tardive dystonia
tardive ulnar nerve palsy
target disorder
Targeted Jobs Tax Credit (TJTC)
targeting, angiographic
Tarlov neurologic function grading system
tarsal arch
tarsal bars
tarsal canal
tarsal coalition
tarsal-metatarsal joint space
tarsal tunnel syndrome
tarsectomy
tarsi, sinus (tarsal canal)
task (see also *test*)
  added purpose
  complex multistep
  repetitive
  sentence closure
  three-step
  word retrieval
Taylor blade
Taylor brain scissors
Taylor dural scissors
Taylor percussion hammer
Taylor spinal retractor blade
Tay-Sachs disease
T-bar
TB montage (transverse bipolar)
TBI (traumatic brain injury)
TBNAA (total body neutron activation analysis)
TC angle
TCA (transcondylar axis)
TCBF (total cerebral blood flow)
TCCK unconstrained knee prostheses
TCD (transcranial Doppler) ultrasonography
TCNB (Tru-Cut needle biopsy)
TCPM pneumatic tourniquet system
TCR (tethered cord release)
TCR (thalamocortical relay) neuron
TCR, rebound excitation of
TCS (tethered cord syndrome)
TCS knee immobilizer
TDD (telecommunication device for the deaf)
TDE (thiamine deficiency encephalopathy)
TE (echo time)
tear
  attritional
  bowstring
  bucket handle
  cleavage
  dural
  fishtail
  flap
  full-thickness
  micro
  radial meniscus
  rotator cuff
  micro
  parrot-beak meniscus
  tendon (types I-IV)
  tibiofibular ligament
teardrop-shaped flexion-compression fracture
Techmedica implant
technetium-99m bicisate (Neurolite)
technetium-99 MDP bone scan
technique (see *operation*; *procedure*)
  activating technique with EEG
  Amspacher-Messenbaugh
  AO/ASIF compression
  Arana-Iniquez intracranial cyst removal

technique *(cont.)*
  Caspar anterior cervical plating
  Coltart fracture
  Cone-Grant
  cuboid squeeze
  cuboid whip
  Deyerle
  dowel graft
  free-floating forehead
  Harmon transfer
  hyperventilation as activating technique during EEG
  Ilizarov
  injection
  Klagsbrun harvesting
  Maquet
  Meyer sublaminar wiring
  minimal incision
  partial saturation technique on MRI
  spin echo technique on MRI
  spray-stretch
  standard pressurized cement
  two-sleeve
  two-strut tibial graft
  xenon washout
technology, work evaluation systems (WEST)
tectal lesions
tectoral ligament
tectospinal tract
tectum
TED hose or stockings (thrombo-embolic disease)
teeth grinding, repetitive
Teflon-coated driver
tegmental tract
tegmentum
  medullary
  midbrain
  pontine
tegmentum mesencephali
tegmentum of midbrain
tegmentum of pons and midbrain
Tegner activity level scale
Tegtmeier hand board
teichopsia
Tekscan in-shoe monitoring device
Tekscan pressure-sensitive insole sensor
tela choroidea
telangiectasia
  ataxia (Louis-Bar syndrome)
  Sturge-Weber
TeleBrailler
TeleCaption TV decoders for the deaf
telecommunication device for the deaf (TDD)
T electrode (temporal) (T_7 - T_{10})
telegraphic speech
telemetry, EEG
teleopsia
telephone electroencephalogram
Tele-Sensor, Cosman ICP
telescope
  Lumina
  Storz
telescoped words
television-induced epilepsy
Telfa bolster
Telfa dressing
Telfa sponge
teloleukoencephalopathy, perinatal
telos radiographic stress device
TEM (terminal extensor mechanism)
temperature discrimination
Temperlite saw blade
template
  broach cutting
  Charnley
  fixator
  hyperthermia
Temple-Fay laminectomy retractor
temporal area
temporal arteritis
temporal artery biopsy
temporal bone fracture
temporal EEG lead
  left anterior (LAT)
  left posterior (LPT)

temporal EEG lead (*cont.*)
  right anterior (RAT)
  right posterior (RPT)
temporal electrode (T_7 - T_{10})
temporal encephalocele
temporal gyrus
temporal horn atrophy
temporal horn neoplasm
temporal lobe contusion
temporal lobe epilepsy
temporal lobe herniation
temporal lobe lesion
temporal lobe seizure
temporal lobe status epilepticus
temporal lobe tumor
temporally
temporal negative sharp transient on EEG
temporal-occipital craniotomy
temporal-occipital junction
temporal pole
temporal positive sharp transient on EEG
temporal region
temporolimbic epilepsy
temporomandibular joint arthralgia
temporomandibular pain and dysfunction syndrome (TMPDS)
temporoparietal aphasia
temporopontine tract
temporozygomatic region
tenaculum
tender, markedly
tenderness
  bony
  joint
  point
  skin-rolling scapular
tendinitis
  bicipital
  calcific
  chronic Achilles
  cuff
  impingement

tendinitis (*cont.*)
  insertional
  noninsertional
  rotator cuff calcific
  tricipital
tendinopathy, insertion
tendinoplasty
tendinosis
tendinosuture
tendinous insertion
tendinum, subsultus
tendo Achillis lengthening (TAL)
tendo calcaneus
tendo (pl. tendines)
tendolysis
tendon
  abductor hallucis
  Achilles
  adductor
  ADQ (abductor digiti quinti)
  APB (abductor pollicis brevis)
  APL (abductor pollicis longus)
  aponeurosis of
  attenuated
  bowed
  bowing in arthritis
  brachioradialis
  bulbous
  collagen fibrils within
  conjoined
  deep flexor
  discontinuity of
  disinsertion of
  ECRB (extensor carpi radialis brevis)
  ECRL (extensor carpi radialis longus)
  ECU (extensor carpi ulnaris)
  EDC (extensor digitorum communis)
  EHL (extensor hallucis longus)
  EIP (extensor indicis proprius)
  elongation of
  EPB (extensor pollicis brevis)
  EPL (extensor pollicis longus)
  EQP (extensor quinti proprius)

tendon *(cont.)*
extensor
FCR (flexor carpi radialis)
FCU (flexor carpi ulnaris)
FDC (flexor digitorum communis)
FDI (first digital interosseous)
FDL (flexor digitorum longus)
FDP (flexor digitorum profundus)
FDQ (flexor digiti quinti)
FDS (flexor digitorum sublimis)
FDS (flexor digitorum superficialis)
FHB (flexor hallucis brevis)
FHL (flexor hallucis longus)
flexor
flexor carpi ulnaris
FPB (flexor pollicis brevis)
FPL (flexor pollicis longus)
fraying of
hamstring
heel
insertion of
interosseous
membranaceous
ODQ (opponens digiti quinti)
open tendon repair
palmaris longus
peroneal
ProCol bovine bioprosthesis
pulled
retraction of
rider's
rotator cuff
rupture of
ruptured Achilles (partial or complete)
slipped
snapping tendon release
sonicated
spontaneous rupture of Achilles
subluxing
subscapular
subscapularis
tenotomized

tendon *(cont.)*
tibial
watershed area of Achilles
Z-lengthening of
tendon dislocation, peroneal
tendon gap
tendon insufficiency
tendon lengthening
tendon of Hector
tendon of Zinn
tendon passer
tendon reflexes, deep (DTRs)
tendon rupture
tendon sheath, ganglionic cyst in synovial
tendon-sheath space infection
tendon sling
tendon stretching exercises
tendon tear (types I-IV)
tendon transfer
tendonitis (see *tendinitis*)
tendonplasty
tendoplasty
tendosynovitis
tendovaginal
tendovaginitis, stenosing
tenectomy
tenets of treatment
teniola
tennis elbow
tennis elbow arm band
tennis leg (plantaris rupture)
tennis shoulder
tennis toe
tenodesis (see *operations*)
tenodesis action
tenographic study
tenography
"tenoids" (see *ctenoids*)
tenon
tenonitis
tenontodynia
tenosynovial injection

tenosynovitis
  de Quervain stenosing
  flexor
  hypertrophic infiltrating
  stenosing
  suppurative
tenotome, Ryerson
tenotomized tendon
tenotomy
  adductor
  extensor
  flexor
  percutaneous
  percutaneous adductor
TENS (transcutaneous electrical nerve stimulation)
TENS unit, microcurrent
tense fontanelle
tensile strength
tensile stretch resistance
Tensilon test for myasthenia gravis
tensing of muscle
tension band wiring
tension headache
tension migraine headache
tension myositis syndrome (TMS)
tension pneumocephalus
tensioned cross-pin
tensioner
  cable
  dynamometric wire
  wire
tensioning device
tensor fasciae latae anchovy
tenth cranial nerve (vagus nerve)
tentorial edge
tentorial herniation
tentorial incisura
tentorial meningioma
tentorial notch herniation
tentorii, incisura
tentorium
  cerebellar
  cerebelli
  incisura of
tentorium cerebri
tentorium of cerebellum
Tenzel elevator
teratoma, suprasellar atypical
teres test
terminal
  axon
  axonal
  nerve
  presynaptic
terminal stance of gait
terminal tremor
terminalis, stria
terminus, rostral
territory of artery
terror, night (pavor nocturnus)
Terry fingernail sign
Terry nails
Terson syndrome
tertiary syphilis
tertius, peroneus
tesla (T)
test, Test
  abduction stress
  Abnormal Involuntary Movement Scale
  Achilles squeeze
  Action Research Arm (ARA)
  actual leg length
  Adams position
  adduction stress
  adductor sweep
  Adson
  AFP (alpha-fetoprotein)
  Alberts Famous Faces
  Allen
  alpha fetoprotein
  amobarbital sodium
  Amsler grid visual
  anterior drawer (ADT)
  anterior innominate
  antibody to VZ (varicella-zoster)
  antigen to *H. influenzae* in CSF
  antigen to meningococci in CSF

test *(cont.)*
- antigen to pneumococci in CSF
- anvil
- APACHE II
- Apley grinding
- Apley scratch
- apparent leg length
- apprehension
- arm abduction
- Ashworth Scale
- axial manual traction
- B-cell surface marker of neoplasm
- BAER (brain stem auditory evoked response)
- ballistic dynamometer
- Barlow hip instability
- Barthel ADL Index
- Behavioral Inattention (BIT)
- Bekhterev sitting
- belt
- Benton Visual Retention
- bentonite flocculation (BFT)
- big toe
- BIT (Behavioral Inattention)
- Blessed Dementia Rating Scales
- Blessed information-memory-concentration
- blood level of anticonvulsant drugs
- blood level of illicit drugs
- blood screen for drugs
- Booth
- Boston Classification system
- Boston Diagnostic Aphasia Examination
- Boston Naming
- bounce home
- box and block tendon of arm disability
- bracelet
- Brunnstrom-Fugl-Meyer (BFM) arm assessment
- Bunnell-Littler
- Burns bench
- calculations

test *(cont.)*
- Callaway
- caloric response
- caloric stimulation
- caloric test for vestibular function
- Cambridge battery
- Caregiver Strain Index
- carotid Amytal procedure (CAP)
- carotid balloon occlusion
- CFQ-for-others
- chest expansion
- Childress duck waddle
- city and state
- Clifton Assessment Procedures for the Elderly
- cognitive failures questionnaire
- cold water calorics
- colloidal gold tendon of CSF
- comb your hair
- complement fixation (CF)
- complex thematic pictures
- compression
- concealed straight leg raising
- Conceptual Series Completion mental status
- confrontation naming
- confrontational visual
- construct validity of rehabilitation testing
- content validity of rehabilitation testing
- continuous performance
- copy geometric designs
- copy intersecting pentagons
- cortical
- Cotton ankle instability
- count backwards from 100
- counterimmune electrophoresis of CSF
- cover-uncover
- Cowdry-type intranuclear inclusion bodies
- COWS (cold to the opposite, warm to the same)

test *(cont.)*
- Cozen
- Cram
- cranial nerve I (olfactory)
- cranial nerve II (optic)
- cranial nerve III (oculomotor)
- cranial nerve IV (trochlear)
- cranial nerve V (trigeminal)
- cranial nerve VI (abducens)
- cranial nerve VII (facial)
- cranial nerve VIII (vestibulo-cochlear)
- cranial nerve IX (glossopharyngeal)
- cranial nerve X (vagus)
- cranial nerve XI (accessory)
- cranial nerve XII (hypoglossal)
- Crawford small parts dexterity
- criterion-related validity of rehabilitation testing
- cross leg/straight leg raising
- crossed leg raising
- crossed straight leg raising
- CSF cryptococcal antigen titer
- CSF-serum HSV antibody ratio
- CUWD (cold up, warm down)
- Cybex
- cytotoxic leukocyte
- D'Ambrosia
- day of month
- dexamethasone suppression (DST)
- Dexter hand evaluation
- Deyerle sciatic tension
- digit repetition
- digit reversal
- digit span
- digit symbol
- distraction
- DNA flow cytometry
- doll's eyes
- dorsal drawer
- double leg raise
- double Maddox rod
- double simultaneous stimulation
- draw a clockface

test *(cont.)*
- draw a house
- draw a picture from memory
- Dreyer
- drop-arm
- drug screening
- duck waddle
- Dugas
- Eden
- Edinburgh Rehabilitation Status Scale
- Edinburgh-2 Coma Scale
- edrophonium chloride (Tensilon)
- elbow flexion
- electroencephalogram (EEG)
- electromyogram (EMG)
- electrophysiologic
- Elihorn Maze
- ELISA (enzyme-linked immuno-sorbent assay)
- Ely heel-to-buttock
- ENA (extractable nuclear antigen)
- end point of
- ESR (erythrocyte sedimentation rate)
- everyday memory questionnaire
- Examining for Aphasia
- external rotation-recurvation
- face validity of rehabilitation
- face-hand
- facial recognition
- femoral nerve stretch
- femoral nerve traction
- fibular squeeze
- 50-hole peg
- finger count
- finger-to-finger
- finger-to-nose (F to N)
- Finkelstein
- Fist-Palm-Side
- Fist-Ring
- fluorescent treponemal antibody (FTA)
- forced duction

test *(cont.)*
- forearm ischemic exercise
- forefoot adduction correction
- formal caloric
- formal visual field
- forward digit span recall
- Fournier ataxic gait
- Frenchay Activities Index
- Frenchay Aphasia Screening (FAST)
- Frenchay Arm (FAT)
- FTA (fluorescent treponemal antibody)
- Functional Ambulation Categories
- Functional Independence Measure
- Functional Limitation Profile
- Functional Status Questionnaire
- fund of information
- fungal culture of CSF
- Gait Abnormality Rating Scale
- Galveston Orientation and Awareness (GOAT)
- Gilchrest
- Gillis
- Glasgow Coma Scale
- glucose level of CSF
- gluteal maximus tensing
- gluteal punch
- Gram stain of CSF
- grimace
- grip pinch
- Guthrie bacterial inhibition
- Hachinski ischemia score
- Halstead-Reitan Battery
- Halstead-Wepman Aphasia Screening
- Hamilton
- Hamilton ruler
- Hauser ambulation index
- Hawiva
- Health Care Questionnaire
- heel walk
- heel-to-knee
- heel-to-shin

test *(cont.)*
- Helfet
- hemagglutination inhibition (HI)
- hemispheric Wada
- herpes simplex antibody titer in CSF
- hesitation
- Hibbs
- hip abduction stress
- HIV viral antigen
- Hodkinson Mental (HMT)
- Hoffa
- hook
- Hoover
- Hughston
- Hughston knee
- hyperemia
- hyperextension
- ice and warm water
- ice water calorics
- iliac compression
- iliopsoas
- immediate memory
- in-a-chair
- India ink examination of CSF
- Ingram-Withers-Speltz motor
- interpretation of proverbs
- intracarotid amobarbital speech
- intracarotid sodium amytal perfusion
- intracranial amobarbital procedure (IAP)
- ischemic forearm exercise
- isolated cold stress (ICST)
- isometric muscle strength
- isotope cisternography
- isotope transfer
- Jackson compression
- Jacob shift
- Jamar grip
- Jebsen hand function
- Jebsen-Taylor hand function
- Johnson-Zuck-Wingate motor
- jugular venous oxygen saturation

test *(cont.)*
- Katz ADL Index
- Kenny ADL Index
- Kenny Self-Care Evaluation
- Kleiger
- knee drop
- knee flexion stress
- kneeling bench
- Kohs block
- Kveim
- Lachman
- lactate level of CSF
- lactic dehydrogenase level of CSF
- Lambeth Disability Screening Questionnaire
- laser Doppler fluxmetry
- lateral pinch
- lateral pivot-shift
- latex particle agglutination
- Laugier
- LDH level of CSF
- LE prep (lupus erythematosus preparation)
- letter cancellation
- Lewin-Gaenslen
- Lewin punch
- Lewin reverse Lasègue
- Lewin snuff
- Lewin standing
- Lewin supine
- lick your lips
- Life Satisfaction Index
- light touch
- line bisection
- Lippman
- locking-position
- logical memory (paragraph recall) (after head injury)
- LOS (Lincoln-Ogeretzky Scale)
- Ludington
- lumbar puncture
- Lyme antibody
- lymphocytes in CSF
- Lysholm knee

test *(cont.)*
- Maddox rod
- Magnuson
- manometric
- Mantoux
- manual muscle (MMT)
- manual percussion
- Marval
- maximum cervical compression
- maximum grip strength
- McDowell Impairment Index
- McIntosh
- McMurray
- Memory for Designs
- memory for digits
- mental status examination
- metatarsal
- mid-tarsal movement
- Milgram
- Miller-Fisher
- Mills
- mini mental status
- Minnesota rate of manipulation
- Minnesota Test for Differential Diagnosis of Aphasia
- Minnesota Test of Aphasia
- misplaced objects
- modified anterior drawer
- modified Ashworth Scale for spasticity
- month of year
- Motor Assessment Scale
- Motor Club Assessment Test
- motor performance
- Motoricity Index
- multi-item
- multiple sleep latency (MSLT)
- Murphy punch
- myelin basic protein
- Myers-Briggs Type Indicator (MBTI)
- MyoForce
- Naffziger
- name the date

test *(cont.)*
- naming common objects
- near card vision
- neck compression
- nerve conduction study (NCS)
- neuro-ophthalmological
- neuropsychologic battery of
- neuropsychological
- neuropsychometric
- neutralization antibodies to St. Louis encephalitis
- Nine Hole Peg (NHPT)
- Northwick Park Index of Independence in ADL
- Nottingham Extended ADL Index
- Nottingham Health Profile
- Nottingham Ten-Point ADL Scale
- number 3 traced on patient's palm
- Nylen-Bárány
- O'Connor finger dexterity
- Ober
- obturator
- ocular tilt reaction (OTR)
- oculovestibular
- OKN (optokinetic nystagmus)
- OMC (orientation-memory-concentration)
- optokinetic drum
- oral potassium loading
- orientation-memory-concentration (OMC)
- Oxford Scale
- Paced Auditory Serial Addition (PASAT)
- Pandy
- paragraph recall (logical memory) (after head injury)
- Parquetry Block
- passive head rotation
- patellar apprehension
- patellar inhibition
- patellar retraction
- patellar tap
- Patrick

test *(cont.)*
- pattern reversal visual evoked response
- peg test of arm disability
- pelvic-rock
- pencil test for Morton neuroma
- percussion
- perimetry
- Perkins
- peroneal tunnel compression
- Perthes
- photometrazol
- pinch strength
- pinprick
- pinwheel
- pivot-shift
- polymorphonuclear leukocytes in CSF
- popliteal press
- Porch Index of Communicative Ability (PICA)
- Porteus Maze
- positive relocation
- posterior drawer
- Pratt test
- praxis
- preoperative balloon occlusion
- preoperative Wada
- Progressive Matrices
- pronator reflex
- protein in CSF
- proverb interpretation
- proverbs
- provocative test for epilepsy
- PRP capsule of *H. influenzae* in CSF
- psychometric
- punch
- pupillary light
- Q angle
- quadrant-position
- Queckenstedt
- Rand Functional Limitations Battery

test *(cont.)*
- Rand Physical Capacities Battery
- Rand Social Health Battery
- random letter
- Rankin Score
- read a sentence
- recall 5 items after 5 minutes
- recall of information
- recent memory
- Reciprocal Coordination
- remote memory
- reverse digit span recall
- reverse pivot shift
- reversed straight leg raising
- Rey Auditory Verbal Learning
- Rey Osterrieth Complex Figure
- RF (rheumatoid factor)
- rheumatoid arthritis agglutinin
- Rinne hearing conduction
- Rivermead ADL
- Rivermead Mobility Index
- Rivermead Motor Assessment
- Rivermead Perceptual Assessment Battery
- Romberg
- Rose-Waaler
- rotatory instability
- RPS (reverse pivot shift)
- Ryder
- Sabin-Feldman dye test for congenital toxoplasmosis
- sacroiliac resisted abduction
- sacroiliac stretch
- scalenus anticus
- sciatic stress
- sciatic stretch
- Selective Reminding
- Semmes-Weinstein monofilament hair test of sensory loss
- sensory extinction
- Sentence Repetition
- sentence closure
- serial sevens
- serial threes

test *(cont.)*
- seriation
- sharp versus dull sensory
- Sharp-Purser
- short orientation-memory-concentration (OMC)
- shoulder compression
- shoulder depression
- shoulder rock
- Sicard
- Sickness Impact Profile
- similarities
- similarities mental status
- Simmonds
- sit-and-reach flexibility
- sitting SLR
- Slocum
- SLR (straight leg raising)
- Smith-Petersen
- Speech Questionnaire
- spell a word backwards
- spell backwards
- sponge
- Spurling
- squat
- squeeze test in syndesmosis ankle sprain
- standing balance
- star-cancellation (SCT)
- Steinmann
- step-second
- straight leg raising (SLR)
- supported Adams
- supraselective Amytal
- supraspinatus press
- swinging flashlight
- swinging light
- systolic toe/brachial index
- talar-tilt
- tandem Romberg
- tandem walking
- tapping
- thematic picture
- Thomas

test *(cont.)*
Thomas flexion
Thompson calf squeeze
three-point pinch
three-stage command
thumb-finding
thumb-finger-approximator
timed walking
tip toe
Tobey-Ayer
toe index
Token test for aphasia
tourniquet
Trail Making
Trendelenburg
tripod
trunk control test
Tufts Quantitative Neuromuscular Exam
two-part Apley
two-point discrimination
two-quarter
understanding of similarities
urine for drug screen
urodynamic (in multiple sclerosis)
valgus extension
valgus stress
varus stress
varus-valgus stress
vertical stress
vestibular caloric
Visual Pattern Completion
visual choice reaction time
visual evoked response
visual field
Visual Neglect
visual threat
VrE (varus extension)
VZ (varicella-zoster) antibody titer
Wada (intracarotid amobarbital speech)
WAIS-R Block Design
wall chart vision
Watson

test *(cont.)*
waving hand threat
Weber two-point discrimination
Wechsler Memory Scale
well-leg straight leg raising
Wide Range Achievement
wiggle this finger
Wisconsin Card Sorting
word retrieval
write a sentence
xenon skin clearance
Yergason

tester
Disk-Criminator sensory
Fitnet joint

tetani, Clostridium
tetanus booster shot
tetanus immunization
tetanus immunoglobulin
tetanus-prone wound
tetany
tether, spinal cord
tethered cord syndrome
tethered spinal cord
tethering of nerves
tetraparesis, dense
tetraplegia
tetraspasticity
Texas Scottish Rite Hospital (TSRH)
TFA (thigh-foot angle)
TFA (tibiofemoral angle)
TFC (theaded fusion cage)
TFCC (triangular fibrocartilaginous complex)
TFCQ (Toronto Functional Capacity Questionnaire)
TGA (transient global amnesia)
TGF-B (transforming growth factor-beta)
THA (total hip arthroplasty)
THA (transient hemisphere attack)
Thackery operation
Thackray hip prosthesis
thalamectomy, stereotactic

thalamic components of limbic system
thalamic deficit
thalamic disorder
thalamic fracture of the calcaneal
thalamic hemorrhage
thalamic hyperpathia
thalamic infarct
thalamic inhibitory interneuron
thalamic lesion
thalamic neural deficits
thalamic nucleus
  associational
  nonspecific
  specific
thalamic pacemaker cell
thalamic pain syndrome
thalamic projection system, diffuse
thalamic syndrome
thalamic ulnar nerve
thalamocaudate artery
thalamocortical pathway
thalamocortical relay (TCR) neuron
thalamofrontal fibers
thalamoperforate artery
thalamostriate vein
thalamotomy
  parafascicular (PFT)
  stereotactic
  stereotaxic
  ventrolateral
thalamus
  dorsal medial nucleus of the
  intralaminar
  lateral
  nonspecific activating nuclei of the
  parafascicularis of the
  thalamic
thallium polyneuropathy
T-handled awl
Tharies hip replacement
THARIES (total hip articular replacement by internal eccentric shells)
theater symptom
thecal injection
theca, spinal
thecal sac
thecoperitoneal shunt
thematic picture test
thenar eminence
thenar groups
thenar muscle
thenar space abscess
theory
  corticoreticular
  facultative pacemaker
Thera-Back back support
Thera-Band progressive weights
Thera-Band Resistive Therapy System
Thera-Bite wafer
Thera-Ciser Light Exercise System
Thera-Ciser Therapeutic Exercise System
Therabite jaw exerciser
therapeutic aspiration
therapeutic recreation (TR)
therapeutic shoe
therapeutic ultrasound for tendon healing
therapist
  language
  occupational
  physical
  speech
TheraPulse bed
therapy
  adjuvant
  Bragg-peak photon-beam
  brisement
  deliberate
  electric differential (EDiT) (lowercase *i*)
  electrical stimulation
  electron beam
  fad (spurious)
  fomentation
  hot fomentation
  interferential
  occupational

therapy *(cont.)*
  outpatient physical
  PEMF (pulsed electromagnetic field)
  perioperative antibiotic
  physical
  Polar Wrap cold
  pool
  prophylactic antibiotic
  range of motion
  spinal manipulative
  steroid
  trial of conservative
  ultrasound
Therex programmable drug pump
thermistor (used in EEG)
  nasal
  oral
thermocoagulation, bipolar
thermography, liquid crystal contact (LCT)
thermometer, low-reading
thermoplastic elastomer (TPE)
thermoplastic knee-ankle-foot orthoses
thermoregulatory sweating of the face
thermorhizotomy
Thermosport hot/cold wrap
theta activity on EEG
theta bursts on EEG
theta frequency band on EEG
theta index
theta pattern on EEG
theta rhythm on EEG
theta slowing, bilateral, on EEG
theta wave bursts
theta wave on EEG
theta waveform
thick bones
thigh-foot angle
thigh-high antiembolic stockings
thin-section CT
thinking
  abstract
  concrete

thinking *(cont.)*
  disorganized
  forced
T1 (spin-lattice or longitudinal relaxation time)
T2 (spin-spin or transverse relaxation time)
T1-weighted image (short TR/TE) (MRI scan)
T2-weighted image (long TR/TE) (MRI scan)
toward the cord
third compartment
third cranial nerve (oculomotor nerve)
third nerve mononeuropathy, diabetic
third nerve palsy
third ventricle tumors
Thomas buckle sling
Thomas fixator
Thomas flexion test
Thomas frame
Thomas half-ring splint
Thomas heel, reverse
Thomas leg splint
Thomas rigid collar
Thomas sign
Thomas sling
Thomas suspension splint
Thomas test
Thomas traction
Thompson calf squeeze test
Thompson carotid clamp
Thompson femoral neck prosthesis
Thompson rasp
Thomsen disease
Thomsen dystrophy
thoracic component of scoliosis
thoracic inlet (Pancoast) syndrome
thoracic outlet syndrome (TOS)
thoracolumbar region
thoracolumbar scoliosis
thoracolumbar spine
thoracolumbosacral orthosis (TLSO)
Thorazine shuffle gait

thought processes, concrete
thought, stream of
thousand-hands Kannon universal
headframe
THR (total hip replacement)
thread length
three-dimensional (3-D) Fourier transform imaging
three-finger spica cast (Dehne cast)
three-phase bone scan
three-phase bone scintigraphy (TPBS)
three-point pinch testing
three-point skull clamp
threes test, serial
threshold
pain
perception
seizure
stimulus
thrills (murmurs)
throat clearing, repetitive
thrombectomy
thrombectomy/embolectomy
thrombi (pl. of thrombus)
thromboembolic stroke
thromboendarterectomy
thrombolectomy
thrombophlebitis, cerebral
thrombosis
cavernous sinus
central
central retinal vein
cortical vein
deep venous (DVT)
dural sinus
intracranial sinus
large-vessel
sagittal sinus
septic cavernous sinus
thrombotic microangiopathy
thrombotic stroke
thrombotic thrombocytopenic purpura (TTP)
thrombus (pl. thrombi)
anterograde extension of

thrombus *(cont.)*
peroneal obliterative
tibial obliterative
thrower's elbow
throwing-arm injury
thumb
adductor sweep of
bowler's
cortical
floating
gamekeeper's
low-set
opposable
skier's
spring swivel
trigger
triphalangeal
unopposable
thumb-finding test
thumb-finger-approximator test
thunderclap headache
thyrocervical trunk of subclavian artery
thyroid myopathy
thyromegaly
thyrotoxicosis
TI (inversion time) (MRI scan)
TIA (transient ischemic attack)
Ti-BAC II hip prosthesis
tib-fib (tibia-fibula)
tibia coordinate system (TIBIACS)
tibia, lip of
TIBIACS (tibia coordinate system)
tibial aligner
tibial crest
tibial flare
tibial jig
tibial obliterative thrombi
tibial plafond
tibial plateau
tibial sesamoid ligament
tibial spacer
tibial tendon
tibial torsion

tibial tuberosity
tibialis sign of Strümpell
tibiarum, anxietas
tibio-astragalocalcaneal canal of Richet
tibiocalcaneal fusion
tibiocalcaneal joint complex
tibiocalcaneal ligament
tibiocalcaneal space
tibiofibular diastasis
tibiofibular fracture
tibiofibular ligament tear
tibiofibular overlap
tibiofibular syndesmosis
tibiofibular synostosis
tibionavicular ligament
tibiotalar angle
tibiotalar joint
tibiotalar ligament
  anterior
  posterior
tibiotalocalcaneal fusion
tic
  articulatory
  facial
  motor
  vocal
TICA (traumatic intracranial aneurysm)
tic douloureux, trigger zones for
tick-borne encephalitis
tick-borne viral encephalitis
tick paralysis
Ti-Cron (or Tycron) suture
Tiemann Meals tenolysis knife
tier, Adson knot
Ti-Fit modular hip system
tight heel cord
tightener
  band
  Kirschner
  Loute wire
  Parham band
  Rhinelander wire
  wire
Tikhoff-Linberg radical arm resection
Tikhoff-Linberg shoulder resection
Tilastin hip prosthesis
Tillaux-Kleiger fracture
tilt
  bent knee pelvic
  head
  patellar
  pelvic
  posterior pelvic
  talar
  valgus
  varus
Tilt and Turn Paragon bed
tilt board
time
  floating, in gait
  interpulse
  nerve conduction
  neuromuscular transmission
  retinocortical (RCT)
  total tourniquet
time sense
timed walking tests
time/money/number concepts
TiMesh
Tindall scissors
tinea pedis
Tinel percussion sign
tingle, tingling
tingling in extremities
Ti-Nidium alloy
Ti-Nidium surface harding process
tinnitus
tip
  Adson brain suction
  Cloward drill
  drill
  Ferguson brain suction
  Fragmatome
  Frazier suction
  occipital
  Rhoton suction
  Sachs brain suction

tip *(cont.)*
  sucker
  suction
  uninsulated electrode
tip of screw
tiptoe gait
tiptoe, stand on
tiredness
TIRR foot-ankle orthosis
Ti6A14V alloy for prosthesis
tissue
  adipose
  devitalized soft
  exuberant granulation
  fibrils of connective
  fibrocartilaginous
  fibrocollagenous connective
  granulation
  grumous
  intertrabecular soft
  isointense soft tissue (on MRI)
  myofascial muscular
  nociceptive
  ossification of soft tissue (on x-ray)
  prevertebral soft
tissue expander
titanium alloy rod
titanium grommet
titanium hip prosthesis
titanium mesh
titanium microsurgical bipolar forceps
titanium microsurgical needle holders
titanium plate
titanium staple
titer, Toxoplasma
titubation
TJ (triceps jerk)
TJTC (Targeted Jobs Tax Credit)
TKA (total knee arthroplasty)
TLE (temporal lobe epilepsy)
TLSO (thoracolumbosacral orthosis)
TMA (transmetatarsal amputation)
TMA (transmetatarsal angle)
TMA (true metatarsus adductus)
TMA pressure
TMA-thigh angle (transmalleolar axis)
TMB (transient monocular blindness)
TME (trapezium-metacarpal eburnation)
TMPDS (temporomandibular pain and dysfunction syndrome)
TMS (tension myositis syndrome)
Tobey-Ayer test
tobramycin-impregnated PMMA implant
Todd motor paralysis
Todd motor weakness
Todd palsy
Todd paralysis (postepileptic)
Todd-Wells guide
Todd-Wells stereotactic frame
toe, toes
  clawing of
  cock-up
  congenital overlapping
  curly
  downgoing
  fanning of
  floppy big
  hammer
  jammed
  lesser
  mallet
  marathoner's
  overlap of
  overlapping
  overriding
  searching
  splaying of
  stoved
  striatal
  tennis
  turf
  unilaterally upgoing
  upgoing
  V-Y plasty correction of varus
toe box of shoe
toe cap
toe-drop

toe flexion
toe flexors
toeing-in gait
toeing in, toeing out
toeing-out gait
toenail
  circumferential
  ingrowing
toe-off phase of gait
toe range of motion
toe separator
toe splint, New Mind Set
toe-straight device
toe systolic pressure
toe-walking gait
Toennis-Adson dissector
Toennis dissecting scissors
Toennis dura dissector
Toennis dura hook
Toennis dura knife
Toennis tumor forceps
Token Test for aphasia
Tolosa-Hunt syndrome
Tom Thumb, repeat the word (during EEG)
Tommy bar
Tommy trapeze bar
tomogram
tomography
  automated computerized axial (ACAT)
  computerized cranial
  fludeoxyglucose F 18 positron emission
  positron emission
  hypocycloidal ankle
  plain
  positron emission (PET)
  positron emission transaxial
  sellar
  single photon emission computed (SPECT)
tomomyelography
tone
  arteriolar muscle
  muscle
  postural
  symmetrically depressed
tone-reducing ankle-foot orthosis (TRAFO)
tongs
  Barton skull traction
  Cherry traction
  Cone skull traction
  Crutchfield-Raney skull traction
  Crutchfield skeletal traction
  Crutchfield skull traction
  Gardner-Wells skull
  Gardner-Wells traction
  Mayfield
  Raney-Crutchfield skull
  Raney-Crutchfield traction
  Reynolds skull traction
  skull
  skull traction
  sugar
  traction
  Trippi-Wells
  Vinke
tongue
  beefy
  deviated to left
  deviated to right
  magenta
tongue and trough bone
tongue and trough technique
tongue biting during seizure
tongue deviation
tongue protrusion, repetitive
tongue thrusting, repetitive
tongue-type fracture
tongue writhing, repetitive
tonic-clonic movements
tonic-clonic seizure
tonic desynchronizing input
tonic deviation of eyes
tonic neck reflex (primitive)

tonic phase-spike on EEG
tonic posturing
tonic pupils
tonic seizure
tonohaptic pupil
tonohaptic reaction of pupil
tonsil, herniated cerebellar
tonsilla cerebelli
tonsillar herniation
tonus
  arterial
  decreased
  increased
  muscular
Tool, Gore Smoother Crucial
tophaceous material in gout
topognosis
topographic mapping (on EEG)
topographical agnosia
topography of wave
Toradol
torch, saline
torcular
torcular Herophili
Torkildsen shunt procedure
tornado epilepsy
Toronto Functional Capacity Questionnaire (TFCQ)
Toronto Medical CPM exerciser
Toronto orthosis
Toronto parapodium
TORP (total ossicular replacement prosthesis)
torque converter, subtalar joint as
torque stress
torsion
  cable twisters as treatment for internal tibial
  femoral
  internal tibial
  internal tibiofibular
  lateral femoral
  malleolar
  tibial
  tibiofibular
torsional abnormalities
torsional alignment
torsional impaction force
torsion bar
torsion spasm
torticollis
  spasmodic
  static
torula (spheroid bodies in cryptococcosis)
Torula histolytica (earlier name for *Cryptococcus neoformans*)
TOS (thoracic outlet syndrome)
total body neutron activation anaylsis (TBNAA)
total contact cast
total cortical blindness
total hip arthroplasty (THA)
total hip replacement (THR)
total pituitary ablation
total synovectomy
total tourniquet time
Total Gym rehabilitation system
Toti trephine drill
touch
  dull
  light
  sharp
Tourette syndrome
tourniquet
  Accuflate
  arthroscopic
  Bodenstab
  Digikit finger
  digital
  finger
  Kidde
  Medi-Quet
  pneumatic
  pneumatic ankle
  Profex arthroscopic
  proximal thigh
  Stille
tourniquet test

tourniquet time, total
towel curls (postoperative exercises)
towel
  moist
  wound
Townley TARA prosthesis
Townsend knee brace
toxic amblyopia
toxic-confusional state
toxic delirium
toxic encephalopathy
toxic hypoxia
toxic nystagmus
toxic retinoneuropathy
toxic synovitis
Toxoplasma gondii
Toxoplasma titer
toxoplasmosis
  acquired
  central nervous system
  cerebral
  congenital
  CSF
  glandular
  Sabin-Feldman dye test for congenital
TPBS (three-phase bone scintigraphy)
TPE (thermoplastic elastomer)
TPE ankle-foot orthosis
TPE biomechanical foot orthosis
TP electrode (temporal-posterior) (TP_7-TP_{10})
TPL-6 total hip replacement
TPR ankle prosthesis
TQNE (Tufts Quantitative Neuromuscular Examination)
TR (repetition time) (MRI scan)
TR (therapeutic recreation)
TR-28 total hip replacement
trabecular bone
tracing
  EEG (electroencephalogram)
  flattening of
Tracker-10 catheter
Tracker-18 catheter
Tracker vascular access system
tracking of movements, visual
tracking, patellar
tract
  anterior corticospinal
  anterior spinocerebellar
  anterior spinothalamic
  ascending
  brain stem pyramidal
  central tegmental (CTT)
  cerebellar
  cerebral fugal
  corticobulbar (CBT)
  corticospinal (CST)
  Dejerine aberrant pyramidal
  dermal sinus
  descending
  dorsal spinocerebellar
  frontopontine
  Gudden
  lateral corticospinal
  lateral spinocerebellar
  lateral spinothalamic
  long
  long spinal white matter
  mamillothalamic
  nerve
  occipitotemporopontine
  olivocerebellar
  optic
  pilonidal
  posterior spinocerebellar
  pyramidal
  reticulospinal
  reticulovestibulospinal
  rubrospinal
  segmental tract of trigeminal
  sensory long
  sinus
  spinocerebellar
  spinocuneocerebellar
  spino-olivary
  spinoreticular

tract *(cont.)*
  spinotectal
  spinothalamic
  tectospinal
  tegmental
  temporopontine
  ventral spinocerebellar
  ventral spinothalamic
  vestibulospinal
traction
  axial
  balanced suspension
  bidirectional
  Bremer halo crown
  Bryant
  Buck
  Buck skin
  cervical
  Cotrel
  Dunlop
  floating
  halo
  inline
  intermittent
  Kuhlman cervical
  leg
  lumbosacral
  mechanical
  pelvic
  pin
  pounds of
  Quigley
  Russell
  skeletal
  skull tong
  supine cervical
  Thomas
  well-leg
traction exostosis
traction tongs, Cone skull
tractus solitarius nucleus
TRAFO (tone-reducing ankle-foot orthosis) trajectory
Trail Making Test
training
  concentric muscle
  eccentric muscle
  gait (for the pronated foot)
  transfer
trains of flashes
trains of waves
traits, premorbid
trajectory
  foot
  lower extremity
tramline calcification
trampoline
tram track pattern on x-ray in Sturge-Weber syndrome
trance, hysterical
trance states
Trans Q 1 iontophoretic drug delivery system
transcallosal
transchondral talar fracture
transchoroidal approach
transclival approach
transcondylar axis (TCA)
transcortical aphasia
  motor
  sensory
transcranial approach
transcranial Doppler (TCD) ultrasound
transcutaneous electrical nerve stimulation (TENS)
transcutaneous oxygen determination ($TCPO_2$)
transducer
  Camino subdural
  ergonomically-designed
  Gaeltec catheter-tip pressure
transected segment
transection of nerve
transection of spinal cord
transection, traumatic cord
transethmoidal encephalocele

transfer
  Brooker-Jones tendon
  Bunnell tendon
  Chandler tendon
  flexor tendon
  free toe
  free-tissue
  independent in bed
  Mustard iliopsoas
  nerve
  pivot
  split posterior tibial tendon
  Sutherland tendon
transfer lesion
transfer skills
transfer training
transfer ulcer
transfibular approach for arthrodesis
transfibular arthrodesis
transfixing screw
transforming growth factor-beta (TGF-B)
transfusion, intraoperative autologous (IAT)
transient, transients
  benign epileptiform
  frontal sharp
  high-amplitude
  multifocal sharp (MST)
  nonepileptiform sharp
  occipital negative sharp
  polyphasic
  positive occipital sharp (POSTs)
  rolandic dip
  rolandic sharp
  sharp
  sleep
  spiky
  temporal negative sharp
  temporal positive sharp
  vertex sharp
transient global amnesia
transient hemisphere attack (THA)
transient ischemic attack (TIA)
transient paresthesia
transient states of depersonalization in migraine
transient vertigo
transients of sleep, benign epileptiform (BETS)
transillumination of head
transition, sitting
transitional shear
translation exercise
transmalleolar axis (TMA)-thigh angle
transmetatarsal amputation (TMA)
transnasal biopsy
transosseous technique
transpedicular approach
transpedicular fixation
transplantation
  adrenal medulla
  autoadrenal
  fetal substantia nigra
transscaphoid perilunate dislocation
transsection, spinal cord
transsphenoidal approach
transsphenoidal cryohypophysectomy
transsphenoidal encephalocele
transsphenoidal hypophysectomy
transsyndesmotic screw fixation
transtemporal approach
transtentorial herniation
transtentorially
transverse arch of foot
transverse carpal ligament
transverse cord lesion
transverse ligaments of the atlas
transverse magnetization
transverse myelitis
transverse orientation
transverse plane forces
transverse rotation of the lower extremity during locomotion
transverse tarsal joint
trap, finger
Trap Strap (to improve trapezius posture)

trapeze bar
trapezial saddle
trapeziometacarpal joint
trapezioscaphoid joint
trapeziotrapezoid joint
trapezium (greater multangular) bone
trapezium, os
trapezoid (lesser multangular) bone
trapezoid body
trapezoid ligament
trapezoideum, os
Traube-Hering-Mayer waves of
  cerebrospinal fluid
Traube percussion hammer
trauma
  cerebral
  closed head
  craniocerebral
  distortion
  fracture
  head
  high-energy
  occult head
trauma-related causalgia
traumatic brain injury (TBI)
traumatic cord damage
traumatic disruption
traumatic encephalopathy of boxers
traumatic injury
traumatic intracranial aneurysm
traumatic meningeal hemorrhage
traumatic neurosis
traumatic osteoarthritis
traumatic periostitis
traumatic shearing of white matter in
  head injury
traumatic spondylolisthesis
  (grades 1-4)
traumatic tap (lumbar puncture)
Trautmann chisel
traversing the fracture
tray
  DiChiara hand
  hand

tray *(cont.)*
  pattie
  surgical hand
Treace microdrill
Treacher Collins syndrome
treatment
  adjustive (chiropractic)
  cable twisters for internal tibial
    torsion
  communication/cognition
  daily
  gate control pain
  outpatient communication/cognition
  rehabilitation
  tenets of
  vasopneumatic
treatment frequency
treatment program
tree, lower extremity arterial
Trélat-Charlin neuralgia
tremor
  action
  benign essential
  cerebellar outflow
  counting-money
  dystonic
  emotional stress precipitating
  endpoint
  essential cerebellar
  familial
  flapping
  head and neck
  hepatic encephalopathy (asterixis)
  heredofamilial
  hysterical
  intention
  kinetic
  metabolic
  no-no
  oscillating
  parkinsonian
  perioral
  physiologic
  physiological

tremor *(cont.)*
pill-rolling (of parkinsonism)
positional
postural
progressive cerebellar
rest
resting
rubral
senile
static
striatocerebellar
terminal
to-and-fro
tongue
voice
volitional
wing-beating
writing
yes-yes
tremulous movement
tremulousness
Trendelenburg gait
Trendelenburg position of weightbearing leg
Trendelenburg test
trephination
trephine
biopsy
bone biopsy
D'Errico skull
DeVilbiss skull
Galt hand
Galt skull
iliac crest
Michele vertebral body
Polley-Bickel biopsy
Rochester bone
Scoville skull
skull
Stille
Turkel bone biopsy
winged
Treponema pallidum
Trevor disease
triad
Charcot
terrible
Triad hip prosthesis
Triad, O'Donohue's Unhappy (OUT)
trial prosthesis
trial reduction of prosthesis
triangle
aponeurotic
Codman, on x-ray
Guillain-Mollaret
insular
Kager
Mollaret
myoclonic
paramedian
posterior
triangular ankle fusion frame
triangular external ankle fixation
triangular ligament
triceps jerk (TJ)
Trichinella spiralis meningoencephalitis
trichinosis
trichopoliodystrophy
tricipital tendinitis
Tricodur compression support bandage
Tricodur Epi (elbow) compression bandage
Tricodur Omos (shoulder) compression bandage
Tricodur Talus (ankle) compression bandage
Tricon-M patellar prosthesis
Tricophyton metagrophytes fungus
Tricophyton rubrum fungus
tricorrectional bunionectomy
tricylic antidepressants
trifurcation of middle cerebral artery
trigeminal cavity
trigeminal hemangioma
trigeminal nerve (fifth cranial nerve)
mandibular division
maxillary division
nucleus of

trigeminal nerve *(cont.)*
ophthalmic division
segmental tract of
spinal tract of
trigeminal neuralgia
trigeminus, porous
trigger a seizure
trigger finger release
trigger point injection
trigger point neuralgia
trigger point therapy
trigger points in paravertebral muscles
trigger thumb release
trigger zones for tic douloureux
triggering conditions
triggering event
triggering mechanism
triggering stimulus
trigone of lateral ventricle
trigonocephaly
trihelical collagen fibers
Trillat osteotomy
trimalleolar fracture
Trimline knee immobilizer
trimlines for ankle-foot orthoses
trimmer, meniscal
Trinkle drill
trio, radial
triorthocresylphosphate poisoning
triphalangism
triphasic slow wave (EEG) activity
triphasic wave complex
tripod test
tripoding maneuver
Trippi-Wells tongs
triquetrohamate joint
triquetrohamate ligament
triquetrum, bone of wrist
tri-radial resector blade
trismus
trisomy 13
trisomy 18
trisomy 21
triton tumor
trocar
brain
Frazier brain
McCain TMJ
Paulus
pyramidal
sharp
trochanter
flare of
greater
lesser
trochanter wire
trochanteric
trochlear nerve (fourth cranial nerve)
Troemner percussion hammer (Trömner)
Troemner sign
troika, aponeurotic
Tronzo elevator
Tronzo VLC cannulated compression screw
trophic skin changes
trough and peak levels
trough level of drug
trough of wave on EEG
trousers, medical (or military) anti-shock (MAST)
Trousseau sign
Troyer syndrome
True/Flex intramedullary nail
Tru-Support EW (elastic wrap) bandage
Tru-Support SA (self-adhering) bandage
true aphasia
true metatarsus adductus (TMA)
true ratio measures in rehabilitation testing
true vertigo
truncal ataxia
truncal instability
trunk
basilar artery
brachiocephalic

trunk *(cont.)*
  costocervical
  nerve
  thyrocervical
trunk control test
Trunkey fracture classification system
Trypanosoma gambiense
T (temporal)
TSPP rectilinear bone scan
TSRH (Texas Scottish Rite Hospital)
TSRH Crosslink
TSRH hook-rod
TSRH spinal instruments
TSRH fixation system
TSRH hook
TSRH pedicle fixation device
TSRH rod
TSRH screw
TSRH universal instrumentation system
TSRH vertebral screw
Tsuge tendon repair (silent *t*)
TTAP-ST acetabular prosthesis
TTR (tarsal tunnel release)
TTS (tarsal tunnel syndrome)
tub bench
tube
  Adson brain suction
  Baron suction
  blocked shunt
  brain suction
  cement
  Cone suction
  Dawson-Yuhl suction
  feeding
  Ferguson brain suction
  Ferguson-Frazier suction
  guide
  Hardy suction
  Hemo-Drain wound
  Jergesen
  Kam Vac suction
  ligament sizing
  Mason suction
  neural

tube *(cont.)*
  New York Glass suction
  obstructed shunt
  pressure-sensitive valve in shunt
  Pribham suction
  Rhoton-Merz suction
  Sachs brain suction
  Schwann cell
  shunt
  suction
  Vidicon vacuum chamber pickup
  Yankauer suction
  Yasargil suction
tuber cinereum
tubercle
  Chaput
  Lister
  tibial
tuberculoma
tuberculosis of spine
tuberculosis, spinal (Pott disease)
tuberculous arthritis
tuberculous meningitis
tuberculum sellae
tuberosity
  calcaneal
  greater
  lesser
  navicular
  tibial
tuberous sclerosis
Tubigrip bandage
Tubigrip dressing
Tudor-Edwards bone cutting forceps
Tuffier laminectomy retractor
Tuffier-Raney retractor
Tuffier rib spreader
tuft fracture
tuft of synovium
Tufts Quantitative Neuromuscular
  Examination (TQNE)
tulip probe
tumbler flaps
tumbler grafts

tumor
- acidophilic pituitary
- acoustic nerve
- ACTH-producing pituitary adenoma
- anaplastic astrocytoma
- anterior cingulate gyrus
- astrocytic
- astrocytoma
- astroglial
- atypical giant cell
- ball-valve
- basal
- basicranial
- basiocciput
- basophilic pituitary
- blood vessel
- bone-forming
- brain stem glioma
- brown
- calcified glial
- capillary hemangioma
- cavernous hemangioma
- cerebellopontine angle
- cerebellum
- chondromyxoid fibroma
- chordoma
- choroid plexus papilloma
- chromophobe adenoma
- chromophobe pituitary
- classic Kaposi sarcoma
- clivus meningioma
- CNS (central nervous system)
- Codman
- colloid cyst
- corpus callosum
- craniopharyngioma
- cystic brain
- debulking of
- decompression of
- deep-seated
- dermoid
- dumbbell neurofibroma
- eccrine angiomatous hamartoma

tumor *(cont.)*
- eighth nerve
- embryonal
- ependymoma
- epidemic Kaposi sarcoma
- epidermoid
- epilepsy-causing brain
- extension of
- extirpation of
- extracompartmental
- extradural
- extramedullary hemangioma
- fatty
- finger of
- flocculonodular
- fourth ventricle
- frontal lobe
- gasserian ganglion
- germ cell (GCT)
- giant cell
- giant cell malignant tumor of soft tissue
- glial
- glioma
- glomus
- glomus jugulare
- granular cell
- growth-producing pituitary
- hemangioblastoma
- hematogenous spread of
- high-grade astrocytoma
- hourglass tumor of the cord
- hypothalamus
- incomplete
- infratentorial brain
- infratentorial Lindau
- inoperable brain
- internal capsule and basal ganglia
- intracompartmental
- intracranial
- intradural extramedullary
- intramedullary
- intramedullary spinal cord
- intrasellar

tumor *(cont.)*
- intraspinal
- invasive malignant sheath
- juxta-articular osteoid osteoma
- juxtacortical sarcoma
- low-grade astrocytoma
- low-grade malignant histiocytoma
- malignant glioma
- medullary
- meningeal
- meningeal spread of
- meningioma
- metastatic
- metastatic (to the brain)
- metastatic (to the spinal cord)
- microglioblastoma
- midbrain
- mixed
- nerve sheath
- neurilemmoma
- neuroectodermal
- neurofibroma
- nongerminomatous germ-cell
- nonglial
- nonneoplastic
- occipital lobe
- occipital neuroblastoma
- oligodendroglioma
- optic chiasm
- optic glioma
- optic pathway
- orbital pseudotumor
- osteoblastic
- papilloma of the fourth ventricle
- parasagittal
- parasellar
- parietal lobe
- parosteal osteoma
- parosteal sarcoma
- perineurial fibroblastoma
- peripheral nerve
- peripheral neuroectodermal
- pilocytic
- pineal gland

tumor *(cont.)*
- pineal region
- pinealoma
- pituitary gland
- pituitary microadenoma
- plantar malignant melanoma
- plasma cell myeloma
- pontine glioma
- poorly differentiated
- posterior fossa
- posterior lobe
- Pott puffy
- primary brain
- primary sarcoma
- primitive neuroectodermal (PNET)
- prolactin-secreting adenoma
- pseudomalignant, nonneoplastic
- osseous soft tissue
- radiosensitive
- round cell
- sacrococcygeal remnant
- sarcomatous
- Schwann cell
- secondary brain
- seeding of
- skull-base
- solid
- solitary brain
- sphenoid ridge
- spinal cord
- spread of
- subfrontal meningioma
- subtotal removal of
- subungual
- subungual amelanotic melanoma
- suprasellar extension of
- supratentorial brain
- temporal lobe
- third ventricle
- triton
- vascular hamartoma
- von Hippel
- well-circumscribed

tumor-bearing bone

tumor bed
tumor blush on cerebral angiography
tumor boundary
tumor cleavage plane
tumor debulking
tumor exophyte
tumor extirpation
tumor marker
tumor matrix
tumor of the infundibulum
tumor psyche
tumor resection
tumor staining, on cerebral angiography
tumoral calcinosis
tumor of the epiconus of the spinal cord
tuning
tunnel
- carpal
- cubital
- fascial
- fibro-osseous
- Guyon
- tarsal
- tibial

tunneler, Gude
tunnel view
tunnel vision
Tuohy lumbar puncture needle
Tupper arthroplasty
Tupper hand-holder and retractor
turbo-whisker
turcica, sella
Türck degeneration
Turco clubfoot operation
Turco posteromedial release operation
Turco repair of talipes equinovarus
Turcot syndrome
turf-toe
Turkel bone biopsy trephine
turkey-claw instrument
turnbuckle distractor
turned-down tendon flap
Turner marginal gyrus
turnip planter's palsy
turricephaly
Turyn sign
Tuwave (programmed waveform TENS treatment)
twelfth cranial nerve (hypoglossal nerve)
twig
- arterial
- nerve

twilight state
twister
- Batzdorf cervical wire
- Cooley-Baumgarten wire
- orthotic twister to treat internal or external rotation
- wire

twitch, twitching
- facial
- focal
- involuntary
- muscle
- rhythmical

two-part Apley test
two-point discrimination test
two-poster cervical orthosis
two-quarter test
two-sleeve technique
two-strut tibial graft technique
T wrench
Tycron suture
Tyler-Gigli saw
tylosis
tympani, chorda
Tyndall effect seen in cerebrospinal fluid
typhus, murine (meningoencephalitis)
tyramine diet
tyramine reaction (cheese, red wine)
Tyrell hook
tyrosinemia, neonatal

U, u

U approach
UBC (University of British Columbia)
  brace
UBP (universal bone plate) system,
  Haid
UCB (unilateral calcaneal brace)
UCB foot orthosis
UCB shoe insert
UCI (University of California, Irvine)
UCI ankle prosthesis
UCL (ulnar collateral ligament)
UCLA anatomic shoulder arthroplasty
UCP compression plate
U-drape
UE (Ulex europaeus) antibody
UE lectins
Uematsu shoulder arthrodesis
UEs (upper extremities)
UHMWPe (ultra-high molecular
  weight polyethylene)
Uhthoff phenomenon
Uhthoff sign
Uhthoff syndrome
UJ (uncovertebral joint)
ulcer
  decubitus
  ischemic foot
  mal perforant diabetic
  stasis
  trophic
ulceration
  neuropathic
  venous
  chronic leg

ulceration *(cont.)*
  periulcer venous channels in
  venous stasis
  venous stasis
Ulcus, Comfeel (occlusive dressing)
Ulex europaeus (UE) antibody
Ullman line
ulnar abutment syndrome
ulnar bursa
ulnar collateral ligament of elbow
ulnar crease of hand
ulnar deviation of hand in rheumatoid
  arthritis
ulnar extensor
ulnar facing of metacarpal heads
ulnar nerve entrapment at the elbow
ulnar nerve lesion
ulnar nerve palsy
ulnar nerve paralysis
ulnar palsy
ulnar sesamoid bone, of hand
ulnarward
ulnocarpal arthrodesis
ulnocarpal ligament
ulnolunate ligament
ulnotriquetral ligament
Ulrich bone-holding clamp
Ulrich bone-holding forceps
Ulrich-St. Gallen forceps
Ultra-Cut instruments
Ultra-Drive bone cement removal
  system
Ultra-Flex orthopedic bed
Ultra ultrasonic aspirator

Ultra-X external fixation system
ultrahigh molecular weight polyethylene (UHMWPe)
ultrasonic assessment of ankle injuries
ultrasonography
  B-mode
  cranial
  CUSALap
  duplex carotid
  pulsed
  Sonicator portable
  therapeutic, for tendon healing
  transcranial Doppler (TCD)
ultrasound-guided stereotactic biopsy
ultrasound scanning, high-resolution, for foreign bodies
ultrasound therapy
ultrastructural changes in wound healing
uncal gyrus
uncal herniation syndrome
uncinate aura
uncinate gyrus
uncinate processes
uncinate region of temporal lobe
uncinate seizure
uncommitted metaphyseal lesion
unconscious
unconsciousness
unconstrained elbow devices
unconstrained knee prostheses
uncotomy
uncovertebral joint (UJ)
uncovertebral spurring
uncus, arachnoid of
uncus corporis
uncus of hamate bone
uncus of temporal lobe
under direct vision
undercorrection
understanding of similarities test
undersurface of patella
undisputed axonopathic neurogenic thoracic outlet syndrome
unequivocal diplopia
unfused physis
ungual tuberosity
unguis incarnatus
Unhappy Triad of O'Donoghue (or O'Donoghue's Unhappy Triad)
UNI-SHUNT hydrocephalus shunt
unicameral bone cyst
unicameral brain
unicompartmental knee prosthesis
Unicondylar Geomedic Hemi-Knee system
unicortical screw
Unidose drug delivery system
Unifix, Ace
uniformly progressive deterioration
Unilab Surgibone bone replacement material
unilateral Babinski sign
unilateral carotid artery occlusion
unilateral carotid stenosis
unilateral enophthalmos in migraine
unilateral facial weakness
unilateral focus of EEG activity
unilateral fragmentation of the apophysi (on x-ray)
unilateral hallux valgus (HV)
unilateral hyperreflexia
unilateral lesion of the cerebellum
unilateral neglect, organic
unilateral paralysis
unilateral Raynaud phenomenon
unilateral spastic leg
unilateral supranuclear disease
unilateral visual neglect
unilaterally fixed, dilated pupil
unilaterally upgoing toe
unilateral seizure
Unilink system
uninhibited ankle motion
uninhibited flexion
union
  bony
  delayed

union *(cont.)*
  delayed fracture
  osseous
  secondary
unit
  AME microcurrent TENS
  Autoflex continuous passive motion (CPM)
  Bovie coagulating
  Cadwell 5200A somatosensory evoked potential
  CPM (continuous passive motion)
  Cybex Torso Rotation Testing and Rehabilitation
  Dial Away Pain 400 electrotherapy
  diathermy
  Eclipse TENS
  gamma
  gravity traction
  Hounsfield
  Hydra-Cadence gait-control
  intermittent compression
  Leksell gamma
  linear accelerator
  Magnatherm diathermy
  Maxima II TENS
  musculotendinous
  neurological intensive care (NICU)
  neurological critical care (NCCU)
  postanesthesia care (PACU)
  Sheffield gamma
  TENS (transcutaneous electrical nerve stimulation)
  Wright Care TENS
Unitek steel crown
univalve cast
univalved
universal proximal femur (UPF) prosthesis
Universal drill point
Universal hip prosthesis
University of Florida LINAC (linear accelerator)
unkempt appearance
unleveling, pelvic
unmyelinated nerve fibers
Unna boot
Unna boot cast
Unna boot wrap
Unna paste
unopposed
unplicated sheaths
unreactive pupils
unresponsive state
unresponsive to environment
unresponsiveness, psychogenic
unroof
unroofing of nerve
unshunted hydrocephalus
unstable fracture
unsteadiness of gait and station
unsustained clonus
untether
Unverricht disease
Unverricht-Lafora disease
Unverricht-Lundborg disease
Unverricht-Lundborg myoclonus epilepsy
Unverricht-Lundborg syndrome
Unverricht syndrome
unvoiced speech
U1-L1 cephalometric measurement
U1-NA cephalometric measurement
up-beat nystagmus, coarse
up-beating nystagmus
UPF prosthesis (universal proximal femur)
upgaze, conjugate
upgoing toes
upper limits of normal
upper median palsy
upper motor neuron disease
upper motor neuron impairment
upper motor neuron paralysis
upper motor neuron signs
upper motor neuron symptoms
Upper 7 head halter
UPPP (uvulopalatopharyngoplasty)

uptake, radioisotope (in vascular brain tumors)
urarthritis
urate crystal
uremic amaurosis
uremic aseptic meningitis
uremic encephalopathy
uric acid crystal
urinary incontinence
urinary or fecal incontinence
urodynamic testing in multiple sclerosis
Urschel first rib rongeur
U.S. Army bone chisel
U.S. Army gouge
U.S. Army osteotome
U.S. Army retractor
useless hand syndrome
U-shaped incision
U-shaped retractor
Uslenghi plate
Utah artificial arm
utensil
  one-handed kitchen
  Spork
uveitis, juxtapapillary
uveomeningoencephalitis
uveomeningoencephalic syndrome
uvula, cerebellar
uvula cerebelli
uvula vermis
uvulopalatopharyngoplasty (UPPP)

V, v

vaccine, duck embryo (for rabies)
Vac-Pac pad
Vacu-Mix cement pump
vacuo, hydrocephalus ex
vacuolation of ganglion cells
vacuum headache
VAD (voluntary anterior drawer) sign
vagal attack
vagal dysarthria
vagal nerve implant
vaginal ligament of hand
vagus nerve (tenth cranial nerve)
Vainio arthroplasty
Vairox high compression vascular stocking
Valenti arthroplasty
Valentine splint
valgus
  adolescent hallux
  hallux (HV)
  hindfoot
  metatarsus
  pes
valgus deformity
valgus foot
valgus heel
valgus hindfoot
valgus index
valgus instability
valgus stress
valgus stress test
valgus tilt
validity of rehabilitation testing
  construct
  content

validity of rehabilitation testing *(cont.)*
  criterion-related
  ecological
  face
Valin hemilaminectomy retractor
Valleix, puncta dolorosa (trigeminal neuralgia)
Valls hip prosthesis
Valpar component work sample series
Valsalva maneuver
valsalva'd (coined past tense verb form)
value
  absolute band (on EEG)
  attenuation, on MRI
  relative band (on EEG)
valve
  Codman slit
  Cordis Orbis Sigman shunt
  dual-chamber flushing
  flushing
  Heyer-Schulte bur hole
  low-profile
  Mishler flush
  pressure-sensitive shunt tube
  Pudenz flushing
  Sophy programmable pressure
vamp of shoe
van Bogaert encephalitis
van Bogaert leukoencephalitis
Van Beck nerve approximator
Van Buren sequestrum forceps
Vandenbos and Bowers procedure
V-angle, femoral torsion
Vanghetti prosthesis

Van Ness procedure
Vanzetti sign
Vari-weights
variabilis, Dermacentor
variable screw placement (VSP)
Varian LINAC (linear accelerator)
variant
  fast alpha
  petit mal
  slow alpha
varicella-zoster (VZ) virus
varicella zoster encephalomyelitis
varicosities, superficial
Varikopf hip prosthesis
varix (pl. varices), cerebral
Varney acromioclavicular brace
Varney pin
varus
  metatarsus
  rearfoot
  subtalar
  tibial
varus angle
varus deformity
varus heel
varus metatarsophalangeal (MTP) angle
varus tilt
varus-valgus adjustment screw
varus-valgus instability
varus-valgus stability
vasa nervorum
vascular accident
vascular anomaly
vascular blush of tumor (on carotid angiography)
vascular cord damage
vascular hamartoma
vascular invasion
vascular occlusion
vascular supply
vascularity, tumor
vasculitis
  giant cell
  rheumatoid
vasculitis *(cont.)*
  Takayasu
  temporal
VA shunt (ventriculoatrial)
vasocoolant sprays
vasodepressor syncope
vasomotor changes
vasomotor headache
vasomotor instability
vasopneumatic compression
vasopneumatic treatment
vasospasm
  cerebral
  symptomatic
vasospastic attacks
vasovagal reflex
vasovagal syncope
Vastamaki paralysis
vastus lateralis muscle
vastus medialis advancement (VMA)
vastus medialis obliquus (VMO)
Vater-Pacini bodies
VATER syndrome
  V vertebral abnormality
  A anal imperforation
  TE tracheoesophageal fistula
  R radial, ray, or renal anomaly
vault, plantar
VBI (vertebrobasilar insufficiency)
V blade plate
V capsulotomy
VDRL (Venereal Disease Research Laboratory)
VDS (ventral derotating spinal)
VDS compression rod
VDS hex nut
VDS screw
VDS screwdriver
VDS wrench
VE (vocational evaluation)
vector
VEDA (Vestibular Disorders Association)
vegetative patient
vegetative state

vehicle, all-terrain (ATV)
vehicular accident
vein
- aneurysmal
- anterior terminal (ATV)
- basal vein of Rosenthal (BVR)
- bulb of internal jugular
- common facial
- diploic
- external jugular
- Galen cerebral
- great cerebral vein of Galen
- internal cerebral (ICV)
- intussusception of
- jugular
- Labbe
- medullary
- meningeal
- palmar cutaneous
- posterior terminal (PTV)
- Rosenthal basal
- saphenous
- Schlesinger
- septal
- thalamostriate
- vermian

Velcro fitting
Velcro immobilizer
Velcro splint
Velcro strap
Veleanu-Rosianu-Ionescu technique
Veley headrest
velocimetry, laser Doppler
velocity
- motor conduction
- motor nerve conduction (MNCV)
- muzzle velocity in handgun injury
- nerve conduction (NCV)
- orthodromic
- peak height
- push-off
- saccade (on EMG)
- sensory conduction
- sensory nerve conduction (SNCV)

Velpeau bandage
Velpeau cast
Velpeau dressing
Velpeau plaster
Velpeau shoulder immobilizer
Velpeau shoulder sling
velum
vena comitans (pl. venae comitantes)
Venable plate
Venable-Stuck nail
Venable-Stuck pin
Venable-Stuck screw
Venezuelan equine encephalitis
Venezuelan equine viral encephalitis
venography
- epidural
- intraosseous
- vertebral

venous plexus
venous pump of the foot
venous reflux
venous stasis ulcers
venous thromboembolic disease (VTED)
venous ulceration
ventilation, mechanical
ventral cochlear nucleus
ventral spinocerebellar tracts
ventral spinothalamic tracts
ventricle
- absent
- atrium of
- ballooned floor of
- cerebral
- compensatory enlargement of
- dilatation of the
- dilated
- effacement of
- elongation of
- enlarged
- enlargement of
- floor of
- fourth
- frontal horn of lateral

ventricle *(cont.)*
  lateral
  loculate
  outflow of
  papilloma of the fourth
  roof of
  shift of the
  single large
  sixth
  slit
  temporal horn of lateral
  third
  tiny
  trigone of lateral
  Verga
ventricular cannula, Ford Hospital
ventricular dilatation
ventricular drain
ventricular drainage
ventricular enlargement
ventricular reservoir
ventricular shift
ventricular size
ventricular space
ventricular span
ventricular system
ventricular tap
ventricular wall
ventriculitis
ventriculoatrial (VA) shunt
ventriculogram
ventriculography
  intraoperative
  metrizamide
ventriculomegaly
ventriculoperitoneal (VP)
ventriculoperitoneal drain
ventriculoperitoneal shunt
ventriculoscope
ventriculostomy
ventriculovenous shunt
VEP (visual evoked potential)
VER (visual evoked response)
verbal (or semantic) paraphasia
verbal command
verbally-mediated functions
verbigeration
Verbrugge bone-holding forceps
Verbrugge clamp
Verbrugge forceps
Verbrugge-Hohmann bone retractor
Verbrugge needle
Verdan technique
Veress needle
Verga ventricle
vergence, downward
vermian medulloblastoma
vermian veins
vermicular movements
vermis (midline cerebellum)
  cerebellar
  dysgenesis of
  folium
  hypoplastic
  superior
  tuber
  uvula of
Vermont spinal fixator (VSF)
Vernet syndrome
vernier calipers
Verocay body
verruca
  mosaic plantar
  single plantar
verruca plantaris
Versa-Fx femoral fixation system
VersaPulse holmium laser
VersaWrist wrist splint
version, internal and external
Versi-Splint
versive seizure
vertebra (pl. vertebrae)
  arch of
  codfish
  displaced
  facet surface of
  fractured
  fused

vertebra *(cont.)*
  last normal (LNV)
  midbody of
  olisthetic
  pear-shaped
  scalloping of
  subluxed
  transitional
  transverse process of
  wedging of olisthetic
vertebra plana fracture
vertebral ankylosis
vertebral artery dissection
vertebral artery endarterectomy
vertebral artery occlusion
vertebral artery stenosis
vertebral body impactor
vertebral collapse
vertebral column
vertebral endarterectomy
vertebral endplate
vertebral steal phenomenon
vertebral steal syndrome
vertebral system of veins
vertebrectomy
  Bohlman anterior cervical
  cervical
  subtotal
vertebrobasilar circulation
vertebrobasilar disease
vertebrobasilar distribution stroke
vertebrobasilar insufficiency (VBI)
vertebrobasilar ischemia
vertebrobasilar occlusion
vertebrobasilar system
vertex of cranium
vertical nystagmus
vertical talus (rockerbottom flatfoot)
vertiginous seizure
vertiginous sensation
vertigo
  benign functional
  benign paroxysmal
  benign paroxysmal positional

vertigo *(cont.)*
  cervical
  disabling
  episodic
  labyrinthine
  motion-induced
  objective
  ocular
  paroxysmal
  positional
  post-traumatic
  postural
  proprioceptive
  psychogenic
  reversible
  rotational
  subjective
  transient
  true
  visual
vesalianum of vertebral body
Vesely-Street nail
Vesely-Street splint
vesical paralysis as response to spinal injury
vesicles (blisters)
vessel, vessels
  collateral
  feeding
  perforator
  pial
vest
  Bremer AirFlo halo
  halo
  Minerva
  Vitrathene
vest-over-pants technique
vestibular apparatus
vestibular division of the eighth cranial nerve
vestibular end-organ nystagmus
vestibular nerve disorder
vestibular neuronitis

vestibular nuclei of cerebellum
  inferior
  lateral (Deiter)
  medial
  principal (Schwalbe)
  spinal
  superior (Von Bechterew)
vestibular nucleus
vestibular nystagmus
vestibular oculocephalic response
vestibular schwannoma
Vestibular Disorders Association (VEDA)
vestibulocerebellar ataxia
vestibulocochlear nucleus
vestibulogenic epilepsy
vestibulo-ocular maneuver
vestibulo-ocular reflex (VOR)
vestibulospinal reflex
vestibulospinal tract
veterinary approach
VHL (von Hippel-Lindau) syndrome
VHTS (volumetric hyperthermia treatment system)
viability
Vibram rockerbottom shoe
vibration perception
vibration sensation
vibration sense
vibration sensitivity
vibration syndrome
vibratory sense
vibratory threshold
Vibrio fetus meningitis
VICON three-dimensional gait analysis system
Vicq d'Azyr, stripe of (in brain)
Vicryl figure-of-8 suture
Vicryl suture
Victorian brace
Vidal-Adrey modified Hoffmann device
video-EEG monitoring and split-screen recording
video fluoroscopy
  swallowing mechanism
  spinal
vidian nerve neuralgia
Vidicon vacuum chamber pickup tube
Vi-Drape
Vieussens
  annulus of
  ansa of
  loop of
view
  AP (anteroposterior)
  apical
  apical lordotic
  axial sesamoid
  axillary
  baseline
  Beath
  Boehler calcaneal (Böhler)
  Boehler lumbosacral
  Breuerton
  Brodan
  carpal tunnel
  Carter-Rowe
  cine
  clenched fist
  coalition
  coned-down
  cross-table
  dens (cervical spine)
  dorsiflexion
  dorsoplantar
  Dunlop-Shands
  Ferguson
  frogleg lateral
  Harris
  Harris-Beath
  Hobb
  Hughston
  infrapatellar view of knees
  intraoperative
  inversion ankle stress
  Jones
  Jude pelvic

view *(cont.)*
  lateral bending view of spine
  lateral oblique
  Merchant
  mortise
  Neer lateral
  Neer transscapular
  nonstanding lateral oblique
  notch
  oblique
  odontoid
  open-mouth
  outlet
  plantar axial
  plantarflexion
  push-pull ankle stress
  push-pull hip
  Schüller
  serendipity
  skijump
  skyline
  spot
  standing dorsoplantar
  standing lateral
  standing weightbearing
  Stenver
  sunrise
  sunset
  swimmer's
  tangential
  true lateral
  tunnel
  von Rosen
  Waters
  weightbearing
  weightbearing dorsoplantar
  x-ray
vigil, coma
vigilance (concentration)
Vigilon dressing
Vigorimeter, Martin
Villaret-Mackenzie syndrome
villi, arachnoidal
villonodular synovitis
villous proliferation
villous synovitis
villus formation in rheumatoid arthritis
VIM (ventral intermedius nucleus) stimulation
vimentin antibody
vimentin immunostain
vinculum
vinculum breve
vinculum longum
Vinertia implant metal
Vinke skull traction tongs
Vinke tongs
viral encephalitis (pl. encephalitides)
viral intracerebral arteritis
viral leukoencephalitis
Virchow law of skull growth
Virchow-Robin spaces of the brain
Virtullene brace material
virus
  ECHO (enteric cytopathic human orphan)
  encephalitis
  herpes zoster
  slow virus infection of the nervous system
  SV-40
  varicella-zoster (VZ)
visceral tendon sheath layer
viscoelastic action
viscoelastic property of muscles
viscoelastic stability
Viscoheel K heel cushion
Viscoheel K orthosis
Viscoheel N heel cushion
Viscoheel N orthosis
Viscoheel SofSpot heel cushion
Viscoheel SofSpot orthosis
Viscolas heel pain and disability
Viscolas orthotic
vise
  AlloGrip bone
  bone
  mechanic's pin

VISI (volarflexed intercalated segment instability)
VISI deformity
vision
  blurred
  blurring of
  darkening of
  foveal
  hemifield of
  loss of
  sudden loss of
  tubular
  tunnel
vision disorder in migraine, cinematographic
Visiting Nurse Association (VNA)
visor, Georgiade
Vistec x-ray detectable sponge
visual acuity
visual agnosia
visual amnesia
visual blurring
visual disturbance
visual epilepsy
visual evoked potential (VEP)
visual evoked response (VER)
visual field constriction
visual field cut
visual field defects
visual field disturbance
visual field exam
visual field test
visual impairment
visual memory
Visual Neglect Test
Visual Pattern Completion Test
visual prodrome
visual radiations
visual seizure
visual-spatial distortion
visual symptoms
visualized
visuospatial disorientation
Vitallium implant metal
Vitallium Küntscher nail
vitamin B_{12} deficiency
Vitox alumina ceramic material in prosthesis
Vitrathene vest
Viva shoes
VJ (ventriculojugular) shunt
VMA (vastus medialis advancement)
V medullary nail
VMO (vastus medialis obliquus)
V nail plate
vocational evaluation (VE)
vocational rehabilitation (VR)
Vogt disease
Vogt-Koyanagi-Harada syndrome
Vogue arm sling
volar carpal ligament
volar, volarly
volar wrist
volarflexed intercalated segment instability (VISI)
volarly
volarward
volitional movement
volitional saccade
Volkmann bone curet
Volkmann bone hook
Volkmann ischemic contracture
Volkmann rake retractor
Volkov-Oganesian external fixation
voltage (on EEG)
  calibration
  high
  low
  medium
  very low
volume
  cerebrospinal fluid
  intracranial vascular
volume element (voxel)
volume imaging
volumetric hyperthermia treatment system (VHTS)
voluntary hysterical overbreathing

voluntary anterior drawer (VAD) sign
voluntary posterior drawer (VPD) sign
Volz total wrist arthroplasty
Volz-Turner reattachment technique
Volz wrist prosthesis
Vom Saal pin
vomer
vomiting, projectile
von Bahr screw
von Bekhterev reflex
von Ebner glands
von Economo disease
von Economo encephalitis lethargica
von Eulenberg disease
VonFrey hair test of sensory loss
von Gierke disease
von Hippel-Landau disease
von Hippel-Lindau (VHL) syndrome
von Lackum transection shift jacket
von Langenbeck periosteal elevator
von Recklinghausen disease
von Recklinghausen syndrome
von Rosen cruciform splint
von Rosen view
von Schwann, law of
von Economo influenza
von Hippel tumor
von Lackum surcingle
Voorhoeve disease
VOR (vestibulo-ocular reflex)
Voshell sign
Vostal classification of radial fracture
V osteotomy, Japas
voxel (volume element)
V phenomenon
VP (ventriculoperitoneal) shunt
VPL thalamic electrode (ventro-posterolateral)
VR (vocational rehabilitation)
VrE (varus extension) test
VSF (Vermont spinal fixator)
VSF clamp
VSF fixation system
VSF rod
VSF screw
V-shaped incision
VSP (variable screw placement)
VSP fixation
VSP plate
VSP screw
VTED (venous thromboembolic disease)
Vulpian-Bernhardt spinal muscular atrophy
Vulpius Achilles tendon reconstruction
Vulpius-Compere gastrocnemius lengthening
Vulpius equinus deformity operation
V waves on EEG
V-Y advancement flap
V-Y plasty
V-Y quadricepsplasty
VZ (varicella-zoster) virus

W, w

WACH shoe (wedge adjustable
  cushioned heel)
wad, flexor
Wada test, hemispheric
Wada valve prosthesis
Waddell Chronic Back Pain Disability
  Index
Waddell sign
wadding
  cotton
  cotton sheet
waddle, duck
waddling gait
Wadsworth unconstrained elbow
  prosthesis
wafer, Thera-Bite
Wagner classification of diabetic foot
  ulcers
Wagner classification of forefoot
  gangrene
Wagner distraction device
Wagner external fixator
Wagner fixer
Wagner frame
Wagner line
Wagner modification of Syme
  amputation
Wagner retractor
Wagner-Schanz screw apparatus
wagon wheel fracture
Wagoner cervical technique
Wagstaffe fracture
Wainwright plate
WAIS-R Block Design Test
waist of the scaphoid
waist of the phalanx
Wakefield Self-Assessment Depression
  Inventory
wakeful
wakefulness
  epochs of
  quiet
  resting
waking attacks (epilepsy)
waking frequency on EEG, dominant
walk, walking
  heel
  heel and toe
  nonweightbearing crutch
  toe
walker
  Cam Walker leg
  Cam Walker ankle
  Castaway ankle
  Castaway leg
  four-point
  Hi-Top foot/ankle
  ORLAU swivel
  Rolator
  rubber wedge
  swivel
Walker disk curet
Walker-Murdoch wrist sign

Walker ruptured disk curet
walking aids
walking cast
walking components
  energy conservation
  progression
  standing stability
walking cycle
walking footprints classification
"walking up the thighs" (Gowers sign)
walking with support
walking without support
wall
  aneurysmal
  cyst
  cystic
  ventricular
Wall stent biliary endoprosthesis
Walldius knee prosthesis
Wallenberg lateral medullary syndrome
wallerian degeneration
Walton cartilage clamp
Walton-Liston bone rongeur
Walton maneuver
Walton meniscus clamp
Walton-Ruskin bone rongeur
Walton-Ruskin forceps
Walton scissors
Walton wire-pulling forceps
Wangensteen needle holder
Ward periosteal elevator
Ward triangle
Warm Springs brace
warmth, joint
Warner-Farber ankle fixation technique
Warren-Marshall classification
Warren White Achilles tendon lengthening operation
wart
  mosaic plantar
  mother-daughter type plantar
  satellite plantar
  single plantar
Wartenberg neurological pinwheel
Wartenberg reflex
Wartenberg sign
washboard effect on myelography in cervical spondylosis
washer
  oval
  resin
  slotted
  toothed
washing out of accumulated metabolites
wasp-tail deformity in Duchenne dystrophy
Wassel classification of thumb polydactyly
Wassel type IV thumb duplication
Wasserstein fixation device
wasting
  muscle
  muscle fiber
wasting of hypothenar eminence
wasting of muscles
wasting of thenar eminence
Watanabe classification of discoid meniscus
Watco brace
Watco 2001 knee immobilizer
water, deionized sterile
water intoxication
water jet tissue cutter
water on the brain
water signal on MRI scan
Water-Pik
Waterman osteotomy
waterpick
Waters x-ray view
watershed area of Achilles tendon
watershed infarct
watershed infarction
watershed area paresis
watershed areas between main arterial territories
Watkins fusion technique
Watson-Cheyne technique

Watson-Jones ankle tenodesis
Watson-Jones bone gouge
Watson-Jones classification of spinal fractures
Watson-Jones fracture repair
Watson-Jones navicular fracture
Watson-Jones tenodesis
Watson test
Watson-Williams intervertebral disk rongeur
Watson-Jones approach
Waugh ankle prosthesis
Waugh knee prosthesis
wave, waves
  A
  alpha
  alpha spindles
  amplitude of
  anterior predominance of
  aperiodic
  apiculate
  arch-shaped
  arrhythmical repetitive
  asymmetric
  asynchronous
  asynchronous delta
  asynchronous slow
  B
  beta spindles
  bilateral
  bilaterally synchronous
  bilaterally synchronous slow
  biparietal hump
  biphasic
  bisynchronous
  bisynchronous delta
  bisynchronous slow
  brain
  bursts of delta
  bursts of theta
  C
  centroparietal slow
  cerebrospinal fluid
  clipping of

wave *(cont.)*
  complex of EEG
  cone
  configuration of
  contoured
  delta
  diphasic
  distribution of
  duration of
  EEG
  epileptiform
  F
  fast
  flattened top of EEG
  focal sharp
  focal slow
  frequency of
  frontal sharp
  frontocentral slow
  generalized asynchronous slow
  generalized fast
  generalized slow
  harmonics of
  high-amplitude
  ictal focal slow
  in-phase
  independent
  interictal focal epileptiform
  interictal focal slow
  interictal generalized epileptiform
  interictal paroxysmal sharp
  interictal paroxysmal spike
  intermittent temporal slow
  intracranial pressure B
  irregular
  lambda
  lambdoid
  larval spike-and-slow
  local ictal slow
  local slow
  localized
  low-amplitude
  low-voltage
  M

wave *(cont.)*
  monomorphic
  monophasic
  monorhythmic
  monorhythmic frontal delta (MFD)
  morphology of
  O
  occipital
  out-of-phase
  paroxysmal rhythmical
  peak of
  periodic
  periodic generalized sharp
  periodic slow
  persistence of
  phase reversing slow
  plateau
  polarity of
  polymorphic
  polyphasic
  polyrhythmic
  positive occipital spike-like sleep
  positive sharp
  posterior predominance of
  postictal bisynchronous slow
  pulse volume
  quadriphasic
  quasi-periodic
  regularity of
  repetitive
  rhythmical
  rhythmical repetitive
  rhythmical slow
  rhythmicity of
  saw-tooth
  saw-toothed
  shape of
  sharp
  sharply contoured
  shut eye
  simultaneous
  sine
  sinusoidal
  slow

wave *(cont.)*
  spike-like
  sporadic
  sporadic generalized slow
  spread of
  symmetry of
  synchronous
  synchrony of
  temporal predominance of
  theta
  topography of
  trains of
  Traube-Hering-Mayer cerebrospinal fluid
  triangular
  triphasic
  troughs of
  unilateral
  V
  vertex
  very slow
wave discharge on EEG
waveform (or wave form)
waveform amplitude
waveform superimposed on waveform
wavelength
waves of youth, posterior slow
wax, bone
waxy flexibility
Wayne laminectomy seat
WBCS (white blood cell scintigraphy) with indium-111
W/C (wheelchair)
WCh (wheelchair)
WCS (Wisconsin Compression System)
weakness
  asymmetric
  breakaway
  central origin
  facial movement
  flaccid
  focal
  hemifacial

weakness *(cont.)*
 infranuclear
 left-sided
 motor
 myopathic
 nuclear
 central origin
 peripheral origin
 progressive
 proximal
 right-sided
 supranuclear
 Todd motor
 unilateral facial
 upper motor neuron
weakness of one side of the face
 central origin
 peripheral origin
wear-and-tear
wearing-off effect of L-dopa in parkinsonism
Weary brain spatula
Weary cordotomy knives
Weary nerve hook
Weary nerve root retractor
weave, Pulver-Taft
Weaver-Dunn acromioclavicular technique
weaver's bottom
web
 finger
 thumb
web-area of hand
web-border of hand
Webb-Andreesen condylar bolt
Webb stove bolt
webbed toes
webbing of fingers
Weber-Brunner-Freuler-Boitzy technique
Weber C fracture
Weber, circle of
Weber esthesiometer
Weber sign
Weber syndrome
Weber two-point discrimination test
Weber-Vasey traction-absorption wiring technique
Webril bandage
Webril dressing
webspace
Webster meniscectomy scissors
Webster needle holder
Wechsler Memory Scale (WMS)
Weck clip
Weck osteotome
wedge
 bed
 compensatory
 Duo-Cline bed
 Hapad heel
 heel
 heel to toe medial shoe
 lateral (for sole or heel of foot)
 medial heel
 shoe
 tibial
 Yancy cast
wedge excision
wedge flexion-compression fracture
wedged shoes
wedge osteotomy, supratubercular
wedging of olisthetic vertebra
wedging of vertebral interspace
weekend athlete
weekend diarrhea (migraine equivalent)
Wegener granulomatosis-associated peripheral neuropathy
Wehrs incus prosthesis
weight acceptance (of gait)
weightbearing (also weight-bearing)
 partial
 progression to
 progressive
 spinal x-ray with
 touchdown
weightbearing crutches

weightbearing dome of acetabulum
weightbearing radiograph
weightbearing rotational injury
weightbearing with crutches
weightbearing x-ray
weight loading, axial
weight-relieving calipers
weight shift
weight shifting
weight-training program
weight transfer
weights
  hand-held (HHW)
  progressive
  Thera-Band progressive
weights and pulleys
Weil-Blakesley intervertebral disk rongeur
Weil-Felix reaction
Weil pelvic sling
Weinberg rib spreader
Weiss amputation saw
Weiss sign
Weiss spring
Weit-Arner retractor
Weitbrecht cord
Weitbrecht ligament
Weitlaner-Beckmann retractor
Welander disease
Welander distal muscular atrophy
well-leg cast
well leg straight leg raising test
well-leg traction
Well-Being, Index of (IWB)
Weller cartilage forceps
Weller cartilage scissors
Wells traction
Wenger plate
Werdnig-Hoffmann disease
Werdnig-Hoffmann spinal muscular atrophy
Werdnig-Hoffmann syndrome
Wernicke aphasia
Wernicke area
Wernicke dementia
Wernicke encephalopathy
Wernicke-Korsakoff encephalopathy
Wernicke-Korsakoff syndrome
Wernicke-Mann predilection paralysis
Wernicke-Mann spastic hemiplegia
Wernicke region
Wernicke syndrome
Wertheim splint
West and Soto-Hall patella operation
West bone chisel
West bone gouge
West hand dissector
West Nile encephalitis
West Nile viral encephalitis
West osteotome
West syndrome
WEST (work evaluation systems technology)
western equine encephalitis
western equine viral encephalitis
Westfield acromioclavicular immobilizer
Westfield envelope sling
Westin tenodesis
Westin-Turco category
Westphal-Edinger nucleus
wet gangrene
wet smear for parasites and fungi in meningitis
WFC (World Federation of Chiropractic)
Wheaton brace
wheel
  Carborundum grinding
  grinding
  pin
  Wartenberg pin
wheelchair (W/C)
  Amigo mechanical
  confinement to
  electric
  HiRider motorized/lift

whiplash
  acute
  chronic
  reflex rebound component of
whiplash injury
whiplash syndrome
Whipple disease
whipstitch
whirlpool bath
whisker shaver
Whitcomb-Kerrison laminectomy rongeur
white blood cell scintigraphy (WBCS) with indium-111
Whitecloud-LaRocca cervical arthrodesis
white commissure of spinal cord
white count with left shift
White epiphysiodesis
white fibers (type II muscle fibers)
white matter of central nervous system
white migraine
Whitesides-Kelly cervical technique
Whitesides Ortholoc II condylar femoral prosthesis
Whitesides tissue pressure determination
Whitesides total knee prosthesis
Whitfield ointment and pumice stone
whitlow
  herpetic
  melanotic
Whitman femoral neck reconstruction
WHO (World Health Organization)
WHO classification of astrocytoma
WHO Handicap Scales
  economic self-sufficiency
  mobility
  orientation
  physical independence
  social integration
whole body hyperthermia
whole bone transplant
Wiberg, CE angle of
Wiberg classification of patellar types
Wiberg periosteal elevator
Wiberg type II patellar contour
wick, saline-soaked cotton
wicket rhythm on EEG
wicket spike on EEG
wide-based gait
wide toebox shoe
Wide Range Achievement Test
widened sulci (on scan)
widening
  growth plate
  interspinous
widening of crural cistern
widening of joint
widening of the ankle mortise (demonstrated on x-ray)
Wiet cup forceps
Wiet graft-measuring instrument
Wiet otologic scissors
Wigmore plaster saw
Wilberg bone staple
Wilco ankle exerciser
Wilco ankle machine
Wilde ethmoid forceps
Wilde intervertebral disk rongeur
Wilke boot
Wilkins classification of radial fracture
Willauer-Gibbon periosteal elevator
William Harris hip prosthesis
Williams exercise program
Williams-Haddad technique
Williams screwdriver
Williger bone curet
Williger bone mallet
Williger periosteal elevator
Willis, arterial circle of
Willis headache
willow fracture
Wilmington jacket
Wilmington scoliosis brace
Wilson-Burstein (DF80) hip prosthesis
Wilson convex frame
Wilson disease
Wilson double oblique osteotomy
Wilson frame

Wilson-Jacobs tibial fracture fixation
Wilson-Johansson-Barrington cone
  arthrodesis
Wilson-McKeever arthroplasty
Wilson-McKeever shoulder technique
Wilson procedure for extra-articular
  fusion of elbow
Wilson rib spreader
Wilson sign
Wiltberger anterior cervical approach
Wiltberger spinous process spreader
Wiltse-Bankart retractor
Wiltse fixation system
Wiltse-Gelpi retractor
Wiltse osteotomy of ankle
Wiltse rod
Wiltse screw-rod
Winberger line
wince, wincing
windlass mechanism
window, cortical
windowshade pulled down on visual
  field
windup injury
wing-beating tremor of Wilson
  disease
wing
  iliac
  sphenoid
  sphenoidal
winged iliac crest trephine
winged scapula
Wingfield frame
winging of the scapula
wing of ilium
wing of sphenoid bone
wink, anal
wink reflex, anal
Wink retractor
Winograd technique for ingrown nail
Winquist-Hansen classification of
  femoral fracture
Winston-Lutz for LINAC-based
  radiosurgery
Winter-King-Moe scoliosis
Winter spondylolisthesis technique
wire, wiring
  Babcock stainless steel
  band
  bayonet-point
  beaded transfixion
  bone suturing
  braided
  Brook
  Bunnell pull-out
  calibrated guide
  cerclage
  chisel-tip
  circular
  Compere fixation
  compression
  conical-point
  crossed
  crossed Kirschner
  diamond-point
  double-strand
  double-stranded
  double-twisted
  Drummond
  encircling
  figure-of-8
  fixator
  gauge of
  Ilizarov
  interfragment
  interfragmentary
  interspinous
  Isola
  K (Kirschner)
  lead
  Luque
  Luque cerclage
  Magnuson
  monofilament
  ninety-ninety (90/90) intraosseous
  Nitinol flexible guide
  nonthreaded
  oblique

wire *(cont.)*
olive
Oppenheimer spring
percutaneous Kirschner (K)
pull-out
Schauwecker patellar tension
Selby I
sharp-pointed
smooth transfixion
stainless steel
steel
sublamina
suture
tension band
Thiersch
threaded
transfixion
transosseous
triple
trocar-point
trochanter
unthreaded
Wisconsin interspinous
Wisconsin spinous process
wire crimper, Caparosa
wire cutter
wire driver
Hall Micro E
Micro Series
Orthairtome
wire fixation
Wirth-Jager tendon technique
Wisconsin button
Wisconsin Card Sorting Test
Wisconsin Compression System (WCS)
Wisconsin interspinous wire
Wisconsin-Luque instrumentation
Wisconsin spinal fracture system
Wisconsin spinous process wire
Wisconsin wire fixation
Wissinger rod
Wister wire/pin cutter
withdrawal
alcohol
drug
withdrawal movements
withdrawal seizures
Wits cephalometric measurement
witzelsucht
Wixson hip positioner
WMS (Wechsler Memory Scale)
Wolf arthroscope
Wolfart-Kugelberg-Welander syndrome
Wolfe-Boehler cast breaker (Böhler)
Wolfe-Boehler cast remover
Wolfe-Boehler mallet
Wolfe-Kawamoto bone graft
Wolff headache
Wolff law (bone structure)
Wolin meniscoid lesion
Wolman disease
Wood alloy
wood screw
Woodson dissector
Woodson dural separator-spatula
Woodson elevator
Woodson separator
Woodward technique
wool, lamb's
woozy, feeling
word blindness
word deafness, pure
word, difficulty finding the right
word-finding ability
word-finding difficulty
word-finding skills
word retrieval tasks
word retrieval test
word substitution
words
inappropriate (paraphrasia)
nonsensical (neologisms)
telescoped (festinant quality in parkinsonian speech)

work evaluation systems technology (WEST)
work hardening
Work Seat driving simulator
Workers' Compensation
working orthopedic surgery film
workplace
World Federation of Chiropractic (WFC)
World Health Organization (WHO)
wormian bone
wound
  ballistic
  clean
  closed
  contaminated
  craniocerebral penetrating
  cross-irrigation of
  depths of
  exit
  gunshot (GSW)
  high-energy gunshot
  high-velocity gunshot
  incised
  open
  plantar puncture
  puncture (types I through IV)
  stab (arthroscopy entry portal)
  tetanus-prone
Wound-Evac drain
wound towels
woven bone
W-plasty
WR nerve stimulator
wrap (bandage)
  Ace
  Coban
  Dura-Kold
  Elasto-Gel shoulder therapy
  Electro-Link joint
  gauze
  joint
  Kerlix
  neck
wrap *(cont.)*
  Nylatex nylon-latex
  Thermosport hot/cold
  Unna
  Unna boot
wraparound splint
wrapping
  compressive centripetal
  stump
wrapping of aneurysm
wrench
  Allen
  box-end
  cannulated
  conical nut
  Fox
  Harrington flat
  hex
  Key-loc
  locknut
  Mueller (Müller)
  open-end
  socket
  VDS (ventral derotating spinal)
wrenched knee
wrestler's ear
wrestler's elbow
Wright-Adson test
Wright Care TENS unit
Wright plate
Wrisberg cardiac ganglion
Wrisberg, intermediate nerve of
Wrisberg ligament
wrist
  gymnast's
  palmar
  SLAC (scapholunate arthritic collapse)
  volar
  Volz
wrist capsule
wristdrop (sign of radial nerve paralysis)
WristJack (see *Agee-WristJack*)

wristlet, elastic
Wrist Pro wrist support device
wrist rest splint
writhing
  limb
  sinuous
  tongue
wryneck (torticollis)
W-sitting position
Wu bunionectomy
Wurzburg plate
Wurzburg screw
Wyburn-Mason arteriovenous
  malformation
Wynne-Davies joint laxity technique

X, x

x (by)
x (times)
xanthochromia of cerebrospinal fluid
  (CSF)
xanthochromic spinal fluid
xanthoma, malignant fibrous
xanthomatosis, cerebrotendinous
xenon skin clearance test
xenon washout technique measurement
Xenophor femoral prosthesis
Xeroform gauze dressing
xerography
xeroradiography
XIP (x-ray in plaster)
xiphoid process
x-irradiation
X-linked recessive adrenoleuko-
  dystrophy
XMB tibial reaming guide
Xomed NIM-2 (nerve integrity
  monitor)
XOP (x-ray out of plaster)
x-ray
  AP (anteroposterior)
  AP inversion stress
  brow-down skull
  brow-up skull
  coronal bending
  CTLV (cross-table lateral view)
  dorsiflexion stress ankle
  dorsoplanar

x-ray *(cont.)*
  FCS (full cervical spine)
  full length
  Harris-Beath axial hindfoot
  hip-to-ankle
  intraoperative
  lateral
  lateral anterior drawer stress
  lateral tilt stress ankle
  mortise
  mortise view
  nonweightbearing
  patellar skyline
  plain
  plantarflexion stress ankle
  postoperative
  preoperative
  prereduction
  standing
  stress
  stress Broden
  stress eversion
  stress inversion
  weightbearing
x-ray tray, Bucky
x-ray view (see *view*)
X-TEND-O knee flexer
XXX syndrome
XXY syndrome
XYY syndrome

Y, y

Yale brace
Yamanda myelotomy knife
Yancy cast wedge
Yankauer periosteal elevator
Yankauer suction tube
Yasargil arachnoid knife
Yasargil artery forceps
Yasargil bayonet forceps
Yasargil bayonet scissors
Yasargil carotid clamp
Yasargil clip-applying forceps
Yasargil dissector
Yasargil elevator
Yasargil hypophyseal forceps
Yasargil knotting forceps
Yasargil Leyla retractor arm
Yasargil ligature carrier
Yasargil ligature guide
Yasargil microclip
Yasargil microcuret
Yasargil microdissector
Yasargil microforceps
Yasargil microrasp
Yasargil microscissors
Yasargil microvascular knife
Yasargil needle holder
Yasargil pituitary rongeur
Yasargil rasp
Yasargil scissors
Yasargil scoop
Yasargil spring hook
Yasargil suction tube
Yasargil tissue lifter
Yasargil tumor forceps
Yasargil vessel clip
Y bone plate
Y connector, universal
Yeager test
Yee posterior shoulder approach
yellow fever encephalitis
yellow fever viral encephalitis
Yergason sign
Yergason test of shoulder subluxation
Y fracture
Y incision
Y line
YIS knee prosthesis
Yoke transposition procedure
Y osteotomy
Young hinged knee prosthesis
Young-Vitallium hinged prosthesis
Yount procedure
Y plate
Y-shaped incision
Y-T fracture
Yucca board

Z, z

Zadik foot procedure
Zadik total nail bed ablation
Zahn, line of
Zancolli procedure for clawhand deformity
Zaricznyj ligament technique
Zarins-Rowe ligament technique
Zaufel-Jansen bone rongeur
Zazepen-Gamidov technique
Z disk
zebra body myopathy
Zeier transfer technique
Zeiss OPMI surgical microscope
Zellballen
Zellweger syndrome
Zenith chiropractic table
Zervas hypophysectomy kit
zeugmatography, Fourier transformation
Z fixation nail
Zickel fracture classification system
Zickel intramedullary nail
Zickel nail fixation
Zickel nail
Zickel subtrochanteric fracture fixation
Zielke derotation level
Zielke distraction device
Zielke gouge
Zielke instrumentation for scoliosis spinal fusion
Zielke rod
Zielke VDS (ventral derotating spinal) implant
zigzag finger incision
Zimalite implant metal
Zimaloy implant metal
Zimaloy prosthesis
Zimfoam head halter
Zimfoam padding
Zimmer CAPE (continuous anatomical passive exerciser)
Zimmer caudal hook
Zimmer Cebotome bone cement drill
Zimmer gouge
Zimmer knee immobilizer
Zimmer low viscosity adhesive
Zimmer low viscosity cement
Zimmer microsaw
Zimmer Osteo Stim bone growth stimulator
Zimmer Y plate
Zimmerman pericyte
Zim-Zap rib belt
zinc peroxide powder
Zinco ankle orthotic
Zinco CAM walker brace
Zinco Castaway D walker
Zinco short high top D walker
Zinco tall walker
Zinco thumb-wrist immobilizer
Zinn, tendon of
Zirconia femoral head prosthesis
Zirconia orthopedic prosthetic heads
zirconium oxide ceramic prosthesis
Z lengthening of tendon
Zlotsky-Ballard classification of acromioclavicular injury
ZMS intramedullary fixation system

Zoellner rasp
Zollinger leg holder
zona compacta
zona incerta of subthalamus
zone
  dorsal-route entry
  epileptogenic
  fracture
  root entry
  root exit (REZ)
  trigger (for tic douloureux)
zone of denervation
zone phenomenon
zoom disorder of visual perception in migraine
Zoroc plaster
zoster
  geniculate herpes
  herpes
Zostrix
Z-plasty
  Cozen-Brockway
  four-flap
Z-plasty closure
Z-plasty incision
Z-plasty local flap graft
Z-plasty release
Z-plasty tenotomy
Z plate
Z slide lengthening in hallux limitus
Z stent prosthesis
Zuckerkandl convolution
Zucker splint
Zuelzer awl
Zuelzer hook plate
Zung Self-Rating Depression Scale
Zweymuller cementless hip prosthesis
Zyranox zirconia material in prosthesis